A TEXTBOOK
OF
RADIOLOGICAL DIAGNOSIS

A TEXTBOOK

OF

RADIOLOGICAL DIAGNOSIS

(formerly 'A Text-Book of X-ray Diagnosis')

FIFTH EDITION

Published under the auspices
of the President and Council
of the Royal College of Radiologists

VOLUME 2

THE CARDIOVASCULAR SYSTEM

Edited by JOHN B. PARTRIDGE, MB.BS, MRCP, FRCR,

Cardiac Radiologist, The Prince Charles Hospital, Brisbane, Australia
Lately Consultant Cardio-Radiologist, Leeds Regional Cardio-Thoracic Unit,
Killingbeck Hospital, Leeds

With over 900 illustrations in 569 figures

W. B. SAUNDERS COMPANY
PHILADELPHIA · TORONTO

1985

First Published ('A Text-Book of X-ray Diagnosis') (3 volumes) . 1938/39
Second Edition (4 volumes) 1950/51
Third Edition (4 volumes) 1957/62
Fourth Edition (6 volumes) 1969/73
Fifth Edition ('A Textbook of Radiological Diagnosis') . . 1984/

©

H. K. LEWIS & Co. Ltd.
1985

ISBN 0-7216-1621-6

Exclusive North American distribution rights
assigned to W. B. Saunders Company, West
Washington Square, Philadelphia, Pa. 19105

PRINTED IN GREAT BRITAIN FOR H. K. LEWIS & Co. Ltd.
BY HAZELL WATSON & VINEY LTD,
MEMBER OF THE BPCC GROUP,
AYLESBURY, BUCKS

PREFACE

Ten years have elapsed since the last edition of 'A Text-Book of X-ray Diagnosis' was published. In its early days in the 1930s, 1940s and 1950s, it was an institution. Not only was it the standard textbook of radiology in Britain but it was the only comprehensive British textbook of radiology. The vision of the original editors, Dr E. W. Twining of Manchester, Dr S. Cochrane Shanks of University College Hospital, London and Sir Peter Kerley of the Westminster Hospital, London was confirmed, and their faith and that of the publishers amply justified. Drs Shanks and Kerley are to be commended for updating and producing subsequent editions. They dedicated the rights of any future editions to the Royal College of Radiologists.

This edition is a completely new set of books in six volumes, each with its own volume editor, a recognised expert in the field. The relevant modern diagnostic imaging procedures are incorporated in the approach to each clinical radiological problem. Some of the newer techniques such as nuclear magnetic resonance and digital vascular imaging have been included though it is recognised that these methods of investigation are not widely available at the present time.

In preparing the new edition the philosophy has been that practising radiologists and radiologists in training require a comprehensive and authoritative review of problems that may be encountered in their daily work. The references given provide the reader with suitable further reading should he wish to pursue a particular subject.

The general format has been changed. The printed text on each page appears in two columns as is the modern practice rather than spreading across the whole page. Illustrations are produced as negatives, rather than as positives which was the practice in previous editions. This latter step brings it in line with modern British and American practice.

It is believed that this entirely new textbook will find favour amongst English-speaking radiologists and will enjoy the popularity and serve as useful a purpose as did the original 'A Text-Book of X-ray Diagnosis' published in 1938.

October 1982   Professor Sir Howard Middlemiss
                                                                                              Editor-in-Chief

Following the unexpected death of Professor Sir Howard Middlemiss on 27 April 1983, the responsibilities of Editor-in-Chief have been assumed by the Council of the Royal College of Radiologists. The Council wishes to express its deep appreciation for the efforts Sir Howard made to ensure continuity of production of these important additions to the radiological literature.

February 1984

CONTRIBUTORS TO THIS VOLUME

Leon M. Gerlis, MB.BS, MRCS, LRCP, FRCPath, Consultant Cardiac Pathologist, National Heart Research Fund and Honorary Consultant Pathologist, Killingbeck Hospital, Leeds, England.

Alan E. Hugh, MB.BCh, FRCPEd, FRCR, DMRD, Consultant Radiologist, North Staffordshire, Royal Infirmary, Stoke-on-Trent, England.

M. Lea Thomas, MA, PhD, FRCP, FRCR, Senior Physician in Radiology and Lecturer, United Medical Schools of Guy's and St Thomas's Hospitals, London.

M. V. Merrick, MA, MSc, BM, BCh, FRCR, Consultant in Nuclear Medicine, Western General Hospital, Edinburgh.

Eric N. C. Milne, MD, FRCR, Professor of Radiological Sciences, University of California College of Medicine, Irvine, California, U.S.A.

John Partridge, MB.BS, MRCP (UK), FRCR, Consultant Cardio-Radiologist, Leeds Regional Cardio-Thoracic Unit, Killingbeck Hospital, Leeds, England.

Ronald B. Pridie, MB.BS, FRCR, FACC, Consultant Radiologist, Harefield Hospital, Middlesex, England.

Maurice J. Raphael, MA, MD, FRCP, FRCR, DMRD, Consultant Radiologist, The National Heart Hospital and The Middlesex Hospital, London.

E. Rhys Davies, MA, MB, BChir (Cantab), FRCPE, FRCR, Hon FFR (RCSI), Professor of Radiodiagnosis, University of Bristol, England.

M. S. T. Ruttley, MB, FRCP, FRCR, Consultant Radiologist, University Hospital of Wales, Cardiff.

John K. Walker, MD, FRCR, Radiologist to Cardiac Unit, Groby Road Hospital and Leicester Royal Infirmary, Leicester, England.

CONTENTS

		PAGE
PREFACE	. . . .	vii
CHAPTER		
1. THE NORMAL HEART – PART I. THE CARDIAC OUTLINE AND CHAMBER ANATOMY	. . . .	1
2. THE NORMAL HEART – PART II. APPLIED ANGIOGRAPHY; CORONARY ARTERIES	. . . .	33
3. PULMONARY PATTERNS IN HEART DISEASE	. . . .	42
4. CARDIAC ULTRASOUND	. . . .	74
5. NUCLEAR CARDIOLOGY	. . . .	92
6. ISCHAEMIC HEART DISEASE	. . . .	105
7. ACQUIRED VALVAR DISEASE AND CARDIAC TUMOURS	. . . .	126
8. PACEMAKERS AND REPLACED VALVES	. . . .	163
9. DISEASES OF HEART MUSCLE	. . . .	171
10. ACQUIRED DISEASES OF THE AORTA	. . . .	178
11. DISEASES OF THE PERICARDIUM	. . . .	194
12. CONGENITAL HEART DISEASE: BASIC PRINCIPLES	. . . .	201
13. SIMPLE CONGENITAL HEART DISEASE	. . . .	211
14. COMPLEX CONGENITAL HEART DISEASE	. . . .	235
15. CONGENITAL DISEASES OF THE GREAT VESSELS AND SURGERY FOR CONGENITAL HEART DISEASE	.	254
16. DISEASES OF THE PERIPHERAL ARTERIES	. . . .	289
17. PHLEBOGRAPHY OF THE LIMB VEINS	. . . .	331
18. DIAGNOSTIC IMAGING OF THE LYMPHATIC SYSTEM	. . . .	370
INDEX	. . . .	396

A TEXTBOOK
OF
RADIOLOGICAL DIAGNOSIS

CHAPTER 1

THE NORMAL HEART—PART I
THE CARDIAC OUTLINE AND CHAMBER ANATOMY

John Walker

The heart is the most open and the most secret object in all radiology. Surrounded by alveolar air (its natural contrast) its outline dominates the chest X-ray. The lung vessels, responding to any change in function, are openly displayed, but within the heart borders the X-ray shadow is obscure and its parts invisible; moreover its vital purpose, movement, is not seen.

This hollow muscular organ is conical, its apex points downwards, forwards and to the left at 60° to the midline. It is roughly 12 cm in length and weighs about 350 g. The main vessels enter and leave at the base posteriorly. Its apex is free within the serous cavity of the pericardium but its base is fixed by vessels and by the pericardial reflexions which surround them. The embryonic dorsal mesopericardium between arteries and veins breaks down to give the transverse sinus which frees the heart posteriorly, and the reflexions around the pulmonary veins form a blind sac, the oblique sinus, which opens to the left.

All is enclosed by fibrous pericardium and occupies the anterior mediastinum at the level of the 6th–9th dorsal vertebrae from which it is separated by the oesophagus, aorta and spinal muscles. It rests on the central tendon of the diaphragm and laterally the right and left lungs envelop it over more than two thirds of its surface (Netter, 1969).

THE CARDIAC SKELETON

Basic to the structure of the heart is the fibrous framework which holds the chambers and vessels together, preventing them from being torn apart by forces generated with every beat (Walmsley & Watson, 1978). The skeleton is the fibrous rings of the tricuspid, mitral and aortic valves bound together by a tough central fibrous body. The tricuspid and mitral rings are in the same vertical plane running from right anterior to left posterior, at 45° to the sagittal. The aortic ring is tilted forwards at an angle of 30° to this plane (Fig. 1.01).

The pulmonary ring is separated from the other valve rings by the right ventricular conus and is joined by a thin conal ligament running in its posterior wall. It is directed upwards and backwards at 45° to the coronal plane.

The inner margins of the aortic and pulmonary rings give attachment to the semilunar valve cusps, whilst outside are attached the ventricular myocardium and the elastic walls of the aorta and pulmonary arteries.

The more complex atrioventricular valves are supported by chordae tendinae and papillary muscles and are also attached to the inner aspect of their rings. The atrial and ventricular myocardium is firmly attached to the outer aspect (see Fig. 1.14 (c)).

RADIOGRAPHIC TECHNIQUE

A practical routine widely accepted is a 'cardiac series' of three films taken erect, with a focus-film distance of 6 feet (180 cm):

(1) The Normal Soft Tissue PA Film

This is principally concerned with demonstrating pulmonary vessels. A low kV is used, no grid and only the upper dorsal vertebrae are to be seen (Fig. 1.02).

(2) Penetrated PA View

This is obtained by doubling the MAS, raising the kV by 10 and employing a fine high ratio grid. It obliterates the lung vessels but gives the heart a sharper outline, and permits some intrapericardial structures to be seen (Fig. 1.03).

(3) The Lateral View

This is necessarily a penetrated view using the grid and the kV is raised by a further 10. It demonstrates the cardiac silhouette, the main vessels and the air-filled trachea. Only gross pulmonary vascular changes can be seen (Fig. 1.04).

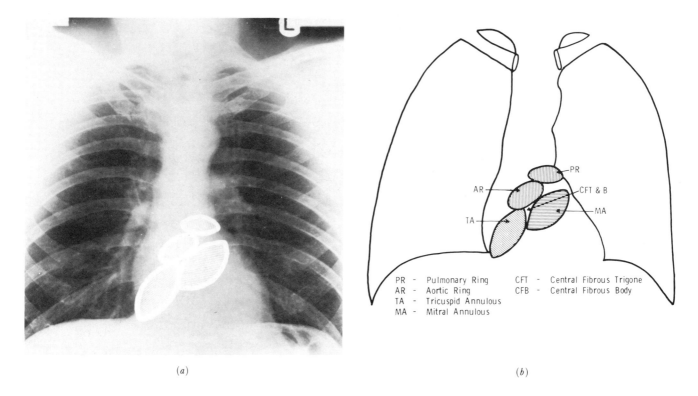

(a)   (b)

FIG. 1.01. The fibrous skeleton of the heart. The mitral, tricuspid and aortic rings are firmly bound together. The pulmonary ring is loosely connected by the conus ligament. (a) PA view of the heart with the skeleton superimposed. (b) Explanatory diagram. (c) Lateral view with the skeleton superimposed. (d) Explanatory diagram.

(c)   (d)

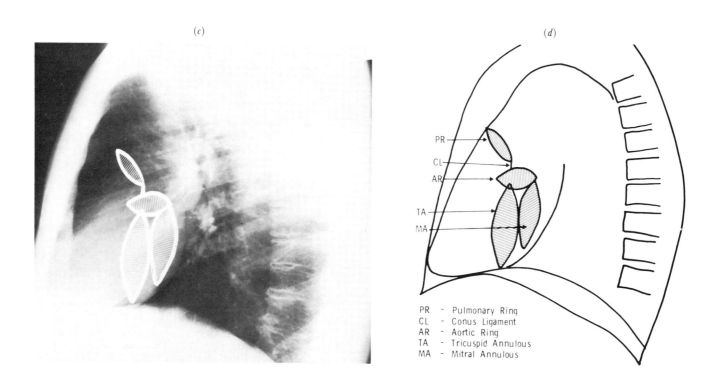

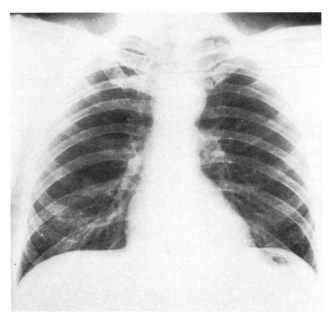

FIG. 1.02. Cardiac series. PA view of chest, low penetration showing cardiac outline and pulmonary vessels.

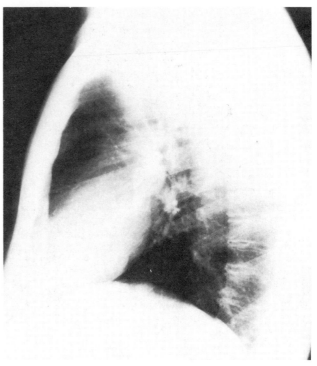

FIG. 1.04. Lateral view showing anterior and posterior heart borders.

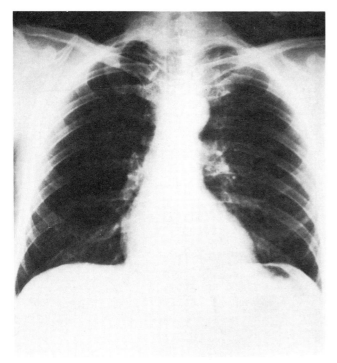

FIG. 1.03. Penetrated PA defining the cardiac outline clearly but obliterating the pulmonary vascular pattern.

HEART SIZE

The heart size in a normal subject follows a distribution curve similar to that of any other physical parameter, e.g. weight, height, blood pressure, pulse rate. A standard deviation from over 15% to as little as 5% depends on measurement technique.

Ultimately only two modes of cardiac dysfunction exist:

(1) Mechanical abnormality
(2) Myocardial dysfunction

Both can cause cardiac enlargement.

Starling's Law here applied shows cardiac dysfunction expressed as an increase in heart size, and this has proved to be the most respected and useful radiological sign. A small heart is never a sign of heart disease but is seen secondary to wasting, of which starvation, carcinomatosis and Addison's disease are classic examples. Obstructive airways disease causes the heart to appear small relative to an increased lung volume.

The difficulties of measuring the heart have been overstated but they are real. They include standardisation for cardiac cycle and respiratory phase, the definition of the exact cardiac border, magnification in two planes and the fact that the heart is not a regular body by geometrical definition.

None of these is insuperable and a simple protocol can make valid readings practicable. It is easy, with care, to determine heart volume and still easier to measure frontal area or a single diameter. If the same method is used on the same individual many variables become constant, and over a series of examinations the normal variation is reduced 4-fold, so that even the single diameter becomes more exact. Definition is improved by comparing heart size with body size (somatic parameter) and a correlation coefficient of $r = 0.6$ will reduce scatter by one third. The three main methods of measurement are one, two and three dimensional.

One Dimension. This is popular and widely used as the cardiothoracic ratio. The widest heart diameter is expressed as a percentage of the widest diameter of the lung shadow. It is simple to carry out and practical, because *All* the information is present on the one film, Fig. 1.05. In the adult the normal range is between 39% and 50% but this is exceeded in childhood and old age (Danzer, 1919).

Two Dimensions. The area of the cardiac silhouette is either traced by plainimeter or calculated from the long and broad axes (Schwarz, 1946). The formula $A = L*W*0.735$ where L is the long diameter from the top of the right atrium on the right heart border to the apex, and W is the width—W(1)+W(2). W(1) is a perpendicular from L to the right cardiac phrenic angle and W(2) is the perpendicular to the top of the left ventricle on the left heart border (Hilbish & Morgan, 1952) (Fig. 1.06).

The use of area versus the transverse diameter will improve accuracy by 50% for very little extra effort, and might be more widely used if it could be expressed as succinctly as the CT ratio. The corresponding CA—T_2 ratio would be 16% in adults (Walker, 1956). A better correlation is cardiac area (CA) with body surface area (Ungerleider & Gubner, 1942).

Three Dimensions (Fig. 1.07). The cardiac volume is derived from frontal area times depth. The depth diameter in the lateral view is a horizontal from the posterior sternum to the posterior extent of the heart shadow. Using the formula $V = L*W*D*K$ where $K = 0.44$ and is a constant which takes account of the shape of the heart and radiographic magnification (Keats & Enge, 1965). Somatic parameters may be those found on the chest film. Better, but requiring more data, is body surface areas, oxygen uptake, blood volume, red cell volume and others.

The sensitivity of each method may be expressed as the minimal enlargement that it will detect with certainty; two standard deviations (a one in twenty chance) is acceptable. Each method is consistent whatever the somatic comparison:

   (1) Single diameter—45%
   (2) Frontal area—30%
   (3) Cardiac volume—20%

When cardiac volume is measured total accuracy is the aim. Posture, the cardiac cycle and respiration as well as somatic factors are critical. By ingenuity and care an

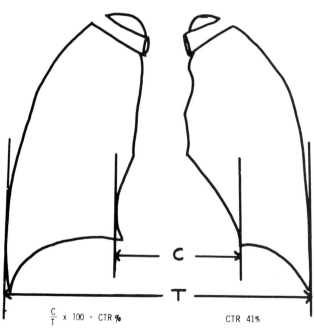

$$\frac{C}{T} \times 100 = CTR\% \qquad CTR\ 41\%$$

FIG. 1.05. Single dimensional cardiac measurement—the cardiothoracic ratio—CTR. C is the maximal transverse diameter of the heart. T is the maximal transverse diameter of the lungs.

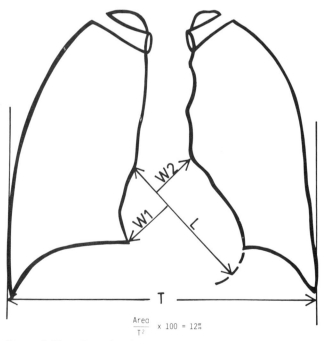

$$\frac{Area}{T^2} \times 100 = 12\%$$

FIG. 1.06. Two dimensional cardiac measurement. L is the long axis of the heart. W1 + W2 is the maximal short axis of the heart. Area = L*W*0.735.

enlargement of as little as 11% can be recognised (Lind, 1950).

Because sensitivity is increased with serial examination, in practice the CT ratio has a value beyond its statistical merit. Habit, the ease of carrying it out and the beguiling belief that the limit of normal is 50% all add to its popularity.

Few centres use cardiac volumes routinely and fewer still take the results so seriously as to challenge an informed subjective impression (Jefferson & Rees, 1980).

Compared with generalised cardiac enlargement selective chamber enlargement seen as a deformity of the silhouette is less definitive. This applies particularly to the thick walled closely apposed ventricles where enlargement may be evident, but where it is difficult to distinguish left from right. The thin walled elastic vessels, the aorta and the pulmonary artery, are easy to identify; likewise the atria 'balloon out' characteristically under increased pressure. Chamber and vessel enlargement in these circumstances are a valuable diagnostic sign, and knowledge of the contribution each makes to the general outline is needed (Roesler, 1943).

The standard PA and lateral films are reproducible and are the most useful views. Oblique views, once popular, vary; they are less reproducible, and less often used in this context.

In each view the heart has two borders, in the PA right and left, and in the lateral and oblique views, anterior and posterior.

THE POSTERO-ANTERIOR (PA) VIEW

The right heart border is shared equally by the superior vena cava above (a straight vertical line overlying the tips of the transverse processes) and the right atrium below (a slight outward bulge) (Fig. 1.08). The right cardiophrenic angle (between the right heart border and the diaphragm) is commonly crossed by a short straight line; this is the inferior vena cava as it enters the right atrium.

After the age of 45 it is normal for the unfolded ascending aorta to encroach upon the superior vena cava and even produce a slight shallow bulge (Fig. 1.09).

The left heart border is also divided roughly equally. The upper half lies vertically over the tips of the transverse processes and is subdivided into three unequal parts. The uppermost, the aortic knuckle, is the left side of the aortic arch. It is the largest and most conspicuous bulge (Fig. 1.10).

Below the aortic knuckle is the pulmonary arc, smaller, shallower and consisting of the main pulmonary trunk and the left main pulmonary artery. Below this and still smaller is the pulmonary bay, a shallow hollow between the pulmonary arc above and the left ventricle. This bay is always occupied by the anterior tip of the

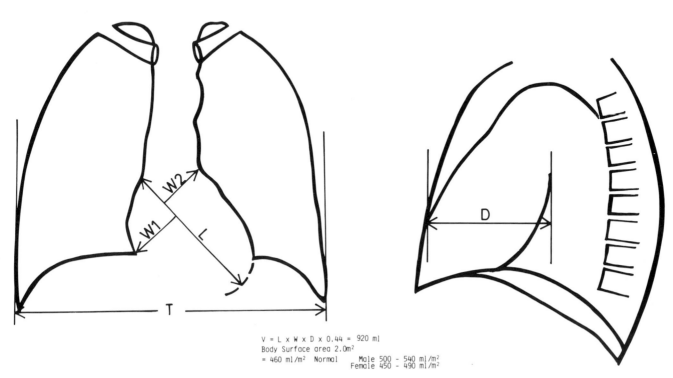

V = L x W x D x 0.44 = 920 ml
Body Surface area 2.0m²
= 460 ml/m²   Normal   Male 500 - 540 ml/m²
                        Female 450 - 490 ml/m²

FIG. 1.07. Three dimensional cardiac measurement. D between the posterior border of the sternum where it abuts on to the cardiac silhouette and the most posterior extent of the posterior border. Volume = L*W*D*0.445.

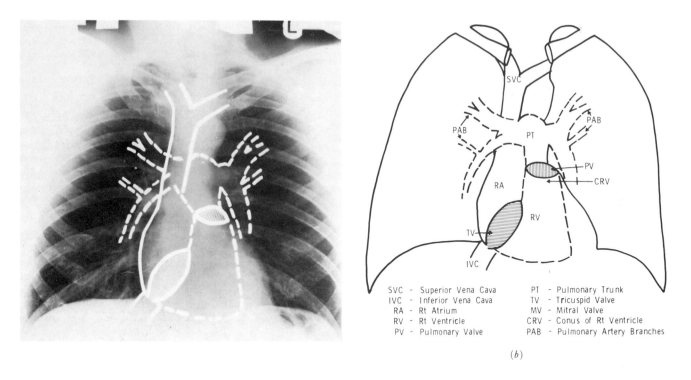

SVC - Superior Vena Cava   PT   - Pulmonary Trunk
IVC - Inferior Vena Cava   TV   - Tricuspid Valve
RA   - Rt Atrium   MV   - Mitral Valve
RV   - Rt Ventricle   CRV - Conus of Rt Ventricle
PV   - Pulmonary Valve   PAB - Pulmonary Artery Branches

(b)

FIG. 1.08. The position of the great veins and right heart structures in the PA view. The accompanying angiograms illustrate the site of the right atrium, the right ventricle and the pulmonary artery. The veins are demonstrated by reflux. TV Tricuspid Valve, PA Pulmonary Artery, RV Rt. Ventricle, SVC Superior Vena Cava, IVC Inferior Vena Cava, PV Pulmonary Valve. (a) PA View C with superimpositions of chambers and vessels. (b) Explanatory diagram Rt. atrium with reflux into the great veins. (c) Angiogram from the Rt. atrium with reflux into the great veins. (d) Angiogram from the Rt. ventricle showing the pulmonary artery. (*By courtesy of Dr J. B. Partridge.*)

(c)   (d)

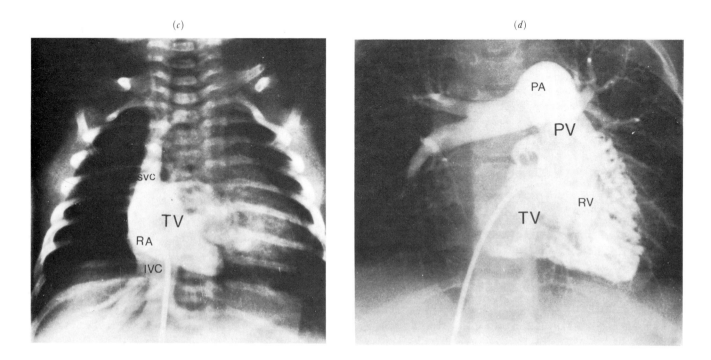

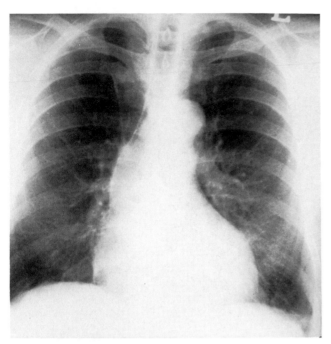

FIG. 1.09. The PA view of an elderly subject with the upper right heart border taken over by the curved bulge of the ascending aorta.

left atrial appendix and in about half of subjects this shows as a small bulge (Jacobson & Weidner, 1962). The whole of the lower half of the left heart border is the arc of the left ventricle, a shallow curve directed outwards and downwards at an angle of 45° to the midline and intersecting the left diaphragm less than half way across.

The upper fifth of the mediastinal shadow is variable. It is straight and formed by the right brachiocephalic and internal jugular veins on the right side, and the left subclavian artery and internal jugular vein on the left.

The right ventricle makes no contribution to the cardiac outline in this view.

LATERAL VIEW

The two borders, anterior and posterior, are less well seen than those of the PA view.

The anterior border is the sharper but its lower third abuts on the anterior chest wall and is obscured. It slopes backwards at 75° to the horizontal in two curves. The upper third is the anterior aortic arch, the lower two-thirds the anterior surface of the right ventricle, the right ventricular outflow tract and a small part of the pulmonary trunk (Fig. 1.11).

The posterior border is more complex. The lower half (the heart itself) is the most clearly seen. The upper three-quarters of this is the left atrium, its edge blurred by incoming pulmonary veins. Below, the right atrium

and inferior vena cava are normally the border, but the left ventricular margin is very close and runs at an angle of less than 45° to the diaphragm. Slight enlargement or rotation may bring it into view (Fig. 1.12 & 1.21).

Above the atrial shadow the aortic arch is well seen behind and discontinuous with the left atrium. The translucent space below the arch is crossed by the pulmonary trunk which divides midway into right and left main branches, the right is seen foreshortened as a dense shadow within the main artery (Fig. 1.23).

OBLIQUE VIEWS

The oblique position was originally used to bring a selected chamber into optimal relief on the heart border and in this respect it still has a use, but its main value today is in angiocardiography.

Right Anterior Oblique View

The right anterior oblique view is taken with the saggital plane at 45° to the beam and the right anterior chest next to the film.

The anterior border can be divided into three. The smaller shallow upper arc is the anterior edge of the ascending aorta. The middle and largest arc is the right ventricular outflow tract and the pulmonary trunk, whilst the lower arc is the apex of the left ventricle (Fig. 1.13).

The posterior border is less conspicuous and is not entirely outlined by air. It may be defined by barium in the oesophagus, its immediate posterior relation, and divided into upper third and lower two-thirds (Fig. 1.14).

The upper third is vertical and has the prominent backward indentation of the posterior aortic arch above. Below this is a smaller arc formed by the right main pulmonary artery as it crosses the origin of the left main bronchus.

The lower two-thirds is a smooth arch curving forwards towards the diaphragm at about 60° to the horizontal. Its upper and larger part is the left atrium. The smaller and lower is the right atrium and the contribution of each can be changed by altering the obliquity.

Left Anterior Oblique View

The left anterior oblique view is taken with the saggital plane at 60° to the beam or until the posterior border clears the spine and with the left anterior chest next to the film.

The anterior border has two equal parts. The upper, vertical and straight, is formed by the superior vena cava with the anterior aortic arch projecting slightly at its centre. The lower is a slightly more prominent arc running forwards at 70° to the horizontal and formed in its upper part by the right atrial appendix and in its

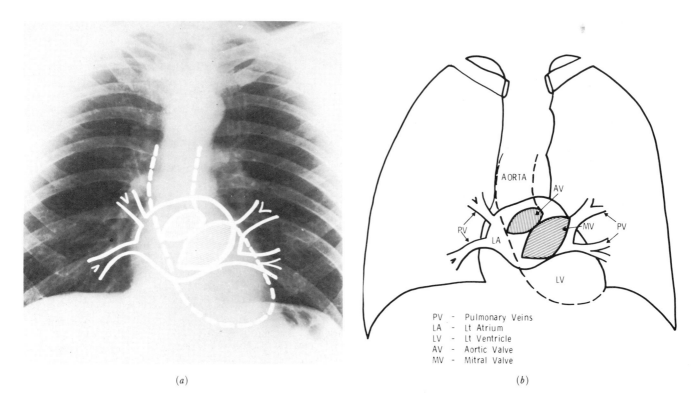

(a)   (b)

FIG. 1.10. Outline of left heart structures as seen in the PA view and illustrated by angiography. LA Left Atrium, MV Mitral Valve, AV Aortic Valve, PV Pulmonary Vein, LA Lt. Atrium, M The negative shadow of the mitral valve caused by inflow of non-opaque blood. (a) PA view with superimposition of chambers and vessels. (b) Explanatory diagram. (c) The filling of the pulmonary veins and Lt. Atrium from a pulmonary arteriogram. (d) The demonstration of the Lt. ventricle and aorta from a Lt. ventricular angiogram.

(c)   (d)

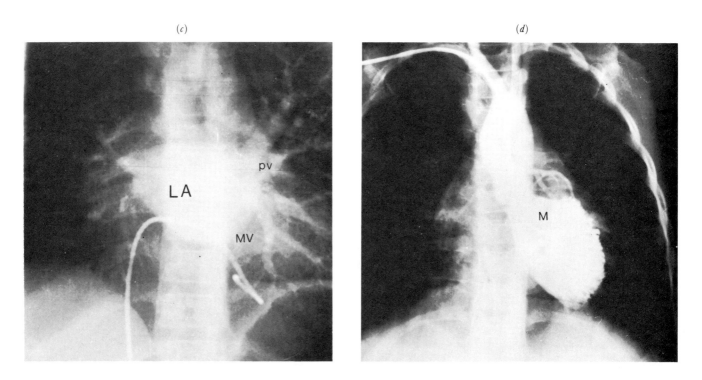

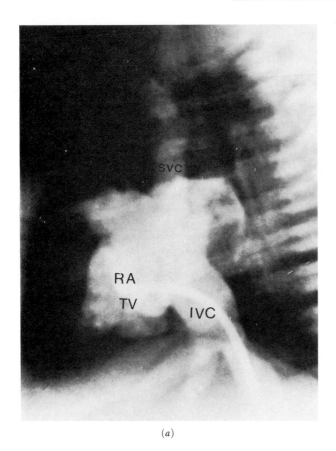

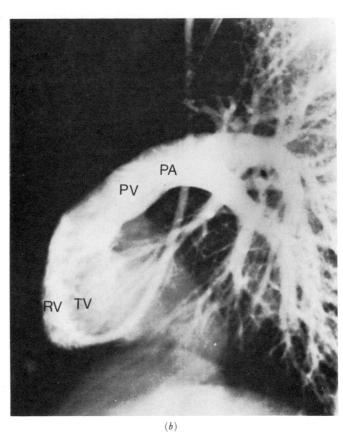

(a)

(b)

FIG. 1.11. The lateral view of right heart structures as illustrated by angiography. The great veins are filled by reflux from the right atrial injection. RA Right Atrium, TV Tricuspid Valve, PV Pulmonary Valve, RV Right Ventricle, C Crista, IVC Inferior Vena Cava, SVC Superior Vena Cava. (a) Angiogram from the Rt. Atrium. (b) Angiogram from the Rt. Ventricle. (c) Explanatory diagram.

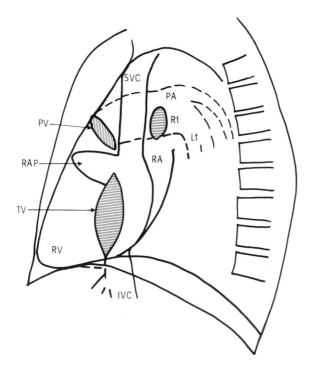

(c)

SVC - Superior Vena Cava
IVC - Inferior Vena Cava
PA   - Pulmonary Artery
PV   - Pulmonary Valve
Rt   - Rt Main Branch of Pulmonary Artery
Lt   - Lt Main Branch of Pulmonary Artery
RAP - Rt Atrial Appendix
RA   - Rt Atrium
RV   - Rt Ventricle
TV   - Tricuspid Valve

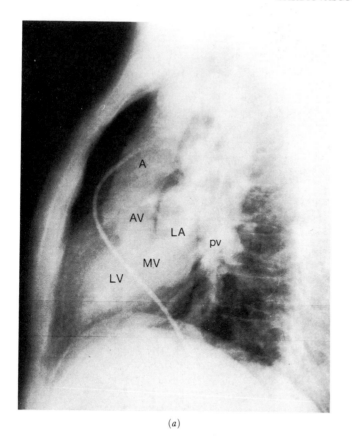

(a)

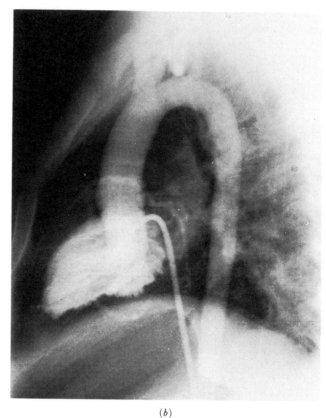

(b)

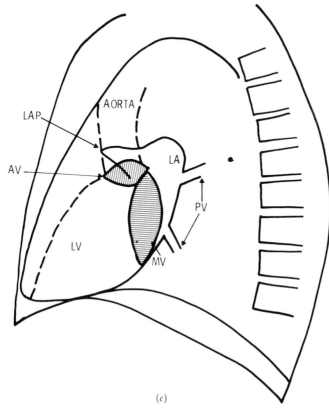

(c)

FIG. 1.12. Position of left-sided structures in the lateral view, as illustrated by angiography. LA Left Atrium, MV Mitral Valve, LV Left Ventricle, AV Aortic Valve, A Aorta, PV Pulmonary Vein. (a) Lt. sided structures demonstrated from a pulmonary arteriogram. (b) Lt. Ventricle and Aorta demonstrated by Lt. ventricular angiogram. (c) Explanatory diagram.

LAP - Lt Atrial Appendix
LA - Lt Atrium
LV - Lt Ventricle
PV - Pulmonary Veins
MV - Mitral Valve
AV - Aortic Valve

lower part by the right ventricle and right ventricular outflow tract (Fig. 1.15).

The posterior border has two disconnected parts almost vertical and equal. The upper and larger is the posterior descending aorta which overlies the shadow of the spine. The lower and sharper border is the posterior surface of the left ventricle and is anterior to it.

This view shows the right and left ventricles in optimal relief and is used to assess individual ventricular enlargement. Caution is needed in that the two ventricles are intimately related and thick walled; enlargement of one may be mimicked by enlargement of the other. The aortic arch is open and through the translucent 'aortic window' can be seen the pulmonary trunk and the left pulmonary artery.

All views are used in fluoroscopy to identify calcium and fat and to assess movement.

INDIVIDUAL CHAMBER ANATOMY

Direct injection of contrast media by catheter into a selected chamber or vessel demonstrates detail as no other method can (Kjellburg *et al.*, 1958). The right heart is entered from peripheral veins and except with some cases of aortic valvular disease the left ventricle can be entered retrogradely via the aorta.

In adults the left atrium is difficult to reach. Transseptal and thoracic puncture carry a risk and retrograde passage from the left ventricle is chancy. In young children the left atrium is usually entered via the right atrium through the foramen ovale.

Right Atrium

The right atrium is a thin walled chamber in two parts; the posterior is smooth walled and receives the main veins. The superior vena cava enters the upper posterolateral margin. The inferior vena cava enters the lower posterolateral margin with the coronary sinus medial to it. On its medial wall is the fossa ovalis. The venous valves, of which the Eustachian valve of the inferior vena cava is the largest, are anterior to the main venous orifices.

The posterior right atrium is derived from the sinus venosus and separated above by a small ridge, the crista terminalis, from the trabeculated anterior part. This anterior part connects with the right ventricle via the tricuspid valve and extends forwards and upwards as the large right atrial appendix which lies on the right anterior heart border in the atrioventricular sulcus.

Angiographic Anatomy. *The PA View* shows the rounded body of the right atrium. The tricuspid valve occupies the lower anteromedial wall and the superior and inferior vena cava are identified by reflux (Fig. 1.08).

In the *lateral view* the tricuspid valve is anterior and visible when closed in systole. It disappears as the cusps open in diastole. The right atrial appendix extends forwards and upwards and overlies the right ventricular outflow tract (Fig. 1.01).

Right Atrial Enlargement. *PA view.* Of all four cardiac chambers the right atrium was the last to have radiological enlargement described. This could be because moderate enlargement rotates the whole heart to the left. The right heart border with the superior vena cava is displaced medially to expose the dorsal spine above, and make the expected bulge of the lower right heart border inconstant (Fig. 1.16).

In the *lateral view* right atrial enlargement obliterates the upper retrosternal space by the dilated right atrial appendix (Fig. 1.17).

Gross dilatation of the right atrium does cause outward bulging of the lower right heart border in the PA view. It is lower, more tethered to the diaphragm and bulges less freely than the left atrium.

Right Ventricle

The right ventricle may also be divided into two parts, the inflow and the outflow tracts; this is clearly seen on angiography (Fig. 1.08, 1.11, 1.13 & 1.15).

The inflow tract is conical, heavily trabeculated and the trabeculae are coarse. Its base, the tricuspid valve, is posterior and opens anteromedially.

A large muscular orifice connects the posterior inflow and the anterior outflow tract. Above it is the prominent crista supra-ventricularis which merges with the septal and parietal bands, thick ridges of muscle which run along their respective ventricular walls.

Inferiorly the septal band continues as a large trabeculum, the moderator band, and completes the circle by joining the tip of the parietal band on the right anterior wall.

The tricuspid valve has a large anterior cusp, a divided posterior cusp and a small variable medial cusp. It has a large constant anterior papillary muscle arising at the point where the moderator band joins the parietal band and it is demonstrable angiographically. The posterior papillary muscles are many, variable and difficult to define. The medial papillary muscle is small but constant and arises where the crista merges with the septal band.

The outflow tract has the free wall of the heart anteriorly and the crista and inflow tract posteriorly. It is triangular in the PA view and semilunar laterally. It connects above with the pulmonary artery via the pulmonary valve.

About a third of its length, the infundibulum, is above the inflow tract and the wall becomes progressively smoother as it approaches the pulmonary valve.

Angiographic Anatomy. *In the PA view* the triangle of the outflow tract dominates the shape of the right ventricle but the tricuspid valve, a shallow concavity, is the lower right border and the septum the left. Entirely

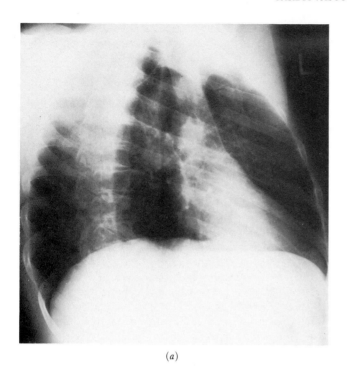

(a)

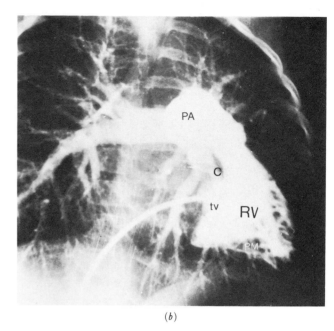

(b)

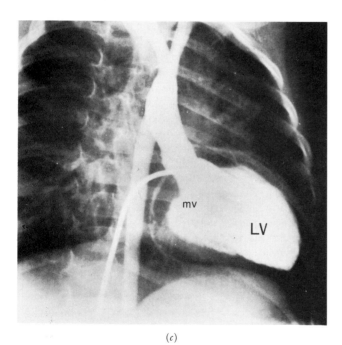

(c)

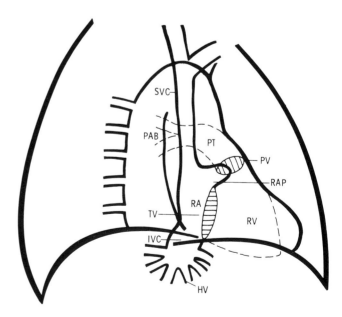

(d)

Fɪɢ. 1.13. The right anterior oblique view with illustrations of the **right-sided and left-sided structures by ventricular angiography of both right and left ventricles.** C Crista, PM Papillary Muscles. (*a*) **Normal Rt. anterior oblique view.** (*b*) Rt. Ventricular angiogram. (*c*) **Lt. Ventricular angiogram.** (*d*) Explanatory diagram Rt. side. (*e*) Explanatory diagram Lt. side. (*By courtesy of Dr J. B. Partridge.*)

SVC	–	Superior Vena Cava	PAB	–	Pulmonary Artery Branches
PT	–	Pulmonary Trunk			
PV	–	Pulmonary Veins	RAP	–	Right Atrial Appendix
RA	–	Right Atrium	TV	–	Tricuspid Valve
RV	–	Right Ventricle	HV	–	Hepatic Veins
IVC	–	Inferior Vena Cava			

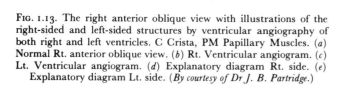

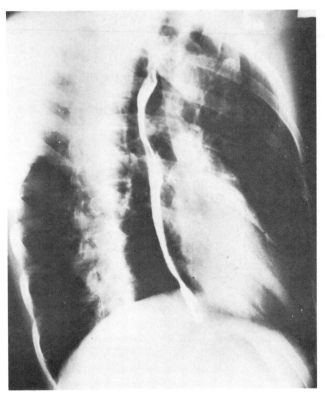

Fig. 1.14. The right anterior oblique view of the heart with the oesophagus outlined by barium and defining the posterior border.

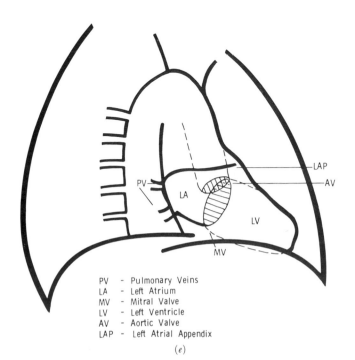

PV - Pulmonary Veins
LA - Left Atrium
MV - Mitral Valve
LV - Left Ventricle
AV - Aortic Valve
LAP - Left Atrial Appendix

(e)

within the silhouette the right ventricle has no part of the heart border in the frontal view. Its apex is the pulmonary trunk, but the pulmonary valve *en face* is hard to define (Fig. 1.08).

The lateral view shows the right ventricle forming the anterior border of the heart. Posteriorly the crista supra-ventricularis is conspicuous above and in front of the tricuspid valve, and from it the infundibulum passes upwards and backwards to be continuous with the pulmonary trunk (Fig. 1.11). The pulmonary valve is seen well in profile.

The crista supra-ventricularis is the dominant feature. The septal and parietal bands are visible but less clear and the moderator band is usually lost among the trabeculae. The anterior papillary muscle may also be seen (Fig. 1.08, 1.13 & 1.15).

The pulmonary valve. The cusps of the pulmonary valve are simple and support each other in apposition when closed in diastole. Each cusp is associated with its pulmonary sinus—a dilatation at the base of the pulmonary artery. These are identified as right anterior, left anterior and posterior.

Right Ventricular Enlargement. *PA View.* (Fig. 1.18). When the right ventricle enlarges it is almost always accompanied by right atrial enlargement and it also rotates the heart to the left. In the PA view the right ventricle takes over the left heart border from below upwards. With moderate enlargement the left ventricle still forms the apex which is characteristically 'turned up' above the diaphragm. When severe it takes over the whole left heart border which becomes straight and barely distinguishable from left ventricular enlargement (Jefferson & Rees, 1980).

In the *lateral view* the anteroposterior diameter is increased, there is obliteration of the retrosternal space from below upwards and the inferior vena cava is displaced backwards.

Backwards displacement of the posterior heart border can mimic left ventricular enlargement but the bulge is higher, above the diaphragm.

Indirect signs of right ventricular enlargement are prominence of the azygos vein (Fig. 1.22) and of the right atrial appendix in the lateral view.

Left Atrium

The left atrium is the most posterior part of the heart. It lies posteromedially and slightly above the right atrium from which it is divided by the interatrial septum. Its wall is thicker.

Normally two pulmonary veins, upper and lower, enter from either lung and are seen well on follow-through angiography. Variations do occur. Pericardial reflexions bind the left atrium closely to the anterior spinal muscles and make it the most fixed part of the heart. Like the right atrium it has two parts; the posterior, derived from the primitive common pulmon-

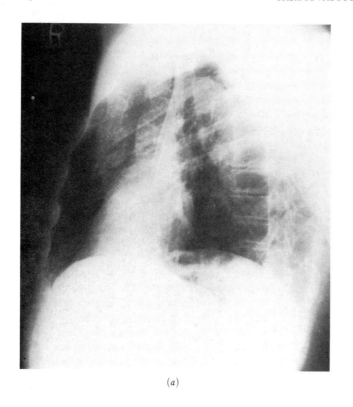

(a)

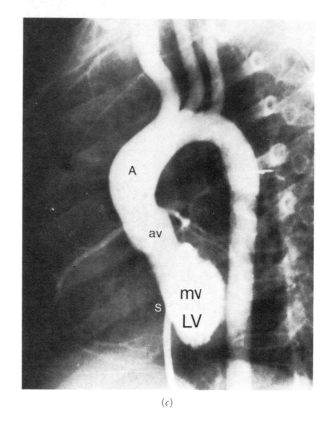

(c)

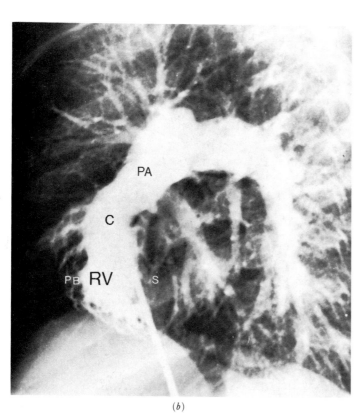

(b)

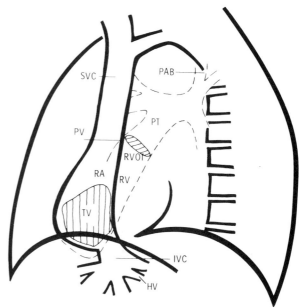

(d)

SVC   –   Superior Vena Cava
RVOT – Rt. Ventricular Outflow Tract
PAB   –   Pulmonary Artery Branches
PV   –   Pulmonary Veins
PT   –   Pulmonary Trunk
RA   –   Right Atrium   IVC   –   Inferior Vena Cava
RV   –   Right Ventricle   HV   –   Hepatic Veins
TV   –   Tricuspid Valve

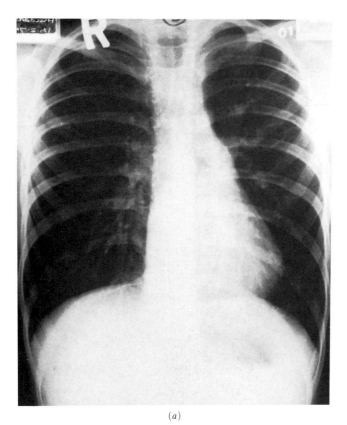

(a)

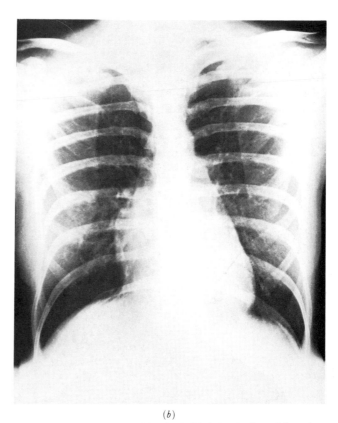

(b)

Fig. 1.16. Right atrial enlargement. (a) With the heart shadow rotated clockwise hiding the right atrial border behind the shadow of the spine. (b) Right atrial enlargement with the heart unrotated showing a bulge on the lower right heart border.

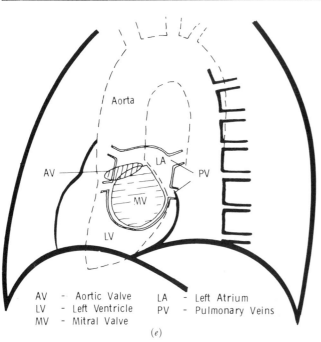

AV	–	Aortic Valve
LV	–	Left Ventricle
MV	–	Mitral Valve

LA	–	Left Atrium
PV	–	Pulmonary Veins

(e)

Fig. 1.15. The left anterior oblique view showing the situation of right and left sided structures and illustrated by right and left ventricular angiograms in systole and diastole. C Crista. PB Pariatal Band. S Inter-Ventricular Septum. (a) Normal Lt. anterior oblique view. (b) Rt. ventricular angiogram. (c) Lt. ventricular angiogram. (d) Explanatory diagram Rt. side. (e) Explanatory diagram Lt. side. (*By courtesy of Dr J. B. Partridge.*)

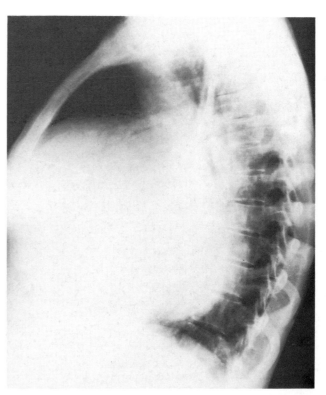

Fig. 1.17. Right atrial enlargement, lateral view. The large right atrial appendix fills the retrosternal space.

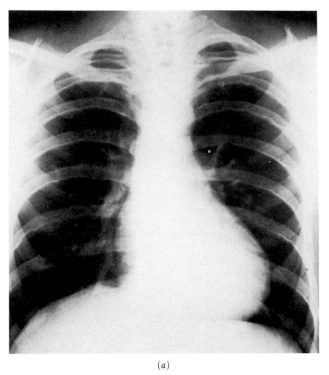

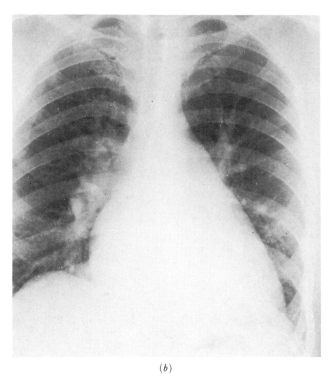

(a)   (b)

FIG. 1.18. Right ventricular enlargement. (a) Moderate. (b) Severe. In (a) the apex of the left ventricle is seen as a high apex on the left heart border. In (b) the grossly enlarged right ventricle has taken over all the lower left heart border.

ary vein, is the bigger and has the valve of the fossa ovalis in its septum. It receives the pulmonary veins (Fig. 1.10 & 1.12). The anterior part derived from the primitive atrium includes the left atrial appendix which forms a tiny but important part of the left heart border. It is trabeculated. Anteriorly the left atrium connects with the left ventricle via the mitral valve.

Angiographic anatomy. In the *PA view* the left atrium is a sphere flattened from front and back. The pulmonary veins enter from the side.

In the *lateral view* it has the mitral valve on its left anterior wall which domes forwards in systole but disappears when the cusps open in diastole. Above it the finger of the appendix points forwards.

Left Atrial Enlargement (Fig. 1.19). *PA view.* Left atrial enlargement is the most characteristic and the easiest to assess. It is first seen on the penetrated PA view as a central rounded density over the base of the heart, touching the left heart border (Jacobson & Weidner, 1962). With further increase the appendix bulges over the left heart border and, to the right, the edge is seen as a contour inside the heart shadow. It may take over the right heart border. The angle of the carina is increased to 90° and more, the left lower bronchus may be compressed, and this may lead to lobar collapse. The descending aorta is displaced to the left as a smooth curve even by moderate enlargement

(Bedford's sign). As left atrial enlargement continues and becomes aneurysmal it forms the whole of the posterior heart, both left and right borders and the angle of the carina approaches 180°.

In the *lateral view*, left atrial enlargement is seen as prominence of the upper curve of the posterior heart border, the lower ventricular curve being directed more acutely forward. Barium in the oesophagus highlights this appearance.

Left Ventricle

The left ventricle is the most predictably regular of the cardiac chambers, it is thick walled, less trabeculated than the right ventricle and the trabeculae are directed towards the apex. Its two valves are situated together at the flattened posteromedial end. They have thick fibrous rings.

The anterolateral and posteromedial papillary muscles are large and constant and arise from the lateral free wall just proximal to the apex. Their chordae tendinae support both cusps of the mitral valve (Fig. 1.13). The anterior cusp is broad. The posterior cusp is narrow but its attachment to the ring is more extensive. The interventricular septum, an anterior continuation of the left ventricular wall, is equally thick and continues upwards towards the mid aortic ring. One centimetre from the ring it ends (the limbus) and

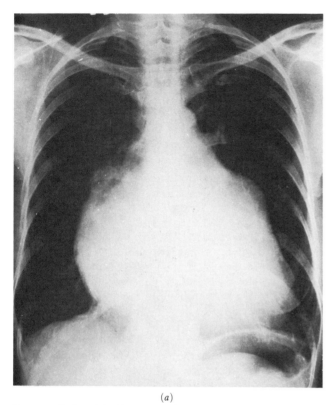

(a)

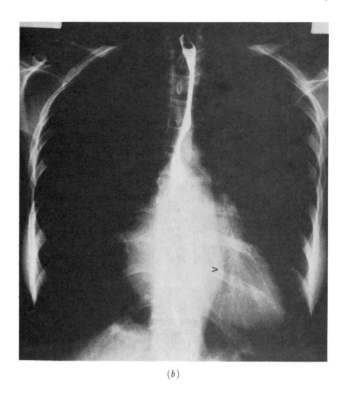

(b)

FIG. 1.19. Left atrial enlargement. (a) PA view showing a bulge on the left heart border and pulmonary venous imbalance. (b) Penetrated view showing lateral displacement of the descending aorta seen through the heart shadow (Bedford's sign) (arrow). (c) Lateral view of moderate Lt. atrial enlargement (arrow). (d) Lateral view of moderate Lt. atrial enlargement with barium in the oesophagus (arrow).

(c)

(d)

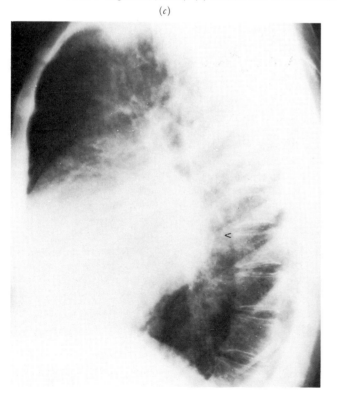

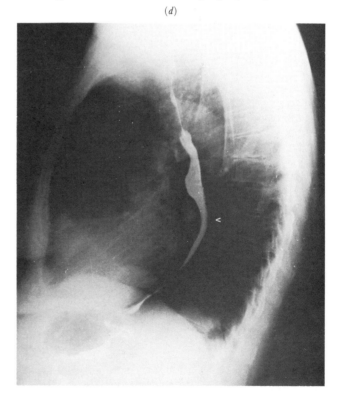

is continued as the membranous septum directed to the right to meet the right edge of the aortic ring.

The membranous septum extends for upwards of 2 cm from the junction of the right coronary and noncoronary cusps of the aortic valve in front to the fibrous trigone behind. On its right side the medial cusp of the tricuspid valve bisects it so that the anterior half separates the right and left ventricles and the posterior half the left ventricle and the right atrium (Walmsley & Watson, 1978).

Angiographic Anatomy of the Left Ventricle. In both PA and lateral views the left ventricle is foreshortened. Its profile is best seen in the right anterior oblique view and it is seen *en face* in the left anterior oblique view (Fig. 1.13).

In the *PA view* the mitral valve is not fully outlined, but can be seen in diastole when opaque medium is trapped behind its cusps. It runs diagonally at 45° from the diaphragmatic surface on the right side to the left heart border (Fig. 1.20). The aortic ring is supromedial to the mitral. The base of the anterior cusp of the mitral valve is adjacent to the left coronary sinus of Valsalva. The aortic valve is less conspicuous than the pulmonary valve having no infundibulum. It forms the upper limit of the left ventricular outline in the PA view. The small left ventricular outflow tract is difficult to identify, but

its short medial border is outlined as the right border of the left ventricle immediately below the aortic valve.

In the *lateral view* the forward dome of the mitral cusp is seen in systole. The aortic ring is anterosuperior to the mitral and the base of the anterior cusp of the mitral valve is adjacent to the left coronary and posterior noncoronary sinus of Valsalva. The aortic valve is best seen during diastole and disappears when the valves open in systole. The two papillary muscles are conspicuous and they appear round and 'end on' (Fig. 1.20).

The right anterior oblique view shows the ellipsoid shape at its best. Posteriorly the mitral cusps are *en profile* and cause flattening or even concavity. The inferior surface is less round than the anterior (Fig. 1.13) and the papillary muscles are well seen.

The aortic valve cusps are similar to those of the pulmonary valve. The aortic sinuses (the sinuses of Valsalva) are identified as anterior, and right and left posterior. They are slightly more prominent than the pulmonary; the right posterior sinus is known as the noncoronary sinus because no coronary artery comes off it. It is lower and larger than the others. The posterior left sinus gives rise to the left coronary artery and the anterior sinus the right coronary artery. These are commonly identified as the left and right coronary sinuses of Valsalva.

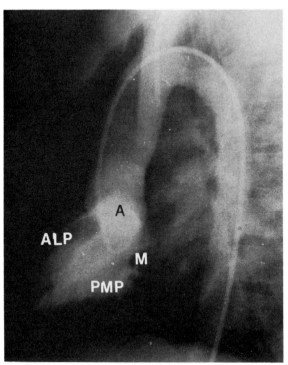

(a) Systole.

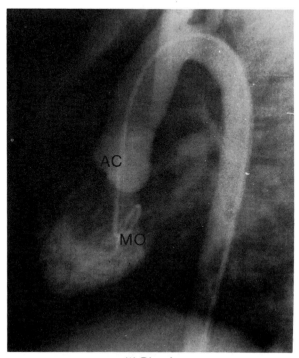

(b) Diastole.

FIG. 1.20. Left ventricle (lateral) in systole and diastole showing the mitral valve opening and the aortic valve closing. (a) Mitral valve closed, A Aortic valve open, ALP anterolateral papillary muscle, PMP posteromedial papillary muscle, (b) MO mitral valve open, AC aortic valve closed.

The left anterior oblique view shows the anterior interventricular septum and the left ventricular outflow tract. It has now been complemented by the 'long axis' view (see Chapter 2).

Left Ventricular Enlargement (Fig. 1.21). Left ventricular enlargement in the PA view is characterised by downward displacement of the apex and elongation of the left ventricular curve on the left heart border. The apex is often below the diaphragm and the pulmonary bay may disappear. As the curve becomes more prominent the whole heart looks big.

In the *lateral view* the depth increases and the lower arc on the posterior border becomes prominent. In a true lateral view, when the posterior border is more than 18 mm behind the inferior vena cava and 20 mm above their point of crossing, left ventricular enlargement is present (Hoffman & Rigler, 1965).

As with the right heart, atrial enlargement and venous changes often accompany or precede signs of left ventricular enlargement.

THE GREAT VESSELS

Systemic Veins

The two main systemic veins, the superior and the inferior venae cavae, carry roughly equal volumes of blood which vary with posture, exercise and respiratory phase.

The superior vena cava is straight, runs vertically downwards from the D4 level and enters the upper lateral margin of the right atrium. Its lower third is within the pericardium. The inferior vena cava, joined by the broad hepatic veins, crosses the diaphragm and runs forwards and medially to enter the right atrium posteriorly; its course within the chest is short. The coronary sinus runs downwards and to the right in the posterior atrioventricular sulcus and enters medial to the orifice of the inferior vena cava.

Systemic Venous Enlargement. With notable exceptions systemic venous enlargement is less useful than radiologists might have hoped. The inferior vena cava is too short to contribute and the superior vena cava is rotated out of view by right cardiac enlargement in most situations where it becomes distended. In this situation enlargement of the azygos vein may show as a shadow in the angle of the right main bronchus (Fig. 1.22). Distally, obstruction of the superior vena cava may cause dilatation and widening of the superior mediastinum.

Pulmonary Arteries

The *main trunk* of the pulmonary artery extends from

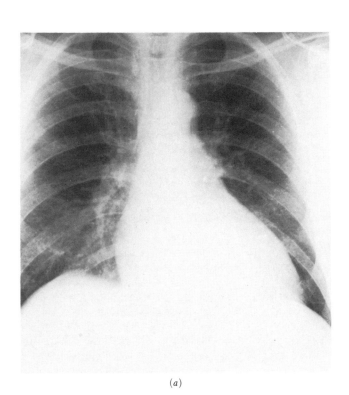

(a)

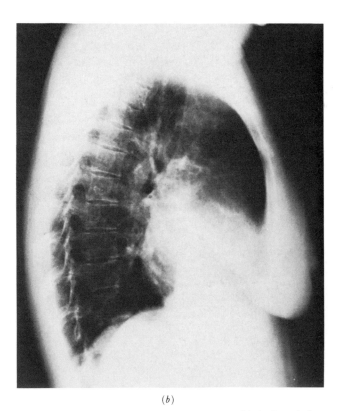

(b)

FIG. 1.21. Left ventricular enlargement. (a) The PA view shows generalised left ventricular enlargement, note the low apex. (b) the lateral view shows the border of the left ventricle bulging behind the right atrium and the inferior vena cava.

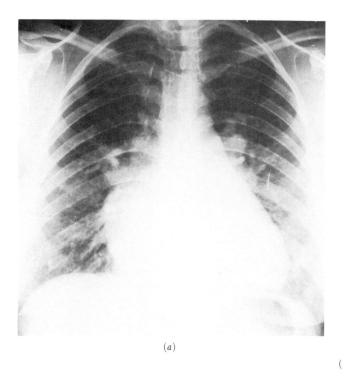

(a)

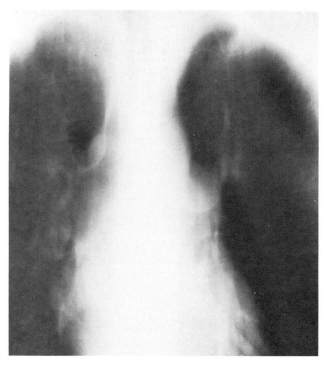

(b)

FIG. 1.22. (a) Prominence of the azygos vein in a patient with an atrial septal defect and generalised systemic venous engorgement. (b) The normal azygos vein as shown by tomography in the supine position. The normal azygos vein is not seen in an erect film.

the pulmonary valve at the level of the third costal cartilage (D7 posteriorly) to its bifurcation into left and right main bronchi. Its direction is backwards and slightly upwards. It is about 4 cm long and almost entirely within the pericardial sac. Behind, below and medial is the ascending aorta. The left coronary artery and the left atrial appendix are lateral. Above and anteriorly is the thymus and the left lung. Medially is the right atrial appendix (Fig. 1.23, 1.08, 1.10, 1.11 & 1.12). The pulmonary artery contributes to the cardiac silhouettes in the PA, lateral and RAO views.

The right main pulmonary artery branches sharply to the right at the D6 level and runs horizontally. The aorta and superior vena cava lie in front, the right pulmonary veins below and both main bronchi and oesophagus behind. Just beyond the origin of the right main bronchus it divides into a small upper lobe branch and a larger lower branch which supplies the middle and lower lobes (Fig. 1.23). These lie lateral to their respective bronchi. The artery to the upper lobe divides segmentally *before* it leaves the mediastinum.

The artery to the lower lobe gives a large branch to the middle lobe and then divides segmentally.

The left main pulmonary artery continues the line of the main trunk outside the mediastinal shadow crossing over the left main bronchus lateral to the oesophagus and descending aorta. It then divides into upper and lower lobe branches which again divide segmentally.

It is the division outside the mediastinum, as well as its high position above the main bronchus, which gives the left hilum a smooth upper margin and characteristic appearance when compared with the right.

Pulmonary Artery Enlargement. Pulmonary artery enlargement in the PA view is commonly seen as straightening of the left heart border when the pulmonary arc, normally smaller than the aorta, takes over. In extreme cases it encroaches on the aortic and left ventricular arcs and obliterates the pulmonary bay (Fig. 1.24).

In marked cases, in the lateral view, pulmonary trunk enlargement will replace the anterior aortic arch border from below upwards.

Pulmonary Veins

The pulmonary veins return oxygenated blood from the lungs. Originating in the alveolar plexus they join their respective segmental veins which at first lie lateral to the arteries. The veins of the upper lobe join those of the middle lobe and lingula segments to make a confluence in the upper mid-lung field lateral to the pulmonary arteries. Because of the low pulmonary venous pressure the upper veins are collapsed in the erect PA chest film but if, for whatever reason, pressure rises, redistribution occurs and they become prominent (Fig. 1.25) (Friedman & Braunwald, 1966).

The lower lobe segmental veins originate laterally

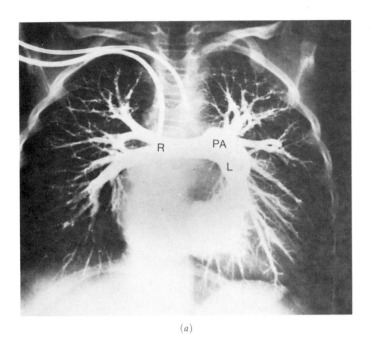

(a)

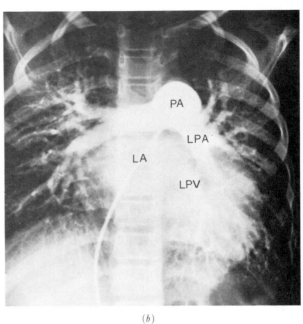

(b)

FIG. 1.23. Diagram of the pulmonary artery and pulmonary veins. Note that in the lower field the veins lie medial to the arteries. (a) Pulmonary arteriogram showing pulmonary arteries only. (b) Pulmonary arteriogram showing filling of both pulmonary arteries and pulmonary veins. (c) The venous phase only of the pulmonary arteriogram showing return to the left atrium. (d) Explanatory diagram. (*By courtesy of Dr J. B. Partridge.*)

(c)

(d)

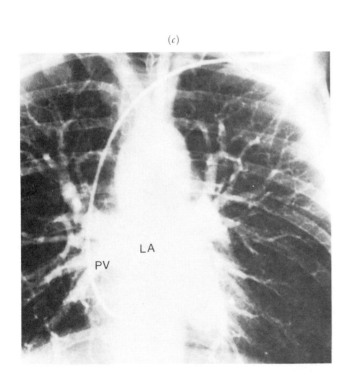

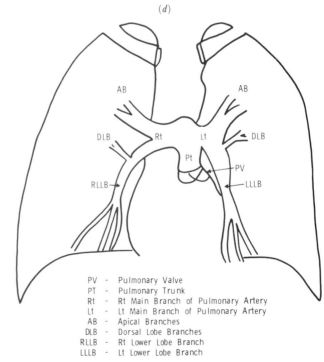

PV – Pulmonary Valve
PT – Pulmonary Trunk
Rt – Rt Main Branch of Pulmonary Artery
Lt – Lt Main Branch of Pulmonary Artery
AB – Apical Branches
DLB – Dorsal Lobe Branches
RLLB – Rt Lower Lobe Branch
LLLB – Lt Lower Lobe Branch

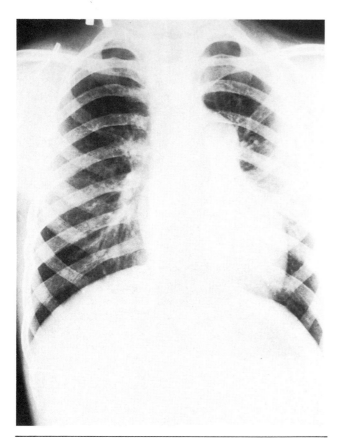

FIG. 1.24. PA view showing pulmonary artery enlargement. The pulmonary arc encroaches on both the aortic knuckle and the pulmonary bay.

but come to lie medially to the arteries as they follow an almost horizontal course towards the left atrium. They criss-cross with the emerging arteries which arise at a higher level, and give shadow which, in the right cardiophrenic angle, may be mistaken for an opacity. The corresponding part of the left lung is hidden by the heart shadow.

The large right lower pulmonary vein is the only pulmonary vein visible on a normal chest film.

The Aorta

The ascending aorta begins as the three sinuses of Valsalva at the level of D8. It runs forwards and upwards to the right heart border with the pulmonary artery and right atrial appendix in front, and the left atrium, the right atrium, the right main pulmonary artery and superior vena cava behind. The right lung and thymus cover the anterior lateral aspect of its upper course, two-thirds of it is within the pericardial cavity.

The aortic arch starts at the level of D5. The aorta arches backwards and to the left and gives off the brachiocephalic trunk. It then continues over the left bronchus, right main pulmonary artery lateral to the

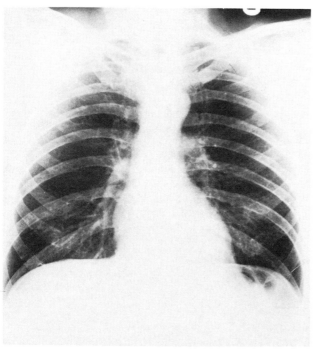

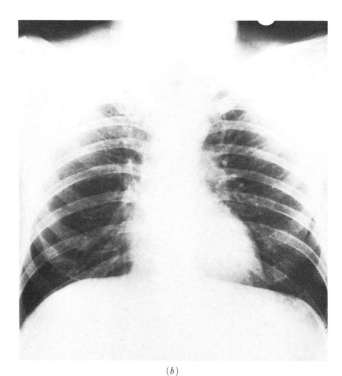

(a)   (b)

FIG. 1.25. Pulmonary veins. Erect and prone views of the same subject showing dilated upper pulmonary veins in the prone film. (a) Erect view. (b) Prone view.

trachea and the oesophagus, giving off the left common carotid artery and the left subclavian artery. Below, the ligamentum arteriosum joins it in front to the pulmonary trunk (Fig. 1.26).

The descending aorta. At this level the arch becomes the descending aorta and runs downwards in front and slightly left of the dorsal vertebra supplying segmental, intercostal and bronchial branches.

Aortic Enlargement. Enlargement of the aorta is either by elongation due to normal ageing with loss of elastic tissue in the media, or dilatation. Dilatation is always pathological.

Elongation. *PA view.* From the age of 40 the normal aorta elongates, becomes tortuous and takes over the upper right heart border as a gentle curve and the aortic knuckle becomes prominent (Fig. 1.09).

Tortuosity of the descending aorta shows as a paravertebral shadow in the lower thorax, usually to the left, but occasionally to the right, and is a shadow within the main heart shadow. The bulge of tortuosity is less smooth and regular than that of left atrial enlargement.

Lateral view. Aortic enlargement is seen as an encroachment on the upper retrosternal space above the right ventricular outlow tract. It is an arc characteristically shallow and contrasts with the upward forward bulge of a dilated right atrial appendix. Posteriorly the arch is not seen, but the tortuous descending aorta may bulge forwards. Tortuosity of the descending aorta carries with it the oesophagus and can make assessment of chamber enlargement by barium swallow misleading.

Dilatation of the Aorta. *PA view.* Dilatation is always pathological. When confined to the aortic root, as in some cases of Marfan's syndrome and medial necrosis, it may be entirely within the pericardium and shows only as a generalised increase in heart size (Keene *et al.*, 1971).

With the greatest degree of dilatation the aorta takes over the whole of the right heart border as a single smooth bulge from the base to the right cardiophrenic angle, well lateral to its normal position, and the aortic valve is displaced inwards (the Shmoo sign) (Fig. 1.27).

Lateral view. Dilatation is seen in the upper retrosternal space, the size of the bulge being consistent with the degree of enlargement.

FACTORS WHICH MODIFY THE NORMAL CARDIAC OUTLINE

Of the circumstances which modify the normal cardiac outline, infancy and age are most commonly met. Deformities of the bony thorax also alter the cardiac outline as does chronic lung disease and cachexia.

Cardiac Outline in Infancy

At birth the heart is relatively larger, and its axis more horizontal, than in the adult. It is globular and the individual chambers and vessels are hard to identify.

The right heart is well developed, the right ventricle being thicker walled and larger by 13% than the left. During the first six months the left ventricle doubles in size whilst the right ventricle increases by only 20%; the heart grows more slowly than the rest of the body, but the right ventricle may remain thicker than the left in normal children up to the age of five. Variation in size is greater than in the adult.

At birth placental circulation ceases whilst the pulmonary resistance persists, so that cardiac output drops and the heart shrinks. The CT ratio is less than 50% and the hilar and lung vessels are small. During the first months, pulmonary resistance falls, output increases, and the normal CT ratio exceeds 55%, from which it gradually falls to approach the adult configuration at about six years. Then it decreases more slowly until the third decade (Elliott & Schiebler, 1979; Maresh & Washburn, 1938) (Fig. 1.28). Pulmonary oligaemia gradually gives way to the normal pattern during the first year of life (Barkwin & Barkwin, 1935).

The thymus gland is large in the infant and obscures the upper cardiac border. It is usually seen more to the right of the upper mediastinum and has a characteristic sharp lower edge (the sail sign) and it rarely, if ever, reaches the lateral chest wall (Fig. 1.29). Uncertainty is resolved by fluoroscopy when the normal thymic shadow is recognised on rotation and disappears on deep inspiration (Grainger, 1970).

The Heart in Old Age

Subject to normal variation the heart maintains its adult configuration until the age of 70 when generalised tissue wasting causes a decrease in the actual mass of the heart. Whilst the heart decreases in size loss of lung parenchyma is even more rapid, the alveoli disappear and pulmonary vascularity and lung volume decrease. Loss of lung volume is accompanied by collapse of the chest wall inwards and this increases the CT ratio to more than 50% even when the heart itself is smaller (Fig. 1.30) (Cowan, 1964).

The replacement of elastic tissues in the great vessels, particularly the aorta, causes unfolding and tortuosity. Loss of peripheral lung vessels leads to increased pulmonary resistance, pulmonary hypertension and prominence of the pulmonary trunk.

Abnormalities of the Chest Wall

Straight Back Syndrome. This is most often seen in young females. The normal dorsal kyphosis is less and the AP diameter of the thorax is decreased, resulting in compression of the heart between the sternum in front

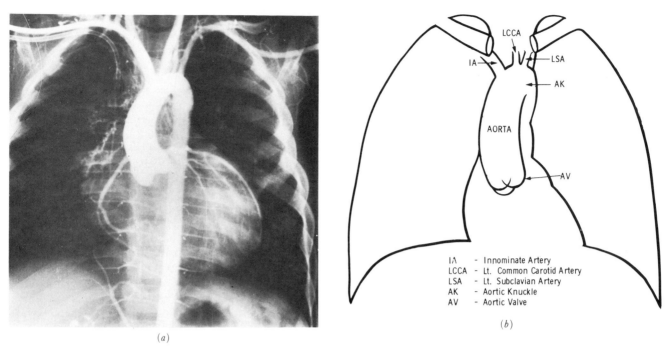

(a)

(b)

IA   – Innominate Artery
LCCA – Lt. Common Carotid Artery
LSA – Lt. Subclavian Artery
AK   – Aortic Knuckle
AV   – Aortic Valve

FIG. 1.26. Angiograms of the aorta in the PA and lateral view. (a) Anterior view. (b) Explanatory diagram. (c) Lateral view. (d) Explanatory diagram. (*By courtesy of Dr J. B. Partridge.*)

(c)

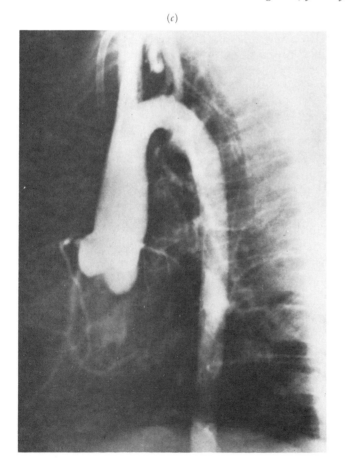

(d)

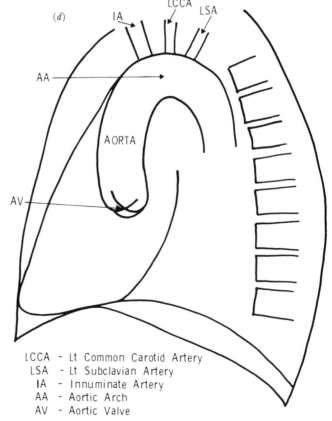

LCCA – Lt Common Carotid Artery
LSA – Lt Subclavian Artery
IA   – Innuminate Artery
AA   – Aortic Arch
AV   – Aortic Valve

and the dorsal spine behind. In the PA view the transverse diameter is increased and the aorta and pulmonary trunk are more prominent (Fig. 1.31).

Sternal Depression. Unlike the straight back syndrome, sternal depression is confined to the lower chest

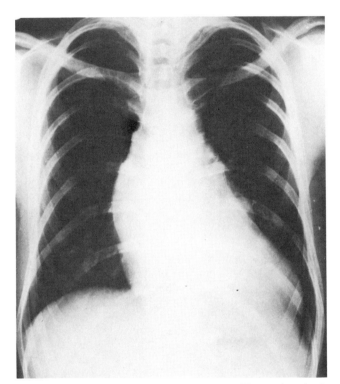

FIG. 1.27. Generalised enlargement of the aorta. The aortic valve is pushed downwards and the shadow of the dilated ascending aorta takes over the right heart border.

immediately above the diaphragm. In the PA film the sternal defect may not be obvious but the posterior ribs are more horizontal than normal and the anterior ribs splayed and angulated downwards. The effect on the heart is to displace it to the left, the right heart border disappears behind the spine and the lower right pulmonary vessels are conspicuous (Fig. 1.32).

Less often the appearance is of generalised cardiac enlargement, this differs from that of the straight back syndrome in that the lower contour is prominent and the great vessels normal or small. Soft tissue may obscure the deformity but in both conditions the lateral view will make the situation clear.

Scoliosis. This deformity is always obvious and frequently it is associated with a lung condition which can cause secondary changes in the heart. Because of the association between congenital skeletal abnormalities and congenital heart disease, the bony thorax must be looked at critically.

Most instances are mild with no effect on the heart, but displacement makes radiological criteria invalid.

The heart, bound closely to the mid-dorsal spinal muscles posteriorly, is rotated into the oblique position corresponding to the convexity of the curve so that rotation to that side (the opposite anterior oblique) 'straightens' the spine and brings the heart back into the PA axis and its contour becomes recognisable. Even so, with such deformity radiological criteria must, as always, be interpreted with caution (Fig. 1.33).

CALCIFICATION

Except in states of abnormal calcium metabolism metastatic calcification never occurs in healthy tissue or

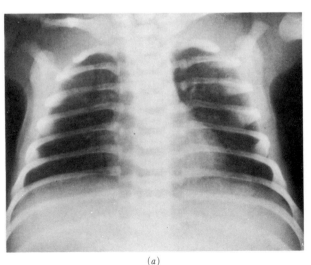

(a)

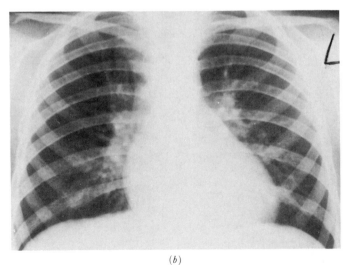

(b)

FIG. 1.28. The chest in childhood. (a) The neonate with a small heart and poor pulmonary vascularity. (By courtesy of Dr D. C. James.) (b) In the year-old infant with the large heart and well vascularised lung fields.

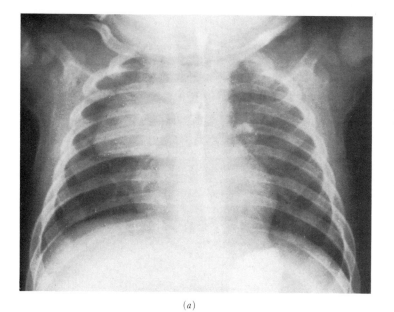

(a)

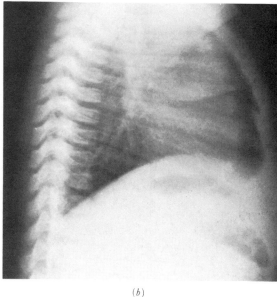

(b)

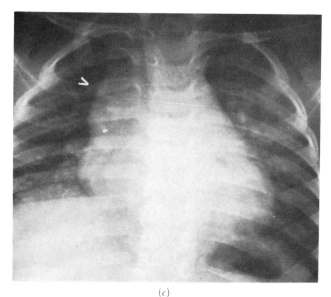

(c)

FIG. 1.29. (a) PA chest of an infant with a prominent but normal thymus gland. (b) Lateral chest of the same child. (c) Normal expiration film of a child showing a prominent thymus gland.

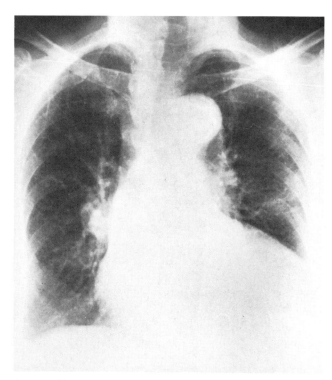

FIG. 1.30. The chest in an old subject showing an apparent increase in the heart size.

within the healthy heart. Yet in persons of over 40 years it is usual and it may be considered a part of radiological anatomy. All tissues continually undergo degenerative change and repair and all calcification seen within the apparently 'normal' heart may be regarded as minimally dystrophic in this sense. The lower wall of the aortic arch near the infundibulum of the ductus is the first site where calcification is seen. This is readily visible partly due to enhancement by foreshortening, and it is so common as to be regarded as normal.

Image intensification will detect deposits of 1 mm in diameter. Fluoroscopy with rotation identifies the site and is helped by inspiration which increases contrast and slows the heart rate. Films are less useful because blurring by movement obliterates all but the largest deposits and these are never 'normal'. Tomograms can be used to show pathological deposits by increasing contrast, but small deposits are blurred out in the long exposure.

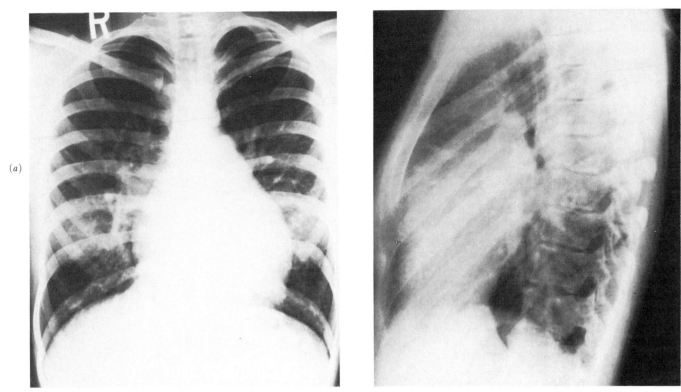

FiG. 1.31. Straight back syndrome, an abnormally straight dorsal kyphosis with a short AP thoracic diameter compressing the heart against the spine and causing it to appear enlarged on the PA view. (a) PA view. (b) Lateral view. (By courtesy of Dr Elizabeth Watkins.)

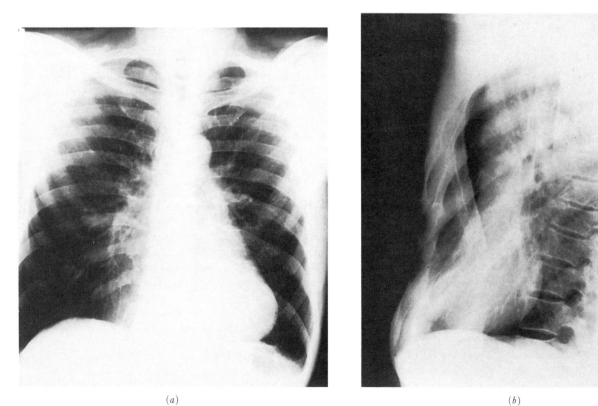

(a)   (b)

FiG. 1.32. A depressed sternum, displacing the heart towards the left and distorting its outline. (a) PA view. (b) Lateral view. (By courtesy of Dr Norah Hudson.)

(a)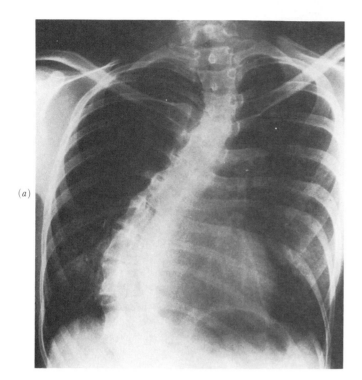

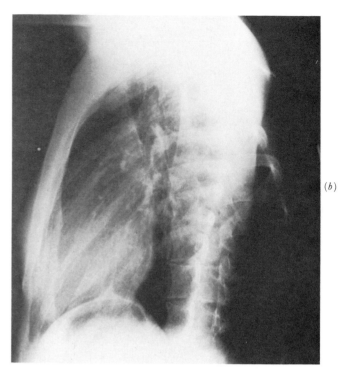 (b)

FIG. 1.33. A subject with scoliosis rotating and distorting the cardiac silhouette. (a) PA view. (b) Lateral view.

Coronary Artery Calcification

Coronary calcification is seen on fluoroscopy in 20% of normal subjects over 50 years and this figure increases rapidly with age. It is not symptomatic and carries no prognostic significance (Hudson & Walker, 1976). Postmortem radiographs with much higher resolution show it to be present in 100% of subjects over 40 (Fink *et al.*, 1970). It is usually punctate and in clusters but sometimes blocks 5–10 mm in diameter are seen. Double lines characteristically seen postmortem are rarely seen at fluoroscopy.

The left main coronary artery at its division, and the proximal LAD branch, are the most common sites. They are best seen fluoroscopically in the RAO view where the AV sulcus meets the left heart border (Fig. 1.34 (a)).

Calcification in the right coronary artery is less common and more difficult to detect. It often occurs further out along the artery and is best seen in the LAO view in the low right AV sulcus (Fig. 1.34 (b)).

Whilst this undoubtedly indicates atheroma, as medial sclerosis has never been reported in coronary arteries, its association with age precludes it from use as an indicator of those at risk of infarction except in the young.

Calcification in the Cardiac Skeleton

Mitral Ring. Metastatic calcification rarely occurs in the fibrous skeleton under the age of 60 and the mitral ring is the commonest site. The free edge is more involved than its attachment and accounts for the typical J or U shape of the shadow. Conditions of abnormal calcium metabolism, of which Paget's disease is characteristic, commonly exhibit this type of calcification (Fig. 1.35). Mitral incompetence may result from the presence of massive deposits when the cusps themselves are normal.

Aortic Ring. Calcification in the aortic ring is rare in the absence of calcific valve disease and when it occurs it is less extensive than in the mitral ring. Spread from a congenitally malformed valve is common and is characteristically massive extending into the interventricular septum where it may interfere with conduction.

Site of Calcification. Guides to identification. The position of the valves can be altered by selective chamber enlargement which override any guides to identification.

(1) In the PA view the aortic valve overlies the spine whilst the mitral valve lies lower and to the left.

(2) In the 60° LAO view the aortic valve is in the middle third of the heart shadow and the mitral valve in the posterior third at a lower level.

(3) In the lateral view a line drawn from the carina to the anterior limit of the diaphragm separ-

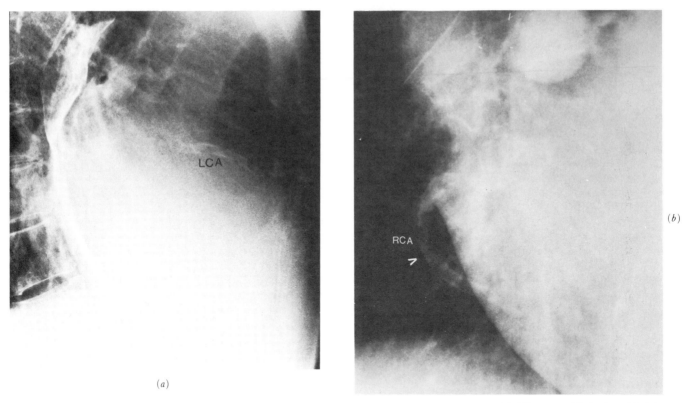

(a)

(b)

FIG. 1.34. Coronary artery calcification. (a) In an elderly subject with severe calcification in the proximal LAD artery. (b) In the mid right coronary artery.

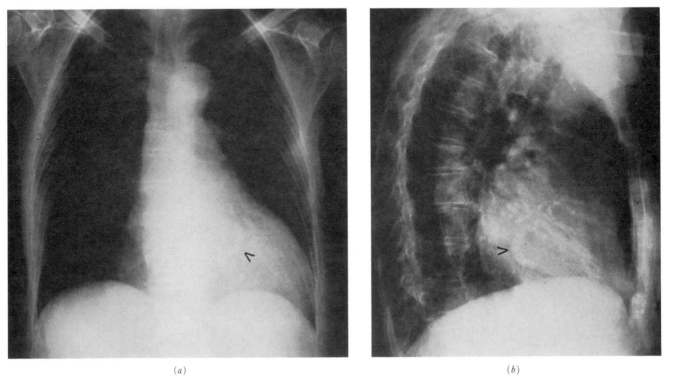

(a)

(b)

FIG. 1.35. Calcification in the normal mitral ring showing the characteristic U shape. (a) PA view. (b) Lateral view.

ates the aortic valve above from the mitral valve below.

Valve Movement. The valve rings are tightly bound together and generally move together. Nevertheless the mitral valve tends to move horizontally and to the left in systole, while the aortic valve moves vertically and counter-clockwise. Attempting to separate the movement of the valve cusps from their ring is unreliable.

Calcification in the pulmonary and tricuspid valves is never seen in the normal. It is rare and mostly associated with raised right heart pressures.

Pericardial Calcification

Whatever its cause pericardial calcification is most likely on the diaphragmatic and right surfaces of the heart and in the atrioventricular sulcus. It is never normal and usually the result of pericarditis of any cause. It is characteristically laminar and seen end-on gives a linear shadow 1 to 2 mm thick (Fig. 1.36). It can be massive—25 mm thick.

Calcification in congenital heart disease is rare and most characteristic in patent ductus arteriosus, but even then occurs in only 5% of cases. It may also be seen in the ligamentum arteriosum so it is of limited diagnostic value (Fig. 1.37).

Post-operative calcification is common and is often seen in prosthetic structures made from biological materials. It may also be seen in material used in the repair of defects and due to tissue damage in bizarre situations.

PERICARDIAL FAT

Fat attenuates the X-ray beam less than do other soft tissues and can be identified. The difference on film is small, and unless exposures are of low KV and short enough to obliterate movement, it is not seen.

Fluoroscopy, cine angiography, or large films with frames of less than 10 milliseconds taken during an optimal phase of the cardiac cycle, overcome this problem (Bergstrand & Szamosi, 1978).

Pericardial fat is either extra- or sub-pericardial.

Extra-Pericardial Fat, outside the fibrous pericardium, is more evident in women than men, increases with age and is related to general obesity. The largest collections occur in the cardiophrenic angle and may give a false impression of an increase in heart size. The

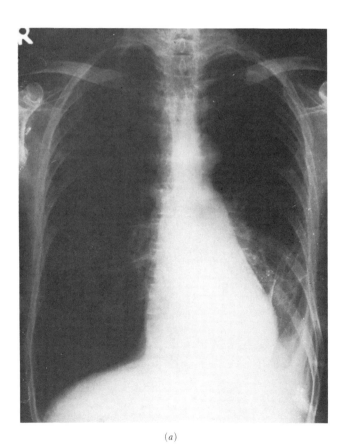

(a)

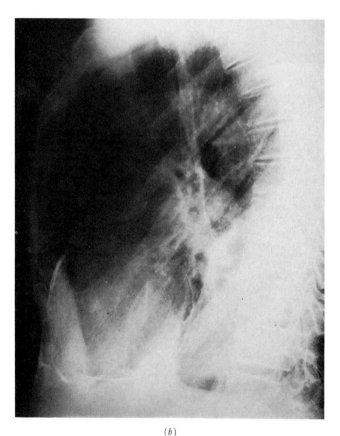

(b)

Fig. 1.36. Pericardial calcification characteristically more in the anterior and right inferior position. (a) PA view. (b) Lateral view.

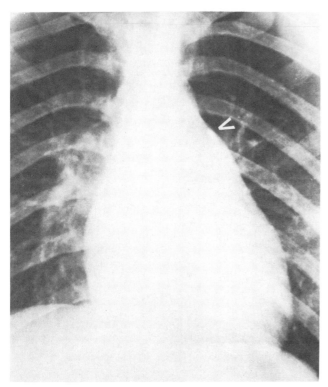

FIG. 1.37. Calcification in a patent ductus in a six-year-old child, the calcification is seen on the left heart border between the aortic knuckle and the pulmonary arch.

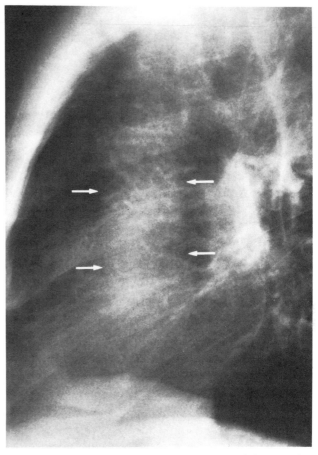

FIG. 1.38. Subpericardial fat delineating the base of the aorta in a normal subject, lateral view. (*By courtesy of Dr A. Szamosi.*)

greater density of the heart itself can be seen within the general outline on a well-taken film.

Sub-Pericardial Fat is constant, even in thin subjects. It predominates in the sulci and increases with age.

Identification of the AV sulcus on fluoroscopy assists the diagnosis of pericardial effusion and sub-pericardial fat around the chambers can be seen as a line moving within the large still pericardial shadow.

In the lateral view the plane between the left atrium and the ascending aorta shows as a thin line. A sensitivity rate of 75% in the older age group is reported (Szamosi, 1981). It can be used in the initial assessment of chamber size and in comparisons of serial films (Fig. 1.38).

REFERENCES

BARKWIN, H. & BARKWIN, R. M. (1935) Body build in infants. Growth of the cardiac silhouette and the thoraco-abdominal cavity. *Amer. J. Dis. Children*, **49**, 861–869.

BERGSTRAND, G. & SZAMOSI, A. (1978) Visibility of the intra pericardial segment of the ascending aorta in conventional lateral chest films. *Acta Radiol.*, **19**, 961–968.

COWAN, N. R. (1964) The heart lung coefficient and the transverse diameter of the heart. *Brit. Heart J.*, **26**, 26–116.

DANZER, C. S. (1919) The cardio-thoracic ratio: an index of cardiac enlargement. *Amer. J. Science*, **157**, 513–522.

ELLIOTT, L. P. & SCHIEBLER, G. L. (1979) *X-ray Diagnosis of Congenital Heart Disease in Infants, Children and Adults.* Springfield, Ill: Charles C. Thomas.

FINK, R. J., ARCHER, R. W., BROWN, A. L., KINCAID, O. W. & BRANDENBERG, R. O. C. (1970) Significance of calcification in coronary arteries. *Amer. J. Cardiology*, **26**, 241–247.

FRIEDMAN, W. F. & BRAUNWALD, E. (1966) Alterations in regional blood flow etc. *Circulation*, **34**, 363–375.

GRAINGER, R. G. (1970) Evaluation of conventional radiology in acquired heart disease. *Brit. J. Radiology*, **43**, 673–684.

HILBISH & MORGAN (1952) Cardiac mensuration by radiological methods. *Amer. J. Med. Sciences*, **224**, 586–596.

HOFFMAN, R. B. & RIGLER, L. G. (1965) Evaluation of left ventricular enlargement in the lateral projection of the chest. *Radiology*, **85**, 93–100.

HUDSON, N. M. & WALKER, J. K. (1976) The prognostic significance of coronary artery calcification. *Clin. Radiol.*, **27**, 545–547.

JACOBSON, G. & WEIDNER, W. (1962) Dilatation of the left atrial appendage by the Valsalva method—an aid to diagnosis of mitral valve disease. *Radiology*, **79**, 274–284.

JEFFERSON, K. & REES, S. (1980) *Clinical Cardiac Radiology*. London: Butterworth.

KEATS, D. E. & ENGE, I. P. (1965) Cardiac Mensuration by the Cardiac Volume Method. *Radiology*, **85**, 850–855.

KEENE, R. J., STEINER, R. E., OLSEN, E. J. G. & OAKLEY, C. (1971) Aortic root aneurysm-radiographic & pathologic features. *Clin. Radiol.*, **22**, 330–340.

KJELLBURG, J. R., MANNHEIMER, E., RUDHE, U. & JONSSON, B. (1958) *Diagnosis of Congenital Heart Disease*. 2nd Ed. New York: Year Book Publishers Inc.

LIND, J. (1950) Heart Volume in Normal Infants; Roentgenological Study. *Acta Radiol. Suppl. 82.* **3**, 127.

MARESH, M. M. & WASHBURN, A. H. (1938) The size of the heart in healthy children. Roentgen measurements. *Amer. J. Dis. Children*, **56**, 33–60.

NETTER, F. H. (1969) *Heart*. Ciba Collection of Medical Illustrations.

ROESLER, H. (1943) *Clinical Radiology of the Cardio-Vascular System.* Springfield, Ill: Charles C. Thomas.

SCHWARZ, G. S. (1946) Determination of frontal plane area from the product of the long and short diameters of the cardiac silhouette. *Radiology*, **47**, 360–370.

SZAMOSI, A. (1981) Radiological detection of aneurysms involving the aortic root. *Radiology*, **138**, (3), 551–555.

UNGERLEIDER, H. E. & GUBNER, R. (1942) Evaluation of heart measurements. *Amer. Heart J.*, **24**, 494–510.

WALKER, J. K. (1956) The radiological appearances of patent ductus arteriosus in children. M.D. Thesis, University of Leeds *Appendix*, 190–193.

WALMSLEY, R. & WATSON, H. (1978) *Clinical Anatomy of the Heart.* London: Churchill Livingstone.

CHAPTER 2

THE NORMAL HEART—PART II
APPLIED ANGIOGRAPHY; CORONARY ARTERIES

John Walker

GEOMETRY

The long axis of the heart is at an angle to that of the body in all three planes and raises interesting radiographic considerations. It lies at 45° to the coronal and sagittal planes and more than 60° to the transverse plane. Moreover, the heart is ovoid so that even with an incident beam perpendicular to one plane the conventional two views at right angles do not preclude foreshortening. The problem is not overcome by simple oblique views, but requires varying degrees of cranial (caudocranial) or caudal (craniocaudal) tube angulation (Bargeron *et al.*, 1977, 1980; Rees, 1981).

Angiography of the left ventricle nicely demonstrates the use of axial views. Enhancement is greater than with other chambers because it is an ellipsoid and prone to foreshortening. The spherical atria are less easily distorted and the right ventricle is too irregular to benefit.

The septum, and particularly the crescentic interventricular septum is better seen by compound angular views than is otherwise possible. The right ventricular outflow tract and proximal pulmonary artery, whilst well seen in the lateral, are foreshortened in the PA view and this is overcome by a 45° caudocranial tilt.

Three views have proved useful:

Four Chamber View—45 LAO, 45 Cranial (Fig. 2.01)

It separates the four chambers and demonstrates well:
(1) Interatrial septum
(2) The posterior interventricular septum and the membranous septum
(3) The cusps of the mitral and tricuspid valves especially the anterior mitral cusp.

Long Axial View—60 LAO, 45 Cranial (Fig. 2.02)

This shows:
(1) The anterior interventricular septum
(2) The left ventricular outflow tract
(3) The cusps of the mitral valve.

PA Axial View—PA, 45 Cranial (Fig. 2.03)

This simple 45° tilt outlines the pulmonary artery in frontal view and demonstrates:
(1) The pulmonary valve

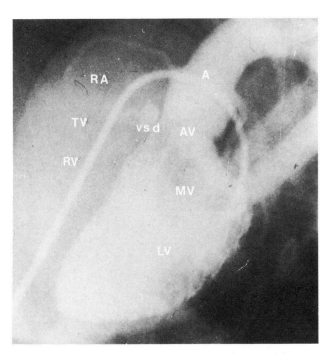

FIG. 2.01. The Four-chamber view. 45 LAO 45 cranial.
LV Left ventricle, RV Right ventricle, LA Left atrium, RA Right atrium, MV Mitral valve, TV Tricuspid valve, A Aorta, AV Aortic valve. VSD Shunt through a Ventricular septal defect.

(2) The division of the pulmonary trunk
(3) The relationship between pulmonary arteries, bronchial arteries and systemic pulmonary collaterals.

THE BLOOD SUPPLY OF THE HEART

The heart receives its only blood supply from the two coronary arteries. The layout and distribution is a girdle in the atrioventricular sulcus encircling the heart, with perpendicular branches in the epicardium running towards the apex and the base. Penetrating branches anastomose in the muscle and the sub-endocardium (Fig. 2.04).

The size and number of the main branches of this arterial girdle is directly proportional to the mass of myocardium and the importance of the part supplied,

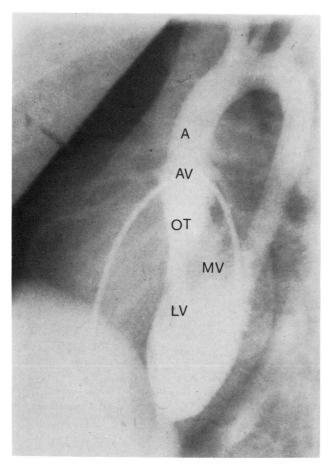

FIG. 2.02. Long axis view. 60 LAO, 45 cranial.
LV Left ventricle, MV Mitral valve, A Aorta, AV Aortic valve, OT
Left ventricular outflow tract.

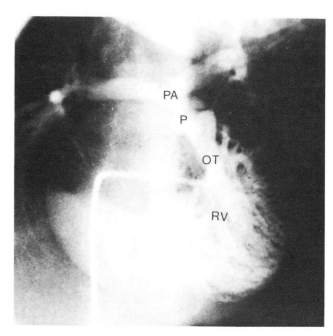

FIG. 2.03. PA axial view. 45 cranial.
RV Right ventricle, PA Pulmonary artery, P Pulmonary valve, OT
Right ventricular outflow tract.

i.e. conducting tissue. Large branches run over the ventricles, especially the left ventricle, and the fewer smaller arteries of the atria are directed to vital parts such as the sinus node. The girdle, part right coronary artery and part circumflex branch of the left coronary artery varies in detail but the pattern is constant.

Collateral Supply. Anatomically the coronary arteries are end arteries but with a vast micro-arteriolar anastomosis within the myocardium which can open instantly as pressure gradients demand (Fig. 2.05).

There is also an anastomosis between the larger branches in the sub-epicardial plane; these appear late, are variable and the factors which cause them to develop are obscure (James, 1970).

Left Coronary Artery

The left coronary artery arises from the left posterior coronary sinus of Valsalva at the level of the free edge of the valve cusp. The main stem runs forwards, upwards and to the left between the pulmonary trunk

in front and the left atrium behind. It varies in length from 4 to 20 mm ending in two large branches. The left anterior descending branch runs in the anterior interventricular sulcus to the apex and the circumflex branch continues round the atrioventricular sulcus (Fig. 2.06, 2.07).

Right Coronary Artery

The right coronary artery arises similarly from the anterior coronary sinus of Valsalva. It runs in the atrioventricular sulcus between the edge of the right atrial appendix, forwards, downwards and to the right, and together with the circumflex branch encircles the heart (Fig. 2.08, 2.09).

The two divisions of the left coronary artery, together with the right are regarded as the three main arteries supplying the myocardium.

Left Anterior Descending Artery—LAD

The left anterior descending branch is the largest and most constant of the three. Its size is determined by the need to supply the interventricular septum and adjacent left ventricular wall, about half the whole myocardial mass. It runs in the anterior interventricular sulcus to the apex.

Its principal branches are:

Septal branches which are straight, parallel and at right angles to the main artery, vary in number; usually four are visible. The first is the largest and its territory

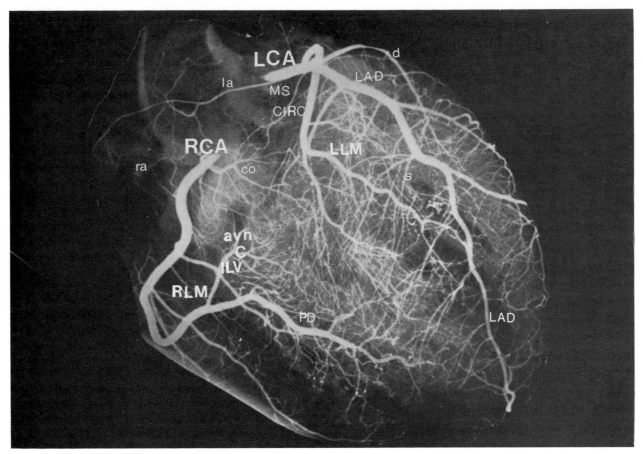

Fig. 2.04. AP postmortem view of the heart with the coronary arteries opacified. The main branches are named LCA left coronary artery, MS main stem, LAD left anterior descending artery, CIRC circumflex artery, D diagonal branch, LLM left lateral marginal branches, S septal branches, LA left atrial branch, RCA right coronary artery, CO conus branch, RA right atrial branch, RLM right lateral marginal branch, AVN atrial ventricular node branch, C crux, PD posterior descending artery. (*By courtesy of Dr V. J. Redding*).

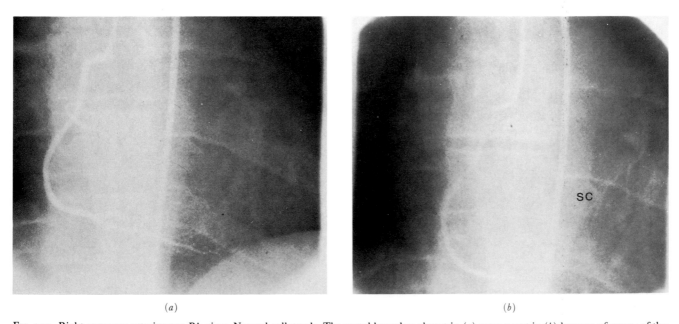

(*a*)   (*b*)

Fig. 2.05. Right coronary arteriogram PA view. Normal collaterals. The septal branches absent in (*a*) are present in (*b*) because of spasm of the LAD proximally. SC Septal collaterals.

Left Coronary Artery

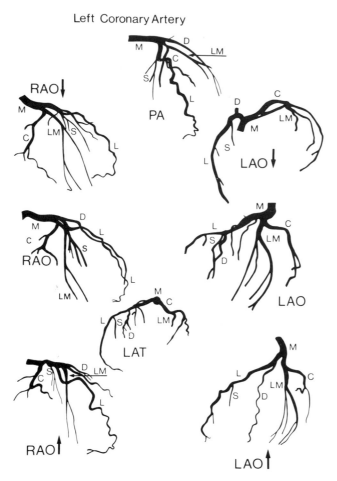

FIG. 2.06. Left coronary artery. Angiographic series. ↑ = cranial angulation, ↓ = caudal angulation. M Main stem, L Left anterior descending branch, C Circumflex branch, S Septal branches, D Diagonal branch, LM Left lateral marginal branch, LA Left atrial branch.

contains the bundle of His together with the proximal right and left bundle branches. The septal branches supply the upper three quarters of the interventricular septum and they are numbered from proximal to distal. As a group they are recognised by their straightness and parallel regularity. They identify the septum.

The diagonal branches are epicardial and supply the anterior wall of the left ventricle. They arise at an acute angle from the left of the main vessel at or just distal to the origin of the first septal branch. They turn towards the apex parallel to the other subepicardial arteries. There may be up to four and they number in the order in which they arise; the first is usually the largest.

Circumflex Artery—CA

The circumflex artery continues in the AV groove and forms the left side of the arterial girdle. It reciprocates with the right coronary artery and if the latter is small it supplies the inferior surface of the left ventricle.

Its main branches are:

The left lateral marginal arteries run towards the apex perpendicular to the main artery. There are usually two and they are numbered in the order in which they arise and are the main supply of the lateral wall of the left ventricle.

The inferior left ventricular arteries continue the series and arise from the circumflex artery when the left coronary artery is dominant and the right coronary artery small. They run along the inferior surface of the left ventricle towards the apex.

Left Atrial Arteries; the circumflex artery gives atrial branches, often two, which are relatively small, divide freely over the surface and anastomose with the atrial branch of the right coronary artery and with each other. In 45% of subjects they supply the sinus node.

Right Coronary Artery—RCA

The right coronary artery is the right side of the arterial girdle and unlike the LCA its major bifurcation is distal where it gives the posterior descending branch. At the point where it meets the coronary sinus and reaches the left ventricle it makes an upward loop, the crux, which is conspicuous in all views.

The Posterior Descending Branch—PD. Like the LAD the PD is constant and in 90% of subjects it is a distal branch of the RCA, usually but not always arising proximal to the crux. It runs in the inferior interventricular sulcus. Where the left coronary artery is dominant it is the terminal branch of the circumflex artery. Just proximal to the apex it anastomoses with the LAD. Normally its only branches are septal; smaller than those of the LAD, they supply the inferior 25% of the septum and are not usually seen on angiography. Small epicardial branches may cross the inferior surface of either ventricle.

The conus branch is the first branch of the RCA and is close to the ostium. It has a separate origin in 25% of subjects. It runs to the left over the conus of the right ventricle supplying it and forming an important anastomosis with the proximal LAD (Vieussen's ring).

The right atrial artery, the second branch, runs to the right and upwards over the surface of the right atrium where it divides and anastomoses with the left atrial artery. In 55% of subjects it supplies the sinus node and is prominent.

The right lateral marginal arteries supply the right ventricle and run in the subepicardial space over its surface towards the apex at right angles to the main artery. One is larger than the others, the acute marginal artery.

The AV node artery is very conspicuous and arises at the apex of the crux. It is straight, runs directly upwards and is about 2 cm long. Its appearance is characteristic and easily recognised. In the 10% of subjects where the

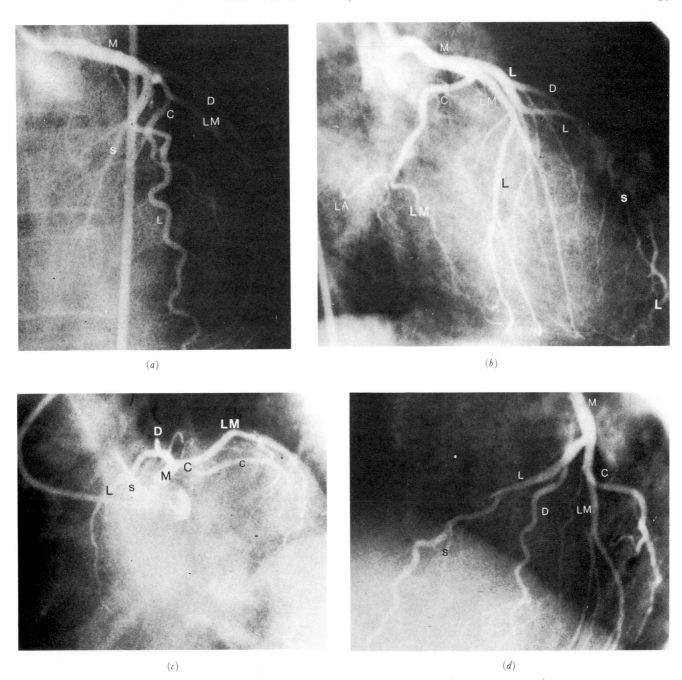

FIG. 2.07. Examples of left coronary artery. (a)—PA. (b)—RAO. (c)—LAO↓ caudal. (d)—LAO↑ cranial.
M Main stem, L Left anterior descending branch, C Circumflex branch, S Septal branches, D Diagonal branch, LM Left lateral marginal branch, LA Left atrial branch.

crux is supplied by the circumflex artery it still retains its characteristic appearance.

The Inferior Left Ventricular Arteries. Beyond the crux the terminal RCA supplies the inferior left ventricular arteries. When dominant its supply extends onto the lateral LV wall. When intermediate it only supplies those nearest the crux.

CORONARY ARTERIOGRAPHY

The most popular method of coronary arteriography is percutaneously via the femoral artery using preformed catheters with an arterial sheath to facilitate change (Judkin, 1968). Brachial arteriotomy (Sones & Shirey, 1962) is used when the iliac vessels are impassable.

Right Coronary Artery

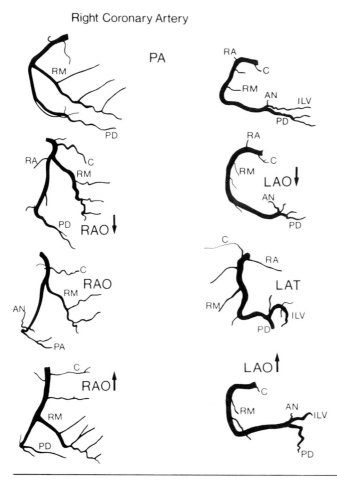

Safety demands vigilance and attention to a detailed protocol as well as familiarity with resuscitation techniques. The greatest risk is from the consequences of an inadequate demonstration. This requires two views of each part of each branch at right angles and perpendicular to the main X-ray beam, and that the examination be pressed until this is achieved.

Because arteries lie on all the surfaces of the heart, axial as well as lateral tilting is needed.

Six views plus extras are needed to demonstrate all the branches of both arteries. The number may be curtailed when the operator considers the arteries normal or when the whole artery is occluded.

Standard Views of Both Right and Left Coronary Arteries

PA siting shot—mid LAD, mid circumflex and mid RCA

LAO caudal—for the proximal arteries

LAO cranial—for the distal arteries and the main trunk of the LCA

RAO caudal—left mainstem, LAD, proximal CA, distal RCA and PD

RAO—left mainstem, LAD, mid CA, mid RCA and PD

RAO cranial—left mainstem, LAD, distal CA, proximal RCA and PD (Fig. 2.06, 2.08).

FIG. 2.08. A full series of views of the right coronary artery. C Conus branch. RA Right atrial branch, RM Right lateral marginal branch, PD Posterior descending branch, AN Atrio-ventricular node branch, ILV Inferior Left ventricular branch.

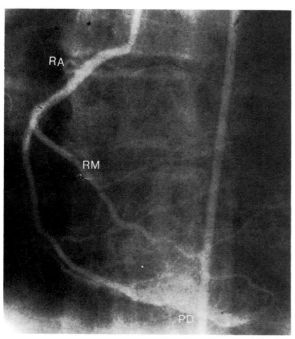

(a)

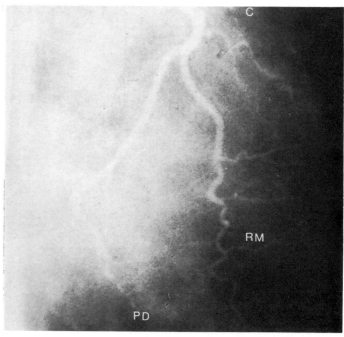

(b)

In the exclusion of unsuspected coronary disease three views of the LCA and one or two of the RCA will suffice.

When studying and reporting on a coronary artery film series it is important to consider only those parts of the artery which are in view, i.e not foreshortened. Failure in this can lead to serious error.

Figure 2.06 shows a full series for the left coronary artery. A left lateral view is included; this can be useful in the separation of the LAD and mid-circumflex arteries and their branches. The straight LAO is less useful.

Figure 2.08 shows two right coronary artery series. Two subjects have been used to exemplify the values of the axial LAO in showing the proximal and the distal

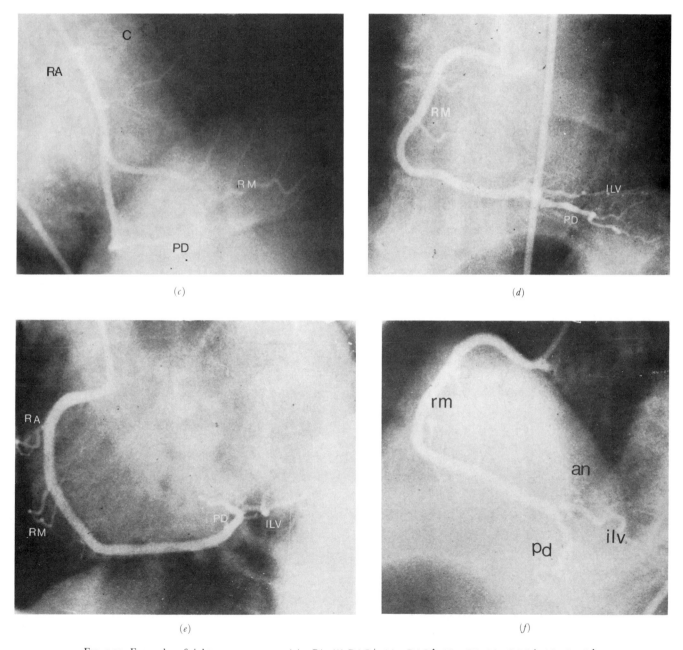

Fig. 2.09. Examples of right coronary artery.(a)—PA. (b) RAO↓. (c)—RAO↑. (d)—PA. (e)—LAO↓. (f)—LAO↑.
C Conus branch, RA Right atrial branch, RM Right lateral marginal branch, PD Posterior descending branch, AN Atrio-ventricular node branch, ILY Inferior left ventricular branch.

artery. The left hand subject illustrates the value of axial RAO views. It has a large right marginal artery which identifies the section of the main trunk which is in view, proximal in the RAO↑—distal in the RAO↓.

Common Variations in Coronary Artery Anatomy

(1) The commonest variation is a separate origin of the conus branch of the RCA from the right coronary sinus (25%) (Fig. 2.10).

(2) The most characteristic variation is the 'so-called' dominant left coronary artery in which the circumflex branch extends beyond the crux and supplies the posterior descending artery, the inferior left ventricular arteries and the AV node artery (10%) (Fig. 2.11).

(3) The three-way division of the main trunk of the left coronary artery to give a large intermediate branch supplying the territory of the diagonal and first left lateral marginal arteries, the ramus intermedius (10%) (Fig. 2.12).

(4) The duplication of the LAD in the anterior interventricular groove, both supplying septal branches. The first two or three septal branches may arise from a single proximal short branch to the right and deep to the main (less than 5%).

(5) A large right lateral marginal branch crossing the anterior and inferior surfaces of the right ventricle and forming the distal posterior descending artery (Fig. 2.08 (a)). In this situation the distal main right coronary artery may be small and the AV node branch supplied from the circumflex (less than 5%).

(6) A long PDA which rounds the apex and joins the LAD in the anterior interventricular groove (less than 5%).

VENOUS DRAINAGE OF THE HEART

The cardiac veins are best seen filled during selective coronary angiography.

Definition depends on the volume of medium and the patency of the arteries.

Injection into either coronary artery will outline the

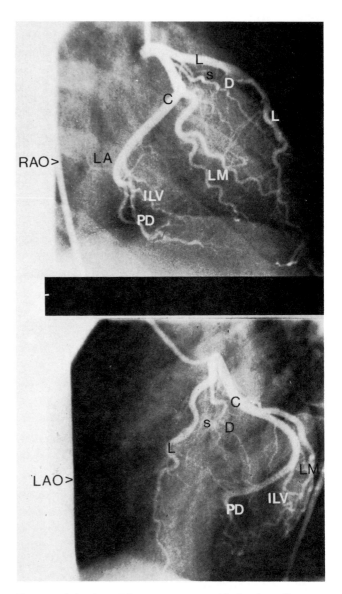

FIG. 2.11. A dominant left coronary artery with the circumflex artery supplying the posterior descending artery.
M Main stem, L Left anterior descending branch, C Circumflex branch, S Septal branches, D Diagonal branch, LM Left lateral marginal branch, LA Left atrial branch, ILV Inferior left ventricular branch.

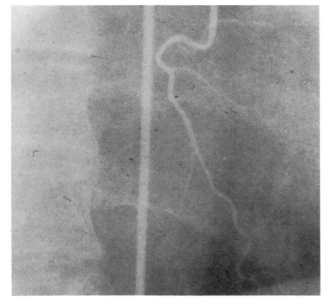

FIG. 2.10. PA The conus branch of the right coronary artery which is seen arising separately. Where this appears the branch is usually larger than normal.

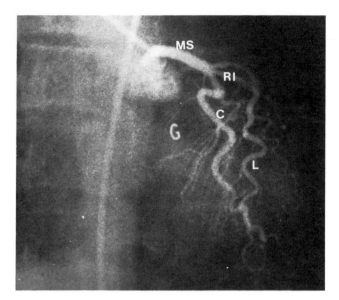

FIG. 2.12. PA Ramus intermedius. In this variant the left main stem divides into three arteries with a large ramus between the LAD and the circumflex.
MS Main stem, RI Ramus intermedius, C Circumflex, L Left anterior descending. (*By courtesy of Dr M. Ruttley*).

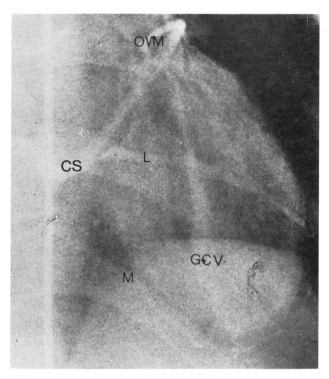

FIG. 2.13. Cardiac veins in the right anterior oblique view showing the venous phase of a left coronary arteriorgram. The small cardiac vein does not fill.
CS Coronary sinus, GCV Great cardiac vein, L Left cardiac vein, OVM Oblique vein of Marshall, M Middle cardiac vein.

whole venous system but the veins draining the left ventricle show better during left coronary arteriography and similarly the right sided veins with right coronary arteriography.

It is a single drainage system converging onto the coronary sinus which runs in the posterior atrioventricular sulcus down from the left heart border towards the right and enters the right atrium posteriorly (Fig. 2.13).

The great cardiac vein originates at the apex, follows the anterior interventricular sulcus to the atrioventricular groove where it runs round the left heart border. There joined by the left cardiac vein and the left atrial vein (the oblique vein of Marshall) it becomes the coronary sinus.

The middle cardiac vein arises at the apex and runs in the inferior sulcus to join the coronary sinus as it enters the right atrium.

The small cardiac vein arises anteriorly in the AV sulcus and runs around the right heart border to join the coronary sinus with the middle cardiac vein.

The anterior cardiac veins are small, arise on the anterior surface of the right ventricle and enter the right atrium separately. The Thebesian veins are not seen in normal subjects.

The author would like to thank the secretarial staff of the Groby Road Hospital and the staff of the photographic department at Leicester Royal Infirmary on whose assistance he depended totally.

REFERENCES

BARGERON, L. M. JR., ELLIOTT, L. P., SOTO, B., BREAM, P. R. & CURRY, G. C. (1977) Axial cineangiography in congenital heart disease. *Circulation*, **56**(6), 1075–1093.

BARGERON, L. M. JR. (1980) Axial cineangiography in congenital heart disease. *Paediatric Cardiovascular Disease*, **2**, 275–291.

GRAINGER, R. G. (1981) Terminology of radiographic projections. *Brit. Heart J.*, **45**, 109–111.

JAMES, T. N. (1970) Distribution of coronary collateral circulation. *Chest*, **58**(3), 183–203.

JUDKIN, M. P. (1968) Percutaneous transfemoral selective coronary arteriography. In *Radiological Clinics of North America*, VI, 3, 467–492.

REES, S. (1981) Terminology of radiographic projections. *Brit. Heart J.*, **46**, 587.

SONES, F. M. JR. & SHIREY, E. K. (1962) Cine coronary arteriography. *Modern Concepts in Cardiovascular Disease*, **31**, 735–738.

CHAPTER 3

PULMONARY PATTERNS IN HEART DISEASE

Eric Milne

INTRODUCTION

Our present ability to analyse the chest radiograph in physiological terms owes much to the pioneering work of several British radiologists. This work includes Kerley's hypothesis on the significance of septal lines, Hodges' treatise on the radiological anatomy of the pulmonary vessels, Lavender's classic work on venous hypertension, Simon's haemodynamic evaluation of pulmonary vessels, and Steiner's numerous papers on the analysis of haemodynamics from the chest radiograph in both acquired and congenital cardiac disease. (Davies *et al.*, 1953; Goodwin *et al.*, 1955; Kerley, 1957; Lavender & Doppman, 1962; Lavender *et al.*, 1962; Lodge, 1946; Simon, 1958, 1963; West *et al.*, 1964; Whitaker & Lodge, 1954). During the same period covered by these papers Leo Rigler in the United States was also emphasising physiological interpretation of the chest radiograph, exquisitely illustrated in his 1959 Caldwell lecture to the American Roentgen Ray Society (Rigler, 1959). It is quite evident that chest radiographs cannot be interpreted adequately by pattern recognition or pathological knowledge alone. Much of the information present on the radiograph will be lost to the radiologist unless his or her knowledge of cardiopulmonary physiology is sufficient to give a clear understanding of the exquisite interrelationships which exist between form and function in the human lung. This chapter has been written in a way which will hopefully help the reader to understand these fundamental interrelationships and to apply this understanding to the interpretation of the chest radiograph in all types of cardiac dysfunction.

VASCULAR ANATOMY

The radiographic pattern of the normal lung is formed almost entirely by pulmonary arteries and veins (Lodge, 1946). The interstitial skeleton of the lung and the smaller divisions of the bronchial tree are not sufficiently radiopaque to be recorded by conventional chest filming techniques. The smallest vessels we can resolve are on the order of 0·5–1·0 mm. These are the conducting vessels by which blood is delivered to the microvascular bed. The capillary bed of the lung has a surface area of approximately 70 m² but contains only 70–100 ml of blood. This is equivalent to spreading two table-spoonsful of blood over a tennis court, giving a layer only one blood cell thick. Despite its vast area the capillary bed contributes only a minor amorphous increase in background density to the chest radiograph.

Although the pulmonary microcirculation cannot be seen on the plain film we can derive clinically valuable information about its functional and organic integrity from a study of the conducting vessels and in particular from the distribution of pulmonary blood flow.

Distinguishing between arteries and veins

It is not usually possible to distinguish between arteries and veins in the periphery of the lung but they can often be separately identified centrally both from their orientation and from slight differences in their individual anatomical characteristics (Fig. 3.01). The main divisions of the right and left pulmonary arteries enter the lung at slightly different levels. In the majority of chest radiographs the upper border of the main division of the right pulmonary artery is seen emerging from the mediastinum between the upper border of the 7th and the lower border of the 8th posterior ribs, while the upper margin of the left pulmonary artery lies at a slightly higher level, between the upper border of the 6th rib and the lower border of the 7th. The difference in level between the right and left main trunks usually equals one rib interspace. Approximately two ribs and one interspace intervene between the entry of the pulmonary arteries into the lung and the exit of the pulmonary veins from the lung, to enter the left atrium. On the right the veins exit between the upper border of the 8th rib and the lower border of the 9th rib. On the left the veins exit at much the same level except that the upper lobe veins enter approximately one rib space higher than on the right. (The entrance of the left upper lobe veins can only be seen on a very well penetrated film). There is some variation in the level of the arteries and veins, depending upon the physical characteristics of the chest. In mesomorphs the vessels tend to lie at a higher level and, in ectomorphs and patients with emphysema, the vessels lie at a lower level. The arteries characteristically taper regularly and with slight sinuosity towards the periphery, branching in a dichotomous fashion to within 1 cm of the pleural surface of the lung. At this point the vessels become too small to resolve and a structureless peripheral zone, (a thin 'cortex' of microcirculation) is seen extending to the pleural surface. In contrast, the pulmonary veins have rather parallel walls and instead of tapering gradually tend to increase their diameter in an abrupt step-wise fashion after each monopodial tributary joins the main stem (Fig. 3.01). It is possible to distinguish one or more veins in 80–90% of normal chest radiographs, the variability resulting largely from variation in radiographic technique. The vein which is most frequently seen courses from the right lower lobe across the cardiophrenic angle to enter the left atrium and can be identified in 80–85% of normal cases. If the film is well penetrated, left lower lower lobe veins can often be identified posterior to the left side of the heart. The upper lobe veins are less commonly seen, partially because of their smaller size in the erect position and partially because they may be obscured, particularly on the left side, by arterial branches to the upper lobes. On the right the upper lobe vein usually lies lateral to the arterial tripod, but on the left the veins may be either lateral to or may overlie the arterial tripod. The ability to distinguish between arteries and veins becomes of importance in assessing pulmonary haemodynamics from the plain chest radiograph.

Clarity of vessel margins. Because the blood-containing vessels are surrounded by air-filled alveoli their margins are quite sharply delineated in the normal lung. This clarity of vessel margins is of diagnostic importance, for example the vessel margins become blurred with the development of pulmonary oedema.

Bronchovascular Bundles and Perivascular/Peribronchial Sheaths

An important exception exists to the statement that the smaller bronchi cannot be seen on the plain film. Bronchi can be visualised if they are seen 'end-on', i.e. parallel to the X-ray beam. In the majority of chest radiographs one or more end-on bronchi can be identified in the perihilar areas, often accompanied by a vessel. The bronchus and accompanying vessel (which is always an artery, since the veins are formed peripherally and do not run with the bronchi) constitute a bronchovascular 'bundle' (Fig. 3.02). This bundle in turn is surrounded by a loose sheath of connective tissue extending from the mediastinal surface of the lung to the periphery where it forms a virtual sac around the pulmonary capillaries and is then prolonged along the pulmonary veins as they travel towards the left atrium. The arterial and venous sheaths are sealed at their points of entry and exit from the lung and do not normally communicate with the mediastinum. This is of some functional significance since accumulation of fluid in the sheaths will result in progressive elevation

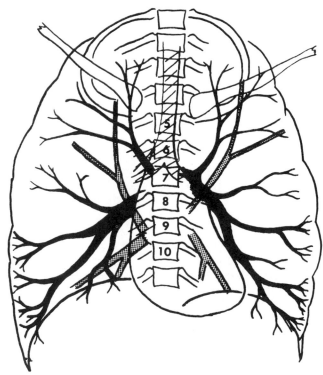

FIG. 3.01. Diagram of the pulmonary circulation. The arteries (in black) enter the lung at a higher position than the veins, taper gradually and branch dichotomously. The veins (in grey) enter the left atrium at a lower level, tend to be parallel-sided and accept tributaries in a monopodial fashion. (See text for a description of the usual anatomical position and degrees of variation of the arteries and veins.)

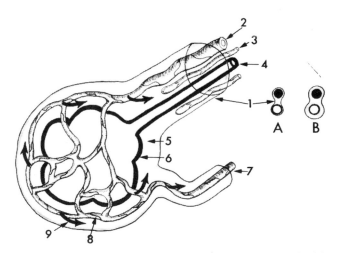

FIG. 3.02. Structure of the peribronchial/perivascular sheath. (1) Peribronchial/perivascular sheath. (2) Arteriole. (3) Lymphatic (does not proceed as far as the alveolar walls). (4) Terminal bronchiole. (5) Interstitial space. (6) Alveolus. (7) Venule (with prolongation of sheath). (8) Capillary endothelial cell junction. (9) Path of fluid from capillary into interstitial space. A. Appearance of a normal bronchovascular bundle seen end-on. B. Peribronchial/ perivascular 'cuffing' due to oedema in the interstitium.

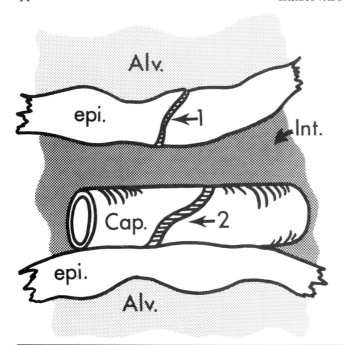

of pressure within the interstitial (perivascular) space. The endothelial cells lining the capillaries within this space have 'loose' intercellular junctions but the epithelial cells which line the alveoli and form the boundaries of the interstitial space have 'tight' junctions (Fig. 3.03). Oedema fluid therefore fills the interstitial space preferentially (rather than passing into the alveoli) and tracks along the peribronchial/perivascular sheaths to present radiologically as a 'cuff' of fluid around the end-on bronchus (Figs. 3.02 & 3.04). The association of blurred vessel margins (due to fluid within the sheaths) and peribronchial cuffing is excellent radiological evidence of the presence of interstitial oedema. When pulmonary oedema is caused by cardiac failure, overhydration, or renal failure, alveolar oedema does not

FIG. 3.03. Diagram of a pulmonary capillary (Cap.) fused on one side (the 'thin' side) to alveolar epithelium (epi). On the other side the interstitial space (Int.) intervenes between the capillary and the alveolus. This constitutes the 'thick' side. The endothelial junction (2) is 'loose', while the epithelial cell junction (1) is 'tight'.

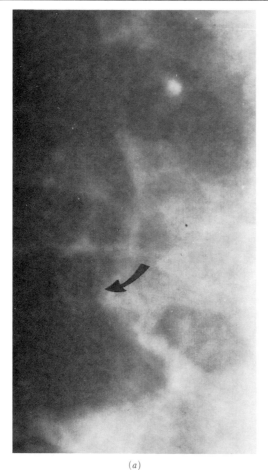

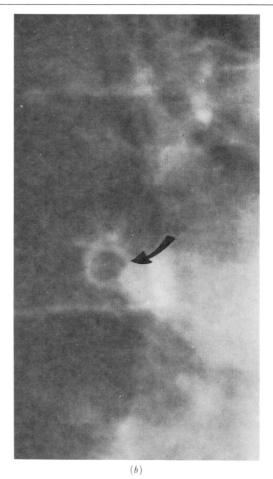

(a)   (b)

FIG. 3.04. (a) Normal 'end-on' bronchus (arrow). (b) The same bronchus following development of interstitial oedema and formation of a peribronchial 'cuff'.

appear to develop until the interstitial space is filled with fluid. It is hypothesised that the pressure within the interstitial space increases until it is too high even for the tight epithelial cell junctions to sustain and at this point rapid alveolar flooding occurs, i.e. the onset of interstitial oedema tends to be insidious but the development of alveolar oedema is abrupt. In contrast to this patients with capillary permeability oedema may sustain direct damage to the alveolar epithelium and alveolar oedema can occur at a much earlier stage.

Lymphatic channels also run within the perivascular/peribronchial space. Occasionally the bronchus and artery may be separated by a distance of several millimetres but remain within the same sheath. In these circumstances the prolongation of the sheath between the artery and the bronchus creates an appearance rather like a small dumb-bell (Fig. 3.05). When oedema develops in the interstitial space the 'bar' of the dumb-bell will widen, providing a subtle but valuable index of early oedema formation.

Bronchial wall thickness. The wall of the normal bronchus is usually thin and quite sharply delineated, as if drawn by a fine-tipped pen. Absolute measurements for bronchial wall thickness are difficult to quote because the normal bronchial wall is so thin that it approaches the limits of resolution of the radiographic imaging system; also, a wall thickness that is normal for a large bronchus would be pathological for a small one. It is therefore more useful in deciding whether pathological change is present to consider the ratio between the external width of the bronchus and the width of its lumen. This ratio should not exceed 1·4, i.e. bronchial wall thickness should not be more than one-seventh of the total width of the bronchus. For example, the wall of a 7·0 mm bronchus should not be more than 1·0 mm in thickness. Fortunately, changes in bronchial wall thickness are readily recognized by the trained eye. These changes include, in addition to a change in thickness, increased density and a blurred outer border (fluid within the peribronchial sheath) so that actual measurement is rarely necessary to confirm or exclude abnormality (Fig. 3.04).

The bronchial circulation. In addition to the pulmonary circulation which takes part in gas exchange, the lungs possess a second blood supply, the bronchial circulation, which is nutrient to the lung. An angiogram demonstrating the size and distribution of a normal bronchial artery is shown in Fig. 3.06. The bronchial arteries are usually too small to be visualised on the chest radiograph without injection of contrast medium but can be seen on rare occasions if they become grossly hypertrophied. This can occur either in association with pulmonary suppuration or with congenital deficiency or absence of the pulmonary circulation. In pulmonary suppuration a single leash of very tortuous vessels may be seen leading towards the infected area (Fig. 3.07).

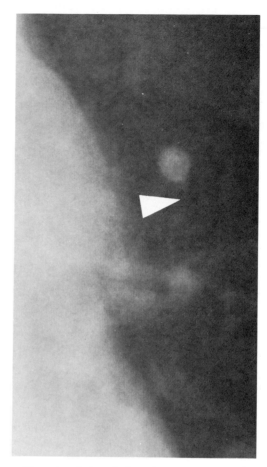

FIG. 3.05. Normal variation of a bronchovascular bundle. The artery and bronchus are separated and the surrounding sheath bridges the gap between them (white arrow) giving a 'dumb-bell' appearance.

On the right side the bronchial arteries enter the lung just above the level of the carina, well above the pulmonary arteries, but on the left side several smaller bronchial arteries usually supply the lung and their levels of origin are inconstant. The hypertrophied vessels, which accompany congenital reduction or absence of pulmonary arterial flow, present in both upper perihilar areas as ill-defined collections of tortuous vessels of much smaller diameter than normal pulmonary arteries. Many of the hypertrophied bronchial vessels may be seen end-on giving the appearance of dense perihilar dots (see Fig. 14.20).

The Vascular Pedicle

In addition to pulmonary vessels some of the largest systemic vessels within the body are seen on the chest radiograph. The large veins draining into the right atrium and the great arteries arising from the aortic arch form respectively the right and left boundaries of

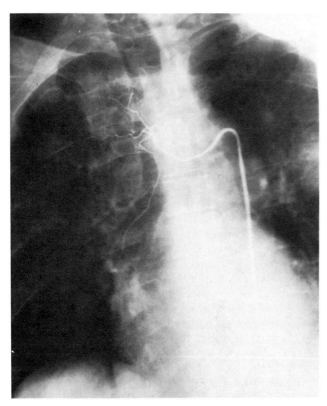

Fig. 3.06. Normal right bronchial arteriogram. The catheter is inserted into the origin of the intercostobronchial trunk (just above the left main bronchus). The bronchial arteries ramify along the course of the bronchi.

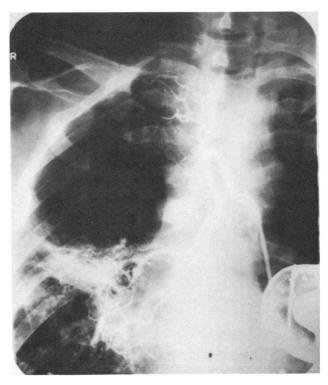

Fig. 3.07. Selective right bronchial arteriogram in a patient with pulmonary suppuration. The bronchial trunk is grossly hypertrophied and there is extensive ramification of the bronchial circulation in the region of the lung abscess.

the mediastinum on the PA film. The heart is virtually suspended within the thorax from these great vessels and this structure has therefore been called the 'vascular pedicle' of the heart (Milne *et al.*, 1982; Pistolesi *et al.*, 1982; Quinke & Pfeiffer, 1871). The right border of the pedicle, formed above by the right brachiocephalic vein and below by the superior vena cava is entirely venous and is therefore very compliant, whereas the left border, formed above the aorta by the subclavian artery, is entirely arterial and is much less compliant (Fig. 3.08).

Vascular pedicle width (VPW) is measured as shown in Fig. 3.08. In normal patients VPW equals 4·8±0·5 cm. While a 70 kg patient of average build will have a VPW of approximately 4·8 cm, a large fat patient will have a normal VPW of 5·3 cm and a small thin patient a VPW of 4·3 cm or less (Milne *et al.*, 1982). VPW is closely related to the circulating blood volume (CBV) and *change* in VPW is very closely correlated with change in CBV (Pistolesi *et al.*, 1982). Each 1·0 mm change in VPW is equal to a change of 200 ml in TBV (i.e. 0·5 cm change in VPW equals a 1·0 litre change in TBV). Because of the greater compliance of the veins bordering the right side of the pedicle, the pedicle will respond to an increase in total blood volume by bulging more to

the right (approximately 70%) then to the left (approximately 30%) (Fig. 3.09). Normal inspiration and expiration has little effect on VPW. On expiration it tends to remain unchanged or to decrease by one or two millimetres reflecting the diminished venous return to the thorax. The right border of the pedicle (the SVC) lies far anteriorly in the chest and the left border (the left subclavian artery) far posteriorly. Changing from the PA to the AP position therefore has little effect on VPW, i.e. in either position one or other of the borders is always close to the film and one further away (Fig. 3.10). Changing the anode-to-film distance from 72–40 ins increases VPW approximately 5% by geometric magnification. Rotation of the patient by more than 10° does have a significant effect on VPW; rotation to the left decreases VPW and rotation to the right increases it (Fig. 3.10). Major changes in VPW are caused by assuming the supine position. A good deal of individual variation occurs, the degree of change varying from 7–40% (mean 17·39±9·4%). Obviously under these circumstances the change in VPW does *not* indicate a change in total blood volume but is caused by a redistribution of CBV giving an increased volume in the upper half of the body. Assessments and comparisons between VPW on successive films should prefer-

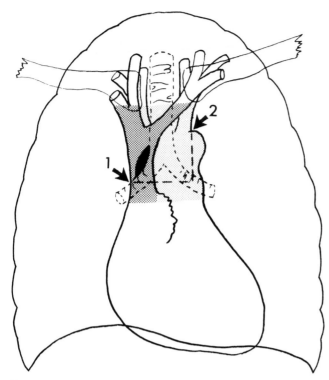

FIG. 3.08. Diagram of the vascular pedicle (shaded area). The right-hand border is entirely venous being formed by the right brachio-cephalic vein and superior vena cava (SVC); the veins are shaded darker. The left border is arterial (left subclavian artery). The vena azygos (black) lies just above the right main bronchus.

Measuring points for the width of the pedicle (VPW) are arrowed. Point 1 is where the SVC crosses the right main bronchus and point 2 where the left subclavian artery takes off from the aorta. VPW is measured along a horizontal from point 1 to a perpendicular dropped from point 2.

ably be made with all of the films being taken either supine or erect and with the patient either non-rotated or rotated to the same degree in both films. The relationship between VPW and CBV is not as good in elderly patients because atherosclerosis may distort the great vessels and artifactually increase VPW; however, even in these patients, the excellent correlation between *change* in VPW and change in CBV remains unaffected. VPW is an easily obtained figure which can give the radiologist excellent data about systemic as opposed to pulmonary haemodynamics and is of considerable value in following the response to therapy of patients with chronic left or biventricular failure and elevated total blood volume.

The azygos vein. The azygos vein runs cranially along the right anterolateral surfaces of the dorsal vertebrae then curves slightly forward over the right main bronchus to enter the back of the superior vena cava. It presents on the frontal chest radiograph as an ovoid opacity lying just above the right main bronchus,

within the shadow of the superior vena cava (Fig. 3.08, 3.09(*b*)). It is bordered by the trachea medially, the right lung superolaterally and the right main bronchus inferomedially. These surrounding structures are all air-containing and the azygos vein can therefore be visualised in approximately 90% of adequately pene-trated chest films. (It tends not to be seen on low kV films). It can be most easily identified by following the right paratracheal stripe downward toward the right main bronchus. The stripe appears to widen inferiorly to 'enclose' the azygos then narrows again below the azygos to form the upper wall of the right main bronchus (Fig. 3.09(*b*)).

Azygos vein size is so variable from individual to individual that there is little value in quoting an average size range. In general if the diameter of the vein from its medial to its lateral border is over 7·0 mm a suspicion of enlargement should be entertained (Heitzman, 1973). Again this is not a very useful measurement since a 7·0 mm azygos may be quite normal in a large individual or in a woman in the mid-trimester of pregnancy. Irrespective of its absolute size on the initial film, *change* in size is of much greater importance in indicating a change in haemodynamic status.

Relationship of azygos vein size to mean right atrial pressure (MRAP) and circulating blood vol-ume (CBV). Many authors have hypothesized that the size of the azygos is related to MRAP and/or CBV but until recently there has been no published work corre-lating azygos measurements with simultaneously meas-ured MRAP and CBV. There is now good evidence that the size of the azygos vein is poorly correlated with CBV but correlates better with MRAP (Pistolesi *et al.*, 1982). The azygos vein can therefore be expected, in a certain proportion of cases, to enlarge in response to elevation of MRAP, for example in right heart failure and following a large pulmonary embolus. Unfortunately the response to increasing MRAP is neither linear nor consistent. In response to the same rise in MRAP, dilatation may be minimal or absent in one individual and very evident in another, possibly because the azygos vein is valvular and a competent valve at its entry point into the SVC may 'protect' it from high pressure. Where a dilated azygos is present it is a good indication that MRAP is elevated but the reverse is not true; the absence of azygos vein dilatation does not exclude the diagnosis of increased MRAP or CBV.

PULMONARY BLOOD FLOW AND PULMONARY BLOOD VOLUME

Since flow and volume within the pulmonary vascular bed are interdependent, they will be considered under the same heading

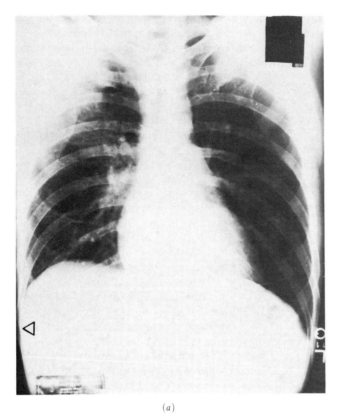 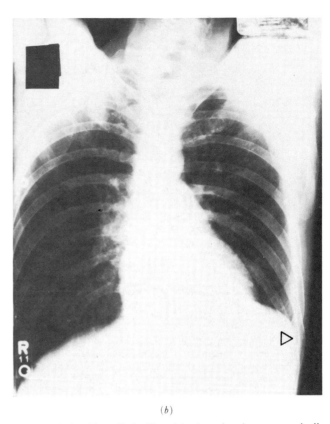

(a)   (b)

FIG. 3.12. (a) Film taken with the patient's right side down (arrow)—(right lateral decubitus film). The right lung has become markedly hyperaemic because of gravitational redistribution of flow, and the left lung oligaemic. (b) Patient in left lateral decubitus position; the right lung is now oligaemic and flow has shifted to the left lung. (Note characteristic behaviour of the diaphragm in Fig. 12(a) & (b) secondary to the change in intra-abdominal pressure gradient.)

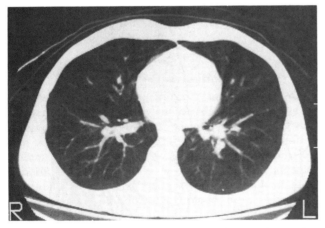

FIG. 3.13. CT scan through the base of a normal chest, patient supine. The dorsal vessels are larger and appear more numerous than the ventral vessels because of the gravitationally induced ventral/dorsal hydrostatic pressure gradient.

recruiting vessels *without* an increase in pulmonary arterial pressure. The pulmonary vascular bed is therefore a circuit of extremely low resistance to flow. Even a very small regional increase in resistance to flow will result in a redistribution of blood flow away from the area of raised resistance to other areas of normal low resistance. While the changes that have led to the regional increase in resistance may be microscopic and impossible to visualise, the resultant redistribution of flow is seen easily and from this the cause of the redistribution can often be deduced.

Relationship between PVBC and PBV

There are many functional and organic causes for changes in either PVBC or PBV. The most important of these are listed in Table 3.1. In Fig. 3.14 the effects of some of these changes on the distribution of flow are shown diagrammatically. It will be seen that as PVBC diminishes to approach PBV (or conversely as PBV increases to approach PVBC) the normal gravitational flow distribution is abolished and a 1:1 ('balanced') flow is seen. Figure 3.15 demonstrates a common organic cause of flow redistribution. In Fig. 3.16 an

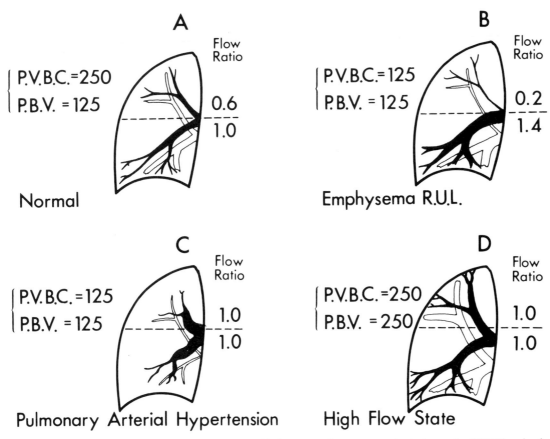

FIG. 3.14. This diagram illustrates several ways in which the relationship between pulmonary vascular bed capacity (PVBC) and pulmonary blood volume (PBV) can be altered and the effects of this on the chest radiograph (arteries black, veins white). (*Reproduced with the author's and publisher's permission from* Radiologic Clinics of North America, *W. B. Saunders Co., Philadelphia.*)

example of functional redistribution is illustrated. PVBC varies according to a patient's size and physical configuration but is not affected by weight gain or loss. Although the redistribution of pulmonary blood flow illustrated in Figs. 3.15 & 3.16 is not caused by cardiac abnormality it is necessary when interpreting cardiac films to be aware of all the possible causes of redistribution, particularly since cardiac disease is very commonly associated with chronic lung disease.

Pulmonary blood volume. In a normal patient the PBV is not constant, being affected by such factors as inspiration and expiration, change in position from erect to supine and by alveolar and interstitial pressure, but obviously there must be a mean baseline value for any given individual in the resting state. Like PVBC this figure is closely related to the patient's size and surface area, but it is also related to his/her adiposity. A small thin patient will have a small pulmonary blood volume, manifested by slender vessels and an easily distinguishable zonal distribution of flow. If the same patient becomes fat, the circulating blood volume will increase, there will be greater filling of the vascular bed

and the gravitational effects will become less obvious. Similarly a tall but thin patient will have a smaller PBV than a tall fat patient. It is therefore necessary, as with vascular pedicle width, to take a patient's physical configuration into consideration when trying to decide if PBV is normal, increased or decreased.

Relationship between PBV and pulmonary blood flow. Pulmonary blood volume is closely linked to right ventricular output (Milne, 1973, 1977, 1978). It is more correct to use the term right ventricular output rather than cardiac output, since in the presence of an anatomical shunt RV and LV output may differ and PBV is not, under these circumstances related to the left ventricular output. The relationship between pulmonary blood flow and pulmonary blood volume is linear (Milne, 1978) but the slope of the relationship varies from individual to individual depending largely upon the compliance of the vascular bed, which can be affected functionally by neurogenic tone, or organically, (for example by endarteritis, emphysema, chronic bronchitis, etc.). Flow through the lungs can increase either by an increase in volume or by an increase in speed of

TABLE.—FACTORS AFFECTING PULMONARY VASCULAR BED CAPACITY (PVBC) AND PULMONARY BLOOD VOLUME (PBV)

I. PULMONARY VASCULAR BED CAPACITY

A. **Functional Changes**
   (1) *Level of inflation* (related to the ability to generate a negative interstitial pressure and therefore affected by chest-wall pain, subdiaphragmatic pathology, pleural pain)
   At T.L.C. (4 zones of flow seen, extreme base tends to become oligaemic)
   At F.R.C. (3 zones—normal flow distribution)
   At R.V. (homogeneous flow, all capillaries recruited)
   (2) *Increased left atrial pressure* (in the normal erect lung leads to basal fluid transudation, less negative interstitial pressure and functional closure—regional 'loss'—of lower lobe vessels
   (3) *Alveolar pressure* (increase)
   General:
      Use of positive end-expiratory pressure
      Valsalva
      Status asthmaticus
      Smoke inhalation (with air-trapping)
   Regional:
      Asthma
      Foreign body
      Mucous plugs
      Mucosal oedema
      Post-obliterative bronchiolitis
      Extrinsic pressure on bronchus
   Alveolar pressure (decrease)
      Mueller manoeuvre
   (4) *Interstitial pressure* (increase: absolute or relative)
   General:
      Inability to move diaphragm (e.g., ascites, abdominal tumour, amyotrophic lateral sclerosis, pneumoperitoneum, corsets, etc.)
   Regional:
      Chest-wall pain or immobilisation

Pleural pain, thickening or effusion
Diaphragmatic paralysis or eventration
Carcinoma or consolidation
Transudation (due to elevated left atrial pressure, osmotic effects or endothelial damage)
   (5) *Pulmonary oedema* (through its effects on compliance, interstitial pressure and oxygenation)
   (6) *Blood gas levels* (e.g., unilateral bronchial obstruction, bronchography, Carlins tube, high-altitude, regional hypoxia, hypercarbia)
   (7) *Pharmacological agents*
(All those entities above which cause functional regional loss of pulmonary vascular bed also cause regional decrease in flow).

B. **Organic Changes (general or regional)**
   (1) *Emphysema**
   (2) *Fibrosis**
   (3) *Embolism** (acute)
   (4) *Sarcoidosis** (direct involvement of vessels)
   (5) *Infiltration** or neoplasm
   (6) *Endarteritis* obliterans**
   (7) *Microembolism/schistosomiasis***
   (8) *Embolism* (chronic)**
   (9) *Veno-occlusive disease***
   (10) *Bodily habitus* (acromegaly, pituitary dwarfism)
   * (In addition to organic change, these conditions also affect PVBC functionally by their effect on pulmonary interstitial pressure)
   ** (Where changes in the pulmonary vascular bed are generalised enough to cause increased pulmonary vascular resistance the PBV may decrease on the venous side while increasing on the arterial and precapillary side)
(All of those entities above which cause organic regional loss of pulmonary vascular bed also cause regional decrease in flow).

II. PULMONARY BLOOD VOLUME

Increased flow causes increased volume: the degree of change in radiological appearance is inversely related to degree of change in transit time.

A. **Functional causes of increased flow.**
   General
   (1) *Exercise*
   (2) *Pregnancy*
   (3) *Pyrexia*
   (4) *Anaemia*
   (5) *Thyrotoxicosis*
   (6) *Renal failure**
   (7) *Overhydration with blood*
   (8) *Overhydration with saline**
   (9) *Pharmacological agents* (bradykinin, isoproterenol, aminophyllin)
   (10) *Polycythaemia*
* Accompanied by increase in extravascular lung water and change in interstitial pressure.

   Regional
   (1) *Gravitational* (e.g., increased flow to apex on inversion)
   (2) Secondary to *increased regional resistance* elsewhere in the lung (e.g., embolus, emphysema, hypoxia, increased alveolar pressure, oedema with increased interstitial pressure, etc.)

B. **Organic causes of increased flow**
   General
   (1) *Intrathoracic L-R shunts*
   (2) *Pulmonary and peripheral arteriovenous anomalies* (including Paget's disease)
   Regional
   (1) *Anomalous venous return*
   (2) *Systemic arterial supply to the lung*
   (3) *Regional bronchial arterial hypertrophy*

   Decreased flow—causes decreased volume:
A. **Functionl causes of decreased flow:**
   General
   (1) *Dehydration* and loss of blood
   (2) *Hypothyroidism*
   (3) *Addison's disease*
   (4) Pharmacological agents (serotonin, histamine, catecholamines)
B. **Organic**
   General
   (1) *Cardiac failure*
   (2) *Valvular disease* (aortic, mitral, pulmonary and tricuspid)
   (3) *Myocardiopathy*
   (4) *Periocardial disease*
   (5) *Endocarditis*

flow (decreased transit time) or by a combination of the two. Healthy individuals tend to increase their pulmonary blood flow on exercise mainly by a decrease in transit time and there is therefore little visible change on the radiograph (Fig. 3.17(a)(b)), whereas people with cardiac disease increase their pulmonary blood flow mainly by increasing the volume flowing per unit time; this change in pulmonary blood volume is easily seen on the chest radiograph. Since, when we are looking at a chest radiograph, we do not usually know the transit times or the compliance of the vessels, we cannot presently quantitate flow in absolute terms from the size of the pulmonary vessels but, since all of these vessels are connected to the same pump (the heart) and

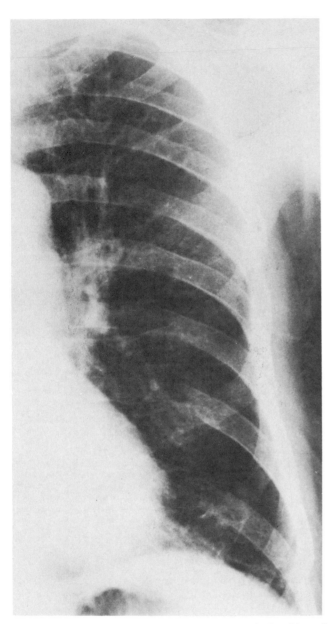

FIG. 3.15. Base-to-apex redistribution of flow caused by basal loss of microvessels from emphysema ('organic' redistribution).

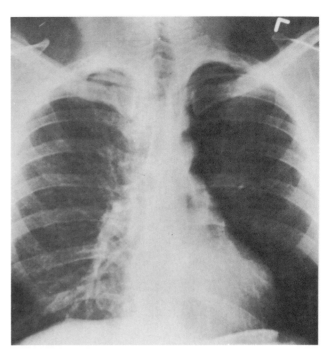

FIG. 3.16. Redistribution of flow from the left lung to the right caused by raised intra-alveolar pressure on the left secondary to old obliterative bronchiolitis in childhood (Swyer-James or McLeod syndrome—'functional' redistribution).

since the relationship between right ventricular output and pulmonary blood volume is linear, we *can* estimate flow in relative terms from one part of the lung to the other. For example, if a pump is connected to two sets of vessels, one of which is either slightly narrower or slightly less compliant than the other then flow will go to the lower resistance vessels and the volume of these vessels will increase indicating the relative increase in flow through them. In the narrower (or stiffer) vessels there will be a lesser increase in volume and the transit time will also be longer so that the relative flow

difference between narrow and wide vessels is even greater than one might suppose from comparing their relative size differences alone.

Where right ventricular output is very high, for example in a large atrial or ventricular septal defect, the pulmonary blood volume is also large and the pulmonary vascular bed becomes completely filled giving a 1:1 flow distribution. Under these circumstances the vascular pedicle is small because left ventricular output is reduced and the systemic blood volume is also small (Fig. 3.18); however, in cases where there is a large increase in cardiac output due to an increase in circulating blood volume, for example renal failure or over-hydration, the vascular pedicle is wide, permitting differentiation between the two conditions (Fig. 3.19). Conversely, in any condition in which circulating blood volume is reduced so that right ventricular output is small the pulmonary blood volume will also be small. This type of oligaemia, due to a low cardiac output can be seen in dehydration and in haemorrhagic shock (Fig. 3.20(a) & (b)). A small pulmonary blood volume may also be found in most cases of compensated aortic stenosis where the cardiac output is very small and in emphysema where several mechanisms are at play, only one of which is the low cardiac output.

In a high flow state, where flow volume through the

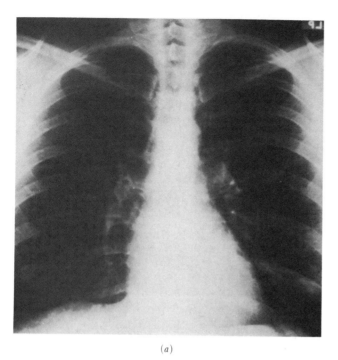

(a)

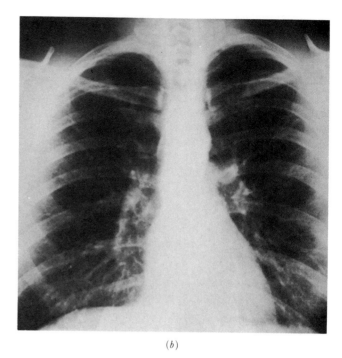

(b)

FIG. 3.17. (a) PA chest film made in the erect position, of a healthy young adult, prior to exercise. (b) The same patient immediately following very vigorous exercise. There is no change in size of the main conducting vessels but the smaller vessels are more easily seen and the lung is denser (probably due to recruitment of microvessels). Note that the heart size is slightly *smaller* immediately after exercise in this healthy male.

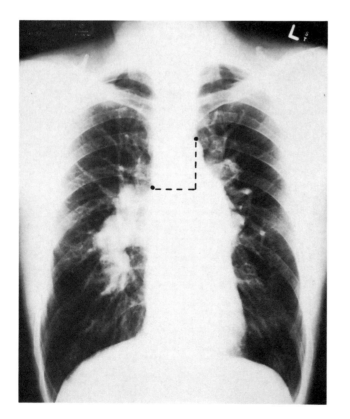

FIG. 3.18. 53-year-old patient with a large ASD. Despite the large pulmonary blood volume (reflecting the huge right ventricular output) the vascular pedicle width (horizontal dotted line) is quite narrow reflecting a small circulating blood volume secondary to diminished left ventricular output.

arteries is increased, flow through the draining veins must also be increased (Fig. 3.19). This is reflected by a concomitant increase in size of the veins. Conversely, when flow is reduced by a diminution in circulating blood volume, for example following dehydration or haemorrhage, the arteries and veins both become smaller and the normal gravitational distribution of flow becomes even more evident (Fig. 3.20(a)). Where pulmonary blood flow is reduced secondary to left heart failure a different mechanism occurs; the CBV is not reduced (and is usually increased if LHF is chronic) and there is also elevation of left atrial pressure. This causes a quite different type of flow redistribution from that seen when flow is reduced but the heart is *not* failing. Since the cause of this redistribution is the development of pulmonary oedema with changes in interstitial pressure it will be discussed under the heading 'Pulmonary Oedema' (*vide infra*).

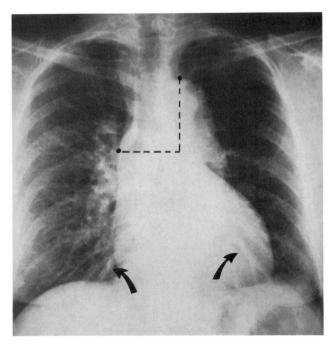

FIG. 3.19. 30-year-old female patient with renal failure causing retention of salt and water and a very large circulating blood volume. As in the case of the ASD (Fig. 3.18) there is a 'balanced' distribution of flow with large arteries and veins (arrowed) indicating a large right ventricular output but, in contrast to the ASD vascular pedicle width is now large indicating the large circulating blood volume. Note the gross enlargement of the vena azygos.

EFFECTS OF ALVEOLAR AND INTERSTITIAL PRESSURE ON PBV AND PBF

The microvessels surrounding the alveoli are directly affected by changes in alveolar pressure (West *et al.*, 1964). As pressure increases the capillaries tend to become flattened, causing a considerable increase in resistance to flow (Fig. 3.21). It should be remembered that while resistance to flow is directly proportional to the change in length of a vessel it is proportional to the fourth power of the *radius* of the vessel (Poiseuilles law) (Rigler, 1959). A very small change in radius therefore produces a large change in resistance. This fact is of considerable significance in explaining why only a small decrease in lung compliance (and therefore in the diameter of the vessels within that portion of lung) will cause a considerable redistribution of blood flow away from that area. Figure 3.16 shows one example of redistribution of flow caused by a local increase in alveolar pressure. Other important pathological causes of increased intra-alveolar pressure include asthma, mucous plugging and valvular obstruction due to a foreign body or pedunculated adenoma, but the commonest cause of altered intra-alveolar pressure is now undoubtedly the use of positive end-expiratory pressure (PEEP). The radiologist must be aware that progressive increase in intra-alveolar pressure causes a progressive decrease in venous return into the thorax, diminishing

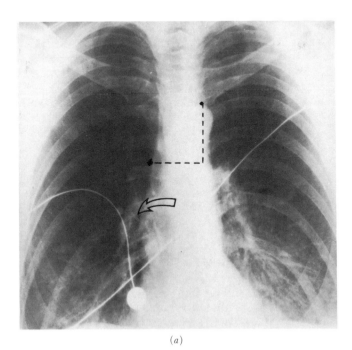

(a)

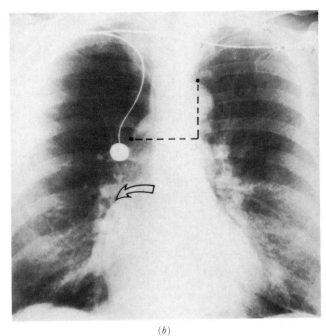

(b)

FIG. 3.20. (a) Patient in Addisonian crisis, severely dehydrated. Note the very small pulmonary veins (arrowed) and exaggeration of normal basal flow predominance. VPW (horizontal dotted line) is very small indicating the very small circulating blood volume. (b) Same patient immediately following rehydration. The pulmonary vessels (arrowed) have increased markedly in size and the VPW and azygos have increased greatly.

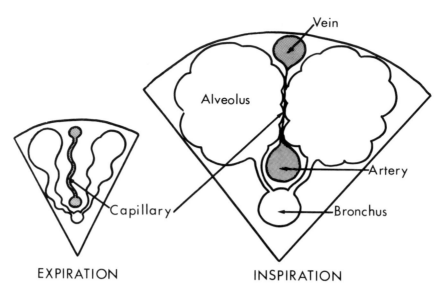

Fig. 3.21. Segment of a lung lobule seen end-on. On expiration the arteriole and venule both reduce in size as the interstitial pressure around them becomes less negative; however, the alveoli between which the capillaries pass are now deflated and the capillaries become shorter and wider.

On inspiration the reverse happens, the conducting vessels increase in size as the interstitial pressure becomes more negative but the capillaries are flattened and elongated between the inflated alveoli causing increased resistance to flow.

the pulmonary blood volume and cardiac output (Fig. 3.22(1) & (2)). Since PEEP is designed to improve ventilation to perfusion ratios there is an optimum level at which ventilation and perfusion are matched; when the pressure becomes so high that perfusion begins to diminish (indicated on the chest radiograph by diminution in pulmonary blood volume) PEEP clearly begins to lose its value.

Since the volume and distribution of blood flow, the width of the vascular pedicle and the appearance of pulmonary oedema are all affected by the degree of lung inflation and by position, it is essential in order to assess and compare films that full details of the patient's position, the X-ray technique used, the type of ventilation and ventilatory pressures employed, be recorded directly on the radiograph. This is of particular importance in cardiac intensive care units where accurate assessment of changes in blood flow, venous and arterial pressures, circulating blood volume and the quantity of oedema can be quite erroneous if the radiologist is unaware that the patient is on artificial ventilation. A simple label of the type shown in Fig. 3.23 provides all of the necessary information and its use should be standard practice in critical care units.

Effects of Interstitial Pressure

The lung is normally held in a partially expanded position by the elastic recoil of the chest wall. The lung itself is always trying to recoil to a smaller volume and

the chest wall to become larger. The result is the development of a negative pressure within the pleural space. This negative pressure is transmitted across the lung, and in association with elastic fibres which surround and tether the vessels and bronchi, creates a negative pressure within the lung interstitium which 'holds' the smaller vessels and bronchi open. During inspiration the interstitial pressure becomes more negative (exceeding minus 30 cm of water) and the vessels and bronchi are pulled open, sucking both air and blood into the lung. On expiration the interstitial pressure becomes less negative, the vessels and bronchi reduce in diameter and air and blood are pumped out of the lung (Fig. 3.21). Any factor which alters the ability of the lungs or chest wall to generate this negative pressure will have an effect on both ventilation and perfusion to the lung. For example, if a patient has strapping applied to the right chest wall to treat a rib fracture so that the right chest cannot expand properly, the vessels on the right will *not* be pulled open on inspiration whereas the vessels on the left will be. The smaller diameter of the vessels on the right will cause a considerable increase in pulmonary vascular resistance and as a result blood flow will redistribute to the left. Any mechanism which causes a change in the compliance of a portion of the lung will also cause a change in the lungs' ability to generate interstitial negative pressure and an alteration in vessel diameter within that area. As indicated above a very small change in vessel diameter will cause a large

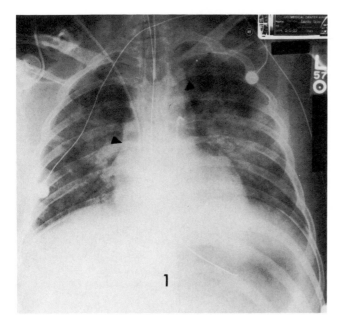

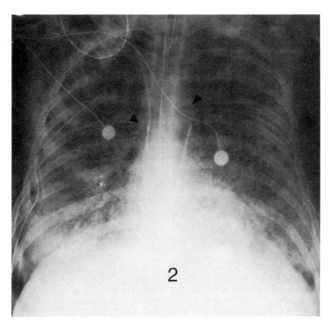

FIG. 3.22. Film (1) shows a 30-year-old male patient with adult respiratory distress syndrome (ARDS). The lung fields show the characteristic patchy distribution of capillary permeability oedema, including the commonly seen air bronchograms. The patient is supine which explains the wide vascular pedicle (arrowed). The patient is on assist-control ventilation (AC) with a peak inflation pressure of 46 cm H2O but is receiving only 5 cm H2O of positive end-expiratory pressure (PEEP). Film (2) shows the same patient several days later. His lung compliance had progressively diminished and his peak inflation pressure was raised to 70 cm H2O. He is now on a PEEP of 25 cm H2O. Note the very marked diminution in VPW (arrowed) even though he is still supine. He now has bilateral interstitial emphysema, pneumomediastinum and bilateral pneumothoraces (treated by chest tubes) as a result of the high inflation pressures. Note the considerable diminution in cardiac volume—the level of pressure is so high that it is causing diminished venous return and a low cardiac output.

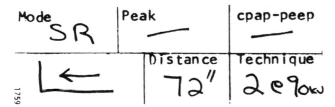

FIG. 3.23. The actual dimensions of this adhesive-backed label are 3×1 ins. *Mode* refers to type of ventilation (S.R. = spontaneous respiration, I.M.V. = intermittent mandatory ventilation and A.C. = assist-control ventilation). *Peak* refers to the maximum inflation pressure used (in cm H2O) and *CPAP-PEEP* indicates whether positive end-expiratory pressure is being used and at what level (cm H2O). The box at the lower left shows the patient's position (straight lines); in this instance the patient is sitting up and the X-ray beam (the arrow) is horizontal and perpendicular to the patient. *Distance* refers to the tube to film distance in inches. *Technique*—the example shown indicates 2 mA at 90 kV.

change in resistance and there will therefore be a redistribution of blood flow away from the affected area. One of the commonest causes for a change in compliance is pulmonary oedema.

Pulmonary Oedema

The ability of a vessel to retain water is dictated by the balance of hydrostatic and osmotic forces within the vessel and within the surrounding interstitium, and by the permeability of the vessel walls. Within the lungs the balance of forces is such that fluid is pushed out of the arterial end of the capillary with a force of approximately 7 mm Hg. At the venous end of the capillary the balance of forces results in a positive pressure of only 3 mm Hg tending to push fluid back into the vessel. Obviously more fluid emerges from the capillary vascular bed than re-enters it. The normal lung is therefore not dry but contains a certain amount of extravascular lung water (EVLW), (approximately 50 ml for every 1000 ml of lung). The excess filtrate (extravascular lung water) is usually taken care of by the pulmonary lymphatics. An increase in left atrial pressure of only a few millimetres will result in a decrease of fluid re-entering the venous end of the capillaries. A further increase in left atrial pressure will cause a complete reversal so that fluid now transudes from both the arterial and venous end of the capillary bed. It is not necessary, as commonly stated, for the left atrial pressure to exceed plasma osmotic pressure (25 mm Hg) before an increase in extravascular lung water occurs. Whether an increase in lung water results in radiologically detectable pulmonary oedema, however, depends upon the ability of the lymphatics to remove the excess water. As with all bodily systems there is considerable biological variation in the size and efficiency of the pulmonary lymphatics and some individuals will manifest pulmonary oedema at much lower left atrial pressures than others. When left atrial pressure is elevated over very long periods of time (such as in mitral stenosis) the lymphatic system hypertrophies greatly and can carry up to 15–20 times its normal burden and left atrial pressures of over 35 mm Hg can be tolerated without visible oedema.

Effect of Oedema on Lung Volume

Since pulmonary oedema causes a loss of compliance it also causes a loss of lung volume, which may be paraphrased by saying that, 'a wet lung should be a small lung'. Left heart failure accompanied by pulmonary oedema usually results in a noticeable loss of lung volume on the chest radiograph. As oedema diminishes with treatment, the lung volume is restored to normal. There is a valuable corollary to this that, if oedema is present but the lung volume is *not* reduced this strongly suggests the presence of air-trapping due to chronic obstructive pulmonary disease.

Effects of Oedema on Flow Distribution

Because of the hydrostatic pressure gradient down the lungs, capillary pressure is considerably higher at the bases than at the apices and as left atrial pressure rises increasing transudation will occur firstly at the bases. This will cause a diminution in lung compliance and a reduction in negative pressure within the interstitium (Hughes *et al.*, 1967; West *et al.*, 1964). With less negative pressure to hold them open, the basal microvessels will become slightly smaller in diameter causing a rise in resistance to flow. As a result, blood will be redistributed from the bases into the apices. Oedema intervening between the pulmonary capillaries and the alveoli will increase the diffusion distance for oxygen and may result in some hypoxaemia. Hypoxaemia is a very potent vasoconstrictor in the lungs and this mechanism may also be responsible for the base-to-apex redistribution which accompanies basal oedema. A neurogenic component has been postulated but has never been proven. It should be noted that the change in interstitial pressure produced by the oedema is not great and the ability to produce redistribution of flow is dependent upon the presence of recruitable vessels in the upper lobes. Should these vessels already be full, for example from an increase in pulmonary blood volume caused by renal failure or by overhydration, base-to-apex redistribution ('flow inversion') cannot take place even in the presence of oedema. Similarly, if the upper lobe vessels have been destroyed by emphysema there will be no vessels available for recruitment and flow redistribution will not be possible.

Flow Redistribution in Mitral Valve Disease and Left Heart Failure

Flow redistribution was first described in association with the elevated left atrial pressure of mitral stenosis and assumes its most dramatic form in such cases where the left atrial pressure can be extremely high (Fig. 3.24) (Kerley, 1957; Lavender *et al.*, 1962; Milne, 1963). In such cases there is a statistically strong relationship between the degree of redistribution and the level of the left atrial pressure, and clinically valuable assessments of left atrial pressure can therefore be made from the plain radiograph in cases of mitral valve disease (Friedman & Braunwald, 1966; Milne, 1963). Redistribution of flow also occurs in left heart failure not associated with valvular disease and prominence of the upper lobe vessels with narrowing of the lower lobe vessels (sometimes called the 'hands-up' sign for obvious reasons) is a valuable radiological indication of left heart decompensation (Kerley, 1957; Lavender & Doppman, 1962; Lavender *et al.*, 1962) (Fig. 3.25). Readily recognizable flow inversion is present in most cases of chronic left heart failure and in many cases of acute LHF, but in a

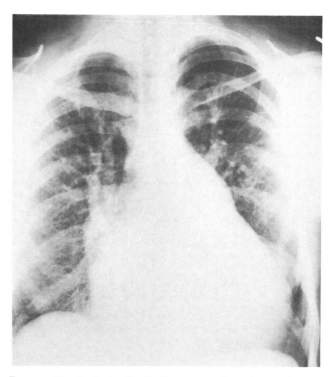

FIG. 3.24. The classical redistribution pattern of a patient with a very high left atrial pressure (in this case 35 mm Hg). Note that the patient has been operated upon; the left atrial appendage has been amputated (obviously from this film the operation was unsuccessful). The VPW is very small, a characteristic finding in mitral valve disease where the cardiac output and circulating blood volume are very small. The small azygos indicates that there is no increase in mean right atrial pressure, i.e. the tricuspid valve is competent and the right heart is not failing.

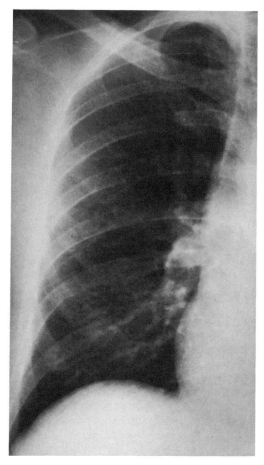

FIG. 3.25. Inversion of flow (base-to-apex redistribution) in a patient with left heart failure.

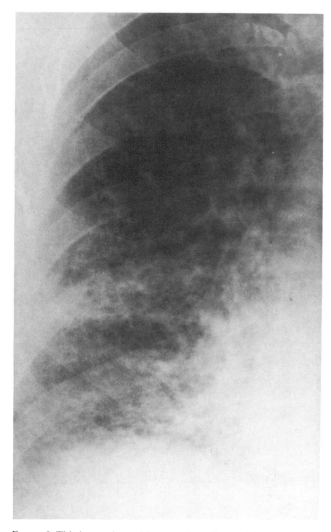

FIG. 3.26. This is a patient with severe lung disease (chronic bronchitis) which has caused randomly distributed damage to the microvascular bed. The patient is now in severe left heart failure but pulmonary oedema has only occurred in those scattered areas where there is still intact microcirculation. The result is a bizarre cystic ('Swiss cheese') appearance which makes it difficult to diagnose left heart failure.

certain proportion of cases, at the first onset of failure, although the upper lobe vessels do become larger and more prominent, the lower lobe vessels do not narrow and there is a balanced (1/1) rather than inverted distribution of flow. The mechanism for this difference in behaviour from chronic left heart failure has not yet been explained.

Many patients with left heart failure also have chronic lung disease, possibly because of the association between smoking and both heart and lung disease, and possibly because chronically wet lungs provide an excellent nidus for bacterial growth. The lung disease causes damage to the vascular bed which may be localised, diffuse or patchy. Since pulmonary oedema can only occur where there are intact capillaries and redistribution can only occur where there are patent recruitable vessels available, lung disease can grossly modify both the distribution of oedema and the pattern of redistribution of blood flow (Hublitz & Shapiro, 1969; Milne, 1972; Milne & Bass, 1969) (Fig. 3.26).

The radiologist is less accurate in assessing left atrial pressure in left heart failure than in mitral valve disease. This is partly because of the differing flow redistribution which occurs in chronic versus acute LHF, partly because the state of compensation or decompensation fluctuates much more in LHF than in mitral disease and partly because of the presence of chronic lung disease.

Distribution of Pulmonary Oedema

Statistical analysis of patterns of oedema in a large number of cases has shown that there are highly significant and diagnostically valuable differences in the distribution of oedema in cardiac failure, capillary

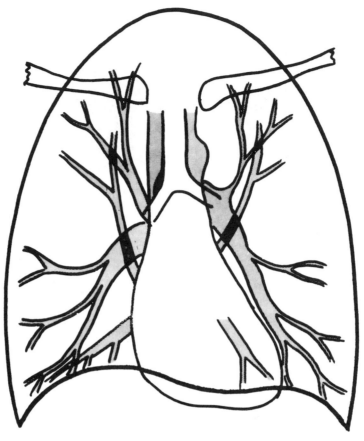

FIG. 3.27

Radiographic Feature	Observation
(1) PBF distribution	Normal
(2) PBV	Normal
(3) VPW	Normal
(4) AW	Normal
(5) Br. Cuffing	Absent
(6) Distribution of Oedema	None Present
(7) Artery/Vein Ratio	Normal
(8) Lung Volume	Normal

Analysis. The normal blood flow distribution tells us that there is no elevation of left heart pressure, and the normal PBV, that there is no increase in right heart output. The normal VPW indicates that the circulating blood volume is within normal limits, which confirms our analysis that there is no abnormality of left or right cardiac output. The normal azygos width indicates there is no elevation of right atrial pressure. The absence of any signs of oedema, plus the normal lung volume further reinforce our conclusion that there is no left heart dysfunction.

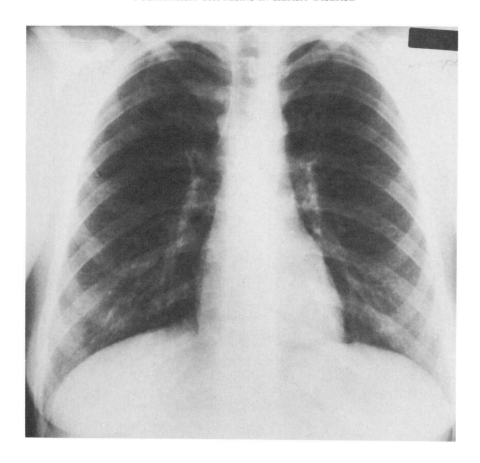

Accompanying radiograph. The findings on the chest film are essentially the same as those on the diagram. The pulmonary veins are somewhat difficult to see in this case but the left lower lobe veins can be seen faintly through the heart and are quite normal.

Conclusion. Normal cardiopulmonary status.

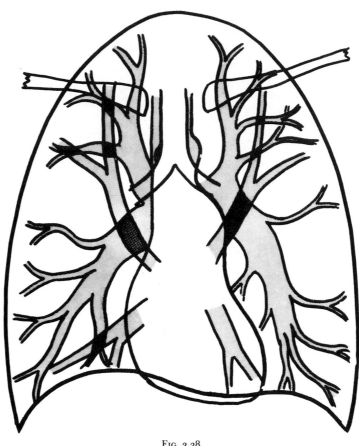

FIG. 3.28

Radiographic Feature	*Observation*
(1) PBF distribution	'Balanced' (homogeneous) flow
(2) PBV	Markedly increased
(3) VPW	Normal to slightly narrowed
(4) AW	Normal
(5) Br. Cuffing	Absent
(6) Distribution of Oedema	No oedema seen
(7) Artery/Vein Ratio	Both arteries and veins are markedly enlarged in the bases and apices but retain a 1/1 ratio.
(8) Lung Volume	Slightly increased

Analysis. The balanced flow, increased PBV and simultaneous increase in size of the arteries and the veins all indicate a high flow state (a large right ventricular output); however the small vascular pedicle indicates a small circulating blood volume commensurate with a small left heart output. Clearly the only circumstance in which the left heart output can be smaller than the right is if a left-to-right shunt is present. The absence of oedema indicates that the heart is not decompensating despite the large output. The enlarged lung volume is common in large left-to-right shunts and appears to be due to 'erection' of the lung by the very large pulmonary blood volume.

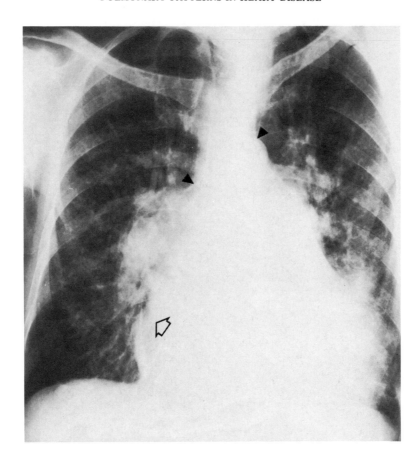

Accompanying radiograph. The accompanying radiograph shows a large ASD, demonstrating all of the features illustrated on the diagram. The contrast between the narrow vascular pedicle and the large heart is striking; its resemblance to a large piece of fruit hanging from a stem has caused this to be called the 'picciolo' (stalk) syndrome.

Conclusion. Left-to-right shunt (not decompensated).

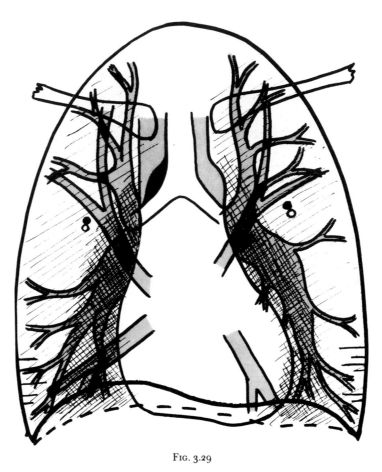

FIG. 3.29

Radiographic Feature	Observation
(1) PBF Distribution	'Balanced' (homogeneous)
(2) PBV	Markedly Increased
(3) VPW	Considerably Widened
(4) AW	Markedly Enlarged
(5) Br. Cuffing	Present
(6) Distribution of Oedema	Principally Central
(7) Artery/Vein Ratio	Costophrenic Angles Spared
(8) Lung Volume	Slightly Increased

Analysis. The blood flow distribution and PBV are identical with the previous case, and the arteries and veins are both enlarged indicating again that there is a large right ventricular output, however in this case the VPW is large indicating that the patient has a large circulating blood volume. The azygos is increased in size indicating some elevation of mean right atrial pressure. The large CBV fits with a large left heart output and there is therefore no evidence here to suggest that there is any intrathoracic shunt. Now it is necessary to consider what kind of mechanism would cause a marked increase in output from both ventricles plus an increased circulating blood volume and pulmonary blood volume. The possibilities are in fact few but certainly include at the top of the list renal failure (with retention of salt and water) or overhydration. Thyro-toxicosis would cause the increased output but not the increased CBV, whereas polycythaemia can give the increased CBV and increased cardiac output; however, there is also oedema present which accords much better with renal failure or overhydration than with polycythaemia. The central distribution of the oedema is highly characteristic for fluid overload due either to renal failure or overhydration. There are no radiological characteristics which would allow us to decide from the film which of the two aetiologies is present (other than the fact that patients with renal oedema are very frequently ambulatory and have their films taken in the upright postero-anterior position, whereas patients who have been overhydrated tend to be in bed in a critical care unit!).

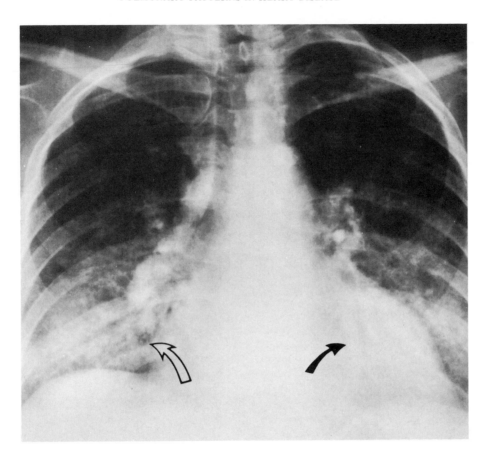

Accompanying radiograph. The accompanying radiograph is, in fact, a PA erect film and belongs to a patient with severe renal failure. Note the large basal vessels (black arrow) which would be *very* uncharacteristic for cardiac failure and the peribronchial cuffing (open arrow).

Conclusion. Renal failure. (It is instructive to compare both the similarities and differences between diagrams 3.29 and 3.28.)

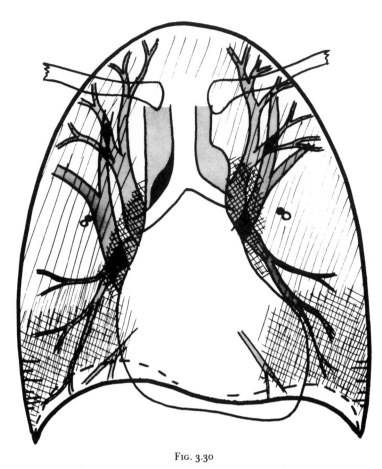

FIG. 3.30

Radiographic Feature	Observation
(1) PBF Distribution	Inverted (base-to-apex redistribution)
(2) PBV	Increased in the upper lungs and decreased in the lower lungs.
(3) VPW	Increased
(4) AW	Increased
(5) Br. Cuffing	Present
(6) Distribution of Oedema	Peribronchial cuffs and basal oedema, homogeneous from the costophrenic angles to the heart (septal lines present).
(7) Artery/Vein Ratio	Normal
(8) Lung Volume	Reduced

Analysis. The inverted flow is strong evidence that there is elevation of left heart pressure (which can be due either to left heart decompensation or to obstruction at the mitral valve level). A consideration of the cardiac configuration would obviously help to decide if mitral valve disease were present; however, the presence of a wide vascular pedicle indicating an increased CBV is not characteristic of uncomplicated mitral valve disease (where the vascular pedicle in fact tends to be narrower than usual (Fig. 3.24)). The presence of the increased CBV and evidence of elevated left heart pressure is strongly suggestive of either chronic left heart failure (with diminished renal perfusion, aldosterone production and an increased CBV) or with biventricular decompensation. (In many cases of *acute* left heart failure the vascular pedicle is normal, correctly reflecting that there is no increase in CBV.) The distribution of the oedema, homogeneously from the costophrenic angles to the heart, is also characteristic of left heart failure. There is often a reduction of lung volume in left heart failure due to the diminished compliance of a wet lung.

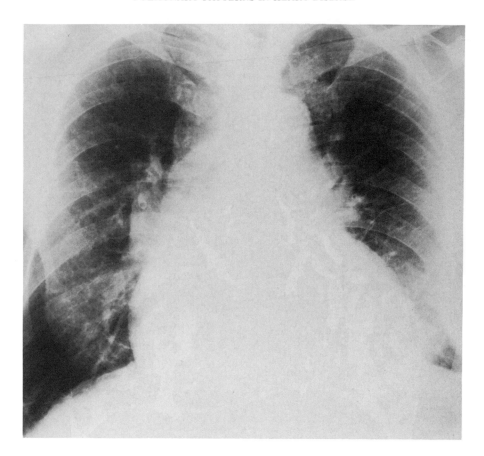

Accompanying radiograph. The accompanying radiograph manifests all of the changes shown in the diagram apart from loss of lung volume. The very large azygos strongly suggests that the mean right atrial pressure is elevated. This patient did indeed have biventricular failure but suffered from mild chronic obstructive pulmonary disease which trapped air and prevented the lung from becoming smaller.

Conclusion. Biventricular cardiac failure.

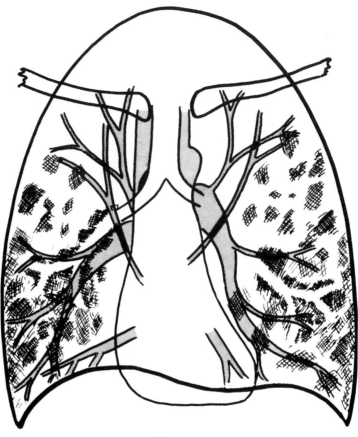

FIG. 3.31

Radiographic Feature	*Observation*
(1) PBF Distribution	Normal
(2) PBV	Normal
(3) VPW	Normal
(4) AW	Normal
(5) Br. Cuffing	Absent
(6) Distribution of Oedema	Patchy, predominantly peripheral—air bronchograms present—no septal lines.
(7) Artery/Vein Ratio	Normal
(8) Lung Volume	Normal

Analysis. The normal blood flow distribution indicates that there is no elevation of left heart pressure and no increase in cardiac output, and the normal VPW indicates that the circulating blood volume is not increased, i.e. there is no evidence of overhydration or renal failure and yet there is oedema present. Since we have already excluded cardiac or renal causes we are left with capillary permeability as a cause (although there are one or two other types of oedema which would have to be considered, for example neurogenic pulmonary oedema and oedema secondary to hypoxaemia, e.g. high altitude and sleep apnoea). In the diagram shown the distribution of oedema is very characteristic for capillary permeability, the presence of air bronchograms and the *absence* of peribronchial cuffing and septal lines all add to the certainty of the diagnosis.

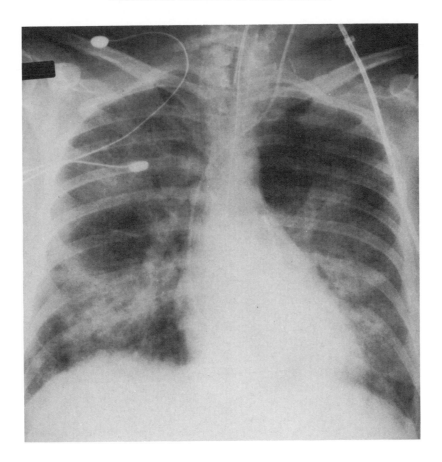

Accompanying radiograph. The accompanying radiograph is of a young Mexican male who inhaled toxic fumes during a fire in his home and developed capillary permeability oedema.

Conclusion. Capillary permeability oedema. (A similar patchy distribution of oedema is seen in Fig. 3.22 where the capillary permeability was caused by fat embolism from trauma to the legs and pelvis. In this case the VPW was increased because the patient was nursed in a supine position because of his injuries.)

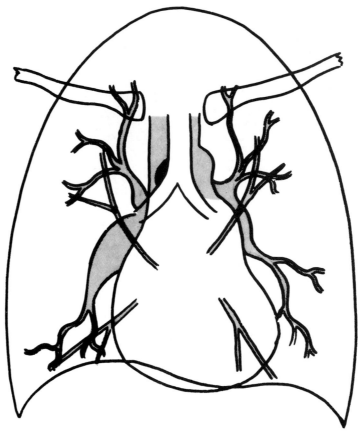

Fig. 3.32

Radiographic Feature	Observation
(1) PBF Distribution	Balanced (homogeneous)
(2) PBV	Increased (centrally only)
(3) VPW	Normal
(4) AW	Normal
(5) Br. Cuffing	Absent
(6) Distribution of Oedema	None present
(7) Artery/Vein Ratio	Markedly Abnormal—arteries large in proportion to veins.
(8) Lung Volume	Normal

Analysis. A balanced distribution of flow would indicate an increased right ventricular output if the arteries and veins were both increased in size, but in this case the veins are *small* indicating that the homogeneous distribution of flow is *not* caused by increased flow but must be due to a loss of vascular bed (PVBC). The reduced vascular bed is completely filled by the normal cardiac output, abolishing the normal gravitational gradient. The PBV at first glance appears to be increased but it is only large on the arterial side; the veins are very small. This sequestration of the PBV on the arterial side can only occur if there is some obstruction proximal to the veins but distal to the arteries, i.e. precapillary pulmonary arterial hypertension. The absence of oedema indicates that there is no left heart decompensation and the normal azygos indicates no elevation of RAP, i.e. no right heart decompensation.

length, placed on the precordium, the whole of the heart. Such phased array machines are more complicated electronically than the mechanical sector scanners and tend therefore to be more expensive. Both types of machine are now produced as reliable tools with good resolution.

All cross-sectional echo beams tend to diverge so that reflections do not necessarily come exactly from in front of the heart but may come from part of the divergent ray. However, the position of the reflection as recorded on the oscilloscope is as if it was coming entirely from a point immediately in front of the transducer. This beam spread thus produces distortion of the image making it appear wider than it is. Only the leading edge of an echo actually denotes the position of the reflected surface and if there is a highly reflected surface the echo may have considerable length on the oscilloscope and the distant end of the echo have no real relationship to the position of the reflecting surface. This becomes important when looking at things like mitral valve orifices on the cross-sectional echo.

Measurements from the single transducer tend to be more reliable than measurements taken from areas on the cross sectional echo machine. Many modern echo machines have a facility which enables an M-mode echo to be recorded through a line which is determined from the cross sectional echo. This overcomes the problem of the unassociated M-mode trace of not knowing exactly at what level and in which direction the echogram has been recorded.

MITRAL VALVE

The mitral valve was the first structure to be studied echocardiographically by Edler. He showed that the normal mitral valve has two opening movements in each cardiac cycle; one at the beginning of diastole and the other after atrial contractions. Between the two, the valve adopts a semi-closed position (Fig. 4.01).

The normal anterior mitral cusp moves forward on opening and the posterior cusp backwards. In health, ventricular filling is completed in the first few milliseconds of diastole. The blood flow produces a Venturi effect which tends to bring the cusps into apposition. Blood entering the ventricle is directed round the walls onto the back surfaces of the cusps and this too tends to close the valve in early diastole. Elongation of the ventricle as it fills tenses the mitral cusps, chordae tendinae and papillary muscles. This pulls them towards a straight line position, away from the ventricular walls and towards the closed position of the valve (Fig. 4.02).

These three mechanisms, all dependent on the left ventricular filling rate, tend to produce a closure rate of the mitral valve which increases and decreases with the ventricular filling rate. Hence in mitral stenosis the

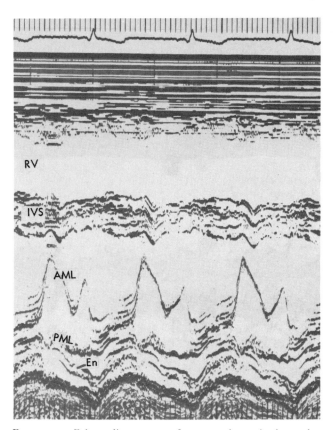

FIG. 4.01. Echocardiograms of normal mitral valve. AML PML = anterior and posterior mitral leaflets. RV = right ventricle. En = endocardium.

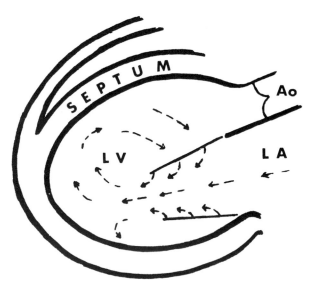

FIG. 4.02. Diagram to show how blood entering the left ventricle tends to close the mitral valve.

diastolic closure rate (DCR) is always reduced (Fig. 4.03). In rheumatic mitral stenosis the anterior and posterior cusps both move forward in diastole, presumably because of the tethering of the cusps at the annular margins (Fig. 4.04).

Because left ventricular filling is dependent on left atrial pressure, the end diastolic pressure of the ventricle and 'compliance' of the muscle as well as valve orifice

size the relationship between DCR and degree of stenosis is not linear, as was considered by early workers. The DCR does, however, give confirmation of mitral stenosis.

The M-mode echocardiogram allows the mobility of the valve and the amount of calcification to be assessed. When subvalvar apparatus is thickened and shortened as in advanced rheumatic disease, the cusps are unable to move more than a few millimetres. The normal amplitude of movement is at least 2·5 cm. When estimating the amplitude of movement, it is essential to position the transducer on the praecordium so that the maximum excursion is achieved. This will only occur when the ultrasound beam is perpendicular to free margin of the mitral cusp. When the correct angulation has been achieved the opening movement of the valve at the beginning of diastole and the closure at the onset of systole will be at least 300 mm/sec (Fig. 4.01).

In the two-dimensional echo all these features are visible with the transducer in the longitudinal plane. The absence of the double opening movement is very obvious and with the transducer rotated to 90° to give the short axis view the failure of the cusps to separate in diastole becomes obvious, producing a fish-mouth type of appearance (Fig. 4.05).

Some workers have tried to correlate the mitral valve orifice by measuring the distance between the anterior and posterior cusp echoes. This is not justified because only the leading edge of each echo actually indicates the

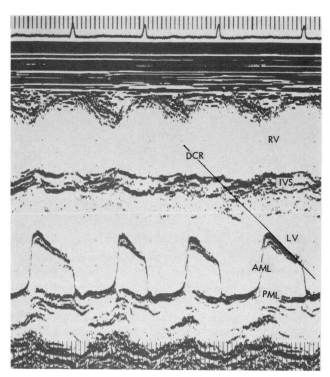

FIG. 4.03. The maximum rate of mitral valve closure (DCR) is reduced in mitral stenosis. The amplitude of movement is normal in this case measuring over 2 cm. RV—Right ventricle; IVS—interventricular septum; AML—anterior mitral leaflet; PML—posterior mitral leaflet.

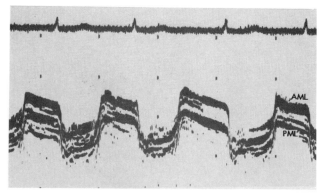

FIG. 4.04. Reduced mitral DCR in mitral stenosis. Anterior and posterior cusps both move forward in diastole and additional echoes indicate calcification.

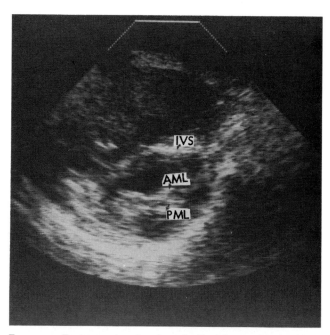

FIG. 4.05. 2D short axis echo through the left ventricle in mitral stenosis showing that the anterior mitral leaflet (AML) and posterior mitral leaflet (PML) do not separate normally in diastole.

reflecting surface so that cusp thickening will produce a spuriously reduced orifice. In addition, beam spread artifactually widens the apparent diameter of any structure lying in the plane of the transducer.

Gibson has shown that a reliable estimate of the rate of left ventricular filling can be obtained from echoes of the left ventricular walls (Fig. 4.20). Normally the rate of separation of echoes from the left side of the interventricular septum and the free wall of the left ventricle will exceed 10 mm/sec. In mitral stenosis of critical severity the rate will usually be well below this level. Occasionally we have discovered patients with tight mitral stenosis with a higher rate of left ventricular diameter increase. These have been in patients with mobile cusps. A possible explanation of this apparent anomaly might be that the whole mitral valve balloons into the ventricle in early diastole so occupying space within the chamber even though the blood is still on the atrial side of the mitral valve (Fig. 4.06). Aortic regurgitation will increase the LV filling rate and make this measurement unreliable for the diagnosis of mitral stenosis.

Calcification is indicated by multiple echoes seen in both diastole and systole (Fig. 4.04). Care must be taken to ensure that the echo intensity is the minimum which will allow a complete recording of the valve throughout the cardiac cycle. If the ultrasound intensity is increased beyond this, multiple echoes can be produced even in the absence of calcification.

The importance of echocardiography in mitral stenosis is not so much in making the diagnosis, although it

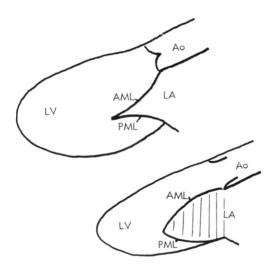

FIG. 4.06. Diagram to show possible explanation of why some patients with pure mitral stenosis appear to fill the left ventricle (LV) more rapidly than expected. The shaded area in the lower diagram in early diastole is blood within the left LV but still contained within the anterior and posterior mitral leaflets (AML and PML) on the left atrial (LA) side of the valve.

can sometimes be useful in differentiation the Austin Flint murmur of aortic regurgitation from a mid-diastolic murmur due to coincidental mitral stenosis and in silent mitral stenosis. The principle value is to enable the clinician to assess the patient's suitability for operation by either an open valvotomy, closed valvotomy or valve replacement.

The size of the left atrium is also important in evaluating a patient with mitral valve disease. The left atrium lies behind the aorta and its width should not exceed that of the aortic diameter in the normal subject (Fig. 4.07).

MITRAL REGURGITATION

In mitral regurgitation unassociated with mitral stenosis the diastolic closure rate of the mitral valve, seen on the M-mode echo, tends to be increased.

In calcific mitral stenosis, however, there will frequently be coincident mitral regurgitation without any increase in the DCR. The left atrium is always increased in size in the presence of significant mitral regurgitation.

Mitral regurgitation associated with mitral valve prolapse can be diagnosed with confidence when separation of the anterior and posterior cusps occurs in systole and when the cusps come together both at the beginning and at the end of diastole. Prolapse may occur at the end of systole alone (Fig. 4.08) or throughout the whole of systole (Fig. 4.09). If the echogram does not show the cusp re-apposing at the end of systole it is impossible to be certain that this is a true prolapse. It may be that during the movement which occurs during the cardiac cycle the reflecting point of the echoes has moved from the free margin of the cusp to a position nearer the mitral ring, where the anterior and posterior cusps are never in apposition. It is often necessary to move the transducer position on the precordium and the angulation small amounts before a definite diagnosis of cusp prolapse can be made. In most patients, where cusp prolapse can be demonstrated, it is also possible to obtain an echo from the adjacent part of the valve where there is no prolapse. This is because usually only a small segment of the valve cusp balloons. Prolapse of the whole of the mitral valve would result in torrential regurgitation. Care should be taken not to over-diagnose this condition. Two-dimensional echoes in mitral valve prolapse are more certainly diagnostic when viewed dynamically. The amplitude of movement of the anterior cusp is increased in anterior cusp prolapse.

In mixed mitral stenosis and regurgitation with a mobile valve which is not unduly thickened there will be a biphasic movement of the anterior mitral cusp. The rate of increase in left ventricle is unhelpful in assessing mixed mitral valve disease. The high left atrial pressure resulting from the regurgitation will tend to

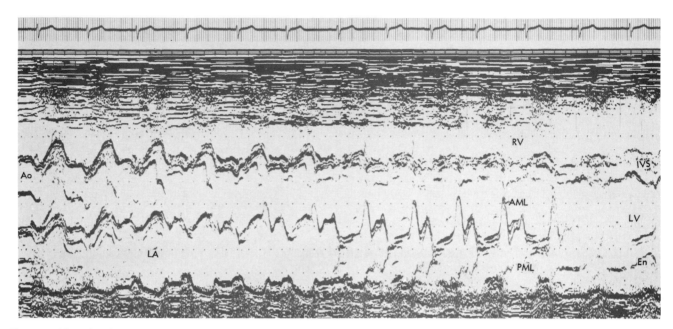

Fig. 4.07. M-mode echo sweep from aorta (Ao) towards the left ventricular apex (LV). The left atrium (LA) lies behind the aorta which is continuous anteriorly with the interventricular septum (IVS) and posteriorly with the anterior mitral leaflet (AML) whose diastolic closure rate appears to be slower at the aortic junction than at the mid LV. Note the DCR of the AML appears to increase as the sweep goes from aorta to apex. PML—posterior mitral leaflet; RV—right ventricle.

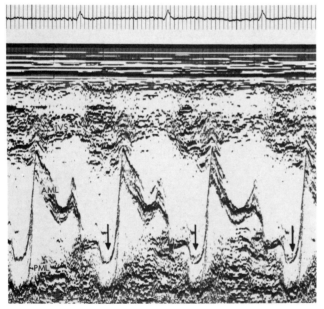

Fig. 4.08. M-mode echocardiogram of the mitral valve with late systolic prolapse (arrows) and separation of the anterior and posterior cusps.

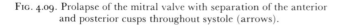

Fig. 4.09. Prolapse of the mitral valve with separation of the anterior and posterior cusps throughout systole (arrows).

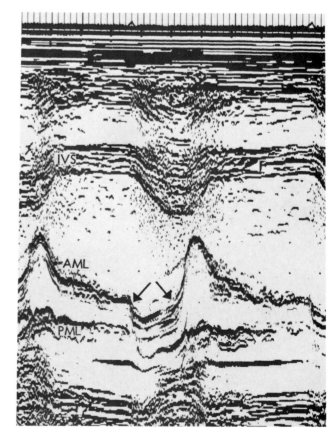

increase the rate of ventricular filling whilst the obstruction at the valve will counteract this. There is no way of assessing where the balance lies.

AORTIC VALVE DISEASE

Chronic aortic regurgitation produces fluttering of the anterior mitral cusp. This rapid oscillation is frequently associated with an Austin Flint murmur. The putative mechanism is that blood regurgitating from the aorta passes anterior to the anterior mitral leaflet and at the same time, blood passes normally from the left atrium to the left ventricle behind the anterior mitral leaflet (Fig. 4.10). These two streams moving on either side of the anterior mitral cusp, which is a thin membrane, set up vibrations which can be seen on the M-mode echo and produce a mid-diastolic murmur (Fig. 4.11). The turbulence thus caused can sometimes produce oscillation of the posterior mitral cusp and vibration of the left side of the septum. The amount of oscillation is not proportional to the extent of the regurgitation, sometimes being seen in trivial regurgitation and absent when the incompetence is severe. Fluttering of the mitral valve will not normally be seen with coincidental mitral stenosis. Occasionally a reduced DCR and mitral fluttering occur together. Fluttering of the mitral valve in aortic regurgitation is often easier to recognise on the M-mode echo than on the two-dimensional echogram.

Aortic regurgitation of acute onset can result in premature closure of the mitral valve. When the aortic reflux is severe and the left ventricle a normal size, the diastolic ventricular pressure will equilibrate with the aortic pressure. As a result, the late diastolic pressure in the ventricle will be greater than the atrial pressure with a consequent closing of the mitral valve. Severe premature closure of the mitral valve is an indication for early surgery (Fig. 4.12).

If acute aortic regurgitation continues the ventricle will dilate so that it can accommodate the refluxed blood without increasing the diastolic pressure above a trial level. Enlargement of the left ventricle will also occur when aortic regurgitation is of chronic onset. Acute regurgitation is seen most often in patients with bacterial endocarditis who suddenly perforate a valve cusp, or in association with an acute dissection of the aorta.

The premature closure of the mitral valve in acute aortic regurgitation occurs before the P wave of the ECG and must be distinguished from closure between the P wave and the QRS which may occur in patients with incipient heart failure of any aetiology and is most often seen when there is a long P-R interval.

AORTIC STENOSIS

The normal aortic valve has a box-shaped configuration on the M-mode echogram (Fig. 4.13).

Echoing the aortic valve in aortic regurgitation is of less value than in aortic stenosis where thickening of the cusps may be seen as well as thickening of the aortic

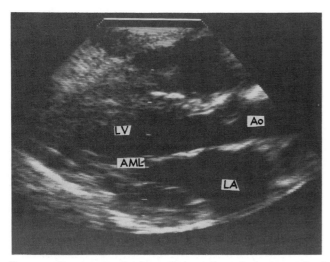

Fig. 4.10. Cross-sectional echocardiogram through the long axis of the heart.

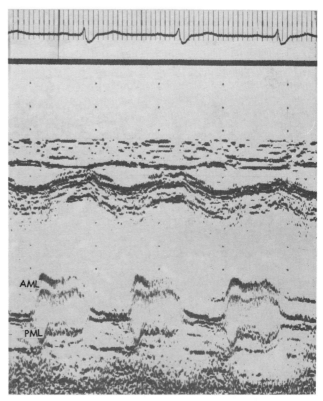

Fig. 4.11. Fluttering of the anterior (AML) and posterior leaflets (PML) of the mitral valve in aortic regurgitation.

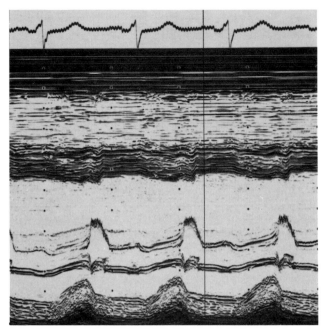

FIG. 4.12. The mitral valve closes before the P wave of the ECG in acute aortic regurgitation. Note also the mitral flutter. Courtesy Dr J. B. Partridge.

roots (Fig. 4.14). Frequently the numerous echoes from the calcium on the aortic wall makes it difficult to actually see cusp movement. In congenital aortic stenosis, doming of the aortic cusps may be appreciated on a long axis two-dimensional echogram (Fig. 4.15). Failure of the aortic valve to open satisfactorily is not often possible to demonstrate on an M-mode echo but can sometimes be seen on the cross-sectional echo although this is difficult to demonstrate except with the moving images. Failure of the aortic cusp to remain fully open throughout systole does not necessarily mean the presence of aortic stenosis but can be seen in any low output state such as severe mitral stenosis (Fig. 4.16).

BACTERIAL ENDOCARDITIS

In addition to producing acute regurgitation, bacterial endocarditis on the aortic valve can lead to the development of vegetations. On the M-mode echo these may be seen as slightly wavy lines that look like extreme thickening of the cusps but moving with the cusps in systole and diastole (Fig. 4.17). The configuration of the valve is usually quite different from that of aortic calcification. When the vegetations grow on an already calcified valve they may be difficult to spot. Cross-sectional echocardiography will often show the thick-

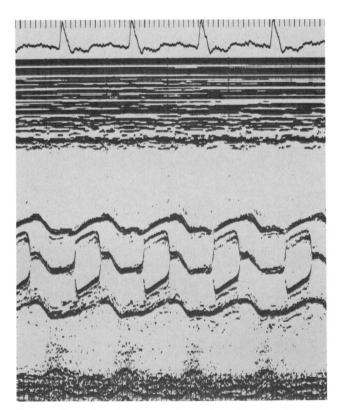

FIG. 4.13. Normal aortic echogram showing box-shaped configuration of the aortic cusps.

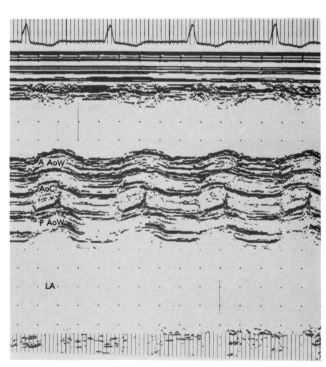

FIG. 4.14. M-mode echogram of the aortic root in calcific aortic stenosis, showing multiple echoes of the aortic walls anteriorly (AAoW) and posteriorly (PAoW) but not quite obscuring the echoes from the aortic cusps, which do not separate more than 1 cm. The left atrium (LA) is also enlarged from mitral valve lesion.

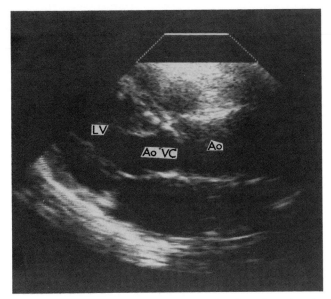

Fig. 4.15. Long axis cross sectional view of a domed aortic valve (AoVC).

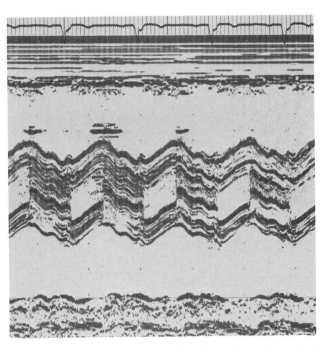

Fig. 4.17. Echocardiogram of the aortic valve and root in a patient with bacterial endocarditis vegetations.

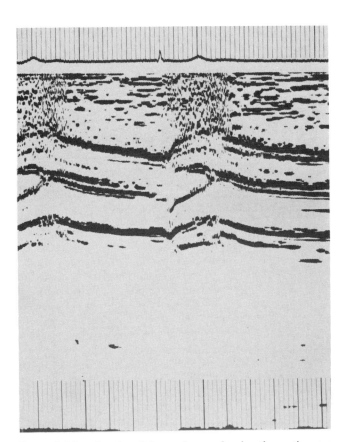

Fig. 4.16. M-mode echo of the aortic root showing the aortic cusps coming together before the end of systole instead of remaining apart. The left atrium below the aorta is enlarged. Both are due to severe mitral stenosis.

ened echoes attached to the aortic cusp and moving with the blood flow; it is necessary to see the picture in its dynamic form in order to make the diagnosis. Stills from the cross-sectional echo merely look like aortic thickening.

The appearances of a flail aortic cusp can look somewhat like a regurgitation on an M-mode echogram (Fig. 4.18) but should be differentiable on the moving cross-sectional echo.

LEFT VENTRICULAR FUNCTION

When an M-mode ultrasonic beam traverses the left ventricle across its lesser diameter, echoes both from the septum and the free wall of the ventricle will be received simultaneously, provided the rays are approximately vertical to the walls (Fig. 4.19). The septum will show as two well defined lines reflected from the endocardium on its right and left sides. Continuous echoes will be received from the endocardial surface of the free left ventricular wall and from its epicardial surface. These appear also as clearly defined lines. If a sweep is made from the aortic root to the apex of the heart the diameter of the ventricle will be found to be maximal just below the mitral valve apparatus and then diminish to a minimum at the apex in the normal subject. It is customary to make left ventricular dimension measurements just below the mitral valve where the diameter is maximal. In the normal the septal and

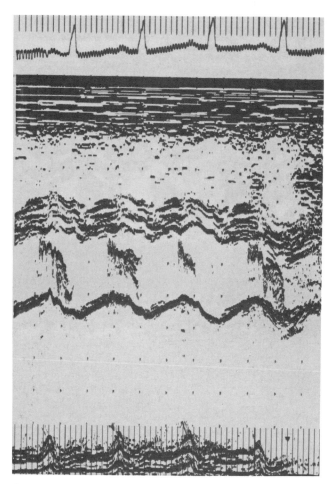

FIG. 4.18. M-mode echogram from a patient with a flail aortic cusp.

free walls of the left ventricle approach each other from the onset of systole with the septum moving backwards immediately after the R wave of the electrocardiogram and the free wall of the ventricle forward. The muscle thickness of the ventricle can be measured from the distance between the endocardial and the epicardial echoes and the distance between the echoes from the right and left side of the septum. Variations in the ventricular size can be followed by serial echoes but because of the difficulty of getting exactly the same obliquity across the ventricle, the same heart rate and output even if the transducer spot is marked on the chest wall, a difference of less than 0·8 cm cannot be considered to be significant. Because the forward movement of the posterior LV wall is not necessarily synchronous with the backward movement of the septum measuring the change in LV diameter can be valuable. For this a digitising instrument is required which, when the pointer or cursor is run along the left side of the septum will enter the co-ordinates of the individual points into a computer.

The co-ordinates of the endocardium of the LV posterior wall are similarly entered and the computer prints out a continuous plot of the left ventricular diameter by subtracting the valve of the Y co-ordinates for each value of X. If suitably programmed, the computer will also calculate the rate of change of diameter (Fig. 4.20).

In patients with mitral stenosis the rate of increase in diameter in early diastole is usually decreased below the normal value of 10 min/sec². Aortic regurgitation will increase the early diastolic filling of the LV so that when AR coexists with mitral stenosis the measurement is of no value.

In patients with right ventricular volume overload (e.g. atrial septal defect) the septum moves paradoxically, that is to say in systole the septum moves anteriorly. The free wall of the left ventricle has to move rather more anteriorly to compensate for this. A similar paradoxical septal movement occurs after most cardiac operations (Fig. 4.21). Dilated ventricles with normal cardiac output will tend to have only a small excursion of movement both of the septum and the free LV wall. Patients with regurgitant valves, either aortic or mitral, will tend to have a large difference between the end systolic and end diastolic diameters and frequently a large absolute measurement to the left ventricular diameter.

A number of workers have shown that there is a correlation between the stroke volume and the difference between the cube of the left ventricular diameters at end diastole and end systole. The relationships hold good only for normally shaped ventricles and the shape of ventricles is difficult to determine accurately by M-mode echocardiography. It is probably better to refer only to the diameters which can be measured rather than calling the difference between the cubes of the EDV and ESV over the cube of the EDV–ejection fraction.

In the presence of coronary artery disease, particularly of the anterior descending artery hypo-function of the septal muscle is likely to occur. This may produce a relatively immobile septum and frequently a compensatory hyperactive free left ventricular wall. Care must be taken not to assume that all immobile septa are due to ischaemia because the ventricle, in addition to contracting down with each beat, also rotates about both the horizontal and the vertical axis and sometimes these movements combine to give an impression of septal immobility which is not genuine. If the left ventricle can be echoed from the adjacent intercostal space and the same appearance of an immobile septum is obtained it is likely that this is due to an organic abnormality.

Localised hypokinesia is more easily and accurately assessed on a two-dimensional echogram where the dynamic movement can be visualised directly. The

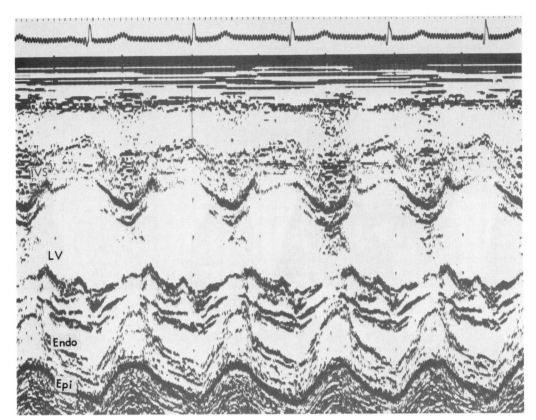

FIG. 4.19. M-mode scan showing the intraventricular septum and the posterior ventricular wall. The endocardium (Endo) and the epicardium (Epi) are visible as a continuous line as well as the left side of the intraventricular septum (IVS).

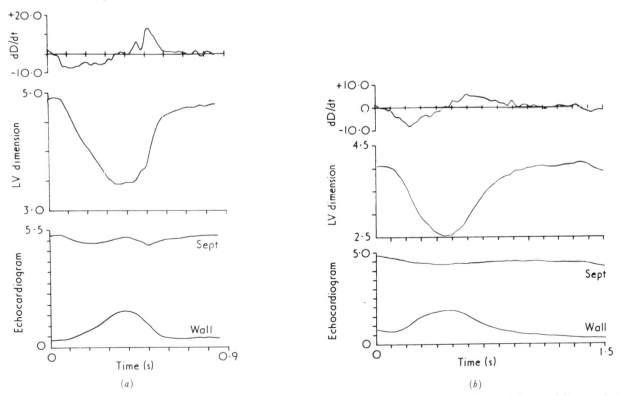

FIG. 4.20. Digitised record of (from below upwards) left ventricular borders, left ventricular diameter and rate of change of diameter in (a) a normal subject and (b) a patient with mitral stenosis.

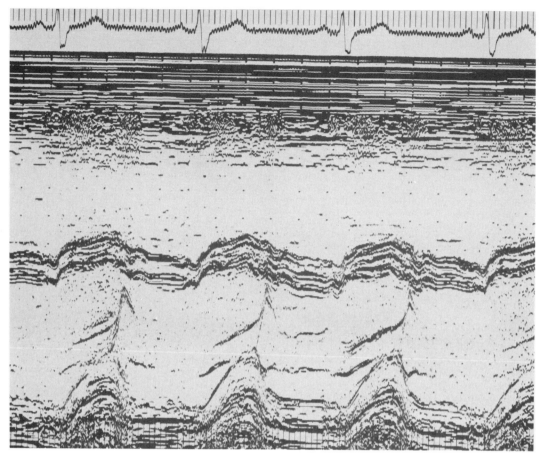

FIG. 4.21. Paradoxical septal motion in a patient with right ventricular volume overload (ASD). The septum (IVS) moves anteriorly in systole.

problem of two-dimensional echoes is the difficulty in measuring the diameters from the screen. The static frames from the oscilloscope tend to look much less satisfactory than the moving image and there is also distortion which occurs because of beam spread and other factors.

Disco-ordinate contraction can be assessed from the M-mode echogram by measuring the time interval between the minimum dimension of the ventricle and the point of opening of the mitral valve. These should coincide. If there is an interval after the left ventricular has started to increase before mitral valve opening occurs it can be concluded that when the part of the ventricle which is being echoed is expanding some other part must be contracting so keeping ventricular pressure above that of the LA. Such inco-ordinate contraction can be visualised on a cross sectional echogram and occurs after cardiac infarction.

CARDIOMYOPATHY

Cardiomyopathies appear in two forms (a) Hyper-

trophic (b) Dilated. The aetiology of heart muscle disease cannot usually be determined by echocardiography. In idiopathic dilated cardiomyopathy it cannot be distinguished from a dilated poorly contracting heart due to generalised myocardial ischaemia. Generalised hypertrophy of the ventricle will be similar whether it be idiopathic or secondary to a known cause such as hypertension.

Despite a recent international committee on nomenclature, to confine the term cardiomyopathy to heart muscle diseases of unknown origin would require a renaming of the condition when and/or if the aeteology of the muscle abnormality is discovered. Two major forms of cardiomyopathy can be recognised echocardiographically, the hypertrophic and the dilated. Both can be either localised or generalised.

Hypertrophic Cardiomyopathy

This was first described in its obstructive form with the clinical presentation of ventricular outflow tract obstruction. The M-mode echocardiogram can be diagnostic. The left ventricle is thickened usually at the septum and frequently at the posterior wall as well. Henry has suggested that the diagnosis can be made whenever the septal thickness/free LV wall thickness exceeds 1·3:1. Such a reversed ratio can be obtained in patients with a horizontal heart so that the echo beam traverses the septum obliquely and the free left ventricular wall perpendicularly (Fig. 4.22). If in doubt, the validity of the ratio can be checked on the two-dimensional echo (Fig. 4.23). Unless the septal thickness measures at least 1·5 cm and/or the free left ventricular wall thickness is at least 2 cm in diastole a diagnosis of hypertrophic cardiomyopathy on this ground alone is probably not justified.

The mitral valve may have an anterior movement of the anterior cusp in systole (Fig. 4.24). The anterior and posterior cusps then separate and this is associated with mitral regurgitation. The probable explanation of the separation of the mitral cusps in systole is that contraction of the papillary muscle occurs normally but shortening of the ventricle does not occur—hence the

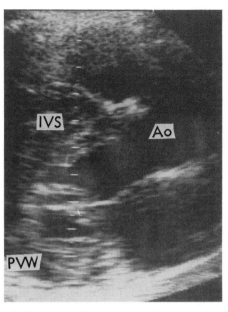

FIG. 4.23. 2 D Echogram of the intraventricular septum (IVS) and posterior ventricular wall (PVW) in hypertrophic cardiomyopathy measuring 2·7 and 1·7 cm in diameter respectively.

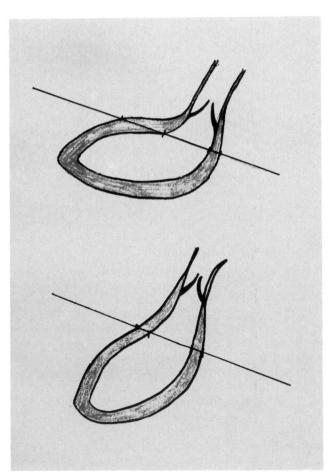

FIG. 4.22. Diagram to explain how an echo beam traversing a horizontal heart can make the septal left ventricular posterior wall thickness ratios appear greater than they are.

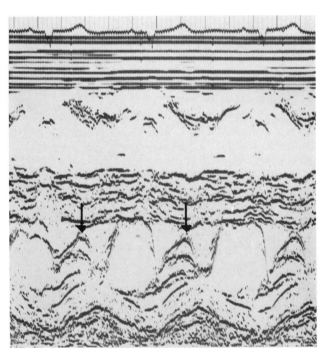

FIG. 4.24. M-mode echogram of mitral valve in a patient with hypertrophic cardiomyopathy showing anterior movement of the anterior mitral cusp (AMC) in systole (arrows). The intraventricular septum (IVS) is thickened and the DCR reduced.

anterior cusp is pulled away from the posterior cusp allowing ventricular blood to regurgitate into the atrium. Wigle suggests that the movement is part of the venturi effect produced by the thick septum bulging towards the posterior cusp so converting the outflow tract of the left ventricle into a tube. However, systolic anterior movement of the mitral cusp is not infrequently seen when there is generalised hypertrophy of the ventricle and no bulging of the septum. Other workers deny that the forward movement frequently seen is due to the anterior cusp claiming it to be part of a hypertrophied papillary muscle.

The rapid diastolic backward movement of the anterior cusp at the beginning of diastole is frequently greatly delayed. Sometimes when the heart rate is rapid the next systole supervenes before rapid diastolic closure can occur. In these patients the administration of beta adenergic blockers will allow a late diastolic closure of the mitral valve and this is associated with an increase in the rapid filling rate of the apex cardiogram and a reduction in the amount of angina. The aortic valve may sometimes show a closing movement in mid systole; this occurs only in patients with the obstructive form of the disease. A second opening movement occurs before final diastolic closure and this is synchronous with the ventricular relaxation and is accompanied by a reduction of the outflow tract obstruction (Fig. 4.25).

A number of cases have been described in which an echogram and clinical and haematological findings indistinguishable from hypertrophic cardiomyopathy have been seen to develop in patients following aortic valve surgery. Echocardiographic changes identical to hypertrophic cardiomyopathy are also seen occasionally in athletes who exhibit no clinical abnormalities but frequently have ECG abnormalities. It would seem reasonable to conjecture that hypertrophic cardiomyopathy is an abnormal response to a number of different stimuli. There is a whole spectrum of changes varying from mere ventricular wall thickening without other haemodynamic effect to full blown picture of the outflow tract obstruction with SAM a slow mitral DCR and aortic systolic closure. Two-dimensional echocardiography, in addition to showing generalised thickening of the muscles will show localised increase in the muscle mass if present and is the most certain way of establishing the diagnosis of hypertrophic cardiomyopathy.

Dilated Cardiomyopathy

Previously these were known as congestive cardiomyopathies, presumably because when first recognised they tended to be in congestive cardiac failure. To the echocardiographer and frequently also the radiologist, the only feature is a dilated left ventricle. The septal thickness and the free left wall thickness is not increased and may be reduced. The amount of movement with

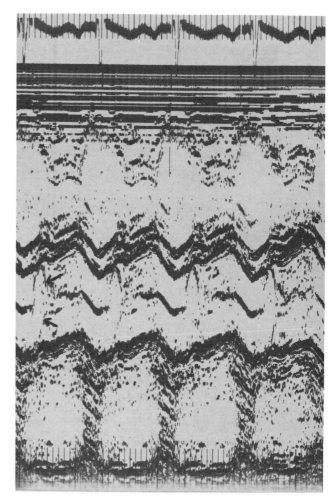

FIG. 4.25. Echogram of the aortic valve in hypertrophic cardiomyopathy showing closure in mid systole (→).

systole and diastole is small. Echocardiographically there is no difference between a dilated cardiomyopathy of unknown cause, a generalised ischaemic cardiomyopathy or a rheumatic cardiomyopathy (Fig. 4.26). If an ischaemic cardiomyopathy is not generalised then the movement of the affected segment will be less than the unaffected segment, which may have a compensatory increase. An M-mode scan can be deceptive in diagnosing localised infarction because movement of the heart within the chest can produce an apparent diminution of septal movement. Cross-sectional echocardiography is much more reliable. There will frequently be mitral regurgitation with enlargement of the left atrium. Localised malcontraction of the left ventricle will frequently produce a delay in mitral valve opening after the left ventricular diameter has started to increase with diastole (Fig. 4.27).

valve replacement, sampling in the same site – when forward flow is clear and undisturbed with no systolic backward flow. The vertical 'blips' reflect the valve sounds.

It can be seen how flow across a valve compliments the image of that valve in giving a much more accurate evaluation.

REFERENCES

Henry, W. L., Clark, C. E. & Epstein, S. (1973) Asymmetrical septal hypertrophy echocardiographic identification of the pathognomic anatomical abnormality of IHSS. *Circulation*, **47**, 225.

Wigle, E. D., Adelman, A. G. & Silver, M. D. (1971) Pathophysiological considerations in muscular subaortic stenosis. In *Hypertrophic Obstructive Cardiomyopathy*. Ed. Wolstenholme, G. & O'Connor, M. London: Churchill. p. 63.

CHAPTER 5

NUCLEAR CARDIOLOGY

Malcolm Merrick

MYOCARDIAL IMAGING

Radiopharmaceuticals

Potassium and its analogues. All living mammalian cells maintain a high intracellular concentration of potassium, balanced osmotically by the extracellular concentration of sodium. When a cell depolarises, potassium is released and replaced by sodium. Repolarisation is associated with active extrusion of the sodium by a 'pump' which can function only if sufficient oxygen is available. Under normal circumstances the blood flow is maintained at a level adequate to supply oxygen requirements.

If a radioisotope of potassium or one of its analogues is added to the blood perfusing a muscle, there is initially a large difference between the intracellular and extracellular isotopic concentration. Because most potassium is intracellular, most of the tracer will become intracellular in the time taken for blood to pass from the aorta to the coronary sinus. The first pass extraction of the potassium isotopes is greater than 70%, despite the absence of any active mechanism for its extraction.

The only radioisotope widely used for myocardial imaging at the present time is thallium-201. The Group 3 metals (beryllium, aluminium, gallium, indium and thallium) are predominantly trivalent, and thallium is unique amongst them in having in addition a stable lower oxidation state. The thallous ion (Tl^+) has an hydrated ionic radius only slightly larger than that of K^+ and at tracer levels cell membranes are unable to distinguish between them.

Tl^+ is a good, but not a perfect, analogue of K^+. The peak extraction rate of both is the same. Cardiac glycosides and beta blockers reduce uptake of both to a similar extent, whilst uptake is increased by such drugs as isoprotenerol or by pyrexia. It is unaffected by ischaemia until irreversible cell damage has occurred. Thallium is, however, released more slowly ($T\frac{1}{2}$ 7–24 hr) than potassium ($T\frac{1}{2}$ 1·5–3 hr).

Uptake depends both on the concentration in the blood, and the amount of blood flowing through the tissue. The blood concentration falls rapidly as extraction by other organs (especially exercising somatic muscles and liver) is almost as high as that by the heart. After the first pass there is a two-way exchange of Tl^+ until, by 10–20 minutes after injection, the blood level reaches a value which subsequently remains constant for many hours as extraction and excretion is balanced by the return of activity from the intracellular to the extracellular fluid compartments.

There is an approximately linear relationship between blood flow and thallium uptake in the range between 10% of normal resting myocardial flow and 200%. At higher flow rates thallium uptake is disproportionately low, possibly because there is insufficient time to establish equilibrium, whilst at very low flow rates the uptake is disproportionately high. Thallium therefore tends to underestimate flow at very high flow rates and overestimate it at low flow rates.

Other myocardial labels. Isotopes of potassium, rubidium and caesium have been used for myocardial imaging but none has ideal physical properties and none is generally available.

Free fatty acids are rapidly taken up by myocardium, the limiting factors being the diffusion gradients and partition coefficients, i.e. the process is essentially passive. ω-iodination does not appear to affect uptake appreciably. The initial uptake and distribution parallel that of potassium and appear to be flow dependent. However the half-time of washout from the myocardium is much faster, about 25 minutes.

Good images have been obtained with [123]I ω-Heptadecenoic and [123]I ω-Hexadecenoic Acids. Wider application is limited by the poor availability of [123]I. Labelling at alternative sites on the fatty acid molecule, or by the iodination of the double bond, produces substances which concentrate less well in the myocardium.

Glucose uptake is coupled to potassium transport and has been studied experimentally in a few centres with positron cameras, using carbon-11 glucose, carbon-11 deoxyglucose or 2-(^{18}F)-Flurodeoxyglucose. None of these agents is likely to be generally available in the foreseeable future.

A number of amino-acids are also taken up rapidly by myocardium. The first pass extraction of taurine in particular is very high. However (apart from carbon-11) no suitable gamma-emitting label of any is yet available.

Technique

A standard ECG (at least 9 leads) is obtained at rest

and examined for contraindications to exercise testing. A physician capable of dealing with a cardiac arrest and the necessary emergency drugs and equipment must be available until exercise has ceased and the pulse rate and blood pressure have returned to normal.

A cannula is inserted into a convenient peripheral vein, but avoiding the neighbourhood of joints because of the risk of displacement when the subject moves. The cephalic vein a few centimetres proximal to the wrist is usually the safest site. The cannula should be kept patent either by filling with heparinised saline or by a continuous slow infusion. The subject then exercises on either a tread mill or a bicycle, with continuous monitoring of the ECG, heart-rate and blood pressure until one of the following end points:

(1) The maximum predicted heart rate for the subject's age and sex have been reached. This criterion may be obscured if the patient is taking β-blockers. Ideally these should be discontinued before stress testing is performed.

(2) Evidence of ischaemia appears on the ECG.

(3) A significant dysrhythmia develops.

(4) The subject develops angina.

(5) There is a sudden fall of 15/20 mm Hg in the systolic pressure with no change in heart rate, indicating that the heart is unable to respond further to stress. This should not be confused with the fall in systolic pressure which is normally associated with a rise in heart rate.

(6) The subject is unable to continue because of dyspnoea.

With adequate reassurance from the physician the last should never be the reason for premature termination of exercise.

As soon as the end point has been reached and whilst the subject is still exercising 2 mCi of thallium-201 (as thallous chloride) is injected through the cannula and flushed with normal saline. Exercise should be continued, if necessary at a lower rate, for a further 30–60 seconds. The patient is then transferred to the gamma camera. Imaging should be started within 5 minutes of the injection to minimise redistribution changes.

A low energy parallel-hole general purpose collimator is generally preferable. Movement negates any advantage of a high resolution collimator, while the distortions caused by converging collimators render interpretation difficult and the magnification they yield is offset by lower contrast, giving no overall advantage. Tomographic views may be obtained by reconstructing images obtained with the 7-pinhole collimator, or a rotating slant-hole collimator. The clinical value of these latter techniques remains unproven, despite enthusiastic advocacy by a few manufacturers.

When not taking tomographic images a minimum of three views must be taken, namely anterior, 45° left anterior oblique and left lateral. Four views are preferable; anterior, 30° and 60° left anterior oblique and left lateral. Sufficient counts must be collected to give a count density of at least 1000 counts per cm² over the myocardium.

Because of the low contrast it is preferable to acquire the views into a data-processing system, so that they may subsequently be displayed optimally. If a magnification facility is available it should be used, as there is no virtue in acquiring counts from extra-cardiac structures. The patient is then discharged for 3–4 hours, during which time no restrictions on eating, drinking or exercise are necessary. When the patient returns the original projections are repeated.

It is important that positioning should be as similar as possible to the initial views. For this reason it is preferable to obtain both sets of projections by moving the camera head around the supine patient, rather than attempting to reposition an erect patient in front of a stationary camera.

Normal Appearances in Views Started Within 5 minutes of Injection during Exercise

There is detectable concentration of isotope in the left ventricular myocardium, to a lesser extent the right ventricular myocardium (Fig. 5.01), and those skeletal muscles which were exercising at the time of injection. Soft tissue background is high, the ratio of count rate in the left ventricular region to that in adjacent areas being between 3:1 and 4:1. Uptake in the lungs is higher in smokers than in non-smokers.

The left ventricle appears circular or elliptical in outline, with a lower count rate centrally, where the cavity is seen indistinctly through the muscle viewed in plan, than peripherally, where there is a greater thickness of muscle seen in profile. The ring of higher count

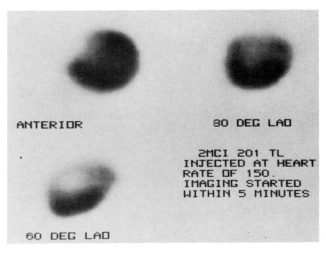

FIG. 5.01. Normal anterior, 30° left anterior oblique and 60° left anterior oblique after injection of ²⁰¹Tl during maximal exercise.

rate is incomplete cranially in the region of the aortic root. In about half the normal population a second defect is visible at the apex. This defect disappears on the systolic frame if multigated studies are performed (Fig. 5.02). For most clinical purposes these are unnecessary.

The anterior and inferior walls and apex of the left ventricle are visualised on the anterior view. Depending on the alignment of the heart the septum is sometimes seen. The septum, posterior wall and free wall of the right ventricle are usually seen in the left anterior oblique projections. In the lateral view the anterior, inferior and posterior walls and apex are visualised. The cavity usually appears symmetrically placed; asymmetry may be evident in some normal subjects in the left anterior oblique projection. The insertion of the papillary muscle may produce an irregular thickening near the mid-point of the posterior wall. A variation of up to 15% in count rate between adjacent areas of left ventricular myocardium in normal subjects is permissible.

The right ventricle is visualised best on the oblique views. It often appears faint, partly because its perfusion is lower than that of the left ventricle, but principally because the muscle is much thinner. In the absence of adequate exercise it may not be visualised at all.

Normal Appearances after Redistribution

The appearance of the normal left ventricle is unchanged. The right ventricle may no longer be visible. The concentration of isotope in the liver and spleen is much greater than after exercise and may be sufficient to partially obscure the inferior border of the heart.

Normal Appearances after Injection into Resting Subjects

The distribution is similar to that found after redistribution of activity injected during exercise. The left ventricle, spleen and liver are clearly visualised but contrast is low, the ratio of count-rate over the ventricle to adjacent lung being in the region of 2:1. The right ventricle is not visible in normal subjects.

Clinical Applications

Ischaemia. The distribution of uptake shortly after injection is principally influenced by the blood flow pattern at the time. Exercise diverts blood away from the splanchnic areas, whilst flow to the myocardium and other exercising muscle groups is increased. Redistribution starts immediately, and continues for many hours. Washout is fastest from well-perfused areas with the highest initial uptake, whereas net accumulation may continue in poorly perfused areas long after net loss is occurring from the well-perfused ones. The distribution seen several hours after injection represents, in effect, the amount of muscle present.

Ischaemic areas appear as defects present in scinti-

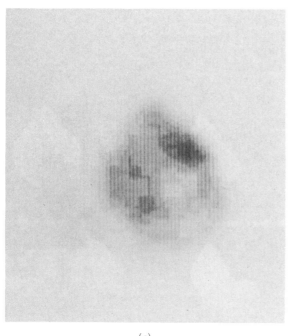

(a)

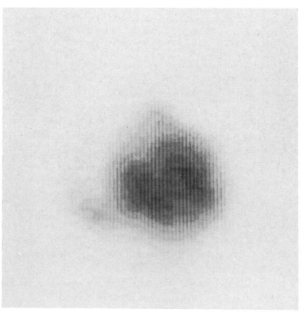

(b)

FIG. 5.02. Two frames from a gated study in the anterior projection. (a) Is in diastole. (b) Is in systole. The apparent large apical defect in the diastolic view disappears in systole.

grams taken after injection during exercise, but absent after redistribution.

There is no simple relationship between the thallium scan and arteriographically demonstrated stenoses. A number of factors contribute to this discordance.

(1) Arteriography demonstrates the stenosis in one plane only. Stenoses commonly do not affect the complete circumference of the arterial lumen; thus, the degree of narrowing estimated from a single projection may underestimate or overestimate the overall effect.

(2) 80% narrowing as estimated arteriographically may be associated with normal resting flow.

(3) The resistance to flow through any tube increases with the square of the length but with the fourth power of the radius. Decreasing the radius of the lumen has relatively little effect until a critical point is reached. This may be such that an adequate flow is maintained at rest, but the increased flow demanded by exertion cannot be met and may actually result in a drop in flow rate if adjacent vessels dilate whereas the stenosed vessel is unable to do so.

(4) The absence of a perfusion defect despite the presence of stenoses may indicate an adequate collateral supply.

(5) Thallium scintigraphy only demonstrates focal asymmetries of flow. When there is a generalised decrease in flow the thallium study may appear normal.

Vasodilators such as ethyl adenosine or isoprotenerol have also been used to demonstrate perfusion differences in the myocardium. They presumably affect only normal vessels, and thus divert blood away from ischaemic areas. The clinical significance of defects demonstrated by these techniques is unclear.

Thus, whereas the arteriogram demonstrates irregularities in the diameter of the arterial lumen, thallium exercise and rest scintigraphy demonstrate areas of myocardium with a significant deficiency of oxygen supply. It is possible to make generalisations about the vascular territories involved, but the actual vessels cannot be identified with sufficient precision for this to be clinically useful. Non-critical stenoses, generalised vascular disease and areas with an adequate collateral supply cannot be detected.

In patients with classical anginal symptoms or with unequivocal electrocardiographic evidence of ischaemia, the probability of coronary arterial stenoses is so high that thallium scintigraphy does not influence clinical management, and is therefore not indicated. The pick-up rate of significant disease in well patients who are totally asymptomatic and have normal electrocardiograms is so low that the test is not cost-effective in this group either.

Thus, the only groups in whom thallium scintigraphy is indicated are those in whom the probability of a coronary artery stricture is neither very low (<20%) nor very high (>80%). This is principally patients with atypical symptoms, and those with atypical or equivocal electrocardiograms.

MYOCARDIAL INFARCTION

There are two techniques of imaging myocardial infarcts:

(a) negative infarct imaging employing tracers which accumulate only in the living myocardium. The infarct therefore appears as an area of reduced count rate.

(b) positive infarct imaging using a tracer which accumulates in infarcted tissue to a greater extent than in normal, the infarcts therefore appearing as areas of increased count rate.

They have different applications and are complementary.

Negative Infarct Imaging

Regions of infarcted myocardium appear as defects on thallium scintigraphy. These defects may be similar on both the early and the redistribution images, or may appear larger on the early views. Infarcts are always detectable when the study is performed within 6 hours of infarction (even if the patient is injected at rest and the exercise study is omitted). The majority of full thickness infarcts are detected in rest studies performed between 6 and 24 hours after infarction, but only about three-quarters of all partial thickness infarcts are clearly detected at this time. After 24 hours has elapsed approximately 80% of larger or transmural infarcts are visualised but only about 50% of small (less than 5 g) or partial thickness ones.

Anterolateral infarction. The perfusion defects should be visible on both the anterior and the left lateral views. It may be concealed in the 45° left anterior oblique because in this projection the anterior wall is viewed *en face* and the infarct is therefore superimposed on normal structures.

An *anterior infarct* may be seen only in the left lateral projection. *Anteroseptal infarcts* are usually visible in all three projections. The degree of septal involvement is best appreciated in the 45° left anterior oblique projection (Fig. 5.03).

Inferior infarcts are also visible on all three views, extending along the inferior wall from the apex. Difficulty may be encountered distinguishing it from a normal apical defect. There are two diagnostic differences:

(1) On a multigated study the normal defect is not visible in systole.

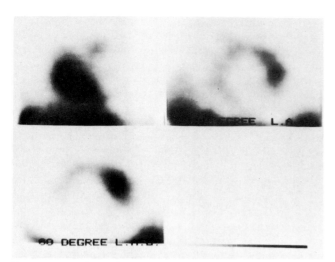

FIG. 5.03. Anterior, 30° left anterior oblique and 60° left anterior oblique projections, following injection at rest of ^{201}Tl in a patient who has suffered a large antero-inferior myocardial infarction.

(2) The normal defect is aligned along the axis of the ventricle whereas the pathological defect is not.

Posterior or postero-inferior infarcts may be seen only on a right lateral decubitous projection, but may sometimes be identified on the left anterior oblique as a defect in the left lower quadrant, or in the anterior view as a defect on the diaphragmatic aspect of the heart.

Right ventricular infarcts cannot be diagnosed directly as the normal ventricle is not visualised on rest scans. Right ventricular infarction may be inferred by the combination of cardiogenic shock, a non-dilated left ventricle and a small inferior wall perfusion defect, often with involvement of the septum.

Cardiomyopathy. Diffuse cardiomyopathies do not produce focal defects on thallium images. With increasing heart failure the ratio of activity in the heart to that in the lungs approaches unity until the heart can no longer be identified from the background. When a cardiomyopathy does produce a defect scintigraphy is of no value in differential diagnosis.

Positive Infarct Imaging

In contrast to the negative infarct scan produced by thallium, which has its highest pick-up rate the sooner scintigraphy is performed after infarction, positive infarct scans with pyrophosphate do not reach their maximal intensity until 36–60 hours after infarction. Infarcts may be visible by 12 hours, but even at this time false positives are not uncommon. Subsequently they fade slowly over a course of several weeks but some remain visible for several months.

Technique. Technetium pyrophosphate is the most widely used radiopharmaceutical. Infarcts have been detected using other bone scanning agents, but they are generally considered to be more likely to miss small lesions. Reliable and reproducible results require meticulous attention to detail. The quality of every dose of technetium pyrophosphate must be checked by thin layer chromatography before administration, as the presence of 1% free pertechnetate in the preparation (which also contains stannous ions) will give rise to labelling of red cells, thus giving a high background in the region of the heart, diminishing the relative difference in count rate between the infarct and the background.

The optimum time for imaging is usually 60–90 minutes after injection, but in older subjects a delay of 90 minutes or more may be preferable. At least 3 projections must be obtained; anterior, at least one anterior oblique and a left lateral. The optimal oblique may be selected using a television or persistence monitor, or one or more standard projections may be taken. High count densities (approximately 1000 counts per cm^2) must be collected using a high resolution collimator.

The sensitivity and specificity is improved if the study is repeated on two occasions, 24 and 72 hours after the suspected infarction, and if a grading system is used when reporting. Grading systems, although essentially subjective, are sufficiently reproducible to be of practical value.

A typical 5-level scale is:

0 – Normal, no myocardial uptake
1 – Minimal or diffuse uptake, probably in blood pool or chest wall
2 – Definite activity in myocardium
3 – Myocardium activity similar to that in ribs or sternum
4 – Myocardial activity greater than bone.

Using this system a grading of 2 or greater is considered a significant abnormality. All three (or more) views must be considered together and the grading is the highest in any one projection. Thus, a thin infarct may be clearly seen in profile (grade 3) but barely visible *en face* (grade 1). The study as a whole would be graded 3.

Accuracy. In centres where there is meticulous quality control of the pyrophosphate and follow-up examinations are performed routinely at 24 and 72 hours, false negative rates of 4% and false positive rates between 8 and 12% have been reported. However, the majority of centres do not achieve this accuracy, finding false negative rates of between 5 and 10% and false positive rates of between 10 and 20%.

The principal cause for false negatives is probably incorrect timing of the examination. This is reduced by repeating all scans after 48 hours. Infarcts involving less than 3 g of muscle cannot be visualised.

The principal causes for false positive scans are:
Rib fractures
Soft tissue damage to the chest wall
Breast tumours
Local inflammation
Unstable angina
Ventricular aneurysms
Valve calcification
Burns (including those due to cardioversion)
Functioning mammary tissue.

Clinical Applications

Negative infarct imaging with thallium will detect infarcts earlier than any other test, before characteristic electrocardiographic or serum enzyme changes are available. However, the routine use of thallium is impracticable because of the cost and its short half-life. It is doubtful whether the routine use of this test would be cost effective.

Positive infarct imaging, although it may detect infarcts at 12 hours, is not reliable until 24 hours have elapsed from the infarct, by which time electrocardiographic and enzyme changes are usually diagnostic. It is, however, useful in selected groups in whom these parameters are uninterpretable, namely:

(1) Perioperative infarction in patients undergoing cardiac or coronary artery surgery.

(2) Infarction in the presence of left bundle branch block.

(3) Subendocardial or right ventricular infarction.

(4) New transmural infarct adjacent to previous infarcts.

Sizing. Positive imaging may complement other methods of infarct siting and sizing. This application is purely of experimental interest at the present time.

Prognosis. Patients in whom the infarct appears as a ring with a less active centre have a higher risk of developing congestive cardiac failure and higher early and late mortality. Patients with persistently positive scintigrams follow a more fulminant clinical course and have a higher mortality and morbidity. Some centres advocate routine follow up infarct scans 3 and 6 months after the initial illness as an aid to improved prediction of prognosis.

MYOCARDIAL PERFUSION

Total myocardial blood flow may be measured by a number of methods:

(1) If a tracer is entirely removed from the blood perfusing an organ on a single passage through that organ the blood flow can be calculated if the uptake, the total amount administered and the cardiac output are known (the Sapirstein principle). Although the extraction ratio for potassium is less than 100% it is sufficiently high for the principle to be applied (with an appropriate correction factor) to an acceptable accuracy, but only during the first passage. The principal disadvantages of this technique are that the first passage is short in duration and ill-defined, so that the accuracy is limited by achievable counting statistics. There is no method of making an accurate background correction except by positron emission tomography.

(2) Radioactive particles injected into the left atrium are also distributed in proportion to blood flow. This technique is only applicable in experimental animals.

(3) The method using carbon dioxide labelled with oxygen-15, originally described for the brain, can in theory be applied to the heart. This technique also requires positron emission tomography.

(4) The most generally used technique measures the rate of washout of an inert radioactive gas such as xenon-133 or krypton-85 following bolus injection of an aqueous solution into a coronary artery. The washout or decay curve is measured using either a simple detector or, preferably, a gamma camera. In theory, this curve should be a simple, single exponential, the slope of which is a measure of the flow per unit mass (or volume). Unfortunately the curve is not a single exponential and cannot be expressed as an unambiguous mathematical function. The results depend very largely on the total duration of observation, and there is a large subjective element in the choice of the slope to be measured. Although this method may be capable of giving accurate results it must be treated with reserve.

CARDIAC OUTPUT

This is most commonly measured utilising the Stuart Hamilton principle, which can be applied to both radioactive and non-radioactive tracers including ^{113}In Cl$_3$, ^{11}CO labelled erythrocytes, technetium or iodine labelled human serum albumin or non-radioactive dyes such as Evans blue or Indicyanin green.

Principle

The requirements of a suitable tracer are:

(1) That it should be non-metabolised.

(2) That none should leave the circulation by diffusion or any other process between the point of injection and the point of measurement.

(3) That there should be, at some point between the injection and measurement, complete mixing.

The average concentration of the tracer is inversely

proportional to the volume of blood with which it has been mixed. The length of time taken for tracer to flow past the mixing point during the first passage indicates the time required for the volume in which it has been diluted to flow past the mixing point. It is therefore necessary firstly to obtain a graph showing how the count rate at some point at or beyond the mixing chamber varies with time during the first pass of the tracer. Secondly, it is necessary to establish the relationship between the amount of activity injected and the count rate actually measured. If the tracer has been mixed with the entire cardiac output, i.e. the blood volume, it will follow that the cardiac output is equal to the activity injected divided by the area under the first pass concentration curve.

Blood volume is measured by measuring the concentration of tracer in a blood sample taken between 5 and 20 minutes after injection and dividing this into the administered activity. The calibration factor for the detector is obtained by counting a phantom containing a known amount of activity in a suitable scattering medium such as a bowl of water.

A typical curve is shown in Fig. 5.04. An ideal tracer

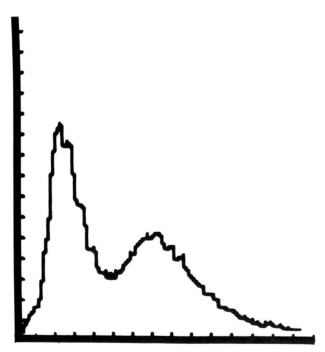

FIG. 5.04. Count-rate curve obtained from a region of interest encompassing both ventricles during the first pass of a bolus injection of tracer. The first peak is due to activity in the right ventricle, the second activity in the left ventricle. In the absence of a shunt the area under both curves is equal. Shunt size may be measured from discrepancies in the areas under the curves. Cardiac output is measured by relating the area under the left ventricular curve to the activity in a blood sample taken at a known time late on in the curve when the activity is changing little with time.

curve starts from and ends at zero. In practice, because the tracer must be non-diffusable and non-metabolised, there is always recirculation. Cardiac output is calculated only from the first pass. An extrapolation of the downslope must therefore be made to approximate to the curve which would have been obtained had there been no recirculation. The greater the difference between the peak and the equilibrium value the more accurately this extrapolation can be made. When cardiac output is low or if a poor bolus injection has been administered, the difference between the peak and the equilibrium value may be too small for this extrapolation to be made accurately. This may be a substantial cause of error.

EJECTION FRACTION AND REGIONAL WALL MOVEMENT

Ejection fraction, i.e. the percentage of the diastolic volume ejected per beat (or the mean percentage ejected per beat) can be measured using non-imaging probes provided that their data acquisition rate is high enough. Accurate positioning of the probes is essential. This may be assisted by ultrasound or by the use of specialised data acquisition systems which indicate when the periodicity of acquisition rate is maximal. A second probe to measure background must also be employed and the position of this probe is equally critical. The cost of the appropriate equipment is much lower than the cost of imaging equipment with its associated data processing, but it is much more restricted in its application and is highly dependent upon the operator. For this reason non-imaging techniques have not been widely accepted.

Whether using imaging or simple probes, two techniques are available, first pass and multigated.

First Pass Studies

The detector or gamma camera is positioned in front of the supine patient. A 30° right anterior oblique projection should be obtained when using the gamma camera. Some centres favour the anterior projection. If the supine position is precluded by orthopnoea or any other cause, it may be necessary to perform the examination with the patient erect. Under these circumstances accurate repositioning is more difficult. A large peripheral vein, e.g. the median basilic vein in the vicinity of the elbow, is selected and a large needle or cannula (at least 19 gauge) attached to a two-way connector is inserted. The activity to be injected is that which gives the highest count rate which the camera or data acquisition system can cope with. The activity must be in as small a volume as possible, certainly less than 2 ml and preferably less than 1 ml. It is injected rapidly and flushed with a 20 ml bolus of normal saline to ensure that it reaches the right atrium as compactly as possible. Once in the right atrium the turbulent flow ensures mixing with the total contents of the chamber.

There are no effective measures which can influence the fate of the bolus after it has entered the right atrium but, if at this point there is a poor bolus, there is no prospect of a diagnostic study more distally.

Radiopharmaceutical. If a first pass study only is to be performed the nature of the radiopharmaceutical is immaterial, provided that it is neither trapped in nor exhaled by the lungs. When using a non-imaging system indium-113m chloride is a useful radiopharmaceutical because its short half-life permits re-examination at fairly frequent intervals. However, its energy is poorly suited to the gamma camera and for this purpose technetium labelled compounds such as Tc DTPA may be used. If the study is to be followed by a multigated study a blood pool label must be employed.

Equipment. For first pass measurement of ejection fraction a gamma camera with a field of view of between 25 and 30 cm is preferable to one with a very large field of view. The latter is more difficult to position as it will project uncomfortably close to the face of the patient. Moreover, it will detect many counts coming from the lung fields, thus increasing the dead-time losses and reducing the number of real counts collected from the cardiac area.

The importance of a camera and data-acquisition system which can handle high counting rates cannot be overemphasised. The number of counts which can be collected from the ventricle greatly influences the quality of the study. As the amount of activity which can be administered depends on the dead-time losses of the data acquisition system, count rate cannot be increased by administering more radioactivity. With the slowest systems, only 100–200 counts may be detected from the left ventricular region of interest during systole. Clearly with such poor statistics the cardiac outline cannot be accurately defined. The fastest systems may be capable of collecting up to ten times as many counts.

Until recently only multicrystal cameras (Bender-Blau cameras) have been capable of very high data acquisition rates. More recently some Anger cameras have achieved similar acquisition rates. However, at the present time all fast cameras have relatively poor resolution at these rates.

A number of specialised collimators have been designed for nuclear cardiology and can be useful. Conventional general purpose parallel hole collimators used in conjunction with a large field of view gamma camera result in the greater part of the field of view being occupied by lung, which is of no interest in this study. Bilateral collimators, in which the septa in the two halves are angled towards each other so that the heart is viewed from two angles simultaneously, permit two studies to be obtained from a single injection.

Data Processing. Data may be acquired in one of two ways. In frame mode a series of images (frames) each of predetermined time (usually 0·025–0·05 sec) are collected starting at the instant of injection and continuing for approximately 30 sec until the bolus has been dispersed from the left ventricle. In list mode the computer records the position and time of arrival of each count over a similar period but the frames are built up subsequently. In practice there is little to choose between the methods, frame mode being in general faster to process but requiring more computer space.

To process results it is first necessary to define regions of interest corresponding to the left ventricle and an adjacent background area. Because of the poor statistics in each frame it is usually necessary to sum a series of frames in order to obtain reasonably clear visualisation of the ventricular outline. Both regions must exclude the aorta, left atrium and pulmonary artery.

In the right anterior oblique projection the right and left ventricles are superimposed upon each other. However, provided a good bolus has been administered, the two are separated in time and it is therefore possible to obtain distinct curves from each ventricle.

These regions are then applied to the consecutive frames to produce a graph as shown in Fig. 5.05. Because of the very poor statistics in each frame systole and diastole are difficult to define. Smoothing, by taking a weighted average of consecutive points on the curve produces a smoother curve on which systole and diastole are easier to identify. However, the averaging process reduces the value of the peaks and increases those of the troughs, thus reducing the calculated value of ejection fraction.

It is therefore necessary to apply a mathematical filter rather than a simple smoothing process. This is a complex technique which attempts to separate random statistical fluctuations in count rate from real differences due to ventricular contraction. The results of filtration are shown in Fig. 5.05. Great care must be taken when accepting filtered curves, as the technique is capable of generating oscillating artefacts.

The validity of correcting for background is questionable. During a first pass study there may be some residual activity in the lungs, particularly in patients in cardiac failure or if there has been a poor bolus, but normally the lung activity should have largely or completely passed into the left atrium. Counts detected outwith the cardiac borders are as likely to be due to scatter from activity within the cardiac chamber as from true background activity. Moreover, there is very little lung between the heart and the detector. It is therefore doubtful whether activity in the lung adjacent to the heart is a valid representation of activity which in any case will not yet have reached other tissues via the systemic circulation.

Ejection fraction is calculated from the ratio of systolic to diastolic counts. It may be averaged over several

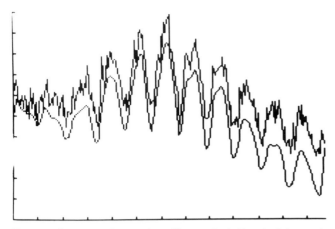

FIG. 5.05. Count-rate from region of interest including the left ventricle. The upper curve is the gross count rate, the lower the count rate after background subtraction and filtration. Use of the raw curve would substantially underestimate the ejection fraction.

beats or the beat to beat variation may be given. In patients with severe dysrhythmia this may be the only valid method of estimating ejection fraction, and it is the only method of measuring the beat to beat variation.

An alternative method is to sum a number of systolic and diastolic frames. Separate systolic and diastolic outlines may be drawn accurately on the summed frames. This should give the same result as that obtained by averaging over several beats. Any discrepancy is likely to be due to errors in the background correction.

Multigated Studies

Using this technique images of the heart are built up over a large number of cycles (usually between 100 and 600) thus giving good statistical data. It depends upon the ability of the data acquisition system to divide up each heart beat into a number of equally timed intervals, usually between 12 and 64. As the study is started, counts are initially accumulated into frame 1. At the end of the preset time interval, counts start to accumulate in frame 2 and so on into successive frames. On detection of a suitable signal the cycle is restarted, more counts being added to frame 1 etc. The whole process is repeated until either a predetermined time, number of beats or number of counts has been accumulated or has elapsed.

The only ECG event which is useful for timing the cardiac cycle is the R wave, which corresponds to end diastole. End systole cannot be identified from the ECG signal but can be defined from the carotid pulse or by phonocardiography. This, however, is usually regarded as an unnecessary complication.

The RR interval is measured over a sufficient number of beats to determine the mean range and standard deviation. The number of frames per cycle should be set to give a time for each frame of between 20 and 30 milliseconds. The number of frames may be limited by the amount of computer memory available, compelling the use of longer frame times. This has the disadvantage that, as end systole lasts only about 50 milliseconds, if the end systolic frame includes part either of emptying or of the filling phase, end-systolic volume will be over-estimated and ejection fraction correspondingly under-estimated.

In practice the error is small provided that the frame times are less than 50 milliseconds but may become appreciable at longer frame times.

There is always some beat-to-beat variation in RR interval. If a new R wave is detected before all of the frames have been 'filled' the computer nevertheless goes back to the beginning of the cycle. Therefore the later frames in the cycle may have been built up from fewer beats, and therefore contain fewer counts than the earlier frames. This variation occurs only during the filling phase, incompleteness of which does not affect the study. If the RR interval is unduly long an excessive number of counts may be added to the last frame of the cycle, or the excess counts may be discarded.

The greatest problem is posed by ectopic beats. These, by altering the filling time both for that and for one or two subsequent beats, may produce a marked disturbance in the pattern of filling and emptying. Most systems have a mechanism for discarding one or two beats after an ectopic. More elaborate systems store the counts for several beats and only include them in the study after the ECG signal has been analysed for the presence of ectopics. Other systems store all the counts in list mode along with the ECG signal and then frame up in retrospect discarding ectopic beats. In patients with severe dysrhythmia this may be the only method of obtaining a diagnostic study. However, it is much more time consuming than 'real-time' multigating.

Projection

The right anterior oblique cannot be used for measurement of ejection fraction in the multigated study as the right ventricle is superimposed over the left. In general the best projection is a 30° left anterior oblique with 10° of caudal tilt, thus projecting the left ventricle clear both of the right ventricle and the left atrium (Fig. 5.09). However, the ventricle is foreshortened in this view, which is therefore not ideal for viewing wall motion. Reproducible positioning can best be achieved by angling the camera with the patient supine. If a large field of view camera is employed this may prove difficult unless a slant-hole or bilateral collimator is available. When the patient is orthopnoeic it may be necessary to perform the examination with the patient erect. Accurate repositioning is more difficult under these circumstances. It is important to choose an ECG lead which gives a well defined positive R wave which is much larger than the T wave, as the trigger is activated by any pulse above a preset voltage, irrespective of the shape of the signal.

Clinical Applications

Ejection fraction is one of the best non-invasive parameters of myocardial function. The isotope methods now used, which measure only the activity within the ventricular cavity, have the great advantage over ultrasound and angiographic techniques that no assumptions about the ventricular geometry are necessary, and the technique is not affected by rotation of the heart or interposition of lung between the heart and the chest wall. The major error is due to estimation of the background correction. Some experience is necessary to obtain reproducible results (Fig. 5.06).

In normal subjects at rest the ejection fraction should be between 40 and 70%. A higher figure is found in erect subjects than in the same subject measured supine. On exercise there should be a further rise in ejection fraction. Failure of ejection fraction to increase, or an actual decrease on exercise, is evidence of impaired myocardial reserves.

When combined with cardiac output many other parameters, including stroke volume, end diastolic volume etc. can be calculated. For most clinical purposes these are unnecessary.

Regional Wall Motion

The individual frames may be replayed in sequence as an 'endless loop' to obtain an impression of cardiac motion. Akinetic and dyskinetic areas, and regions of paradoxical motion may be identified, but this is not a reliable method of detecting focal dyskinesia, principally because of the limitations of the modified LAO projection.

Where regional wall movement is of importance it is necessary to obtain several projections, e.g. LPO, RAO and anterior, and to view them simultaneously. Even so, analogue interpretation of movement is subjective and relatively insensitive.

The most sensitive method of detecting and assessing the severity of regional or global abnormalities is parametric imaging. A parameter is a quantity which is constant in a particular case considered, but which varies in different cases.

Any scintigraphic image could be considered a parametric image as it displays the spacial distribution of the administered radioactivity (a variable) (Fig. 5.07). If a series of images (e.g. a multigated cardiac study) is considered, numerous other variables can be measured, such as the rate of change of activity at each point in the image, the timing of maximum or minimum count-rate, the time at which the rate of change is maximal or minimal, etc. These parameters are calculated and stored by the computer as an array of numbers. How-

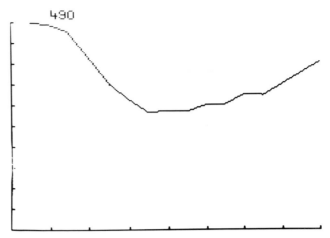

FIG. 5.06. Left ventricular multigated ejection fraction curve. Note that the curve is not symmetrical.

ever, such an array is difficult to assimilate, and the data is much easier to interpret if it is presented as a matrix in which each value is represented by a colour or shade of grey. The term parametric image is usually reserved for this type of display.

A large number of parameters have been calculated from multigated left ventricular studies, amongst the most useful of which are the phase image, the maximum rate of filling and the regional ejection fraction. Experience with this technique is limited and other parameters may prove their value in the future.

The phase image is one of the most important, and one of the most difficult to understand. Production of the image requires very complex mathematics including Fourier analysis (hence the alternative name sometimes used of the Fourier image). Effectively it shows the timing of contraction. In the normal case the whole ventricle contracts synchronously, and therefore appears in the phase image as a uniform colour or shade of grey, which is an index of the mean interval from the R-wave to end systole (Fig. 5.08). This interval is longer in the presence of left bundle branch block, and in hypokinetic, dyskinetic and akinetic segments which therefore appear in different shades. Dyskinetic segments in particular move in phase with the atria rather than the rest of the ventricle, and are demonstrated with striking clarity (Fig. 5.09).

The whole ventricle should fill at the same rate. The parametric image of the maximal rate of filling should therefore show a uniform shade within the ventricular area. Ischaemic muscle relaxes less readily than normal muscle, with a consequent reduction in the maximal rate of filling. It is thus possible to display regional loss of compliance (as evidence of ischaemia) even in the absence of a contraction abnormality.

The regional ejection fraction shows the difference

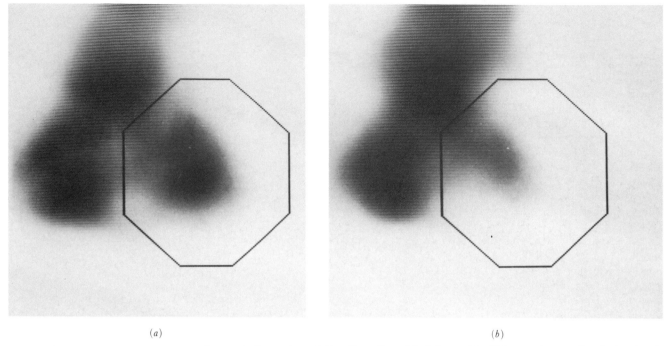

(a)   (b)

FIG. 5.07. (a) end diastole, (b) end systole. The line indicates the end diastolic outline of the left ventricle. This extends somewhat further than is evident on the reproductions.

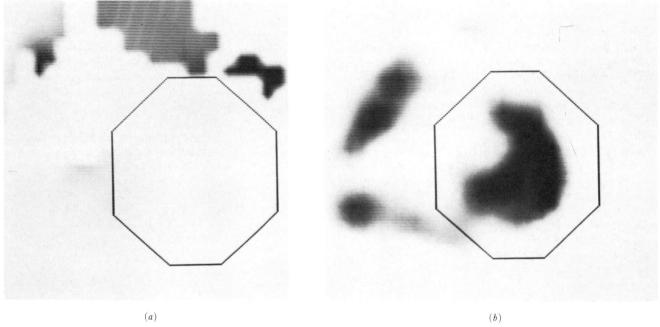

(a)   (b)

FIG. 5.08. (a) The same study as Fig. 5.07, the phase image showing that the entire area within the ventricular region of interest is in the same phase. The left atrium (above) is out of phase. (b) Shows the amplitude of the phase variation which is high and equal throughout the ventricular area.

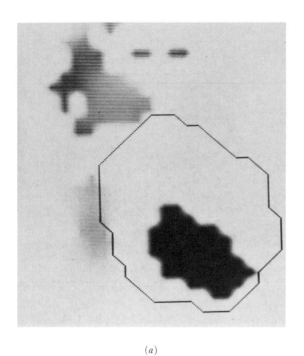
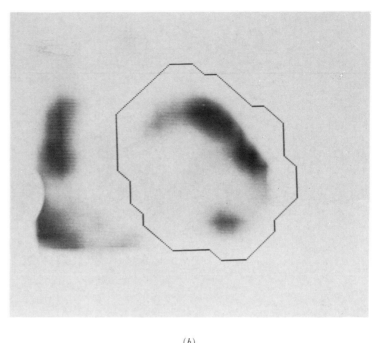

(a)   (b)

FIG. 5.09. Abnormal study. (a) Phase image showing a large area out of phase with the rest of the ventricle. (b) Shows the amplitude of movement at this point is very low.

between the activity in the diastolic and systolic frames expressed as a fraction of the activity in the diastolic frame. In the normal case there should be a uniform thick crescent around the residual volume. Hypokinetic regions are a readily identified lower fraction, displayed as a difference in shade or colour.

A minimum of three studies must be performed; at rest, during stress and after recovery. If an unequivocal abnormality is present on the resting study, it is unnecessary, and possibly dangerous, to stress the subject. The resting study must therefore always be processed before deciding whether or not to perform a stress test.

Supine bicycle exercise, with control of the level of work and monitoring of the heart rate and blood pressure is the most sensitive method, i.e. it has the highest pick-up rate. It is, however, often difficult to prevent patient movement. The cold pressor test is slightly less sensitive than graduated exercise, but is better than sub-maximal exercise, requires little active cooperation and eliminates movement. The choice of examination is ultimately dependent upon available equipment and the clinical assessment of the capability of the patient.

Right Ventricular Function

No method is entirely satisfactory, principally because of the shape and position of the chamber, which on the one hand is difficult to project clear of the right atrium, whilst on the other it is difficult to define the plane of the pulmonary valve.

Relatively little of the free wall of the right ventricle is seen on the LAO, the only projection which can be obtained of it in the multigated study. The RAO gives a much clearer view of regional contraction, but can be used only in first-pass studies. The right ventricle is also routinely displayed in parametric images.

VALVULAR STENOSES AND REGURGITATION

A number of experimental techniques to detect and measure regurgitation through the aortic or mitral valves have been developed, but none is yet sufficiently validated to be accepted into clinical practice. The measurement of stenosis, by definition, requires the demonstration of a pressure gradient and is therefore not amenable to nuclear medicine techniques.

CONGENITAL HEART DISEASE

Right to left shunts may be measured if radioactive microspheres are injected intravenously. Normally these will be trapped only in the lungs. Thus, measurement of extrapulmonary activity indicates the presence of a shunt, and enables its size to be measured. The technique is safe provided that the total number of particles is less than 200,000, and none are greater than 40 μm in diameter.

Left to right shunts can be detected, and their size measured, on first-pass studies. The anatomical detail is in practice insufficient for most clinical purposes, and for this reason the techniques have not been widely adopted. However, the measurements of shunt size remain valid.

SUGGESTIONS FOR FURTHER READING

The following reviews contain extensive bibliographies, and are recommended as a starting point.

BACHARACH, S. L., GREEN, M. V. & BORER, J. S. (1979) Instrumentation and data processing in cardiovascular nuclear medicine: evaluation of ventricular function. *Sem. Nuclear Med.*, **9**, 257–274.

BERGER, H. J., MATTHAY, R. A., PYTLIK, L. M., GOTTSCHALK, A. & ZARET, B. L. (1979) First-pass radionucleide assessment of right and left ventricular performance in patients with cardiac and pulmonary disease. *Sem. Nuclear Med.*, **9**, 275–295.

CHERVU, L. R. (1979) Radiopharmaceuticals in cardiovascular nuclear medicine. *Sem. Nuclear Med.*, **9**, 241–256.

DONATO, L. (1971) Studies of cardiac and pulmonary function. In *Radioisotopes in Medical Diagnoses*. Ed. E. H. Belcher & H. Vetter. London: Butterworth.

GREENFIELD, L. D., VINCENT, W. R., GRAHAM, L. S. & BENNETT, L. R. (1975) Evaluation of intracardiac shunts. *CRC Critical Reviews in Clin. Radiol. Nuclear Med.*, **6**, 217–251.

LEPPO, J. A., SCHEUER, J., POHOST, G. M., FREEMAN, L. M. & STRAUSS, H. W. (1980) The evaluation of ischaemic heart disease: Thallium 201 with comments on radionucleide angiography. *Sem. Nuclear Med.*, **10**, 115–126.

PARISI, A. F., TOW, D. E., FELIX, W. R. & SASAHARA, A. A. (1977) Noninvasive cardiac diagnosis. *New Eng. J. Med.*, **296**, 316–320, 368–374, 427–432.

PARKEY, R. W., BONTE, F. J., STOKELY, E. M., CURRY, G. C. & WILLERSON, J. T. (1975) Measurement of myocardial blood flow. *CRC Critical Reviews in Clin. Radiol. Nuclear Med.*, **6**, 441–458.

CHAPTER 6

ISCHAEMIC HEART DISEASE

Michael Ruttley

INTRODUCTION

Ischaemic heart disease can vary from reversible myocardial ischaemia to myocardial infarction with its many possible complications; it can be clinically silent or characterised by symptoms ranging from angina pectoris to those of congestive cardiac failure, and sudden death can occur at any stage. Myocardial ischaemia reflects an imbalance between oxygen supply and demand and can occur with normal or even enlarged coronary arteries in conditions of extreme left ventricular hypertrophy (e.g. aortic valve disease, hypertrophic cardiomyopathy) but, in the overwhelming majority, ischaemic heart disease is due to obstructive coronary artery disease and this is so commonly a consequence of coronary atherosclerosis that the terms are synonymous in general use. Nonatherosclerotic coronary causes include certain congenital coronary anomalies, coronary artery spasm, coronary artery embolus, arteritis, aortic or coronary dissection, trauma and the mural thickening associated with some inherited disorders such as pseudoxanthoma elasticum and Hurler's syndrome. After all recognised causes have been excluded there remains a very small group of patients with evidence of myocardial ischaemia, even infarction, but normal coronary arteries and no defined underlying disease.

At the present time the vast majority of coronary artery bypass operations are done for the relief of angina pectoris. Only in the case of severe stenosis of the left main coronary artery is it generally accepted that surgical relief of the obstruction improves life expectancy. This may seem remarkable for a disease that is a major cause of death in the developed world; the reason is mainly that studies on the natural history of the subdivisions of ischaemic heart disease only became possible with the advent of coronary arteriography, and were soon frustrated by the inroads made by surgery into the available population. Large series of patients have suggested quite strongly that disease in all three coronary arteries is another situation where surgery may prolong life, but this group contains many patients who have poor ventricular function due to one or more infarcts and this in itself limits the prognosis.

Radiology has an important role in the diagnosis and management of ischaemic heart disease, notably in the investigation of angina pectoris, the monitoring of acute myocardial infarction and the assessment of its non-fatal complications; recent application of catheter techniques to the treatment of ischaemic heart disease has been a progression from Dotter's original work on peripheral arterial dilation (Dotter & Judkins, 1964) made possible by Gruntzig's development of a suitable dilating catheter for coronary stenosis (Gruntzig, 1978).

CHEST RADIOGRAPHS: FLUOROSCOPY

Patients presenting with angina pectoris usually have normal plain chest radiographs apart from the occasional finding of coronary artery calcification; patients admitted to hospital with acute myocardial infarction are about equally divided between those with normal films and those with radiographic evidence of pulmonary venous hypertension and/or cardiomegaly; plain film findings in survivors of acute myocardial infarction depend on the extent of myocardial necrosis and its complications and therefore vary from normality to gross changes of congestive cardiac failure and can include signs almost specific for ischaemic heart disease, i.e. aneurysmal bulge of the left ventricle, left ventricular calcification.

The chest radiograph is one of the first investigations ordered for a patient admitted to hospital with acute myocardial infarction and, while it helps exclude other conditions which can have similar clinical presentation (e.g. dissecting aneurysm of the aorta), its main value is in the assessment of pulmonary venous pressure and heart size; it is therefore surprising that the 'portable' film taken and accepted on the coronary care unit is so often an anteroposterior view of the supine or semi-erect patient which is of very limited value in these respects. It is not prohibitively difficult or dangerous to obtain a good quality erect (sitting) posteroanterior view at the bedside (Lame & Redick, 1970).

Coronary artery calcification indicates coronary artery disease, typically inconsequential in the elderly but associated with significant obstructive lesions (not necessarily at the site of calcification) in patients under 50 years of age (Hamby *et al.*, 1974). A recent review (Green & Kelley, 1980) has emphasised the value of radiographically detected coronary artery calcification as a pointer to ischaemic heart disease in patients with atypical chest pain or cardiomyopathy of unknown cause and as an adjunct to exercise stress testing. Calcification occurs in the left coronary artery, particularly the left anterior descending (LAD) branch, more often than the right and is most commonly proximal. It is rarely so gross as in Fig. 6.01a and b but, despite motion blur, left coronary calcification can be seen on frontal chest radiographs more frequently than is generally accepted if specific search is made in the upper third of the heart shadow to the left of the spine (Souza et al., 1978). Any serious attempt to find coronary calcification must include fluoroscopy where the oblique projections are particularly useful; the sites of the major epicardial arteries are obvious after study of the aortogram and coronary arteriogram illustrations in this volume. The right coronary artery and the circumflex branch of the left coronary artery run in the atrioventricular groove and the LAD runs in the anterior interventricular groove; each of these grooves contains radiolucent fat, a considerable aid to fluoroscopic localisation. Vascular calcification is also one of the plain film signs of coronary arteriovenous fistula (Fig. 6.02),

a congenital malformation which can cause myocardial ischaemia by 'stealing' blood from the coronary circuit into a low pressure chamber or vessel (Fig. 6.03).

Heart size; chamber enlargement. Normal heart size is the typical finding in patients with angina pectoris and no previous myocardial infarction and is seen in about half those admitted to hospital with acute infarct; it does not exclude left ventricular dysfunction. Acute myocardial infarction can occur without plain film evidence of cardiac enlargement even when complicated by papillary muscle rupture, ruptured interventricular septum or even cardiogenic shock because of the limited extent to which previously normal heart chambers can suddenly dilate; the combination of pulmonary oedema and normal heart size suggests rather than excludes such a cardiac cause.

Cardiomegaly in ischaemic heart disease usually indicates left ventricular dysfunction from one or more previous infarcts, even when seen in cases of acute infarction where it carries a poor prognosis with or without accompanying signs of pulmonary venous hypertension (Battler et al., 1980). Diffuse fibrosis from

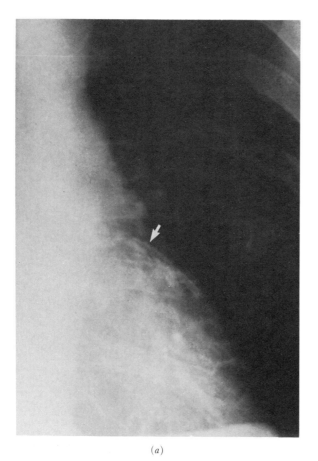

(a)

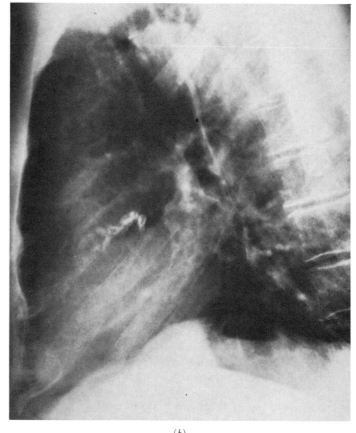

(b)

FIG. 6.01. (a) PA chest radiograph showing typical position of left coronary artery calcification (arrow). (b) Lateral chest radiography of same patient.

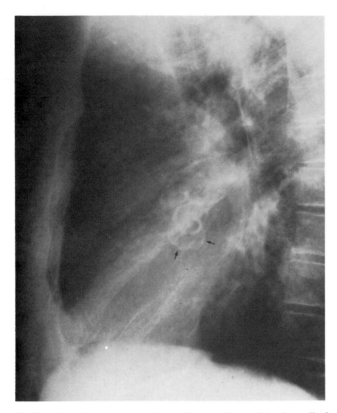

FIG. 6.02. Curvilinear concentric calcification (arrows) in the wall of a coronary arteriovenous fistula.

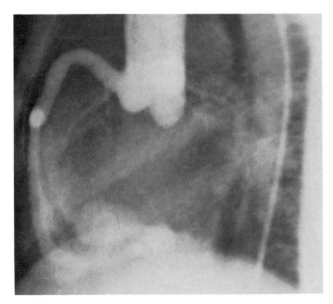

FIG. 6.03. Lateral aortogram showing coronary arteriovenous fistula supplied by a large right coronary artery and draining into right ventricle.

multiple infarcts is a common cause of left ventricular failure and cardiomegaly in this disease and has been termed ischaemic cardiomyopathy (Burch *et al.*, 1970). The early mortality of papillary muscle or septal rupture without surgical repair leaves few survivors to develop chronic cardiomegaly in response to the volume overload of mitral regurgitation or left to right shunt but this is not so for another of the mechanical complications of myocardial infarction, left ventricular aneurysm, which has an incidence variously reported between 3% (Dubnow *et al.*, 1965) and 35% (Cheng, 1971) depending on whether a pathological or angiographic definition is used. The majority of left ventricular aneurysms arise from the anterolateral wall and apex of the ventricle following an infarct due to occlusion of the left anterior descending (LAD) branch of the left coronary artery. The 15% which occur in circumflex or right coronary artery territory are usually inferior and this is also the typical location of the rare false aneurysm formed from a walled-off myocardial rupture. Left ventricular functional disturbance due to aneurysm depends on the size and compliance of the latter and the state of the remaining myocardium: it has been estimated that normal ventricular myocardium can compensate for loss of contractile tissue if this is less than 20% of left ventricular surface area (Klein, 1967) but myocardial work can be wasted if there is systolic expansion of the aneurysm with useless translocation of blood within the overall cavity rather than ejection into the aorta; such paradoxical motion (dyskinesis) is much less common than generally believed (Soulen & Freeman, 1971). Classically associated with a large heart and a localised (Fig. 6.04), sometimes calcified (Fig. 6.05), bulge of the left heart border, left ventricular aneurysm (by any definition) can occur with non-specific cardiomegaly (Fig. 6.06) or even a heart shadow of normal size and shape (Raphael *et al.*, 1972) (Fig. 6.07). An aneurysm clearly recognisable on plain chest radiographs is almost always a well demarcated fibrous sac arising from the anterolateral wall and apex of the ventricle; its lateral position on the frontal radiograph (Fig. 6.08*a*) is no surprise but its appearance as an anterior density on the lateral (Fig. 6.08*b*) can be quite misleading to those expecting it to be placed posteriorly with the ventricle proper, from which of course it has extended. Localised apical aneurysms and particularly inferior aneurysms can be hidden by the diaphragm and an aneurysmal bulge in any position can be obscured if there is associated failure and dilation of the remaining ventricle. Calcification of the wall of an aneurysm is curvilinear and is nearly always seen at the cardiac apex; it should be sought in cases of unexplained cardiac failure which can be due to clinically 'silent' ischaemic heart disease (Fig. 6.09). Cardiac fluoroscopy is of no value in the diagnosis or exclusion of left ventricular aneurysm when the plain radiographs are negative, for

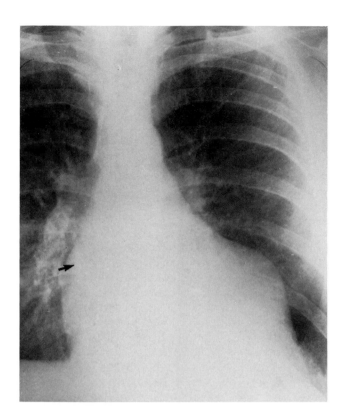

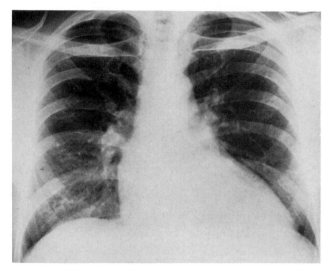

FIG. 6.04. Typical bulge of left ventricular aneurysm. Left atrial enlargement present (arrow).

FIG. 6.06. Left ventricular aneurysm. Non-specific cardiomegaly.

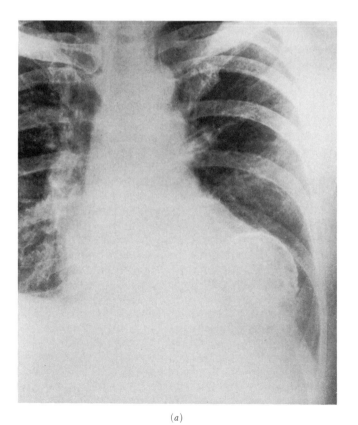

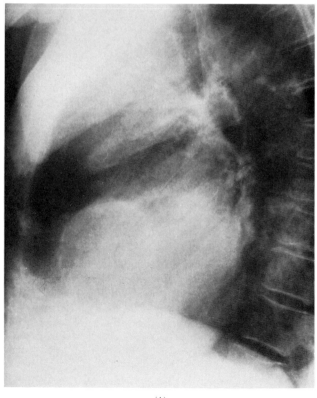

(a)

(b)

FIG. 6.05. (a) PA Chest radiography, curvilinear calcification of left ventricular aneurysm. (b) Lateral chest radiograph of same patient. Note the anterior position of the aneurysm.

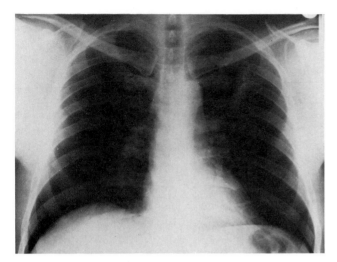

FIG. 6.07. Proven left ventricular aneurysm (apical)!

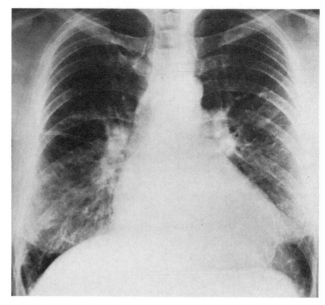

FIG. 6.09. Previously unexplained left ventricular failure. Ischaemic heart disease diagnosed by left ventricular (aneurysm) calcification on chest radiograph.

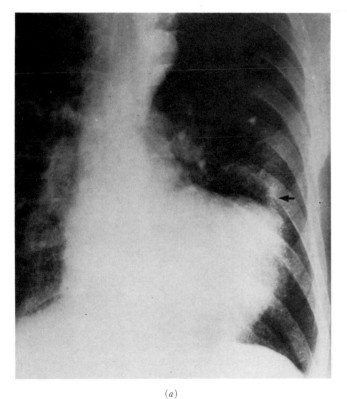

(a)

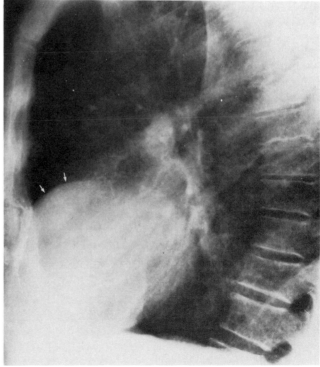

(b)

FIG. 6.08. (a) Left ventricular aneurysm. Pleuropericardial adhesion (arrow). (b) Same patient. Note the high anterior soft tissue density of the aneurysm (arrows).

the results are no better than chance even with experienced observers (Sos *et al.*, 1979). Left atrial enlargement in chronic ischaemic heart disease can indicate left ventricular failure or mitral regurgitation (see Chapter 7) but its absence excludes neither; if present it is rarely more than moderate and usually detected only as the double shadow of the heart to the right of the spine. The causes of its enlargement determine that it is rarely seen without evidence of a large left ventricle or overall cardiomegaly. A bulge easily mistaken for enlargement of the left atrial appendage is that due to coronary arteriovenous fistula arising from the proximal left coronary artery (Fig. 6.10) (a rare lesion but a recognised cause for myocardial ischaemia); visible enlargement of the left atrial appendage itself is unusual in ischaemic heart disease (Green *et al.*, 1982).

Left ventricular failure in ischaemic heart disease has such limited prognosis that it is unusual for chronic pulmonary arterial hypertension and its associated right heart changes to be seen. Occasionally myocardial infarction is predominantly right ventricular and the chest radiograph may then show development of right heart enlargement in the absence of left ventricular failure (Fig. 6.11). Apparent cardiomegaly in ischaemic heart disease can be due to pericardial effusion and though the post-myocardial infarction syndrome of pericarditis with effusion, pleural effusions and pulmonary infiltrates described by Dressler (1959) has recently been brought into question as a distinct entity (Kossowsky *et al.*, 1981) there is no doubt that prolonged pericarditis with effusion can complicate severe myocardial infarction and can be a cause of persistent 'cardiomegaly'.

Pulmonary vascular pattern. Evidence of pulmonary venous hypertension in ischaemic heart disease can reflect the increased filling pressure of a stiff (non compliant) ischaemic left ventricle of normal size (Diamond & Forrester, 1972) or frank left ventricular failure due to loss of contractile tissue from infarction. Other causes are papillary muscle dysfunction (rarely rupture) with mitral regurgitation, ruptured interventricular septum with volume overload from the left to right shunt overwhelming an already compromised ventricle, and left ventricular aneurysm. Radiological signs of pulmonary venous hypertension are usually seen in acute infarction when the left ventricular damage is such as to raise left atrial pressure above 18 mmHg. Exceptions occur and at lower levels of pulmonary venous hypertension the presence of radiological signs is variable; it is also known that these signs, even alveolar oedema, can be seen despite normal pulmonary venous pressure at the time of the radiograph. Such apparent inconsistencies have been attributed to time lags between pressure changes and consequent fluid shifts: radiological changes can lag behind acute elevation of pulmonary venous pressure for many hours,

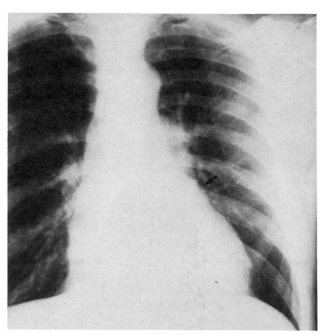

FIG. 6.10. Left mediastinal bulge (arrow) due to coronary arteriovenous fistula simulating left atrial appendage enlargement.

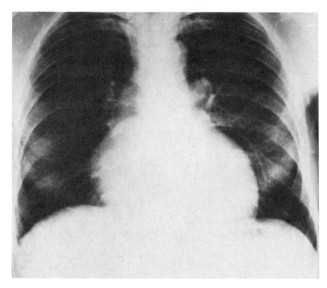

FIG. 6.11. Cardiomegaly due to right atrioventricular enlargement following right ventricular infarction complicated by tricuspid regurgitation.

the 'diagnostic phase lag' (Kostuck *et al.*, 1973) or persist for many days after its return to normal, the 'therapeutic phase lag' (McHugh *et al.*, 1972). It follows that therapeutic intervention in the haemodynamic disturbances of acute myocardial infarction cannot be based on radiographs alone but this is not to deny that the chest film has value: subclinical left ventricular failure diagnosed from admission chest radiographs helps predict those who will subsequently develop clinical failure (Chait *et al.*, 1972) and the presence and severity of the radiological signs correlates with both early and late mortality (Battler *et al.*, 1980), allowing high risk groups to be defined.

Some rise in arterial pressure accompanies pulmonary venous hypertension but it is unusual to become disproportionate in the limited survival time of severe ischaemic left ventricular dysfunction and radiological signs of pulmonary arterial hypertension are rare in this condition.

Lung opacities (other than those of pulmonary oedema), particularly basal band shadows, are common transient findings during the course of acute myocardial infarction and are attributed to pulmonary infarcts; autopsy evidence of major emboli has been reported in 11% of deaths from acute myocardial infarction (Davies *et al.*, 1976). Transmural myocardial infarction has been described as a cause of pleuropericardial adhesions visible as small triangular shadows based on the left ventricle (Groden & James, 1968) (Fig. 6.08*a*).

ECHOCARDIOGRAPHY

Two-dimensional echocardiography can demonstrate coronary artery stenosis (Rink *et al.*, 1982) and aneurysms (Chung *et al.*, 1982) but only in very proximal segments, usually the main left coronary artery alone, and even here with some technical difficulty. Despite its present limitations in study of the arteries themselves, echocardiography is of value in investigating the effects of coronary artery disease for myocardial contraction and relaxation, thickness and, to some extent, even composition can be assessed by both two-dimensional and M-mode techniques. Demonstration of the myocardium in addition to the chamber cavities of the heart is an advantage echocardiography enjoys over both radionuclide and conventional contrast angiography (computed tomography and nuclear magnetic resonance share this advantage but cannot yet be considered readily available alternatives!). Two-dimensional studies utilising all available 'windows' and sections can demonstrate virtually all the left ventricle while M-mode is limited by its single static transducer to relatively small segments of the interventricular septum and posterior wall and an even smaller part of the anterior wall; M-mode does, however, allow more complex time–motion analysis than is yet available for two-dimensional images and complementary information can be gained from the two techniques.

Regional variations in left ventricular wall motion, so typical of ischaemic heart disease and described in the section on left ventriculography, can be shown non-invasively by two-dimensional echocardiography and frozen frames of a gross example, an aneurysm, are shown in Fig. 6.12. Ischaemia not only alters segmental wall motion but can also reduce wall thickness and diminish or even reverse the thickening which normally occurs with systole (Corya *et al.*, 1977) while normal areas of a ventricle in this patchy disease may show exaggerated systolic motion and thickening; altered relaxation patterns may similarly occur in both diseased and normal areas, and such features are particularly well shown by M-mode records (Doran *et al.*, 1978). Fibrosis alters the acoustic properties of the myocardium and areas of scar can be more echogenic though thinner than the normal myocardium (Rasmussen *et al.*, 1977). Assessment of left ventricular volumes and ejection fraction from M-mode measurement of a cavity dimension and its change with the cardiac cycle in necessarily limited areas of the ventricle is suspect in ischaemic heart disease (Teichholz *et al.*, 1976) but the diastolic diameter alone is a guide to ventricular function and the distance between the E point of the anterior mitral cusp and the interventricular septum also has value in this respect (Massie *et al.*, 1977). The anterior cusp echo itself gives evidence of elevated left ventricular end disastolic pressure when the A-C segment is prolonged and notched (Feigenbaum *et al.*, 1976). Emphasis is obviously given to assessment of left ventricular function in ischaemic heart disease and indeed the right ventricle usually shows vigorous motion; if dilated and hypokinetic it has probably suffered infarction (Lorell *et al.*, 1979).

Echocardiography is particularly appropriate to the investigation of the mechanical complications of myocardial infarction, not least because it is non-invasive and can be performed at the bedside. A two-dimensional study can show left ventricular aneurysm (Visser *et al.*, 1982) and allows functional assessment of residual myocardium. False aneurysm due to a contained localised myocardial rupture into the pericardium (Mills *et al.*, 1977) and ruptured interventricular septum (Mintz *et al.*, 1981) can be diagnosed and the value of echocardiography in mitral regurgitation due to papillary muscle damage is indicated in Chapter 7. Intraventricular thrombus complicating infarct or aneurysm is well shown (Stratton *et al.*, 1981) and echocardiography is to be recommended in cases of unexplained arterial embolism (ventricular thrombus is a commoner source than left atrial thrombus or tumour). Pericardial effusion can occur in the acute or recovery stages of myocardial infarction and echocardiography is the investigation of choice when it is suspected. The potential for echocardiography in the investigation of ischaemic heart disease is obvious but its exact place is not yet defined; evaluation of the mechanical complications of myocardial infarction seems its most valued current use.

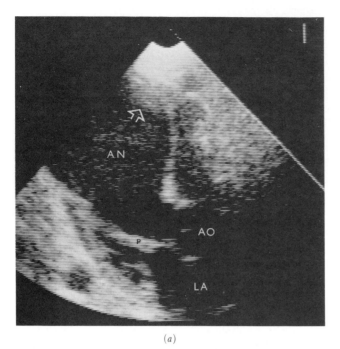
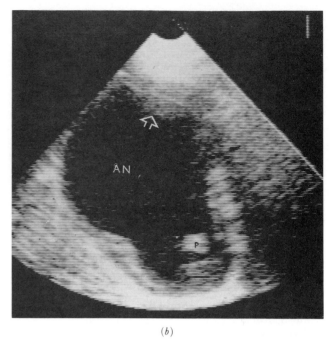

(a)   (b)

FIG. 6.12. Long (a) and short (b) axis parasternal views of left ventricular aneurysm and contained (arrowed) thrombus, confirmed at surgery. AO, aorta; LA, left atrium; P, papillary muscle; AN, aneurysm.

RADIONUCLIDE STUDIES

Those appropriate to ischaemic heart disease have been detailed in Chapter 5; the rapid expansion of available techniques and their importance in diagnosis and management is reflected in the extensive literature of nuclear cardiology, best sampled by the non-specialist through reviews such as those of Donaldson & Ell, 1981 or Berger & Zaret, 1981. In bare summary, myocardial infarction can be imaged in the acute stage as a scintigraphic 'hot spot' following intravenous injection of an infarct avid radiopharmaceutical (e.g. technetium-99 m phosphate) or as an area of decreased uptake of a marker of perfusion (thallium-201) but the latter 'cold spot' imaging at rest does not distinguish between old and new infarcts or even transient rest ischaemia. Decreased thallium-201 uptake immediately following exercise in an area of normal uptake in the redistribution phase 2–4 hours later (equivalent to rest) indicates reversible ischaemia. Left ventricular function can be assessed by radionuclide angiocardiography using first pass studies (with technetium-99 m or, more recently, short half-life radionuclides such as gold-195 m) or multiple gated acquisition at equilibrium (again with technetium-99 m); these techniques provide data, which can include cinefilm images, giving ejection fraction and regional wall motion pattern non-invasively and repetitively, at rest or with stress. Nuclear probe detectors provide a relatively cheap and considerably more port-

able alternative to scintillation cameras in first pass and equilibrium studies and allow estimation of global left ventricular function but, without images, regional wall motion is not defined.

The expense of acute infarct scanning cannot generally be justified but is of value where conventional clinical and laboratory tests are equivocal, for example when electrocardiographic interpretation is hampered by prior abnormality, when clinical presentation is late or when acute infarction is suspected after cardioversion or trauma (including cardiac surgery). The categorization of chest pain as that of myocardial ischaemia by stress testing is most cheaply accomplished by exercise electrocardiography but increased accuracy is gained from radionuclide studies (assessment of changes in ejection fraction, regional wall motion or myocardial perfusion with stress), which are a justified addition when the conventional test is equivocal and a better primary test when resting electrocardiographic changes hamper interpretation or in conditions where false positive electrocardiographic changes are recognised to occur (e.g. mitral valve prolapse). In patients with established ischaemic heart disease, radionuclide study of regional ischaemia can aid evaluation of coronary artery stenoses of doubtful arteriographic significance; pre- and postoperative studies provide a method for assessing efficacy of bypass grafting or angioplasty for coronary disease. Radionuclide angiocardiography in patients with cardiac failure due to the complications of previous myocardial infarction allows selection of those likely to benefit from surgery (e.g. aneurysmectomy) and who therefore require cardiac catheterisation for further assessment; it can obviate the need for such invasive investigation when surgery is clearly inappropriate in cases of severe and diffuse left ventricular dilation and wall motion abnormality. Non-invasive cardiac imaging is a rapidly developing field in which radionuclide techniques currently have pre-eminence for the screening of suspected ischaemic heart disease and the functional assessment of established ischaemic heart disease; given this and the epidemic proportions of the disease in the Western world, nuclear cardiology is seen as an essential facility in specialist centres and desirable in referring hospitals.

CARDIAC CATHETERIZATION: ANGIOCARDIOGRAPHY

The catheter investigation of ischaemic heart disease is often summarised as 'coronary arteriography' but the arteriogram is usually preceded by left ventricular pressure measurement and left ventriculography and these three form the core of an invasive study which may, depending on clinical need or research protocol, also include right heart catheterisation, stress testing such as atrial pacing, transmyocardial blood (aortic and coronary sinus) sampling for markers of ischaemia and various pharmacological interventions. Recent advances in ultrasound, radionuclide and computer enhanced X-ray imaging have eroded the advantages of the high quality cine ventriculography obtained by left ventricular catheterisation to the point where it is hard to justify as an isolated study for ventricular function but selective cine coronary arteriography remains the final arbiter of coronary disease and anatomy.

The procedure is not without risk but continued refinement has reduced this to levels where it is apparently acceptable as a screening test for continued employment in some groups (Froelicher et al., 1977)! A recent collaborative study of the complications of coronary arteriography in patients suspected of coronary artery disease showed a mortality rate of 0·2% and a non-fatal myocardial infarction rate of 0·25% (Davis et al.m 1979); other possible complications include cerebral embolus, arrhythmias and the usual list common to all vascular catheterisations and contrast angiography.

Indications for the study show wide national and international variation, but in general it is undertaken in three broad groups of patients: (1) those with known or suspected ischaemic heart disease (or those in whom it cannot otherwise be excluded) where the benefit of precise documentation or exclusion of disease outweighs the risks of the procedure; (2) those awaiting forms of cardiac surgery for which precise knowledge of coronary disease or anatomy is a prerequisite; (3) those in whom the procedure is part of a therapeutic catheter intervention such as angioplasty or intracoronary thrombolytic infusion. Given these indications, contraindications can be generalised as those circumstances where the procedure carries a risk unacceptable to the patient or physician; these circumstances may relate to the fitness of the patient or of the institution and it should be noted that there has been little dissent from the editorial comment of Judkins & Gander (1974) that coronary arteriography should not be continued in institutions where the procedure carries a mortality greater than 0·3%.

Left ventriculography is preceded by base line pressure measurements and is performed before coronary arteriography because of the adverse effects of intraventricular and intracoronary contrast medium on left ventricular function. Some elevation of left ventricular end disastolic pressure is normal after ventriculography but an increase to 18 mmHg or more after injection of high osmolality contrast medium indicates left ventricular dysfunction (Brundage & Cheitlin, 1973) and has some value as a positive stress test when resting pressures are normal; there is obvious risk of cardiac decompensation where left ventricular function is impaired. Adverse effects are considerably less with the new low osmolality contrast media (Cumberland, 1981; Partridge et al., 1981) and it is a pleasure to sacrifice the stress test in the interests of patient safety quite apart from the markedly better subjective tolerance for the new media.

Cine ventriculography in the right anterior oblique projection (generally preferred for a single plane study as it places the ventricular long axis at right angles to the X-ray beam) shows anterior, inferior and apical wall motion, as judged by their endocardial surfaces, and allows assessment of any mitral regurgitation present. The left anterior oblique projection is necessary to show the posterior wall and septum and should be included if there is biplane facility or added if full ventriculographic assessment is necessary (Cohn et al., 1974a) for example with left ventricular aneurysm. The value of the left anterior oblique is improved by adding 25° caudocranial angulation (Rogers et al., 1982).

The normal left ventricular contraction pattern shown by cine ventriculography was described by Herman & Gorlin (1969) as a 'uniform, almost concentric inward motion of all points along its inner surface during systolic ejection' though an early systolic outward bulge of the high posterior wall can occur (Adams et al., 1972). Normal diastole is more steplike: an initial outward motion in the isovolumic period of early relaxation is usually seen in the anterior and apical regions (Ruttley et al., 1974); this is followed by generalised expansion in the rapid filling phase and finally by a late diastolic expansion due to atrial systole.

Disordered systolic wall motion, asynergy (Harrison, 1965), is seen in ischaemic injury and the ventriculographic appearances were categorized by Herman and his fellow workers as (1) *akinesis*, a total lack of motion of a portion of the ventricular wall, (2) *asyneresis*, diminished motion of a part of the wall, (3) *dyskinesis*, paradoxical systolic expansion of a part of the wall, and (4) *asynchrony*, a disturbed temporal sequence of contraction (Herman *et al.*, 1967); *hypokinesis* was reserved for generalised reduction in left ventricular contraction but, in common use, hypokinesis of a specified area has

replaced the term asyneresis. Dyskinesis, local or general, has been confusingly used in later British literature (Gahl *et al.*, 1978) in substitution for hypokinesis. Regional alterations in relaxation are also present in the asynergic ventricle but require complex analysis (Gibson *et al.*, 1976). Asynergy can be due to ischaemia of viable myocardium, necrosis or subsequent fibrosis and its severity tends to reflect the degree of injury: hypokinesis suggests ischaemia (Fig. 6.13) and akinesis or dyskinesis suggests old or new transmural infarction (Fig. 6.14). Stress (rapid atrial pacing, exercise) and

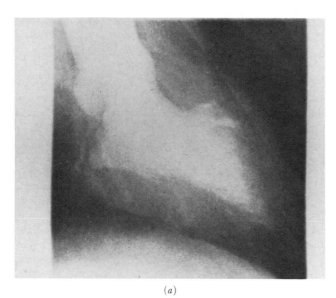

(a)

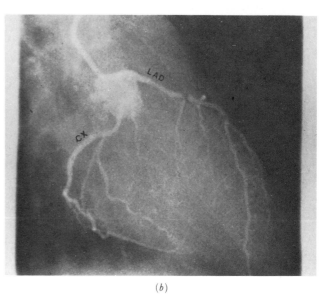

(b)

Fig. 6.13. (a) Left ventriculogram, right anterior oblique projection, end systolic frame showing slight anterior hypokinesis. (b) Same patient. Causative LAD stenosis.

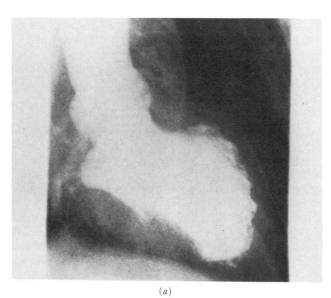

(a)

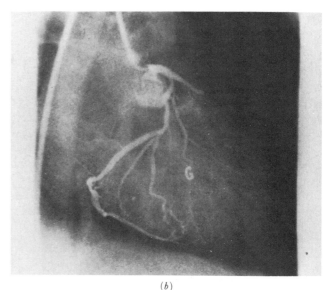

(b)

Fig. 6.14. (a) Same patient as Fig. 6.13. Following anterolateral infarction while on surgical waiting list. End systolic frame showing anteroapical akinetic bulge. (b) Same patient. LAD stenosis has progressed to occlusion.

drugs (notably glyceryl trinitrate) have been used respectively to produce or reduce asynergy in patients with coronary disease (Pasternac *et al.*, 1972; Sharma *et al.*, 1976; Helfant *et al.*, 1974) and such demonstration of reversible ischaemic effect has obvious implication in the assessment of coronary lesions and in choice of surgery; similar information can now be obtained non-invasively (e.g. radionuclide studies), removing the need for multiple catheter ventriculograms but even the standard ventriculogram, with its all too common ventricular extrasystoles, can be of use as a potentiated postextrasystolic beat gives 'free' assessment of improvement in contraction (Dyke *et al.*, 1974). Note must be taken of a patient's drug therapy in evaluation of the left ventriculogram as beta blockade can induce or exaggerate asynergy (Helfant *et al.*, 1971).

The most severe and extensive asynergy is seen with left ventricular aneurysm which, in the most quoted definition, is 'a protrusion of a localised portion of the external aspect of the left ventricle beyond the remainder of the cardiac surface, with simultaneous protrusion of the cavity as well' (Edwards, 1961). Such aneurysms are recognised by pathologists and surgeons as fibrous sacs and at ventriculography appear as large areas of akinesis, less commonly dyskinesis, or a mixture of both, usually associated with a bulge persisting through diastole (Fig. 6.15). The ventriculographic features are not specific to fibrous aneurysms and can be seen in lesser degree with acute or chronic infarcts and even in areas of viable ischaemic myocardium (which more

typically show hypokinesis); these were considered 'functional' aneurysms by Gorlin and his fellow workers and included with fibrous aneurysms in their classic paper (Gorlin *et al.*, 1967). It is not always clear in subsequent literature whether a pathological or ventriculographic definition of aneurysm is used. Their pathophysiological effects relate mainly to size (Klein *et al.*, 1967) and are similar whatever the definition but surgery, if indicated, would differ between resection of a fibrous sac and revascularisation of a 'functional' aneurysm of viable myocardium; distinction is therefore desirable and pointers to fibrous aneurysm are large size, thin wall and sharp demarcation from normal ventricle (Raphael *et al.*, 1972).

False aneurysm is typically inferior or posterior (Fig. 6.16) and has a narrow neck and no overlying coronary arteries (Higgins *et al.*, 1978); such distinguishing features are of value as the lesion has a high incidence of fatal perforation which is rare with true aneurysm.

Intraventricular thrombus occurring in asynergic areas is seen as contained filling defect (Fig. 6.17) separate from the papillary muscles or, when laminar and apical, as amputation of the cavity (Fig. 6.18).

The left to right shunt of contrast medium which occurs with ruptured interventricular septum is easily detected by left ventriculography but the actual site of the muscular septal defect is difficult to locate even in the left anterior oblique projection which profiles much of the septum (Fig. 6.19). It is indirectly located by the

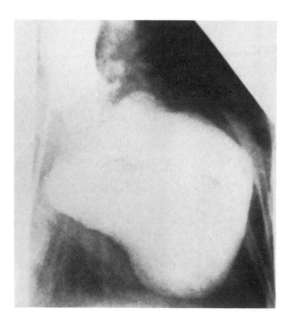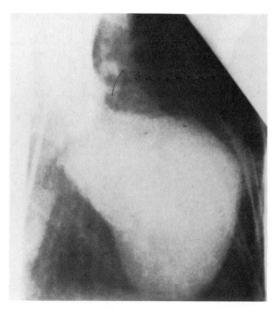

FIG. 6.15. Left ventriculogram, right anterior oblique projection, end diastolic and end systolic frames. Fibrous aneurysm of anterolateral wall and apex.

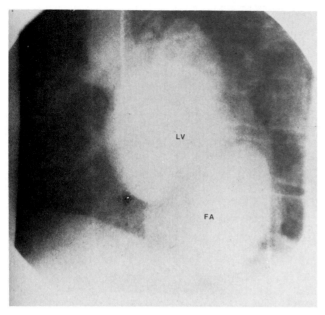

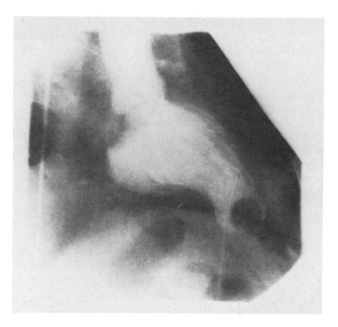

FIG. 6.16. Left ventriculogram, left anterior oblique projection. Two cavities shown, left ventricle (LV) above, false aneurysm (FA) below. Faint left atrial opacity indicates mitral regurgitation.

FIG. 6.17. Left ventriculogram showing a ball of thrombus in a localised apical aneurysm.

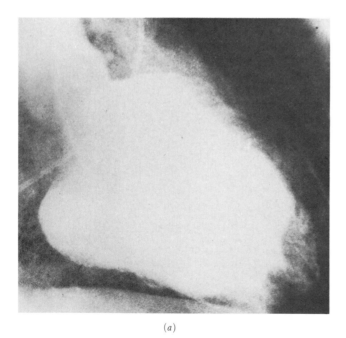

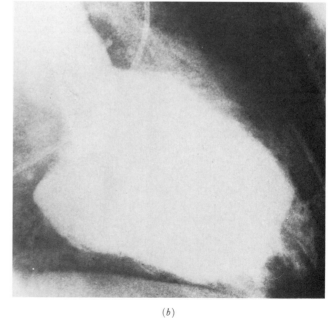

(a)   (b)

FIG. 6.18. Left ventriculogram, right anterior oblique projection, end diastolic and end systolic frames (which is which?). Diffuse gross asynergy (ischaemic cardiomyopathy) with apical cut-off due to contained and laminar thrombus.

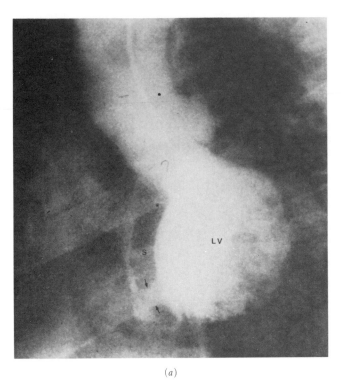
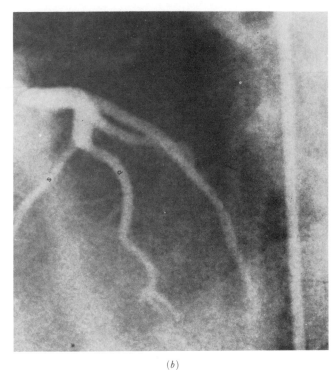

(a)   (b)

FIG. 6.19. (a) Left ventriculogram, left anterior oblique projection. Unusual (localised, small and well shown) acquired ventricular septal defect (arrowed). LV, left ventricle; S, septum. (b) Same patient. Left coronary arteriogram. LAD occlusion shear beyond diagonal (d) and septal (s) branches. Such shear occlusions make for difficult diagnosis.

site of observed asynergy and the known territory of supply of the diseased coronary artery responsible (Miller *et al.*, 1978).

The ventriculographic features of mitral regurgitation in ischaemic heart disease are described in Chapter 7.

Quantitative analysis of the left ventriculogram allows calculation of left ventricular volumes, ejection fraction and many other parameters of left ventricular function; the mathematical basis and techniques involved are beyond the scope of this work and the interested reader is referred to reviews such as those of Dodge (1971) or Rackley (1976). It can be noted here that the most widely applied parameter, ejection fraction (the ratio of stroke volume to end diastolic volume), is easily derived from area (A) and length (L) measurements of the projected end diastolic (ed) and end systolic (es) cavity images by the formula $EF = (A^2_{ed}/L_{ed} - A^2_{es}/L_{es}) \div (A^2_{ed}/L_{ed})$. The ejection fraction has been shown to have importance in predicting the morbidity and mortality of coronary artery bypass surgery (Cohn *et al.*, 1974*b*), and therefore, of importance in the ventriculographic assessment of ischaemic heart disease.

Coronary arteriography now is the selective coronary arterial injection of radiopaque contrast material visualised by indirect radiography through an image

intensification system and permanently recorded on cine film. In the past, non-selective arteriograms were obtained from aortic root injections (Paulin, 1972) and in the future it seems possible that digital subtraction techniques will allow a return to non-selective (or even 'venous') arteriography with obvious patient and economic benefit.

Description of the practical techniques of selective catheterisation, learned by apprenticeship, is not appropriate here and the reader is referred to the originators' descriptions of the brachial arterial cutdown (Sones & Shirley, 1962) and the percutaneous transfemoral (Judkins, 1968) approaches. Multiple radiographic projections are necessary for delineation of the multidirectional coronary arteries: the main left coronary artery and its proximal branches lie to varying degrees in the transverse plane of the patient and the traditional transverse projections give considerable foreshortening and overlap of these important segments (Fig. 6.20); the value of hemiaxial projections to demonstrate lesions otherwise obscured (Fig. 6.21) was recognised in the early 1970's (Bunnell *et al.*, 1973) and led to considerable modification of angiocardiographic equipment, a subject recently reviewed (Guthaner & Wexler, 1980).

The object of coronary arteriography is to document

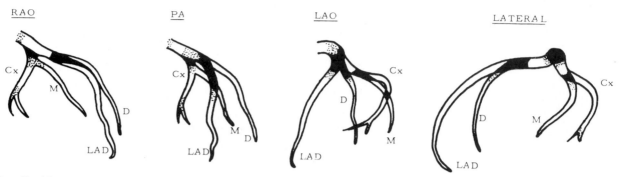

FIG. 6.20. Semidiagrammatic left coronary arteriogram. Severity of overlap/foreshortening indicated by density of shading. Note the persistently 'blind' segment of proximal LAD.

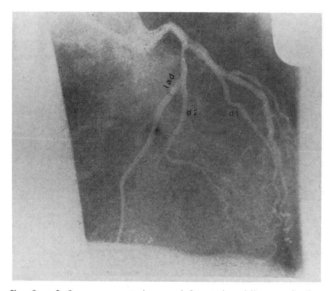

FIG. 6.21. Left coronary arteriogram, left anterior oblique projection with 20° caudo-cranial tilt. Obvious LAD stenosis between first and second diagonal branches (d₁ and d₂). This was completely obscured by foreshortening and overlap (from d₁) in the four standard transverse plane views.

or exclude coronary disease and an incomplete or non-diagnostic examination has been categorised by Judkins & Gander (1974) as a severe complication adversely affecting patient management; the same is true of misinterpretation. The examination must show each segment of the major arteries free of foreshortening and of overlapping branches in at least two projections. Anatomical variants must be recognised (preferably during the examination as aberrant origins from the aorta require separate injection) for they can otherwise result in 'missed' vessels or simulate disease; in rare instances they cause cardiac dysfunction (Cheitlin *et al.*, 1974; Roberts *et al.*, 1982). Myocardial bridging of all

the large epicardial arteries is a frequent autopsy finding manifest less often arteriographically as phasic systolic narrowing strangely confined to one branch, the left anterior descending (Fig. 6.22); its functional significance is uncertain (Kramer *et al.*, 1982; MacAlpin, 1982) and it must be differentiated from spasm and fixed stenosis. Apart from major congenital abnormalities such as coronary artery origin from pulmonary artery and coronary arteriovenous fistula (Edwards, 1958), the arteriographic manifestations of coronary disease are limited to marginal irregularity, filling defect, stenosis and occlusion (fixed or variable), dilation (ectasia) and a visible collateral circulation. All of these can be seen in coronary atherosclerosis which is by far the commonest cause for any one though none is specific for that disease and some alternative causes are listed in the introduction. A stenosis or occlusion that is variable during an examination indicates spasm which may be catheter induced (typically at the catheter tip and asymptomatic), associated with atherosclerosis or a significant isolated finding in otherwise normal arteries.

The haemodynamic significance of occlusion (Figs. 6.14*b* and 6.19*b*) is obvious, that of stenosis (Figs. 6.13*b* and 6.23) or filling defect (Fig. 6.24) depends on the degree of obstruction and that of ectasia (Fig. 6.25) is uncertain (Swanton *et al.*, 1978). A 75% stenosis is generally agreed to be significant though it is often not stated whether this is an estimated cross sectional area or diameter reduction (diameter reduction of 50% = cross sectional area reduction of 75% if the lesion is concentric) and the problem is aggravated by the state of the adjacent 'marker' vessel; can it really be assumed to have the 100% patency by which the stenosis is judged in a disease such as atherosclerosis? Eccentricity (Fig. 6.26), length and multiplicity of stenoses add to the confusion of what must be a subjective assessment. Localised delay in flow of contrast medium across a diseased segment indicates significance as does

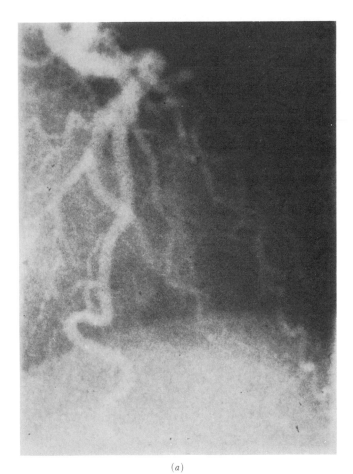

(a)

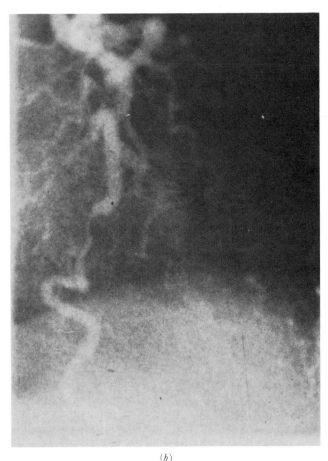

(b)

FIG. 6.22. (a) Left coronary arteriogram, PA projection diastolic frame showing normal LAD. (b) Same study. Systolic frame showing LAD stenosis; typical systolic squeeze due to myocardial bridging (this segment of vessel dipped into the myocardium).

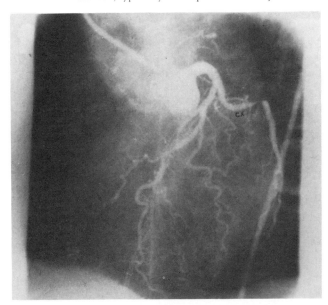

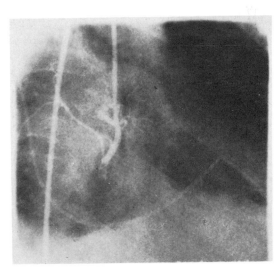

FIG. 6.23. Left coronary arteriogram, standard left anterior oblique projection. Circumflex stenosis. Note right ventricular branch of LAD (arrow), a collateral to a diseased right coronary artery.

FIG. 6.24. Right coronary arteriogram, right anterior oblique projection. Right coronary occlusion with contained filling defect (thrombus) in patient with evolving myocardial infarction.

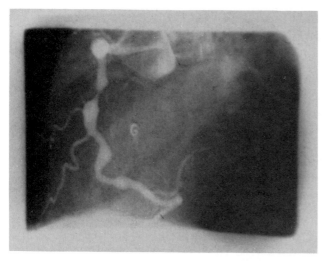

FIG. 6.25. Right coronary arteriogram, left anterior oblique projection. Stenosis and ectasia. 'G' indicates glyceryl trinitrate given.

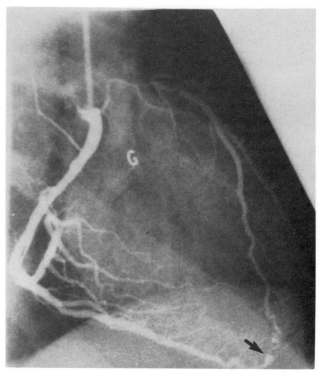

collateral supply to the distal vessel (Figs. 6.23 and 6.27); these features are unusual with lesions of less than 75% diameter stenosis which require other evidence (e.g. ventriculographic, metabolic or radionuclide evidence of ischaemic effect at rest or with stress) before they can be ascribed certain significance. It should be noted of collaterals that though their functional significance is debated (Newman, 1981) their inflow into arteries beyond a severe stenosis or obstruction (typically localised in coronary disease) can be assumed to maintain distal vessel patency and also allows arterio-

FIG. 6.27. Right coronary arteriogram after glyceryl trinitrate ('G'), right anterior oblique projection. Proximal LAD occlusion known from left coronary injection; note collateral filling of LAD to the point of occlusion by apical (arrow) collaterals between the posterior descending branch of the right coronary artery and the LAD.

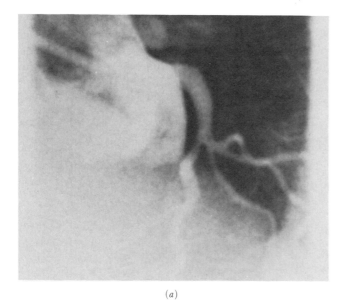

(a)

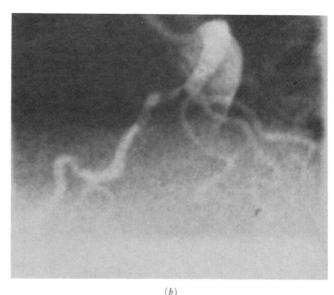

(b)

FIG. 6.26. Left coronary arteriogram in two caudo-cranial projections; (a) left anterior oblique, (b) lateral. The very localised eccentric stenosis was only shown in the lateral caudo-cranial view. Objective evidence of ischaemia in LAD territory present.

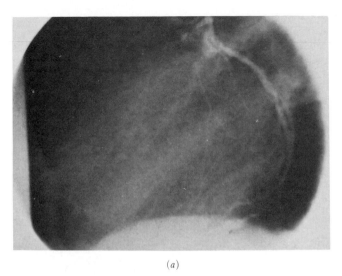

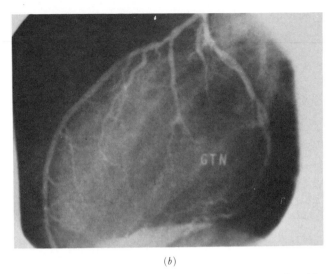

(a)   (b)

Fig. 6.28. Left coronary arteriograms, lateral projection. Spasm superimposed on atherosclerosis giving LAD occlusion which was relieved by glyceryl trinitrate (GTN). Unstable angina!

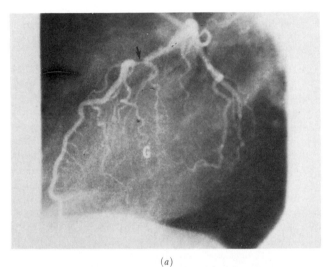

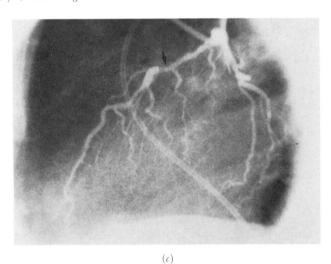

(a)

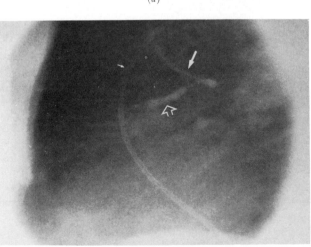

(b)

(c)

Fig. 6.29. (a) Left coronary arteriogram, lateral projection. LAD stenosis (arrow). (b) Gruntzig balloon dilated (open arrow) at stenosis site. Large closed arrow, guide catheter in left coronary ostium. Small arrow, pulmonary artery catheter. (c) LAD after angioplasty (identical appearance shown at 9 months).

graphic assessment of its suitability as a bypass graft recipient. The various collateral pathways seen arteriographically have been elegantly shown by Paulin (1967). The reporting of a coronary arteriogram must indicate an assessment of severity of lesions as well as site and multiplicity and should ideally relate these findings to the myocardium compromised or at risk (which will be influenced by coronary anatomy as well as disease). Scoring systems have been advocated (e.g. Brandt *et al.*, 1977; Gensini, 1983) but none has been universally adopted. Coronary artery spasm in isolation

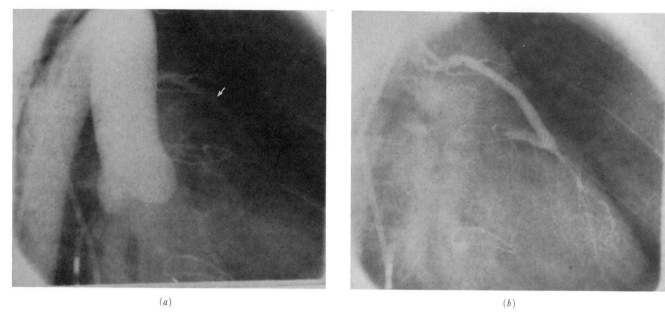

(a)   (b)

FIG. 6.30. (a) Aortogram. Right anterior oblique projection. Aortocoronary vein graft arrowed. (b) Same patient. Selective vein graft injection.

or associated with atherosclerosis is now a recognised cause of myocardial ischaemia (Maseri, 1975), particularly seen in patients with spontaneous angina. It was documented by aortography in 1962 (Gensini et al., 1962) and by selective coronary arteriography a decade later (Dhurandhar et al., 1972). Arteriographic proof of spasm requires recorded abolition or reduction of stenosis or occlusion spontaneously or with a vasodilator, e.g. glyceryl trinitrate (Fig. 6.28), or pharmacological provocation, e.g. by ergometrine (Heupler et al., 1978). It should be noted that ergometrine can also provoke oesophageal spasm, a well-known mimic of cardiac pain (Dart et al., 1980).

Interventional coronary arteriography has progressed beyond pharmacological provocation and the pioneering work of Gruntzig and his colleagues (Gruntzig, 1978) has established percutaneous coronary angioplasty as an effective and widely applied treatment for coronary stenosis (Kent et al., 1982); an illustrative case is shown in Fig. 29. Catheter treatment of ischaemic heart disease also includes intracoronary infusion thrombolysis of the occluding thrombus so commonly found arteriographically in cases of evolving myocardial infarction (Fig. 6.24); this has been combined with angioplasty of the underlying stenosis but such therapies require further evaluation before widespread application (Swan, 1982).

Not all coronary artery bypass graft surgery is successful and the underlying disease process is not abolished by such palliative treatment. Coronary arteriography for postoperative assessment of graft patency is routine in some centres and reserved for symptomatic patients in others. The grafts arise from mid ascending aorta and patency can be established by left ventriculography or aortography (Fig. 6.30a) but selective injection (Fig. 6.30b) is required for complete assessment of the graft and recipient vessel; arteriography of the native arteries is also required to assess disease progress.

OTHER EXAMINATIONS

Computed tomography (Brundage & Lipton, 1982), *nuclear magnetic resonance* (Worthington, 1983) and *digital subtraction left ventriculography* (Tobias et al., 1982) will all command separate and detailed description in the near future but the only commonly applied current application of these exciting developments is assessment of aortocoronary vein grafts by computed tomography; patency can be established with a high degree of accuracy but arteriographic study is still required for symptomatic patients being assessed for further operation.

REFERENCES

ADAMS, D. F., ABRAMS, H. L. & RUTTLEY, M. (1972) The roentgen pathology of coronary artery disease. *Sem. Roentgenol.*, **7**, 319–351.

BATTLER, A., KARLINER, J. S., HIGGINS, C. B., SLUTSKY, R., GILPIN, E. A., FROELICHER, V. F. & ROSS, J. (1980) The initial chest x-ray in acute myocardial infarction. *Circulation*, **61**, 1004–1009.

BERGER, H. J. & ZARET, B. L. (1981) Nuclear cardiology. *New Eng. J. Med.*, **305**, 799–807 and 855–865.

BRANDT, P. W. T., PARTRIDGE, J. B. & WATTIE, W. J. (1977) Coronary arteriography: method of presentation of the arteriogram report and a scoring system. *Clin. Radiol.*, **28**, 361–365.

BRUNDAGE, B. H. & CHEITLIN, M. D. (1973) Left ventricular angiography as a function test. *Chest*, **64**, 70–74.

BRUNDAGE, B. H. & LIPTON, M. J. (1982) The emergence of computed tomography as a cardiovascular diagnostic technique. *Amer. Heart J.*, **103**, 313–316.

BUNNELL, I. L., GREENE, D. G., TANDON, R. N. & ARANI, D. T. (1973) The half-axial projection. A new look at the proximal left coronary artery. *Circulation*, **48**, 1151–1156.

BURCH, G. E., GILES, T. D. & COLCOLOUGH, H. L. (1970) Editorial—Ischemic cardiomyopathy. *Amer. Heart J.*, **79**, 291–292.

CHAIT, A., COHEN, H. E., MELTZER, L. E. & VANDURME, J. P. (1972) The bedside chest radiograph in the evaluation of incipient heart failure. *Radiology*, **105**, 563–566.

CHEITLIN, M. D., DE CASTRO, C. M. & MCALLISTER, H. A. (1974) Sudden death as a complication of anomalous left coronary origin from the anterior sinus of valsalva. A not-so-minor congenital anomaly. *Circulation*, **50**, 780–787.

CHENG, T. O. (1971) Incidence of ventricular aneurysm in coronary artery disease. An angiographic appraisal. *Amer. J. Med.*, **50**, 340–355.

CHUNG, K. J., BRANDT, L., FULTON, D. R. & KREIDBERG, M. B. (1982) Cardiac and coronary arterial involvement in infants and children from New England with mucocutaneous lymph node syndrome (Kawasaki disease). Angiocardiographic-echocardiographic correlations. *Amer. J. Cardiol.*, **50**, 136–142.

COHN, P. F., GORLIN, R., COHN, L. H. & COLLINS, J. J. (1974a) Left ventricular ejection fraction as a prognostic guide in surgical treatment of coronary and valvular heart disease. *Amer. J. Cardiol.*, **34**, 136–141.

COHN, P. F., GORLIN, R., ADAMS, D. F., CHAHINE, R. A., VOKONAS, P. S. & HERMAN, M. V. (1974b) Comparison of biplane and single plane left ventriculograms in patients with coronary artery disease. *Amer. J. Cardiol.*, **33**, 1–6.

CORYA, B. C., RASMUSSEN, S., FEIGENBAUM, H., KNOEBEL, S. B. & BLACK, M. J. (1977) Systolic thickening and thinning of the septum and posterior wall in patients with coronary artery disease, congestive cardiomyopathy, and atrial septal defect. *Circulation*, **55**, 109–114.

CUMBERLAND, D. C. (1981) Hexabrix—a new contrast medium in angiocardiography. *Brit. Heart J.*, **45**, 698–702.

DART, A. M., ALBAN DAVIES, H., LOWNDES, R. H., DALAL, J., RUTTLEY, M. & HENDERSON, A. H. (1980) Oesophageal spasm and angina: diagnostic value of ergometrine (ergonovine) provocation. *Eur. Heart. J.*, **1**, 91–95.

DAVIES, M. J., WOOLF, N. & ROBERTSON, W. B. (1976) Pathology of acute myocardial infarction with particular reference to occlusive coronary thrombi. *Brit. Heart J.*, **38**, 659–664.

DAVIS, K., KENNEDY, J. W., KEMP, H. G., JUDKINS, M. P., GOSSELIN, A. J. & KILLIP, T. (1979) Complications of coronary arteriography from the collaborative study of coronary artery surgery. *Circulation*, **59**, 1105–1112.

DHURANDHAR, R. W., WATT, D. L., SILVER, M. D., TRIMBLE, A. S. & ADELMAN, A. G. (1972) Prinzmetal's variant form of angina with arteriographic evidence of coronary arterial spasm. *Amer. J. Cardiol.*, **30**, 902–905.

DIAMOND, G. & FORRESTER, J. S. (1972) Effect of coronary artery disease and acute myocardial infarction on left ventricular compliance in man. *Circulation*, **45**, 11–19.

DODGE, H. T. (1971) Determination of left ventricular volume and mass. *Radiol. Clin. N. Amer.*, **9**, 459–467.

DONALDSON, R. M. & ELL, P. J. (1981) Nuclear cardiology—a review. *Brit. J. Hosp. Med.*, February, 111–126.

DORAN, J. H., TRAILL, T. A., BROWN, D. J. & GIBSON, D. G. (1978) Detection of abnormal left ventricular wall movement during isovolumic contraction and early relaxation. Comparison of echo- and angiocardiography. *Brit. Heart J.*, **40**, 367–371.

DOTTER, C. T. & JUDKINS, M. P. (1964) Transluminal treatment of arteriosclerotic obstruction. *Circulation*, **30**, 654–670.

DRESSLER, W. (1959) The post-myocardial infarction syndrome. *Arch. Int. Med.*, **103**, 28–42.

DUBNOW, M. H., BURCHELL, H. B. & TITUS, J. L. (1965) Postinfarction ventricular aneurysm. A clinicomorphologic and electrocardiographic study of 80 cases. *Amer. Heart J.*, **70**, 753–760.

DYKE, S. H., COHN, P. F., GORLIN, R. & SONNENBLICK, E. H. (1974) Detection of residual myocardial function in coronary artery disease using post-extra systolic potentiation. *Circulation*, **50**, 694–699.

EDWARDS, J. E. (1958) Editorial—anomalous coronary arteries with special reference to arteriovenous-like communications. *Circulation*, **17**, 1001–1006.

EDWARDS, J. E. (1961) *An Atlas of Acquired Diseases of the Heart and Great Vessels*. Vol. 2. Philadelphia: Saunders.

FEIGENBAUM, H., CORYA, B. C., DILLON, J. C., WEYMAN, A. E., RASMUSSEN, S., BLACK, M. J. & CHANG, S. (1976) Role of echocardiography in patients with coronary artery disease. *Amer. J. Cardiol.*, **37**, 775–786.

FROELICHER, V. F., THOMPSON, A. J., WOLTHUIS, R., FUCHS, R., BALUSEK, R., LONGO, M. R., TRIEBWASSER, J. H. & LANCASTER, M. C. (1977) Angiographic findings in asymptomatic aircrewmen with electrocardiographic abnormalities. *Amer. J. Cardiol.*, **39**, 32–38.

GAHL, K., REES, S., SUTTON, R., CASPARI, P., LAIRET, A. & MCDONALD, L. (1978) Left ventricular contraction in coronary heart disease. *Clin. Radiol.*, **29**, 113–118.

GENSINI, G. G., DI GIORGI, S., MURAD-NETTO, S. & BLACK, A. (1962) Arteriographic demonstration of coronary artery spasm and its release after the use of a vasodilator in a case of angina pectoris and in the experimental animal. *Angiology*, **13**, 550–553.

GENSINI, G. G. (1983) A more meaningful scoring system for determining the severity of coronary heart disease. *Amer. J. Cardiol.*, **51**, 606.

GIBSON, D. C., PREWITT, T. A. & BROWN, D. J. (1976) Analysis of left ventricular wall movement during isovolumic relaxation and its relation to coronary artery disease. *Brit. Heart J.*, **38**, 1010–1019.

GORLIN, R., KLEIN, M. D. & SULLIVAN, J. M. (1967) Prospective correlative study of ventricular aneurysm. Mechanistic concept and clinical recognition. *Amer. J. Med.*, **42**, 512–531.

GREEN, C. E. & KELLEY, M. J. (1980) A renewed role for fluoroscopy in the evaluation of cardiac disease. *Radiol. Clin. N. Amer.*, **18**, 345–357.

GREEN, C. E., KELLEY, M. J. & HIGGINS, C. B. (1982) Etiologic significance of enlargement of the left atrial appendage in adults. *Radiology*, **142**, 21–27.

GRODEN, B. M. & JAMES, W. B. (1968) Radiological abnormalities in patients who have survived a myocardial infarction. Their possible relationship to aneurysm formation. *Brit. Heart J.*, **30**, 236–241.

GRUNTZIG, A. (1978) Transluminal dilatation of coronary artery stenosis. *Lancet*, i, 263.

GUTHANER, D. F. & WEXLER, L. (1980) New aspects of coronary angiography. *Radiol. Clin. N. Amer.*, **18**, 501–514.

HAMBY, R. I., TABRADH, F., WISOFF, B. G. & HARTSTEIN, M. L.

(1974) Coronary artery calcification: clinical implications and angiographic correlates. *Amer. Heart J.*, **87**, 565–570.

HARRISON, T. R. (1965) Some unanswered questions concerning enlargement and failure of the heart. *Amer. Heart J.*, **69**, 100–115.

HELFANT, R. H., HERMAN, M. V. & GORLIN, R. (1971) Abnormalities of left ventricular contraction induced by beta adrenergic blockade. *Circulation*, **33**, 641–647.

HELFANT, R. H., PINE, R., MEISTER, S. G., FELDMAN, M. S., TROUT, R. G. & BANKA, V. S. (1974) Nitroglycerin to unmask reversible asynergy. Correlation with post coronary bypass ventriculography. *Circulation*, **50**, 108–113.

HERMAN, M. V., HEINLE, R. A., KLEIN, M. D. & GORLIN, R. (1967) Localised disorders in myocardial contraction. Asynergy and its role in congestive heart failure. *New Eng. J. Med.*, **277**, 222–232.

HERMAN, M. V. & GORLIN, R. (1969) Implications of left ventricular asynergy. *Sem. Roentgen.*, **4**, 346.

HEUPLER, F. A., PROUDFIT, W. L., RAZAVI, M., SHIREY, E. K., GREENSTREET, R. & SHELDON, W. C. (1978) Ergonovine maleate provocative test for coronary arterial spasm. *Amer. J. Cardiol.*, **41**, 631–640.

HIGGINS, C. B., LIPTON, M. J., JOHNSON, A. D., PETERSON, K. L. & VIEWEG, W. V. R. (1978) False aneurysms of the left ventricle. *Radiology*, **127**, 21–27.

JUDKINS, M. P. (1968) Percutaneous transfemoral selective coronary arteriography. *Radiol. Clin. N. Amer.*, **6**, 467–492.

JUDKINS, M. P. & GANDER, M. P. (1974) Editorial—prevention of complications of coronary arteriography. *Circulation*, **49**, 599–602.

KENT, K. M., BENTIVOGLIO, L. G., BLOCK, P. C., COWLEY, M. J., DORROS, G., GOSSELIN, A. J., GRUNTZIG, A., MYLER, R. K., SIMPSON, J., STERTZER, S. H., WILLIAMS, D. O., FISHER, L., GILLESPIE, M. J., DETRE, K., KELSEY, S., MULLIN, S. M. & MOCK, M. B. (1982) Percutaneous transluminal coronary angioplasty: report from the registry of the national heart, lung and blood institute. *Amer. J. Cardiol.*, **49**, 2011–2020.

KLEIN, M. D., HERMAN, M. V. & GORLIN, R. (1967) A hemodynamic study of left ventricular aneurysm. *Circulation*, **35**, 614–630.

KOSSOWSKY, W. A., LYON, A. F. & SPAIN, D. M. (1981) Reappraisal of the postmyocardial infarction Dressler's syndrome. *Amer. Heart J.*, **102**, 954–956.

KOSTUK, W., BARR, J. W., SIMON, A. L. & ROSS, J. (1973) Correlations between the chest film and hemodynamics in acute myocardial infarction. *Circulation*, **48**, 624–632.

KRAMER, J. R., KITAZUME, H., PROUDFIT, W. L. & SONES, F. M. (1982) Clinical significance of isolated coronary bridges: benign and frequent condition involving the left anterior descending artery. *Amer. Heart J.*, **103**, 283–288.

LAME, E. L. & REDICK, T. J. (1970) A bedside cassette holder for 6 foot posteroanterior chest radiographs in comfort. *Radiology*, **95**, 698–699.

LORRELL, B., LEINBACH, R. C., POHOST, G. M., GOLD, H. K., DINSMORE, R. E., HUTTER, A. M., PASTORE, J. O. & DESANCTIS, R. W. (1979) Right ventricular infarction. Clinical diagnosis and differentiation from cardiac tamponade and pericardial constriction. *Amer. J. Cardiol.*, **43**, 465–471.

MACALPIN, R. N. (1982) Clinical significance of myocardial bridges. *Amer. Heart J.*, **104**, 648–649.

McHUGH, T. J., FORRESTER, J. S., ADLER, L., ZION, D. & SWAN, H. J. C. (1972) Pulmonary vascular congestion in acute myocardial infarction: hemodynamic and radiologic correlations. *Ann. Int. Med.*, **76**, 29–33.

MASERI, A., MIMMO, R., CHIERCHIA, S., MARCHESI, C., PESOLA, A. & L'ABBATE, A. (1975) Coronary artery spasm as a cause of acute myocardial ischemia in man. *Chest*, **68**, 625–633.

MASSIE, B. M., SCHILLER, N. B., RATSHIN, R. A. & PARMLEY, W. W. (1977) Mitral-septal separation: new echocardiographic index of left ventricular function. *Amer. J. Cardiol.*, **39**, 1008–1016.

MILLER, S. W., DINSMORE, R. E., GREENE, R. E. & DAGGETT, W. M. (1978) Coronary, ventricular, and pulmonary abnormalities associated with rupture of the interventricular septum complicating myocardial infarction. *Amer. J. Roentgenol.*, **131**, 571–577.

MILLS, P. G., ROSE, J. D., BRODIE, B. R., DELANY, D. J. & GRAIGE, E. (1977) Echophonocardiographic diagnosis of left ventricular pseudoaneurysm. *Chest*, **72**, 365–367.

MINTZ, G. S., VICTOR, M. F., MOTLER, M. N., PARRY, W. R. & SEGAL, B. L. (1981) Two-dimensional echocardiographic identification of surgically correctable complications of acute myocardial infarction. *Circulation*, **34**, 91–96.

NEWMAN, P. E. (1981) The coronary collateral circulation; determinants and functional significance in ischemic heart disease. *Amer. Heart J.*, **102**, 431–445.

PARTRIDGE, J. B., ROBINSON, P. J., TURNBULL, C. M., STOKER, J. B., BOYLE, R. M. & MORRISON, G. W. (1981) Clinical cardiovascular experiences with iopamidol: a new non-ionic contrast medium. *Clin. Radiol.*, **32**, 451–455.

PASTERNAC, A., GORLIN, R., SONNENBLICK, E. H., HAFT, J. I. & KEMP, H. G. (1972) Abnormalities of ventricular motion induced by atrial pacing in coronary artery disease. *Circulation*, **45**, 1195–1205.

PAULIN, S. (1967) Interarterial coronary anastomoses in relation to arterial obstruction demonstrated in coronary arteriography. *Invest. Radiol.*, **2**, 147–159.

PAULIN, S. (1972) Non-selective coronary arteriography. *Sem. Roentgenol.*, **7**, 369–375.

RACKLEY, C. E. (1976) Quantitative evaluation of left ventricular function by radiographic techniques. *Circulation*, **54**, 862–879.

RAPHAEL, M. J., STEINER, R. E., GOODWIN, J. F. & OAKLEY, C. M. (1972) Cine angiography of left ventricular aneurysms. *Clin. Radiol.*, **23**, 129–139.

RASMUSSEN, S., CORYA, B. C., FEIGENBAUM, H. & KNOEBEL, S. B. (1977) Detection of myocardial scar tissue by M mode echocardiography. *Circulation*, **57**, 230–237.

RINK, L. D., FEIGENBAUM, H., GODLEY, R. W., WEYMAN, A. E., DILLON, J. C., PHILLIPS, J. F. & MARSHALL, J. E. (1982) Echocardiographic detection of left main coronary artery obstruction. *Circulation*, **65**, 719–724.

ROBERTS, W. C., SIEGEL, R. J. & ZIPES, D. P. (1982) Origin of the right coronary artery from the left sinus of valsalva and its functional consequences: analysis of 10 necropsy patients. *Amer. J. Cardiol.*, **49**, 863–868.

ROGERS, W. J., SMITH, L. R., BREAM, P. R., ELLIOTT, L. P., RACKLEY, C. E. & RUSSELL, R. O. (1982) Quantitative axial oblique contrast left ventriculography: validation of the method by demonstrating improved visualisation of regional wall motion and mitral valve function with accurate volume determinations. *Amer. Heart J.*, **103**, 185–194.

RUTTLEY, M. S., ADAMS, D. F., COHN, P. F. & ABRAMS, H. L. (1974) Shape and volume changes during 'isovolumetric relaxations' in normal and asynergic ventricles. *Circulation*, **50**, 306–316.

SHARMA, B., GOODWIN, J. F., RAPHAEL, M. J., STEINER, R. E., RAINBOW, R. G. & TAYLOR, S. H. (1976) Left ventricular angiography on exercise. A new method of assessing left ventricular function in ischaemic heart disease. *Brit. Heart J.*, **38**, 59–70.

SONES, F. M. & SHIREY, E. K. (1962) Cine coronary arteriography. *Modern Concepts of Cardiovascular Disease*, **31**, 735–741.

SOS, T. A., SNIDERMAN, K. W., LEVIN, D. C. & BECKMANN, C. F. (1979) Cinefluoroscopy in evaluating left ventricular contractility and aneurysms. *Radiology*, **133**, 31–37.

SOULEN, R. L. & FREEMAN, E. (1971) Radiologic evaluation of myocardial infarction. *Radiol. Clin. N. Amer.*, **9**, 567–582.

SOUZA, A. S., BREAM, P. R. & ELLIOTT, L. P. (1978) Chest film detection of coronary artery calcification. The value of the CAC triangle. *Radiology*, **129**, 7–10.

STRATTON, J. R., RITCHIE, J. L., HAMILTON, G. W., HAMMERMEISTER, K. E. & HARKER, L. A. (1981) Left ventricular thrombi: in vivo detection by indium—111 platelet imaging and two dimensional echocardiography. *Amer. J. Cardiol.*, **47**, 874–881.

SWAN, H. J. C. (1982) Editorial: thrombolysis in acute myocardial infarction: treatment of the underlying coronary artery disease. *Circulation*, **66**, 914–916.

TEICHHOLZ, L. E., KREULEN, T., HERMAN, M. V. & GORLIN, R. (1976) Problems in echocardiographic volume determinations: echocardiographic-angiographic correlations in the presence or absence of asynergy. *Amer. J. Cardiol.*, **37**, 7–11.

TOBIS, J., NACIOGLU, O., JOHNSTON, W. D., SEIBERT, A., ISERI, L. T., ROECK, W., ELKAYAM, U. & HENRY, W. (1982) Left ventricular imaging with digital subtraction angiography using intravenous contrast injection and fluoroscopic exposure levels. *Amer. Heart J.*, **104**, 20–27.

VISSER, C. A., KAN, G., DAVID, G. K., LIE, K. I. & DURRER, D. (1982) Echocardiographic-cineangiographic correlation in detecting left ventricular aneurysm: a prospective study of 422 patients. *Amer. J. Cardiol.*, **50**, 337–341.

WORTHINGTON, B. S. (1983) Clinical prospects for nuclear magnetic resonance. *Clin. Radiol.*, **34**, 3–12.

CHAPTER 7

ACQUIRED VALVAR DISEASE AND CARDIAC TUMOURS

Michael Ruttley

INTRODUCTION

The many possible causes of heart valve disease vary in importance throughout the world with social and geographic factors. Rheumatic valvulitis predominates by far in the 'developing' countries but elsewhere its falling incidence, together with increased awareness or incidence of other diseases, has diminished its importance. In the United Kingdom rheumatic valvulitis is no longer the leading cause of aortic valve disease or of isolated mitral regurgitation though it still predominates where two or more valves are involved and other causes of mitral or tricuspid stenosis are rare.

Valve disease may cause little haemodynamic disturbance or may result in significant stenosis or regurgitation, in isolation or combination and in one or more valves (isolated single valve lesions, though least common, will be emphasized here for clarity). Stenosis obstructs blood flow with pressure overload of the chamber proximal to the valve. Gradual onset and increase in severity allows compensation by structural and pathophysiological changes in the cardiovascular system, but eventual decompensation with cardiac failure is to be expected. Regurgitation leads to volume overload of the chamber proximal to the valve and of the chamber or great vessel distal to the valve with similar phases of compensation and decompensation in the chronic case. Acute dysfunction (usually regurgitation, though prosthetic valves may suddenly obstruct) can result in immediate failure. Cardiac failure from any cause predisposes to peripheral venous thrombosis and therefore pulmonary embolism is a potential complication of valve disease. A diseased valve may itself be a source of emboli or these can occur following intracardiac thrombosis related to the valve dysfunction and other effects of the underlying disease. Infective endocarditis can complicate diseased or previously normal valves with often profound alteration of haemodynamics and the possibility of septic emboli.

Investigation must determine the severity of the valve fault or faults, the effect on cardiac function and the significance of any associated cardiac disease in order that surgical referral can be made when appropriate with knowledge of operative risk and prognosis; radiology plays an important part in this.

Radiological features will depend on the valve or valves affected, the type and severity of the haemodynamic disturbance and its time scale of development and duration. They may be modified by embolism or infection and there may be specific radiological manifestations of the underlying disease.

AORTIC STENOSIS

Left ventricular outflow obstruction can be at, above or below the aortic valve. Supra and subvalvar stenosis are largely congenital in origin and discussed elsewhere (Chapter 13) but rare cases where aortic atheroma contributes to atheromatous valve stenosis are seen in familial hypercholesterolaemia and subvalvar obstruction occurs in hypertrophic cardiomyopathy (Chapter 9).

Valve stenosis can be congenital (Chapter 13) or acquired but the distinction is confused as the predominant cause of isolated aortic stenosis in adults is the *acquired* stenosis of a *congenitally* bicuspid valve. Despite its known association with another congenital heart disease, notably coarctation of the aorta, a bicuspid aortic valve is not intrinsically stenotic but has a particular propensity to develop this complication (Edwards, 1961). Aortic valve fibrosis with dystrophic calcification is a normal consequence of ageing, but occurs earlier in bicuspid than in normal tricuspid aortic valves. This may have no clinical consequence and may never become radiologically visible but in some cases, for reasons unknown, the process is gross, leading to cusp rigidity and stenosis with clinical presentation typically in the sixth decade. The bicuspid malformation occurs in up to 2% of the population (Davies, 1980) and only a small minority develop stenosis (or the other complications of regurgitation or infection); exact figures are not available. Calcification of a tricuspid aortic valve in old age may be radiologically visible and associated with an ejection systolic murmur. Stenosis is typically minimal ('aortic sclerosis') but progression to gross calcification and severe stenosis can occur. It is not known why some valves are affected and others not, or why this essentially senile disease is sometimes seen at an earlier age. A relationship with Paget's disease has been reported (King *et al.*, 1969).

Rheumatic aortic valve stenosis is characterised by fusion of the valve commissures and a fixed central stenotic orifice. All three commissures are usually involved though fusion of one may occur, resulting in an acquired bicuspid valve. The cusps become thickened but calcification occurs relatively late and is not the prime determinant of stenosis as in the calcific stenoses above. Isolated aortic stenosis is a relatively uncommon manifestation of rheumatic disease; there is usually aortic regurgitation due to cusp retraction and the incidence of associated mitral disease is high.

These three conditions, calcific stenosis of bicuspid and tricuspid aortic valves and rheumatic valvulitis, account for virtually all cases of acquired aortic valve stenosis (an extremely rare cause, ochronosis (Gould *et al.*, 1976), deserves mention here only because of its other radiological features). Their relative incidence depends on the prevalence of rheumatic fever in a given area and also varies with age group and sex. In the United Kingdom calcific bicuspid stenosis predominates overall but rheumatic stenosis is more common below middle age and calcific tricuspid stenosis predominates in patients over 75 years of age (Pomerance, 1972). A recent series suggests that rheumatic valvulitis now accounts for less than 2% of isolated aortic stenosis undergoing surgery in the United Kingdom (Davies, 1980). Male:female ratios are of the order of 2:1 for bicuspid, 1:2 for tricuspid and 1:1 for rheumatic aortic stenosis.

Chest Radiographs: Fluoroscopy

Valve calcification. Aetiological considerations determine that the most important radiological sign in acquired aortic stenosis is aortic valve calcification. Aortic stenosis, a potentially lethal but surgically correctable disease, not infrequently escapes detection in life and aortic valve calcification must therefore always suggest the diagnosis (though it is recognised that a calcified valve is not inevitably stenotic). Conversely a diagnosis of aortic stenosis is highly unlikely without valve calcification in a middle-aged patient and virtually excluded by its absence in the elderly.

Aortic valve calcification originates in the cusps but usually extends to the annulus and may continue into the interventricular septum (with the possibility of heart block) or towards the mitral valve (calcification of the mitral cusps suggests rheumatic disease and degenerative calcification of the mitral annulus frequently accompanies senile calcific aortic stenosis).

A calcified aortic valve may be seen on plain chest radiographs, inevitably blurred by rapid valve motion. It cannot be excluded without fluoroscopy. In frontal projection the valve overlaps the spine, largely above a line drawn from the junction of left atrial appendage and left ventricle to the right cardiophrenic angle (Fig. 7.01). In the more useful lateral projection it is clear of the spine, largely above the mid part of a line

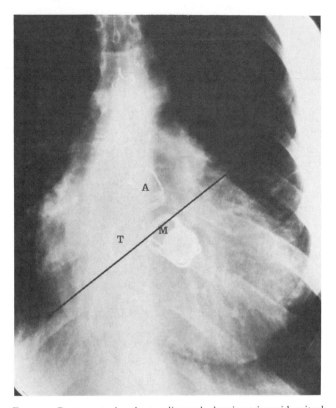

FIG. 7.01. Posteroanterior chest radiograph showing tricuspid, mitral and aortic valve prostheses. The rings of the Starr Edwards mitral (metal ball) and aortic (non-opaque ball) valves indicate the typical calcification sites of native valves.

drawn from the hilum to the junction of anterior chest wall and diaphragm (Figs. 7.02 and 7.03).

Right anterior oblique fluoroscopy readily identifies valve calcification, which is closely related to the usually visible radiolucent stripe of fat in the atrioventricular groove, but differentiation between aortic and mitral valves can be difficult. Aortic is the higher but there is often overlap (Fig. 7.04). Subtleties of motion help differentiate (mitral calcification moves in an axis directed towards the cardiac apex and aortic motion is more vertical) but, having identified calcification, the valves can be distinguished in the left anterior oblique projection where they are well separated, aortic high in the middle third of the heart shadow and mitral lower and to the patient's left (observer's right) (Fig. 7.05).

The extent of calcification can be graded according to its detection: *grade 1*, seen on fluoroscopy only; *grade 2*, suspected on plain film, confirmed by fluoroscopy; *grade 3*, definite on plain film. Where aortic stenosis is present, the extent of calcification correlates well with severity of obstruction (Clancy, *et al.*, 1969).

The importance of the radiological detection of aortic valve calcification cannot be overstressed; in nine of a

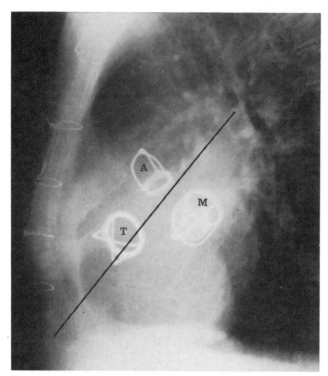

FIG. 7.02. Lateral view of Fig. 7.01.

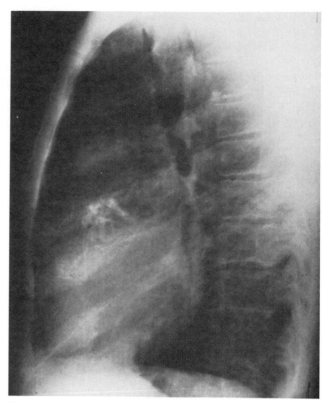

FIG. 7.03. Lateral chest radiograph of a patient with calcific stenosis of a bicuspid aortic valve showing typical calcification site.

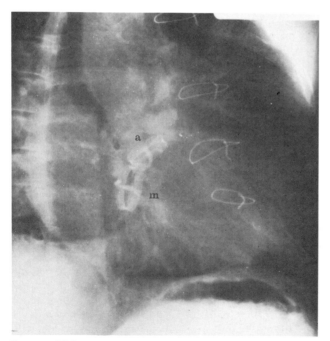

FIG. 7.04. Right anterior oblique chest radiograph with Hall Kaster disc valve prostheses, aortic (*a*) and mitral (*m*), to show valve positions.

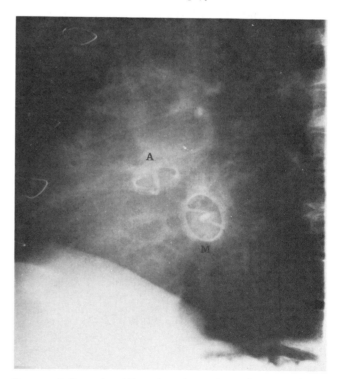

FIG. 7.05. Left anterior oblique view of aortic (A) and mitral (M) Hall Kaster valve prostheses.

group of ten patients with unrecognised severe aortic stenosis referred to a cardiac centre as heart failure of unknown cause, the correct diagnosis of this surgically treatable lesion was reached after detection of aortic valve calcification, seven by lateral chest radiograph and two by fluoroscopy (Morgan & Hall, 1979). Chest radiography in cases of 'heart failure' must not be confined to the all too frequent AP film of a patient in bed.

Detection of coronary artery calcification at fluoroscopy will indicate coexistent coronary disease but has little predictive value for significance in the typical age group of aortic stenosis. Calcified atheroma is most common in the proximal part of the left anterior descending artery; this is foreshortened in the left anterior oblique projection and therefore seen as a ring shadow or nodule to the left of the aortic valve (Fig. 7.06). It can be mistaken for valve calcification (or overlooked in its presence) but should be distinguished in other projections as a 'tramline' shadow near the upper margin of the heart.

Aortic dilation. Post stenotic dilation of the ascending aorta is a valuable sign of aortic valve stenosis, reported in some 90% of adults with isolated disease (Klatte *et al.*, 1979). The dilation results from structural changes in the aortic wall due to turbulent flow and is related to the presence of stenosis, not its severity. It affects the ascending aorta above the sinuses of Valsalva (Fig. 7.07). In frontal projection it is a well defined convex mediastinal bulge to the right, above the right atrial border (Fig. 7.08). The aortic knuckle and descending aorta are not involved but aortic stenosis is predominantly a disease of late middle age and over and coexistent degenerative aortic dilation is frequently present (Fig. 7.09). Age related or hypertensive changes alone seldom give the localised ascending aortic bulge of post stenotic dilation. In lateral projection the dilated ascending aortic shadow encroaches on the retrosternal space, replacing the ill-defined margin of the right ventricular outflow tract and main pulmonary artery with a sharper edged and more vertical aortic shadow (Fig. 7.10).

Heart size; chamber enlargement. Heart size and shape are of limited value in the radiological diagnosis of aortic stenosis. The pressure overload of outflow obstruction results in left ventricular hypertrophy but this cannot be confidently diagnosed on plain films. Increase in left ventricular muscle mass can give an increase in heart size as assessed by frontal area (Lewis *et al.*, 1971) but the cardiothoracic ratio is less than 50% in the majority, rarely much above in the absence of failure and has no relation to severity of stenosis (Klatte *et al.*, 1979). With failure the ventricular cavity will dilate, enlargement should be visible and the cardiothoracic ratio will increase.

An increase in left ventricular end diastolic pressure due to decreased compliance of the hypertrophied

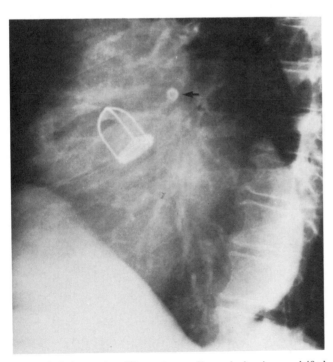

Fig. 7.06. Left anterior oblique chest radiograph showing a calcified left anterior coronary artery seen end-on as a ring shadow (arrow) and its relationship to the aortic valve position (Starr Edwards non-opaque ball prosthesis).

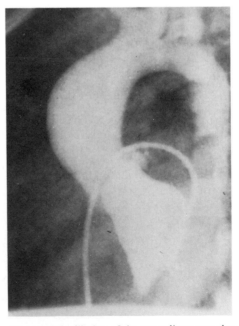

Fig. 7.07. Post stenotic dilation of the ascending aorta shown in left anterior oblique projection. Left ventriculogram (trans-septal catheter) of a child with congenital aortic stenosis.

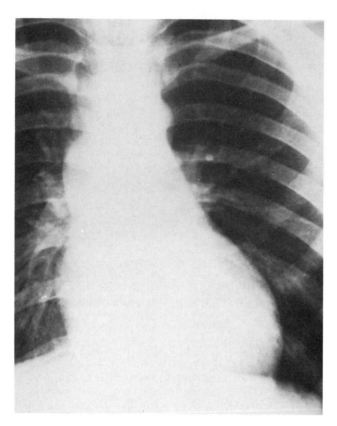

FIG. 7.08. The right mediastinal bulge of post stenotic dilation of the ascending aorta. 40-year-old male with calcific stenosis of a bicuspid aortic valve.

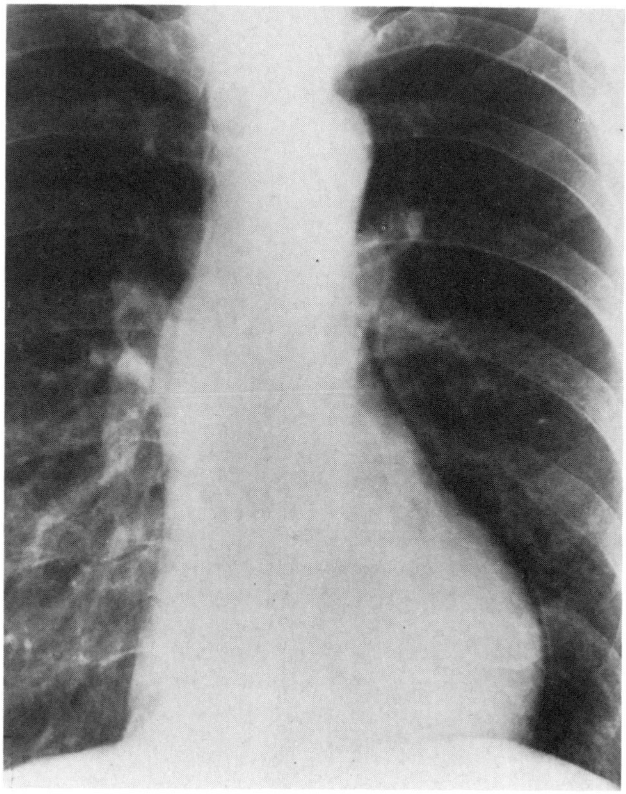

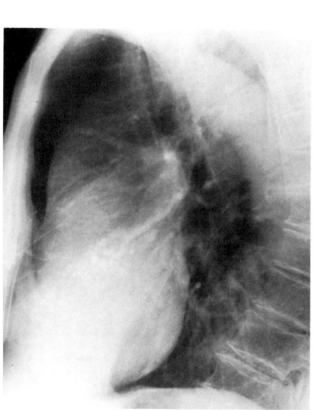

FIG. 7.09. 75-year-old male with calcific stenosis of a tricuspid aortic valve showing post-stenotic dilation of the ascending aorta and age-related dilation of the arch.

FIG. 7.10. Calcific aortic stenosis; calcified valve and post-stenotic dilation of the aorta in lateral chest radiograph.

ventricle of failure or both will influence left atrial pressure. Increased atrial contraction maintains ventricular filling against decreased compliance with minimal elevation of mean atrial pressure and left atrial enlargement is unusual until the ventricle fails and mean left atrial pressure rises significantly. When left atrial enlargement occurs it is no more than moderate and usually only visible on the PA film as the double shadow of the heart to the right of the spine. If other signs of left atrial enlargement are present, particularly enlargement of the appendage, coexistent mitral disease is likely.

The right heart chambers do not enlarge unless the late stage of congestive cardiac failure is reached and are then radiographically indistinguishable in the generally enlarged heart.

Pulmonary vascular pattern is normal until left ventricular failure occurs with resultant elevation of left atrial and therefore pulmonary venous pressure; pulmonary vascular redistribution and, depending on severity, pulmonary oedema will then be seen.

Without corrective surgery the interval between the onset of failure and death is about 2 years in aortic stenosis (Morrow *et al.*, 1968), too short for the development of the lung changes (haemosiderosis, ossification nodules) which may be associated with more chronic pulmonary venous hypertension. Some elevation of pulmonary artery pressure inevitably accompanies pulmonary venous hypertension but it rarely becomes disproportionate in the time available and plain film signs of pulmonary arterial hypertension are unusual in aortic stenosis.

Echocardiography

The diagnosis of acquired aortic stenosis and its quantification can be achieved by ultrasound techniques in the majority of cases. Left ventricular function can also be assessed and the other heart valves examined.

Bicuspid aortic valve can be diagnosed from eccentricity of the valve closure line within the aorta on M-mode echocardiography (Fig. 7.11). Thickened cusps with reduced amplitude of opening strongly suggest stenosis (Fig. 7.12) but quantification by M-mode is unreliable. Severity is better assessed by the two dimensional (real time) echo measurement of systolic cusp separation; a figure of 8 mm or less has a high predictive value for severe stenosis but there are still problems of specificity with this technique (Godley *et al.*, 1981). The pressure gradient across the aortic valve can be calculated from the maximal velocity in the aortic jet measured by Doppler technique with an external probe. The angle between the jet and the ultrasound beam must, however, be known or small enough to be ignored in calculation and this presents technical difficulty in the age group where acquired aortic stenosis typically presents (Hatle *et al.*, 1980).

Despite some present difficulties it seems inevitable that ultrasound techniques, together with other cardiological parameters, will soon replace invasive (catheter) measurement of severity in the majority of cases of aortic stenosis; this is already policy in some cardiac centres.

Cardiac Catheterisation: Angiocardiography

At cardiac catheterisation, aortic stenosis is primarily assessed by haemodynamic data. The degree of valve stenosis constituting significant obstruction is arguable but a peak systolic pressure gradient between left ventricle and aorta of 50 mmHg or more is severe stenosis. Reduction of forward blood flow, as in left

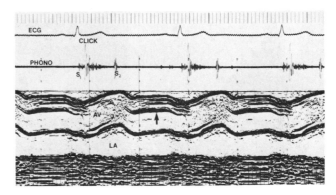

FIG. 7.11. M-mode echocardiogram showing eccentric diastolic closure line (arrow) of a bicuspid aortic valve. The ejection click and murmur are shown in relation to aortic valve opening by the simultaneous phonocardiogram.

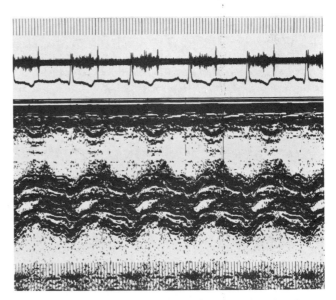

FIG. 7.12. Grossly calcified stenosed aortic valve, M-mode echocardiogram.

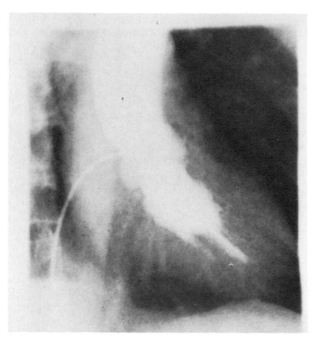

FIG. 7.13. Left ventricular hypertrophy in aortic stenosis. Right anterior oblique left ventriculogram (trans-septal catheter) at end systole. Note the thick wall of myocardium shown between contrast medium in the cavity and the heart-lung interface, the large papillary muscles and the obliteration of the apex.

ventricular failure, may markedly reduce a pressure gradient, masking severe stenosis. The latter can be recognised by calculation of valve orifice area from catheterisation data which take account of both flow and gradient (Gorlin and Gorlin, 1951).

Catheter studies of necessity involve fluoroscopy and usually include left ventriculography and aortography; coronary arteriography may be a routine addition or reserved for certain clinical groups.

Left ventriculography. This is discussed more fully in relation to coronary artery disease (Chapter 6) and mitral disease; it is similarly used in aortic stenosis to assess global and regional ventricular function and any associated mitral regurgitation. The ventricle is typically thick walled, without dilation and shows vigorous contraction (Fig. 7.13). The failing ventricle dilates and shows general impairment of contraction (Fig. 7.14) with reduced ejection fraction. Coexistent ischaemic heart disease is suggested by regional variation in contraction. Mitral regurgitation may be 'functional' (a consequence of left ventricular dysfunction) and is not necessarily indicative of organic mitral disease; distinction may be difficult and takes account of any other mitral valve abnormality, notably calcification, in addition to the extent of left ventricular dilation and contraction abnormality.

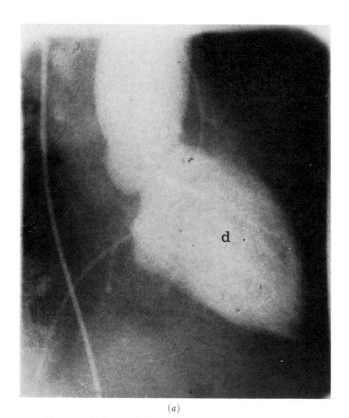

(a)

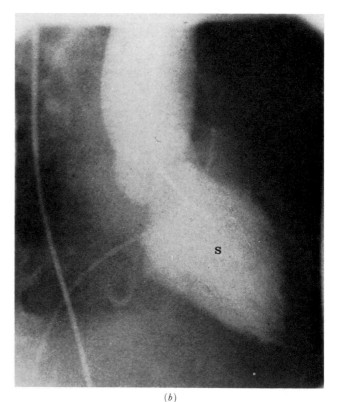

(b)

FIG. 7.14. Left ventricular failure in aortic stenosis. Right anterior oblique left ventriculogram at end diastole (d) and end systole (s).

Aortic valve abnormalities may be seen in the left ventriculogram but are more conveniently described under aortography.

Aortography. The three sinuses of Valsalva of a tricuspid aortic valve are best shown in left anterior oblique projection, where the posterior (or non-coronary) sinus is central and at a lower level than the two coronary sinuses (Fig. 7.15). This is determined by their anatomical relations in the transverse plane of the body and the caudocranial tilt to the left of the valve axis.

The majority of bicuspid valves have only two sinuses, though angiographic demonstration of a third does not exclude the condition (Waller *et al.*, 1973). The two are most commonly a large posterior noncoronary sinus and a smaller anterior coronary sinus. These are superimposed in left anterior oblique projection with the noncoronary sinus extending to a lower level, giving an 'inverted thumb' appearance to the aortic root (Fig. 7.16a), and separated in right anterior oblique projection (Fig. 7.16b). The less common right and left coronary sinus arrangement shows separate sinuses in the left anterior oblique (Fig. 7.17a) and superimposition in the right anterior oblique (Fig. 7.17b). Calcification may so distort the appearances that recognition of separate sinuses is impossible.

Restricted valve opening should be obvious on a cine aortogram; systolic doming indicates abnormality of a tricuspid aortic valve (Fig. 7.18) but is the normal appearance of a bicuspid valve even without stenosis (Baron, 1971). A negative jet into the opacified aorta is good evidence of stenosis (Fig. 7.18); a positive contrast jet is the left ventriculographic counterpart (Fig. 7.19). Post stenotic dilation due to the jet is seen in most cases. Cusp thickening with little or no calcification (as in rheumatic valvulitis) will not be visible unless there is contrast medium above and below the valve (Fig. 7.20), as with aortic regurgitation or in the left ventriculogram. The diameter of the aortic valve annulus can be estimated from the aortogram and may have surgical relevance in the choice of prosthetic valve size.

The several angiographic signs of stenosis have no exact correlation with severity but this is not required where the pressure gradient is available. They may assume negative importance in the rare event of a pressure gradient across the left ventricular outflow being wrongly attributed to valve stenosis; an angiographically normal valve in 'aortic stenosis' raises this suspicion and the left ventriculogram must be reviewed for signs of subvalvar stenosis in such a case.

The usual importance of the aortogram in aortic valve stenosis is in the assessment of any associated aortic regurgitation and in the albeit limited information it gives on the coronary arteries. These are typically large, reflecting the demands of left ventricular hypertrophy, and the major vessels at least should be visible, allowing recognition of dominance pattern and anom-

(a)

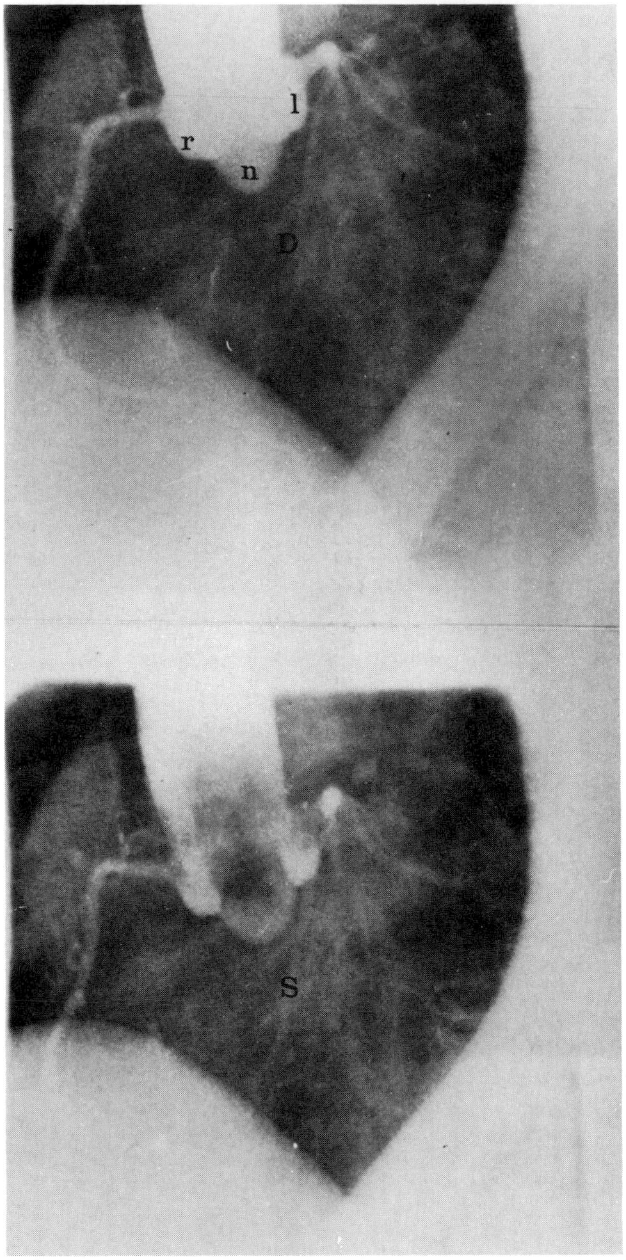

(b)

FIG. 7.15. Normal aortogram, left anterior oblique projection, showing the right (r), left (l) and noncoronary (n) sinuses of Valsalva in diastole (D) and systole (S).

alies of origin. Coronary artery disease may be diagnosed from the aortogram but cannot be excluded or precisely documented without selective coronary arteriography.

Coronary arteriography. The role of this procedure

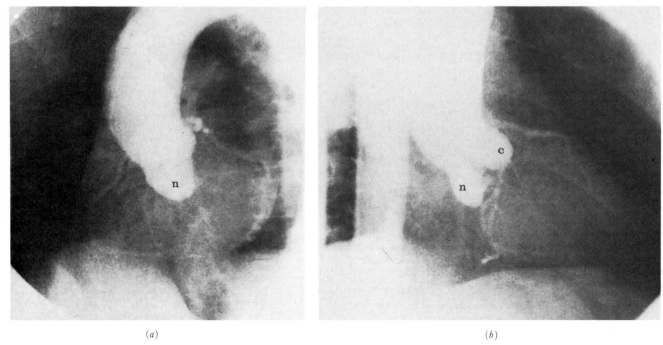

FIG. 7.16. (a) (b). Left and right anterior oblique projections of an aortogram showing a bicuspid aortic valve with coronary and noncoronary (posterior) sinuses of Valsalva.

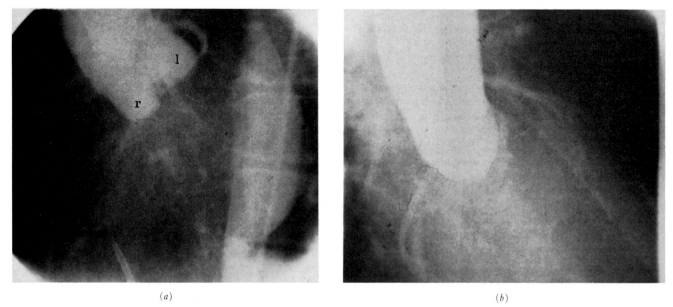

FIG. 7.17. (a) (b). Left and right anterior oblique projections of an aortogram showing a bicuspid aortic valve with right (r) and left (l) coronary sinuses of Valsalva.

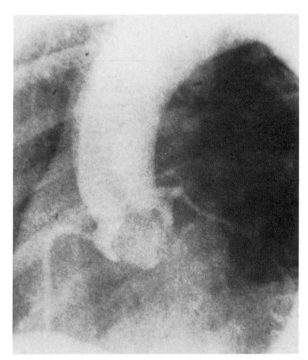

FIG. 7.18. Rheumatic aortic stenosis (tricuspid aortic valve). Left anterior oblique aortogram showing systolic doming of the valve and a negative jet of non-opaque blood in the aorta.

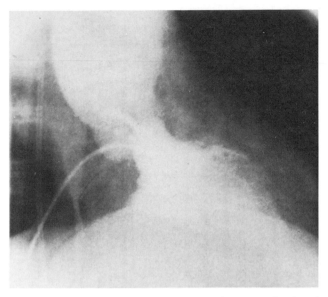

FIG. 7.19. Aortic stenosis. Left ventriculogram (trans-septal catheter) in right anterior oblique projection showing positive contrast jet through the valve orifice into aorta.

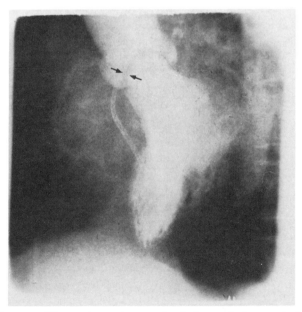

FIG. 7.20. Rheumatic aortic stenosis. Left ventriculogram in left anterior oblique projection showing systolic doming of a thick (arrows) aortic valve.

in aortic stenosis is the determination of coronary anatomy (if not shown by an aortogram) and the assessment of any coexistent coronary disease. Unlike other catheter studies it is therefore unlikely to be replaced by non invasive tests in the preoperative assessment of aortic stenosis at least in the forseeable future.

Left coronary dominance occurs in about 10% of the general population but is significantly increased in association with bicuspid aortic valve (Higgins & Wexler, 1975). Short main left coronary artery is a frequent accompaniment of left dominance and minor anomalies of coronary artery origin are reported to be more common in patients with valve disease than others (Kimbris *et al.*, 1978). Recognition of such variation is important in the preoperative assessment of patients selected for aortic valve replacement, particularly in centres where intraoperative coronary perfusion is used.

A particular relation between coronary atheroma and aortic stenosis is unlikely but age factors alone determine an appreciable coincidence and there is evidence that treatment of significant coexistent coronary disease by bypass grafting at the time of valve replacement improves the surgical outcome in aortic valve disease (Kirklin & Kouchoukos, 1981). Preoperative coronary arteriography is therefore generally agreed to be mandatory in the presence of angina pectoris (albeit a symptom common to both diseases) and has been variously adopted by different centres as a routine in all patients, or in those above a certain age (usually 40 years), regardless of angina. It is accepted that coronary disease cannot be certainly excluded in the individual without coronary arteriography despite the statistical value of noninvasive tests, but the procedure has complications, though rare, and its yield is very low in angina-free patients with no coronary risk factors (Ramsdale *et al.*, 1982). There is, therefore, an argument for its omission in such patients unless positive indication emerges from fluoroscopy or aortography.

There are no arteriographic features peculiar to coronary artery disease in aortic stenosis but the diseased valve must be remembered as one of the causes of coronary embolus (Fig. 7.21). Systolic narrowing of the intramyocardial septal arteries may occur in severe left ventricular hypertrophy from any cause, including aortic stenosis, and can be mistaken for fixed disease if its phasic pattern is not recognised.

Other Examinations

Radionuclide studies may help in the assessment of left ventricular function or myocardial ischaemia in aortic valve disease but have as yet no place in the measurement of aortic stenosis.

Aortic stenosis carries an increased incidence of gastrointestinal bleeding in general and has a recognised association with angiodysplasia (Gelfand *et al.*, 1979). This is of practical radiological importance for if the source of gastrointestinal haemorrhage in a patient with aortic stenosis is not shown by routine studies, angio-

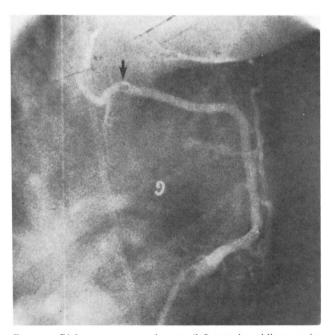

FIG. 7.21. Right coronary arteriogram (left anterior oblique projection). Showing coronary embolus (arrow) in an otherwise normal artery. Patient with calcific aortic stenosis.

dysplasia is the expected diagnosis and *mesenteric arteriography* is indicated.

AORTIC REGURGITATION

Aortic regurgitation generally denotes flow from aorta to left ventricle through a leaking aortic valve but regurgitation can occur around a detached prosthetic valve, can be nonvalvar (sinus of Valsalva aneurysm with rupture into the left ventricle, aorto-left ventricular tunnel) or can be directed into another chamber (right or single ventricle) by coexistent congenital faults.

The normal aortic valve has three semilunar cusps, each concave towards the aorta, based in its own sinus of Valsalva and supported by a fibrous annulus. The cusps meet at commissures, equally spaced peripherally on the sinotubular ridge which separates the sinuses from the aorta above. Diastolic competence is ensured by considerable apposition of the concave cusps above their closure line and by annular and commissural support. Valvar regurgitation can therefore result from disease of the cusps themselves or of the aortic root (a term frequently encountered in the literature and used here to denote the aorta up to and including the sinotubular ridge).

Aortic regurgitation is associated with a multitude of diseases and in many it is rare, trivial or both. The list is formidable; that below is exhausting if not exhaustive but given without apology as many of the diseases have other well known radiological features.

Diseases associated with aortic regurgitation
Aortic stenosis: all types
Aortic valve replacement: prosthetic dysfunction
Aortitis: Ankylosing spondylitis
          Behcet's syndrome
          Giant cell
          Nonspecific
          Psoriasis
          Reiter's disease
          Relapsing polychondritis
          Rheumatoid arthritis
          Syphilis
          Takayasu
          Ulcerative colitis
Bicuspid aortic valve
Dissecting aneurysm of the aorta
Infective endocarditis
Lupus erythematosus
Mucopolysaccharidoses
Myxomatous degeneration of the valve
Noninflammatory aortic root dilation:
   Annuloaortic ectasia (synonyms; idiopathic cystic medionecrosis, idiopathic aortic root dilation)
   Ehlers Danlos syndrome
   Marfan's syndrome
   Osteogenesis imperfecta

Rheumatic valvulitis
Rheumatoid arthritis (valve granulomata)
Sinus of Valsalva aneurysm
Spontaneous valve rupture
Systemic hypertension
Trauma
Ventricular septal defect
Whipple's disease

Various permutations of common—uncommon, congenital—acquired, valve cusp—aortic root disease can be made from this list but the distinctions are often blurred. For practical purposes only those diseases or groups in italics warrant further consideration as causes of isolated severe aortic regurgitation.

Infective endocarditis may involve previously normal or diseased tricuspid or bicuspid aortic valves. Tricuspid and bicuspid are equally common in most series, indicating a greater propensity to infection of the much rarer bicuspid valve. It is worth noting that heavily calcified valves rarely become infected. Regurgitation is a common but not inevitable result of infection and is due to cusp perforation or fibrotic retraction, depending on the virulence of the organism. Involvement of the sinuses of Valsalva may lead to an acquired aneurysm with consequent distortion of the aortic root and increased regurgitation. Infective endocarditis figures highly in any surgical experience of aortic regurgitation and is the commonest cause of acute regurgitation requiring valve replacement.

Bicuspid aortic valve. It has recently been emphasised that isolated severe aortic regurgitation occurs as frequently in noninfected as infected bicuspid valves (Roberts *et al.*, 1981). Regurgitation is unusual at birth and the reasons for its subsequent development in a minority of bicuspid valves are obscure. Calcification is not a factor; many calcified stenotic bicuspid valves allow some regurgitation but calcification is unusual in isolated regurgitation (Glancy *et al.*, 1969). Clinical presentation is typically in young adult life (in contrast to calcific stenosis) with male predominance.

Rheumatic valvulitis causes aortic regurgitation by fibrotic cusp retraction. This is usually accompanied by some commissural fusion (and therefore stenosis) and the incidence of associated mitral involvement is high. Isolated aortic regurgitation is therefore an uncommon manifestation of rheumatic disease.

Noninflammatory aortic root dilation. Annular dilation must separate the valve cusps to some extent and at the extreme there will be no diastolic apposition and inevitable regurgitation; lesser degrees of dilation reduce the support derived from cusp overlap which can result in prolapse and therefore regurgitation. An aggravating factor may be myxomatous degeneration which can occur in aortic or mitral valve cusps in association with cystic medionecrosis.

The condition is typified by Marfan's syndrome and its forme fruste but is seen in other connective tissue disorders. Numerically more important are patients with the aortic changes but no other features or family history of a connective tissue disorder. This group has been variously named and no clear favourite has emerged; annuloaortic ectasia (Ellis *et al.*, 1961) has the advantage of emphasising the annular dilation. Though initially considered rare it is now recognised with increasing frequency as a cause of isolated aortic regurgitation requiring valve replacement. It is unusual below middle age but seen at all ages above with a male preponderance.

Aortitis. Cardiovascular syphilis is typified by a calcified aneurysm of the ascending aorta. Aortic regurgitation is seen with about half of these and may occasionally be seen alone. It is due to aortic root dilation and separation of the commissures, the cusps themselves are not usually involved.

Aortitis and aortic regurgitation associated with arthropathy is rare even in the most quoted example, ankylosing spondylitis. Aortic dilation is typically confined to the root and calcification is unusual. Fibrosis is extensive, involves the aortic valve cusps and often extends beyond to the base of the mitral valve, the atrioventricular node and the interventricular septum (causing heart block). Nonspecific forms of aortitis are commoner than those associated with arthropathy, similar in their involvement of the aortic root and valve cusps but often more extensive throughout the aorta and its branches (with calcification, localised aneurysms, stenoses and occlusions).

Dissecting aneurysm of the aorta. Aortic regurgitation can result when the dissecting haematoma strips down to the valve and is seen in over half of proximal dissections. It may coexist with even distal dissections as both aortic regurgitation and dissecting aneurysm can complicate most forms of aortic dilation, particularly that due to cystic medionecrosis.

It is obvious from this consideration of causative mechanisms and diseases that, in contrast to aortic stenosis, aortic regurgitation may occur in acute or chronic forms; these have important clinical and radiological differences.

Chest Radiographs: Fluoroscopy

Heart size; chamber enlargement. The left ventricle's adaptive response to chronic volume overload is cavity dilation and muscle hypertrophy, with maintenance of a normal ejection fraction in the compensated phase. The extent of hypertrophy is often underestimated in the presence of cavity dilation as the ratio of cavity size to wall thickness can be normal despite a total muscle mass often greater than seen in pressure overload. Considerable left ventricular enlargement and consequent overall increase in heart size can therefore occur in chronic aortic regurgitation in the absence of signs of cardiac failure (Figs. 7.22 and 7.23) and radiographic heart size correlates well with the degree of regurgitation (Lewis *et al.*, 1971).

Acute volume overload does not allow such adaptive response; the left ventricle cannot acutely dilate to any significant degree and instant hypertrophy is impossible. Heart size and shape may therefore be normal in acute aortic regurgitation despite other radiographic evidence of left ventricular failure.

In chronic aortic regurgitation, as in aortic stenosis, left atrial enlargement is rare until left ventricular failure occurs and even then is typically slight. Disproportionate left atrial enlargement must always suggest associated mitral valve disease (almost a certainty if there is a large appendage shadow). The sudden haemodynamic changes of acute aortic regurgitation do not allow time for appreciable left atrial enlargement despite often considerable elevation of left atrial pressure (manifest by the signs of pulmonary venous hypertension in the lungs).

As in aortic stenosis, enlargement of the right heart chambers will only occur if the late stage of congestive cardiac failure is reached and they will then be radiographically indistinguishable in the generally enlarged heart.

Aortic dilation involving the ascending part and the arch (and therefore 'knuckle') is often emphasised as a plain film sign of aortic regurgitation but it is uncommon when the lesion is isolated and due to valve cusp disease (Klatte *et al.*, 1979) (Fig. 7.22). The exaggerated

systolic-diastolic volume changes are, however, manifest by increased aortic pulsatility on fluoroscopy. Aortic root dilation is an essential feature of most of the aortic wall diseases responsible for aortic regurgitation and extends throughout the ascending aorta in many, particularly cystic medionecrosis. Such dilation is obvious radiographically (Fig. 7.23) but more indicative of cause than severity of the leak. Extensive calcification of a dilated ascending aorta is seen in syphilis (Fig. 7.24) but is not a feature of the other aortic wall diseases.

Valve calcification is not an important sign in isolated aortic regurgitation; its presence indicates cusp disease but even in this subgroup it is only seen in a minority, is rarely marked and has no correlation with the severity of regurgitation (Glancy *et al.*, 1969).

Pulmonary vascular pattern is normal until left ventricular failure occurs; the changes of pulmonary venous hypertension are therefore seen late in the natural history of chronic aortic regurgitation but early in acute aortic regurgitation (a cause of pulmonary oedema in the presence of a normal sized heart). As with aortic stenosis (and for the same reason) radiographic signs of pulmonary arterial hypertension are rarely seen in aortic regurgitation.

Echocardiography

The presence of aortic regurgitation is usually indicated by high frequency diastolic flutter of the anterior mitral cusp and less commonly by flutter of the interventricular septum (Fig. 7.25) due to the effect of the regurgitant stream on these structures of the left ventricular outflow tract.

In acute severe aortic regurgitation the regurgitant

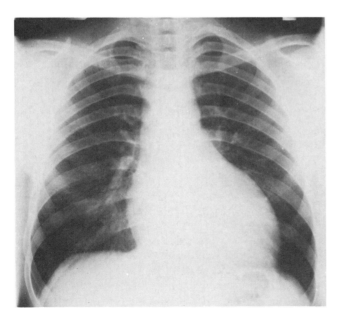

FIG. 7.22. Rheumatic aortic regurgitation. This posteroanterior chest radiograph shows a large heart with a shape suggesting left ventricular enlargement. The aorta is relatively normal. Pulmonary vascular pattern is normal.

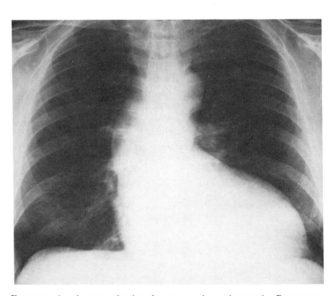

FIG. 7.23. Aortic regurgitation due to annuloaortic ectasia. Posteroanterior chest radiograph showing large heart and large aorta. Normal pulmonary vascular pattern.

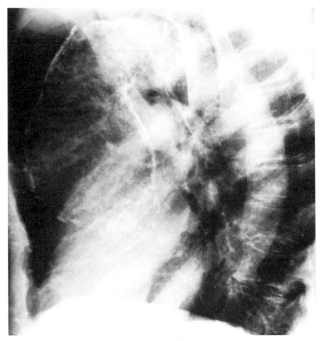

FIG. 7.24. Lateral chest radiograph of syphilitic aortic aneurysm.

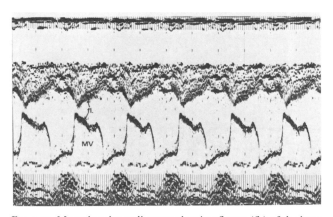

FIG. 7.25. M-mode echocardiogram showing flutter (fl.) of the interventricular septal and anterior mitral cusp echoes in a case of aortic regugitation.

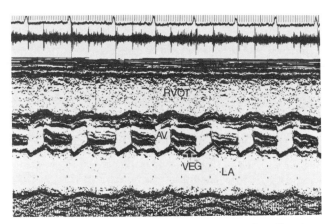

FIG. 7.26. M-mode echocardiogram showing coarse diastolic echoes from vegetations of infective endocarditis on the aortic valve. Right ventricular outflow trast (RVOT), aortic valve opening (AV), the vegetations (VEG) and the left atrium (LA) are labelled.

stream and marked increase in left ventricular end diastolic pressure delay mitral valve opening, reduce both its opening amplitude and its closing E–F slope and bring forward its closure point, all in the presence of normal left ventricular dimensions. In chronic aortic regurgitation the left ventricular end diastolic diameter is increased but with a normal end systolic diameter and no evidence of increased end diastolic pressure in the mitral valve echoes until failure occurs.

The cause of aortic regurgitation may be indicated by the fluttering diastolic echoes of a prolapsed aortic valve cusp in the left ventricular outflow tract or by the coarse diastolic echoes of cusp vegetations there or in the aortic root (Fig. 7.26). Gross enlargement of the aortic root will be seen in cystic medionecrosis.

These valuable signs of presence, cause and effect of aortic regurgitation can be detected by M-mode or two dimensional studies; the former are at present best for measurement and reproduction but the latter provide dramatic diagnostic moving pictures. Doppler study can detect aortic regurgitation and looks promising as a noninvasive measure of its degree (Quinones et al., 1980). A major benefit of echocardiography is that it allows serial noninvasive study of the patient with aortic regurgitation which can be of considerable value in deciding the optimal time for surgery.

Radionuclide Studies

These are of general use in the assessment of left ventricular function and myocardial ischaemia and gated cardiac blood pool imaging has recently been applied to the estimation of valvar regurgitation (Rigo et al., 1979): left and right ventricular stroke counts derived from end diastolic—end systolic count differences are used to give a stroke volume ratio which will be greater than unity in the presence of mitral or aortic regurgitation.

Cardiac Catheterisation: Angiocardiography

The degree of aortic regurgitation is assessed by aortography and its effect on the left ventricle by both pressure measurement (notably left ventricular end diastolic pressure) and ventriculography. Coronary arteriography is not usually a routine but essential in the presence of angina.

Aortography. Aortic regurgitation is most commonly graded by the extent of left ventricular opacification shown by cine radiography when contrast medium is injected above the valve. The left anterior oblique projection is generally preferred for its good view of the valve, sinuses of Valsalva and left ventricular outflow tract but the right anterior oblique gives better demonstration of an opacified left ventricular body and biplane facilities have obvious advantage. Despite the label 'aortogram' the left ventricle and coronary arteries should be fully included in the cine frame. Grade I aortic regurgitation is cleared from the left ventricle in systole, grade II is not cleared but does not perceptibly accumulate in successive diastoles, grade III signifies accumulation and in grade IV there is complete ventricular opacification in the first diastole (after Jefferson & Rees, 1980). Such grading is subjective and influenced by aortographic technique, aortic size and both volume and function of the left ventricle; in left ventricular failure aortography can significantly underestimate underlying valve disease as increased ventricular diastolic pressure reduces the pressure drop across the valve and therefore the leak (Armstrong *et al.*, 1973).

The cause of aortic regurgitation may be shown by the appearances of the valve (Fig. 7.27) or the aortic root (Figs. 7.28 and 7.29). Left ventricular opacification by regurgitation may be sufficient for angiographic assessment of that chamber and the mitral valve without recourse to formal ventriculography. The coronary arteries should be visible but are poorly opacified in significant aortic regurgitation due to rapid dilution of contrast medium in the aortic root by the considerable tidal flow across the valve.

Left ventriculography is required for assessment of ventricular function and any associated mitral regurgitation. In chronic aortic regurgitation the hypertrophied ventricle shows an increased end diastolic volume with normal end systolic volume and ejection fraction until failure occurs; in acute regurgitation the ventricle may be angiographically normal despite considerable elevation of end diastolic pressure. Quantitative analysis of the ventriculogram allows the ventricular stroke volume to be calculated and if the forward stroke volume is known (from cardiac output determination and heart rate) the regurgitant volume is given by their difference (Dodge, 1971).

Coronary arteriography is performed for much the same indications as in aortic stenosis but, perhaps because of the generally younger age group of isolated aortic regurgitation, it is not usually a routine in the absence of angina pectoris. Angina is as much a symptom of aortic regurgitation as it is of aortic stenosis (Graboys & Cohn, 1977) and does not necessarily indicate coexistent coronary disease.

MITRAL STENOSIS

Mitral stenosis is not seen in an initial attack of acute rheumatic fever but develops as a manifestation of chronic rheumatic valvulitis in some patients after a long latent period. In the West it is typically a disease of adults but more rapid progression in 'developing' countries can lead to clinical presentation in adoles-

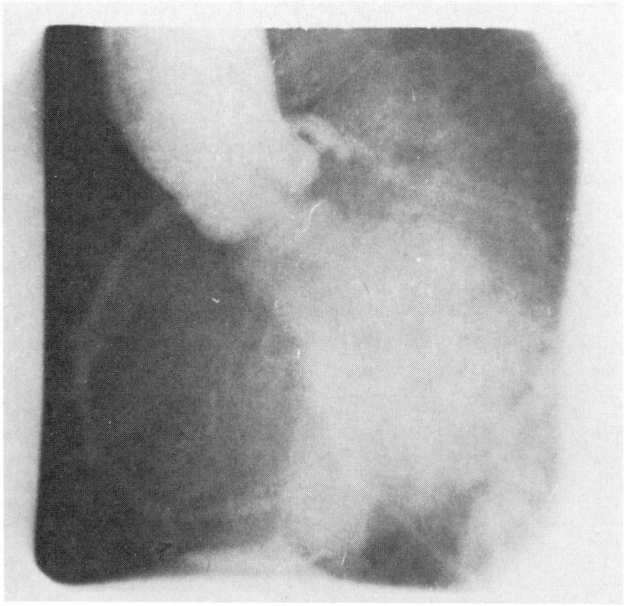

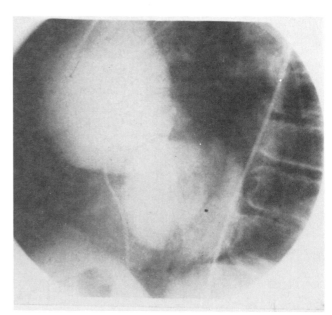

FIG. 7.27. Left anterior oblique aortogram showing aortic regurgitation through a thickened (rheumatic) valve.

FIG. 7.28. Left anterior oblique aortogram: grossly dilated aortic root and ascending aorta (annuloaortic ectasia) with aortic regurgitation.

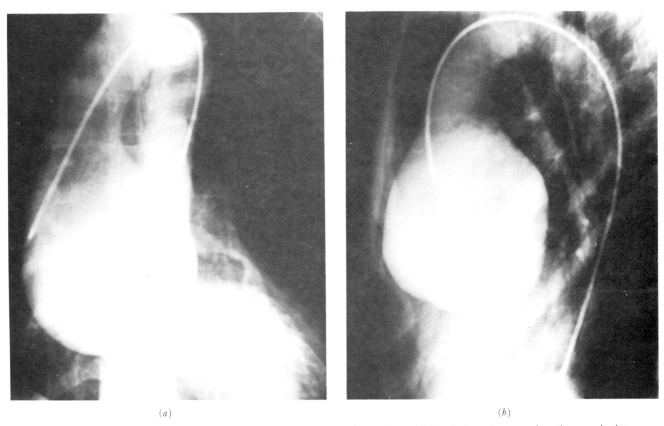

Fig. 7.29. Anterioposterior (a) and lateral (b) views of an aortogram in a patient with Marfan's syndrome and aortic regurgitation.

cence or even childhood. The stenosis is due to one or any combination of (a) commissural fusion, (b) fibrotic cusp rigidity, often exaggerated by later calcification, and (c) fusion of shortened chordae tendineae into a fibrous subvalvar obstruction. Acquired mitral stenosis is, with rare exceptions, generally considered synonymous with such chronic rheumatic valvulitis though a history of rheumatic fever is only found in 50% of cases and there is a female predominance of about 3:1 despite the equal sex incidence of rheumatic fever.

Left atrial myxoma can obstruct the mitral orifice with a clinical presentation similar to rheumatic stenosis; it is rare but a potential cause of sudden death and an important differential diagnosis. 'Ball valve' left atrial thrombus (a rare complication of valvar mitral stenosis) can similarly give fatal obstruction. Other recognised causes of acquired mitral stenosis are systemic lupus erythematosus, mucopolysaccharidoses, carcinoid syndrome and massive mitral annual calcification; in these the stenosis is rare and even when present only a secondary feature in the patient's general clinical condition. Congenital mitral stenosis is considered in Chapter 13; Lutembacher's syndrome is the fortuitous combination of a congenital fault, atrial septal defect, and acquired (rheumatic) mitral stenosis.

Chest Radiographs: Fluoroscopy

Heart size: chamber enlargement. Heart size in mitral stenosis depends on the degree of left atrial enlargement and the extent of pulmonary hypertensive right heart changes; the left ventricle is not enlarged. At clinical presentation a typical case shows a normal cardiothoracic ratio and slight to moderate enlargement of the left atrium (Fig. 7.30).

Significant mitral stenosis is unlikely but not unknown without radiographic left atrial enlargement and though this is usually slight to moderate all degrees can be seen, even the massive left atrium more usually associated with additional mitral regurgitation. The enlargement is determined by the distending effect of left atrial hypertension (consequent on mitral obstruction) and the distensibility of the atrial wall. Reduced atrial wall compliance due to the initial rheumatic carditis is thought responsible for the poor relationship between left atrial pressure and volume in rheumatic mitral stenosis (Chen *et al.*, 1968); particular susceptibility of the appendage to such damage may account for its disproportionate enlargement relative to the atrial body (Fig. 7.31) which is so typical of rheumatic mitral valve disease and uncommon in other causes of left

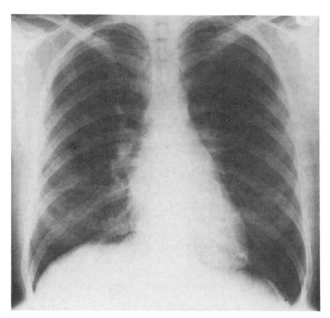

FIG. 7.30. Normal heart size, slight left atrial enlargement (large appendage, double shadow of heart to the right of the spine) and slight pulmonary vascular redistribution in a patient presenting with signs and symptoms of mitral stenosis.

atrial enlargement (Green *et al.*, 1982). Large left atria and atrial fibrillation have a positive association but it is unclear which is cause and effect.

The enlarging left atrium in rheumatic mitral valve disease is as much a space-occupying lesion as any intrathoracic tumour and many of the plain film signs described in Chapter 1 depend on its displacement of other structures, notably the aorta (Figs. 7.32 and 7.37) and bronchi (Fig. 7.33). Oesophageal compression can lead to dysphagia (Whitney & Croxon, 1972), bronchial compression (Fig. 7.32) to obstructive pneumonitis and left recurrent laryngeal nerve compression to hoarseness (Camishion *et al.*, 1966).

Left atrial hypertension is transmitted back through the valveless pulmonary veins and must be accompanied by an appropriate ('passive') rise in pulmonary artery pressure to maintain pulmonary blood flow. In about a third of patients with chronic pulmonary venous hypertension from mitral stenosis there is a further inappropriate ('reactive') elevation of pulmonary artery pressure, sometimes to systemic levels. Development of right ventricular hypertrophy, failure, 'functional' tricuspid regurgitation and right atrial enlargement will depend on the degree and chronicity of these pulmonary hypertensive changes; at the extreme they can lead to a chest radiograph dominated by right heart enlargement (Fig. 7.34) despite the underlying left heart lesion.

Calcification of the mitral valve is common in mitral stenosis, particularly in males, but is of minor diagnostic importance (cf. aortic valve calcification in aortic stenosis) except in the rare case of 'silent' mitral

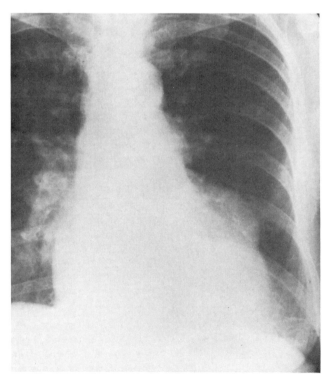

FIG. 7.31. Disproportionate enlargement of the left atrial appendage in rheumatic mitral valve disease. Posteroanterior chest radiograph of a patient with mitral stenosis.

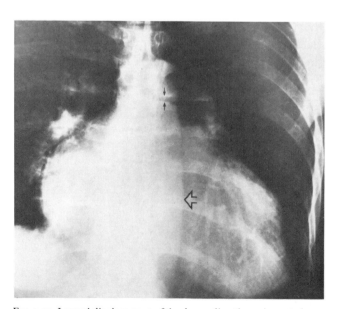

FIG. 7.32. Lateral displacement of the descending thoracic aorta (open arrow) and compression of the left main bronchus beneath the aortic arch (small arrows) due to gross left atrial enlargement in rheumatic mitral valve disease.

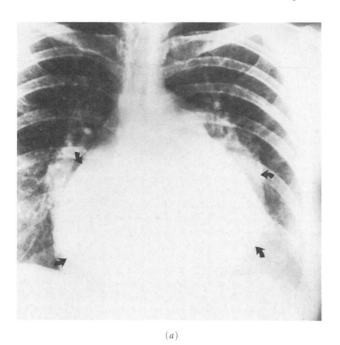

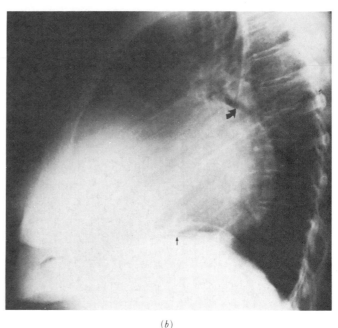

(a)

(b)

Fig. 7.33. Gross left atrial enlargement in rheumatic mitral valve disease (mitral stenosis in this case but more typically seen in regurgitant or mixed lesions). Note that the left heart border is formed partly by the left atrium (body not appendage here) and that there is a double shadow of left atrial enlargement on *both* sides of the chest. The carina is splayed and the lateral view shows that the left main bronchus (curved arrow) is displaced posteriorly and superiorly. The small arrow indicates free subphrenic gas remaining after a Caesarean section!

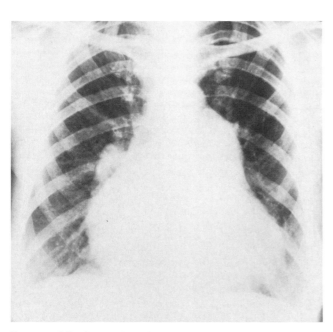

Fig. 7.34. Mitral stenosis with severe reactive pulmonary arterial hypertension. The mediastinal border between aortic 'knuckle' and left ventricle is formed by dilated main pulmonary artery and dilated right ventricular outflow tract (the latter can obscure a large left atrial appendage; in this patient the appendage had been amputated at a previous mitral valvotomy).

stenosis (auscultatory signs masked by low cardiac output) presenting as pulmonary hypertension. In the frontal projection a calcified mitral valve is seen to the left of the spine, largely below a line drawn from the left atrial appendage—left ventricular junction to the right cardiophrenic angle (Figs. 7.01 and 7.35a) in the lateral it is largely below a line from the hilum to the anterior chest wall-diaphragm junction (Figs. 7.02 and 7.35b). It may be suspected, even diagnosed, on plain films but cannot be excluded without fluoroscopy. A calcified valve is a relative contraindication to closed mitral valvotomy and fluoroscopy is therefore of importance in the assessment of mitral stenosis where this operation is contemplated. Fluoroscopic detection is outlined on p. 127; mitral valve calcification can be graded in like manner to aortic valve calcification (p. 127). Rheumatic calcification is of the cusps and commissures and thus distinguished from the partial or complete ring of coarse mitral annual calcification familiar to radiologists as an incidental finding in chest radiographs or barium swallows of the elderly. Such mitral annular calcification is common in old age, particularly in females, and is rarely of functional significance, though it can cause mitral regurgitation, mitral stenosis or, by extension into the conducting system, bradyarrhythmias (Pomerance, 1974). It is considered to be a degenerative 'wear and tear' change and its formation can be accelerated in conditions of left ventricular hypertrophy.

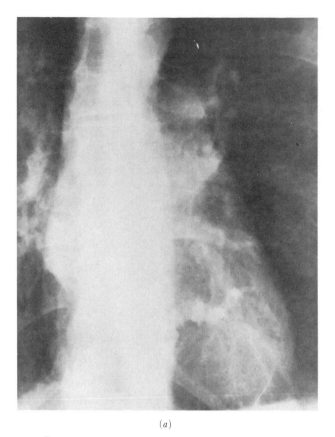

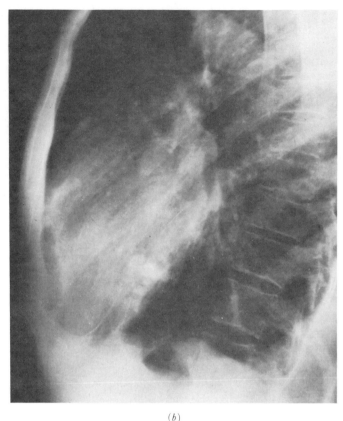

(a)   (b)

FIG. 7.35. (a) and (b). Posteroanterior and lateral views of unusually gross mitral valve calcification in a patient with mitral stenosis.

Calcification of the left atrial wall (rarely of contained thrombus) is seen in a small number of patients, usually females, with isolated mitral stenosis or dominant stenosis in mixed mitral valve disease (Seltzer et al., 1967). Calcification of the free wall (the septum is rarely affected) can be partial or complete and in the latter case the almost immobile atrial shell is seen as a circular shadow in frontal projection (Fig. 7.36a) and as a circle broken anteriorly in lateral projection (Fig. 7.36b). This anterior deficiency is due to the position of the mitral valve which may also be calcified but is blurred by valve motion.

The aortic knuckle is said to be small in mitral stenosis (Jefferson & Rees, 1980) and this may be actual, due to low cardiac output, or merely suggested by increased size of the adjacent pulmonary artery. Mitral stenosis has a positive association with systemic hypertension, presumed due to renal emboli from the left atrium or mitral valve itself (Obeyeskere et al., 1965), and this can lead to an enlarged aortic knuckle; nothing is simple! (Fig. 7.37).

Pulmonary vascular pattern. Pulmonary venous hypertension is inevitable in severe mitral stenosis and is manifest on the plain chest radiograph as pulmonary

vascular redistribution in most cases. Simon has drawn attention to its occasional and unexplained absence (Simon, 1972).

It is generally accepted that elevation of pulmonary capillary pressure above 20–25 mmHg results in pulmonary oedema. This is certainly true of an acute rise, but considerably higher levels of chronic pulmonary venous hypertension (as seen in severe mitral stenosis) can occur without obvious oedema because of two protective mechanisms; thickening of the alveolar-capillary membrane, acting as a barrier to oedema formation, and increased lymphatic drainage of the lung, which may remove oedema as rapidly as it is formed. Acute on chronic increase in pulmonary venous pressure in mitral stenosis is usually manifest as an interstitial oedema pattern on the chest radiograph but alveolar oedema can occur, notably when some additional load such as pregnancy is placed upon the circulatory system.

A 'passive' rise in pulmonary arterial pressure is a necessary accompaniment to pulmonary venous hypertension and is predicted by the radiographic signs of the latter. In about a third of patients with mitral stenosis gross vasoconstrictive and obliterative changes in small

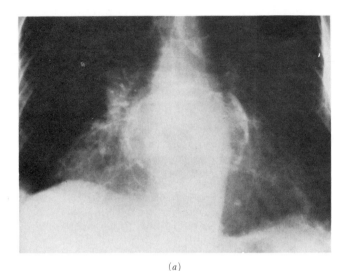

(a)

FIG. 7.36. (a) and (b). Posteroanterior and lateral chest radiographs of a calcified left atrium. Note also the evidence of right atrial enlargent which was due to functional tricuspid regurgitation.

(b)

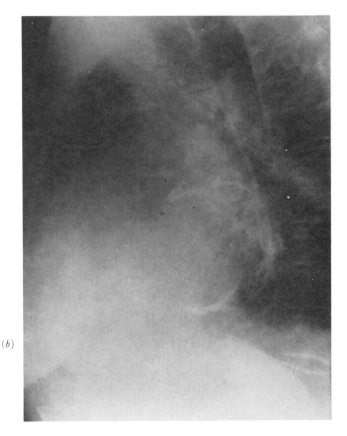

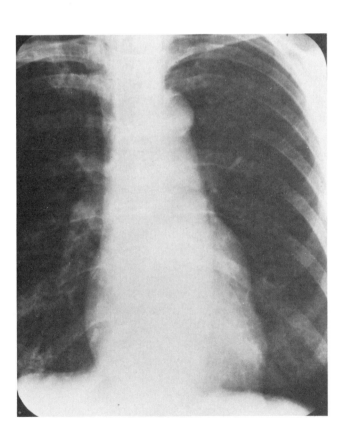

FIG. 7.37. Mitral stenosis and hypertension: the aortic 'knuckle' is large in this patient with both conditions and the aortic enlargement is exaggerated by lateral displacement of the descending aorta by the large left atrium.

muscular pulmonary arteries and arterioles develop in response to the chronic pulmonary venous hypertension and cause additional and severe 'reactive' pulmonary arterial hypertension. This results in reduced right ventricular output and thus diminished pulmonary blood flow with consequent reduction in pulmonary venous pressure, another protective mechanism against pulmonary oedema but one which operates at the cost of low cardiac output. The radiographic signs of such pulmonary hypertension are narrowing of the lower zone segmental arteries and dilation of more proximal arteries, particularly the main pulmonary artery, in the presence of pulmonary vascular redistribution (Figs. 7.34 and 7.39a).

The plain film signs of pulmonary venous and arterial hypertension generally have good correlation with pressures measured at cardiac catheterisation and with the degree of causative mitral stenosis (Chen *et al.*, 1968) but exceptions do occur; severe mitral stenosis can be present with a normal pulmonary vascular pattern, a patient with mitral stenosis may show considerable pulmonary vascular redistribution despite only marginally raised left atrial pressure at catheterisation and main pulmonary artery can be obviously dilated despite near normal pulmonary artery pressure. Such discrepancies are not easily explained but, in respect of the false positives, it must be remembered that pressures recorded at cardiac catheterisation are usually from sedated resting patients receiving optimal medical treatment in hospital. It may be that the chest radiograph is more representative of their haemodynamic state outside hospital; radiological improvement can certainly lag behind haemodynamic improvement and, from observation of patients after successful mitral valve surgery, the radiological signs can be irreversible in some cases.

Pleural effusion can occur in mitral stenosis as a result of pulmonary venous hypertension or right heart failure. Pulmonary infarction is common in mitral stenosis and an additional cause for pleural effusion; persistent unilateral effusion raises the possibility of pulmonary venous thrombosis or vein occlusion by left atrial thrombus.

Pulmonary haemosiderosis is a common pathological finding in mitral stenosis and in some cases the aggregates of haemosiderin-laden phagocytes, resulting from repeated small alveolar haemorrhages due to the high pulmonary capillary pressure, can be large enough to give diffuse nodular lung opacities (Lendrum *et al.*, 1950). The nodules are typically of uniform size, about 1–2 mm in diameter, and most abundant in the mid and lower zones (Fig. 7.38). Accompanying fibrosis can give reticulation and septal lines. These findings are only distinguishable from non-cardiac (primary) pulmonary haemosiderosis by the accompanying signs of heart disease.

Emphasis is given here to pulmonary haemosiderosis in mitral stenosis but it is a consequence of longstanding pulmonary venous hypertension and not the valve lesion *per se*; most other causes of pulmonary venous hypertension are, however, associated with left ventricular dysfunction which usually precludes the longevity needed for development of the lung opacities.

Pulmonary ossification nodules are also associated with the chronic pulmonary venous hypertension typified by mitral stenosis and are due to bone formation in areas of chronic intra-alveolar oedema. They are seen on the chest radiograph as irregular calcific nodules of up to 10 mm diameter, largest and most numerous in the lower zones (Fig. 7.39). The nodules have been described in 13% of patients with mitral valve disease (Galloway *et al.*, 1961) which is similar to the incidence of (radiographic) pulmonary haemosiderosis, though the two are rarely seen together and ossification nodules differ in showing a marked male predominance.

Echocardiography

Ultrasound examination of the heart began with the study of mitral valve disease (Edler & Gustafson, 1957) and it remains an important clinical application of the technique. M-mode studies in mitral stenosis show reduced amplitude of motion of a thickened anterior

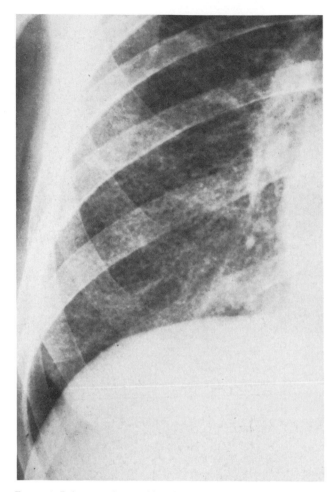

FIG. 7.38. Pulmonary haemosiderosis in a patient with mitral stenosis.

mitral cusp and a reduced early diastolic closing (E–F) slope (Fig. 7.40). Reduced E–F slope was once considered pathognomonic of mitral stenosis and the flattening of the slope was thought to correlate well with the degree of stenosis. It is now recognised as occurring in other conditions of decreased left ventricular filling rate (Layton *et al.*, 1973) and in pulmonary hypertension (McLaurin *et al.*, 1973); its supposed correlation with severity in mitral stenosis has not been substantiated (Cope *et al.*, 1975). Anterior diastolic motion of the posterior mitral cusp echoes (reversal of their normal motion) occurs in mitral stenosis and this parallel movement with the anterior cusp (Fig. 7.40) has been attributed to commissural fusion. Normal motion of the posterior cusp echoes was taken to differentiate other causes of reduced E–F slope from mitral stenosis until the inevitable report of normal motion in approximately 10% of a series of proven mitral stenotics (Levisman *et al.*, 1975). A calcified mitral valve gives dense echoes which are essentially an exaggeration of those seen with

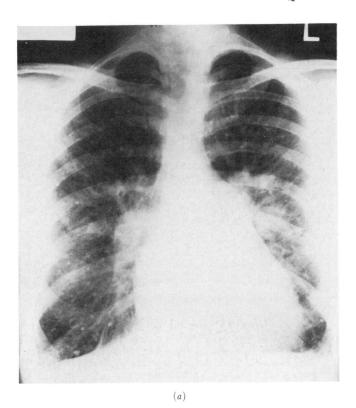

(a)

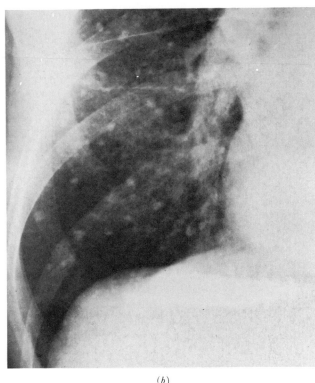

(b)

FIG. 7.39. (a) and (b). Chest radiographs of two patients with pulmonary ossification nodules due to the chronic pulmonary venus hypertension of mitral stenosis. Note the evidence of reactive pulmonary arterial hypertension in (a).

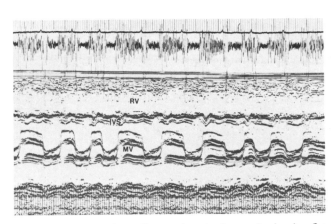

FIG. 7.40. M-mode echocardiogram in mitral stenosis showing flat E–F slope and parallel motion of the echoes of both mitral valve (MV) cusps.

fibrotic thickening alone; differentiation between the two is not always easy and fluoroscopy, albeit less sensitive in the detection of calcification, still has a role here.

Despite individual criticism, the three signs of reduced E–F slope of the anterior cusp, anterior diastolic motion of the posterior cusp and coarse multiple cusp echoes together reliably indicate mitral stenosis. Quantification by the M-mode echocardiogram has been poor and the many proposals of improved M-mode indices now appear outdated by two-dimensional studies which appear reliable and reproducible (Martin et al., 1979). The two-dimensional short axis view cuts across the valve which is seen as an opening and shutting 'fish mouth' (Fig. 7.41c & d); the maximal diastolic orifice can thus be measured but the slice must be taken at the apex of the stenosed valve, with gain settings which do not artefactually alter the orifice.

Doppler technique has been applied to mitral stenosis and, as with aortic stenosis, has been shown able to estimate the pressure gradient across the valve (Thuillez et al., 1980).

It is increasingly apparent that a patient with isolated mitral stenosis and no angina pectoris who is a potential candidate for valve surgery can be adequately assessed before operation by echocardiography without need for cardiac catheterisation. If local policy still demands pre-operative catheterisation, echocardiography should not be omitted or the occasional left atrial myxoma masquerading as rheumatic mitral stenosis will wait on catheter diagnosis, with its attendant risk of induced tumour embolus.

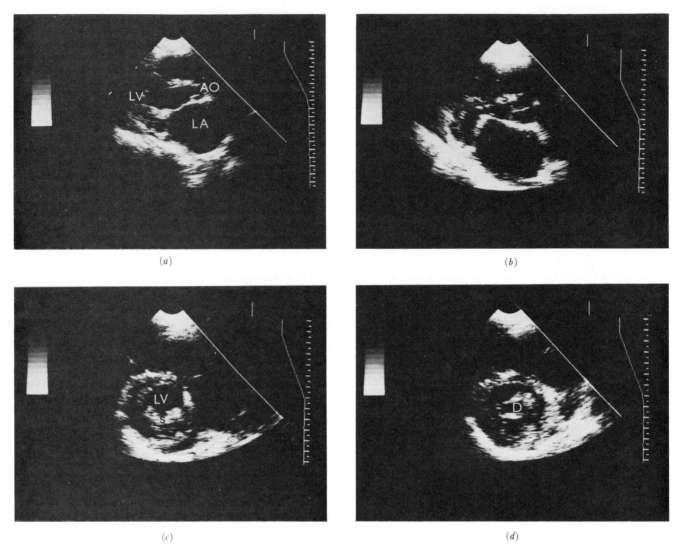

FIG. 7.41. Four views of a two dimensional echocardiogram in mitral stenosis. (a) is a long axis view in systole; the aortic valve cusps are shown open in the aortic root (AO) and the mitral valve between left atrium (LA) and left ventricle (LV) is closed. (b) Shows the same projection (or section) in diastole and the restricted opening of the doming mitral valve is obvious. The corresponding short axis views are (c) and (d) which show the mitral valve closed (S), then open like a 'fish mouth' (D).

Cardiac Catheterisation: Angiocardiography

This is still widely practised in the investigation of mitral stenosis despite a reported 0·8% major complication rate for diagnostic cardiovascular catheterisation (Karnegis & Heinz, 1979) and the known potential of the non-invasive studies discussed above.

The mitral valve gradient is measured at cardiac catheterisation from simultaneously recorded left atrial (or the equivalent pulmonary capillary wedge) and left ventricular pressures. Mitral valve orifice area is calculated from this gradient and other catheter data which give mitral valve flow by the Gorlin formula, first described in 1951 and still, with minor revision (Cohen & Gorlin, 1972), the accepted standard for other quantification of mitral stenosis. The normal calculated valve area is 4 cm² or more; mitral stenosis is severe with an area less than 1 cm², moderate at 1–1·5 cm² and mild above 1·5 cm². Amongst other data obtained at catheter, the pulmonary artery pressure and pulmonary vascular resistance (calculated from the mean pressure difference between pulmonary artery and left atrium divided by flow, the result usually expressed in arbitrary units) are of particular prognostic importance.

Left ventriculography supplements other catheter data with a cine angiographic assessment of left ventricular and mitral valve function and particularly allows exclusion of mitral regurgitation.

The right anterior oblique projection is preferred for a single plane study as it puts the ventricular long axis at right angles to the X-ray beam and gives good separation of the ventricle and left atrium, with the mitral valve in profile between them. In systole the profiled, closed valve sharply defines the junction between the non-opaque atrium and the opacified ventricle (with some overlap from the left ventricular outflow tract). This demarcation is normally lost in diastole as non-opaque blood floods through the open valve, but with mitral stenosis it persists and bulges into the opaque ventricle as the cusps dome forward in their attempt to open (Fig. 7.42); the extent of the bulging motion depends on the pliability of the valve (Demany *et al.*, 1966). A negative jet of non-opaque blood entering the left ventricle may be seen, though the diastolic gradient across even a severely stenosed valve is seldom sufficient to give this sign.

The chordae tendineae extend from the papillary muscle tips to the mitral valve and this distance can be measured from the right anterior oblique left ventriculogram. Chordal shortening and fusion in chronic rheumatic disease can give a significant subvalvar element to mitral stenosis, a contraindication to simple mitral valvotomy which can be predicted from the ventriculogram by the ratio of chordal to ventricular length (Akins *et al.*, 1979).

Mitral regurgitation is a contraindication to simple mitral valvotomy and its presence is confirmed or denied by the left ventriculogram. It is unfortunate that the catheter motion inevitable with a pressure injection of contrast medium into the left ventricle so frequently produces ventricular ectopic beats with disturbance of papillary muscle function and artefactual mitral regurgitation. Such artefact must be recognised at the time and if necessary proved by repeat ventriculography with altered catheter position and reduced injection rate to avoid ectopics.

Left ventricular dysfunction is not a feature of mitral stenosis but the ventriculogram often shows minor abnormalities of contraction—hypokinesis of the posterobasal area, attributed to splinting by the rigid mitral valve complex (Heller & Carleton, 1970), and anterolateral hypokinesis, attributed to a compression effect by an enlarged right ventricle (Curry *et al.*, 1972), with slight reduction of ejection fraction. Occasionally more severe generalised impairment of contraction is present, perhaps due to rheumatic myocarditis. Marked left atrial enlargement can occur in mitral stenosis, mitral regurgitation or any combination of the two, but when stenosis is dominant and left ventricular enlargement is therefore absent or slight, the effect of the large left atrium on the ventricle can be dramatic as shown in Fig. 7.43 where the ventricle is seen to be pushed forward against the chest wall with consequent squaring of its normally ellipsoid shape. This ventriculographic

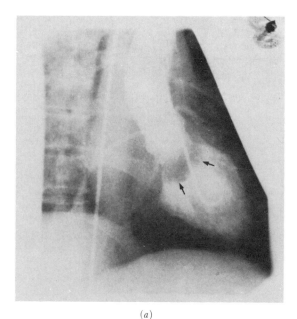
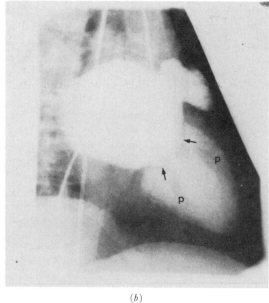

(a)   (b)

FIG. 7.42. (a) Right anterior oblique left ventriculogram in mitral stenosis. This diastolic frame of the cine film shows the mitral valve bulging or doming into the opaque left ventricle, giving a filling defect (arrowed). (b) Shows a left atrial contrast injection in the same patient and same projection. The doming slightly thickened valve is now seen (arrowed) as a curvilinear filling defect between the opaque atrium and ventricle. The other filling defects seen in the ventricle are the papillary muscles (p).

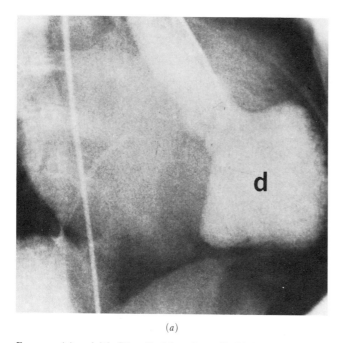
(a)

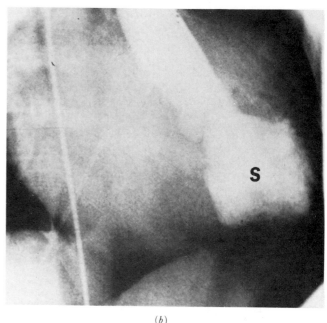
(b)

FIG. 7.43. (a) and (b). Diastolic (d) and systolic (s) frames from a right anterior oblique left ventriculogram in mitral stenosis. Note the forward displacement and 'squaring' of the left ventricle due to the huge left atrium.

finding has been strangely neglected in the literature though a recent echochardiographic study has described it in part (Beppu *et al.*, 1982).

The haemodynamic changes resulting from intravascular injection of conventional (high osmolality) contrast media at left ventriculography have long been utilised in the assessment of severity of mitral stenosis (Rahimtoola *et al.*, 1966); the new low osmolality media have considerably less effect on mitral gradient and pulmonary pressures and their use is to be welcomed despite loss of the ventriculographic 'stress test'.

Aortography. Some degree of rheumatic aortic regurgitation is so commonly associated with mitral stenosis that it is usual to complete a catheter assessment of the mitral lesion with cine aortography; in addition to reassuring the surgeon that significant aortic regurgitation (which would influence surgical technique) has not been missed, some information on the coronary arteries is usually gained.

Coronary arteriography is usually reserved for patients with angina pectoris in addition to the symptoms of mitral stenosis. Coronary embolus (Fig. 7.21) is a recognised complication of mitral valve disease but any disease of the coronary arteries found is more likely to be atherosclerosis. A coronary arteriographic feature almost peculiar to mitral stenosis is the occasional neovascularity of organised left atrial thrombus, with numerous small arterial branches to the atrium, contrast blush in the thrombus and contrast leak into the atrial cavity (Fig. 7.44) (Soulen *et al.*, 1977).

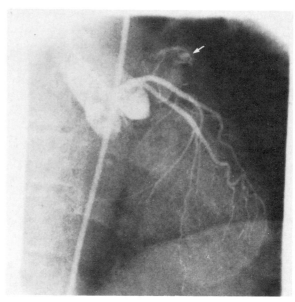

FIG. 7.44. Left coronary arteriogram (shallow right anterior oblique projection) showing neovascularity of thrombus in the left atrial appendage (arrow).

Other Examinations

Pulmonary and systemic emboli are well-known complications of mitral stenosis which may require investigation by the usual radiological methods. If venography or arteriography is required, the radiologist should

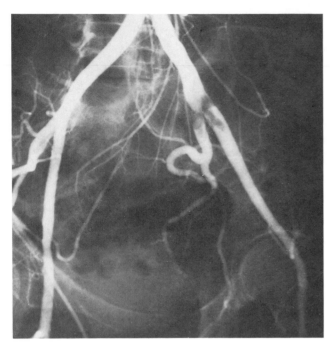

FIG. 7.45. 'Saddle embolus' at the bifurcation of the left common iliac artery. Pelvic arteriogram in a patient with mitral stenosis and systemic embolus.

remember the lesser cardiovascular toxicity of low osmolality contrast media, particularly if there is cardiac decompensation. Systemic embolus (Fig. 7.45) can complicate mitral stenosis of any degree and can even be a presenting feature; the valve lesion is therefore important in the list of potential causes for unexplained arterial occlusion.

MITRAL REGURGITATION

The mitral valve apparatus consists of the annulus, the two cusps, chordae tendineae, two papillary muscle groups (anterolateral and posteromedial) and the left ventricular free wall in which the papillary muscles are based. Dysfunction of any of these elements can result in mitral regurgitation, a haemodynamic fault seen in numerous diseases, many of which are listed below; no doubt the reader can add a favourite rarity. There are obvious similarities with the list given for aortic regurgitation, not least that the valve fault is rare, trivial or both in many of the conditions. Important causes of severe mitral regurgitation are in italics and will be discussed further.

Diseases associated with mitral regurgitation
Carcinoid syndrome
Cardiomyopathy: dilated or hypertrophic
Congenital mitral valve disease

Ehlers Danlos syndrome
Infective endocarditis
Ischaemic heart disease
Left atrial myxoma
Lupus erythematosus
Marfan's syndrome
Mitral annular calcification
Mitral valve replacement: prosthetic dysfunction
Mucopolysaccharidoses
Ostegenesis imperfecta
Primary mitral valve prolapse
Pseudoxanthoma elasticum
Rheumatic valvulitis
Rheumatoid arthritis
Spontaneous rupture of chordae tendineae
Trauma: blunt or penetrating

Mitral regurgitation resulting from the annular dilation or papillary muscle distortion which can occur in any severe left ventricular dilation is termed 'functional' and brings virtually all causes of left ventricular disease into the list.

Primary mitral valve prolapse. Systolic prolapse of floppy mitral cusps into the left atrium is characterised pathologically by myxomatous degeneration of the cusps and clinically by a mid systolic click followed in many cases by a mitral regurgitant murmur. It can be seen in the collagen diseases listed above but is most common in a primary (idiopathic) form which affects a surprisingly high percentage of the 'normal' population, at least 6% (Darsee et al., 1979; Procacci et al., 1976); this is to be remembered when noting its numerous reported associations but there is no doubt of its true association with the skeletal deformities of depressed sternum and the straight back syndrome (Bon Tempo et al., 1975). Symptoms, other than those of mitral regurgitation, are atypical chest pain, usually of undetermined cause, though coronary artery spasm has been implicated (Mautner et al., 1981), and palpitations (arrhythmias are a recognised feature). Complications include rupture of chordae tendineae (also involved in the myxomatous process), infective endocarditis and emboli; the neuroradiologist should note its implication as a cause of stroke (Kostuk et al., 1977) and amaurosis fugax (Wilson et al., 1977). The mitral regurgitation is typically trivial but progresses to severity in some cases (Mills et al., 1977) and may be acutely and massively increased by chordal rupture. Though relatively few people with mitral valve prolapse suffer its potentially fatal complications it is now one of the major causes of isolated mitral regurgitation requiring mitral valve replacement (Waller et al., 1982).

Ischaemic heart disease is probably the commonest cause of mitral regurgitation and though the percentage of cases with severe regurgitation is small, the very numbers involved ensure prominence in any list of causes for mitral valve replacement. Papillary muscle dysfunction with mitral regurgitation (Burch *et al.*, 1968) can be transient in an episode of myocardial ischaemia or persistent when there is infarction of papillary muscle or adjacent left ventricular free wall. Left ventricular aneurysm can involve a papillary muscle base and also alter its alignment to the valve, with consequent regurgitation. The generalised left ventricular dilation of ischaemic cardiomyopathy can cause functional mitral regurgitation.

Mitral regurgitation rarely dominates the clinical picture in ischaemic heart disease unless rupture of a papillary muscle during myocardial infarction produces acute massive leak.

Infective endocarditis can involve a normal or diseased mitral valve and may produce regurgitation by destruction of cusps, abscess formation in the annulus or rupture of chordae tendineae.

Rheumatic valvulitis. Mitral regurgitation can be clinically audible in acute rheumatic fever, usually as a consequence of annular dilation, but rarely has haemodynamic importance until the stage of chronic rheumatic disease is reached. It is then typically combined with stenosis but fibrotic cusp retraction and chordal shortening occasionally occur without fusion of these elements, giving isolated regurgitation.

Chest Radiographs: Fluoroscopy

Radiological signs in mitral regurgitation are determined by the magnitude of the leak and its mode of onset. In general, severe acute regurgitation shows a normal or slightly enlarged heart with pulmonary oedema while chronic regurgitation shows cardiomegaly with large left heart chambers, particularly the atrium, but relatively slight changes of venous hypertension in the lungs.

Heart size: chamber enlargement. The limited distensibility of previously normal heart chambers allows only slight enlargement in acute mitral regurgitation (Fig. 7.46) despite considerable volume overload of the left ventricle and both volume and pressure overload of the left atrium. In chronic regurgitation the left ventricle adapts by dilation and hypertrophy and the left atrium shows either moderate dilation (with significantly raised left atrial pressure) or massively enlarges to accommodate even gross regurgitant volumes with little or no increase in pressure (Braunwald & Awe, 1963). Thus, in chronic mitral regurgitation the overall heart size is increased, left ventricular enlargement is usually detectable and the left atrium is either moderately or grossly enlarged (Figs. 7.47 and 7.48). The largest atria are usually seen in rheumatic disease and rheumatic carditis is presumably a factor; it is again worth noting that a disproportionately large appendage strongly suggests rheumatic aetiology (Green *et al.*, 1982).

Pulmonary vascular pattern of course varies with

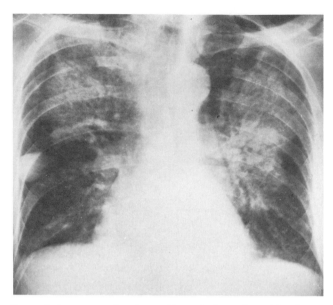

FIG. 7.46. Anteroposterior chest radiograph of a patient with pulmonary oedema (and locculated right pleural effusion) due to acute mitral regurgitation.

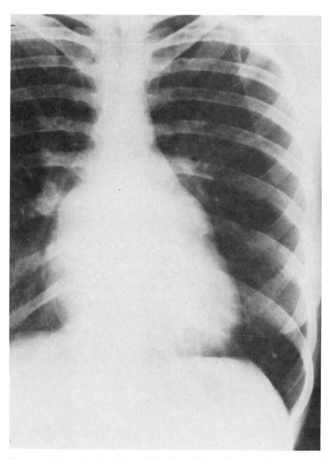

FIG. 7.47. Chronic mitral regurgitation with moderate enlargement of the left atrium.

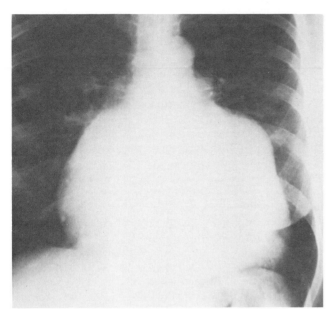

FIG. 7.48. Chronic mitral regurgitation with gross enlargement of the left atrium.

the severity of the haemodynamic fault but is considerably influenced by the compliance of the left atrium (Braunwald, 1969). In severe acute regurgitation (e.g. ruptured chordae or papillary muscle) with a virtually normal-sized atrium, the high left atrial pressure is transmitted into the pulmonary vasculature with immediate and gross changes of pulmonary venous hypertension (Fig. 7.46). Survivors of the acute insult (which has a high mortality) develop severe reactive pulmonary hypertension in months rather than the years taken for this development in mitral stenosis; pulmonary arterial enlargement occurs but is relatively slight. In severe chronic mitral regurgitation those cases with moderate left atrial enlargement (the majority) have significant left atrial hypertension and the plain film signs of pulmonary venous hypertension (Fig. 7.47). These are typically less than those seen in mitral stenosis, as the mean left atrial pressure is higher with mitral obstruction than with a comparable degree of regurgitation. Severe left atrial hypertension will supervene in this as in any type of mitral regurgitation when the left ventricle fails; life expectancy is then limited. Reactive pulmonary arterial hypertension, haemosiderosis and ossification nodules are all rare in isolated mitral regurgitation, presumably reflecting the differences in degree and chronicity of venous hypertension in mitral regurgitation compared with mitral stenosis. The less common type of chronic mitral regurgitation associated with a huge left atrium shows relatively little plain film evidence of pulmonary venous hypertension (Fig. 7.48) until the stage of left ventricular failure.

Calcification of the mitral cusps generally indicates a rheumatic cause for the mitral regurgitation. Mitral annular calcification is usually massive in the rare instance when this common degenerative condition of old age is associated with significant mitral regurgitation. Left atrial calcification is rare in isolated mitral regurgitation.

Echocardiography

M-mode and two-dimensional echocardiography are of limited value in detection and quantitation of mitral regurgitation; pulsed Doppler has been shown to have a high diagnostic accuracy but as yet offers no reliable quantitation (Quinones et al., 1980). However, considerable information on the cause of known mitral regurgitation is given by both M-mode and two-dimensional studies. Rheumatic valvulitis is characterised by thickened cusps (multiple echoes) and restricted motion, whereas the common non-rheumatic causes usually show thin cusps and, even if there is some thickening due to myxomatous degeneration, hypermobility. Mitral valve prolapse is classically detected by later systolic posterior movement of the cusp echoes in M-mode (Fig. 7.49) but in some causes the movement is pansystolic and distinction from similar but less marked pansystolic motion shown by many normal valves can be difficult (Sahn et al., 1977). As might be expected, two-dimensional echocardiography can detect mitral cusp prolapse into the left atrium (Cohen, 1978) but there is still some difficulty in distinguishing minor degrees of prolapse from normality. A flail cusp due to ruptured chordae or papillary muscle shows marked posterior motion into the left atrium on M-mode and two-dimensional studies and is often associated with fluttering cusp echoes in diastole and systole (Child et al., 1979). Vegetations on the valve cusps may be detected in mitral regurgitation associated with infective endocarditis and can be particularly striking in two-dimensional images (Fig. 7.50).

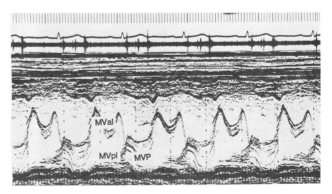

FIG. 7.49. M-mode echocardiogram of mitral valve prolapse showing the posterior systolic motion (MVP) of the posterior cusp. The accompanying phonocardiogram shows the mid-systolic click.

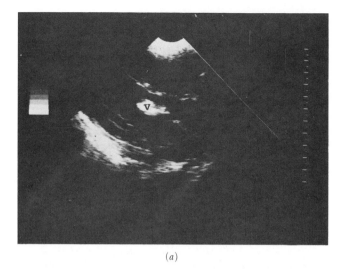

(a)

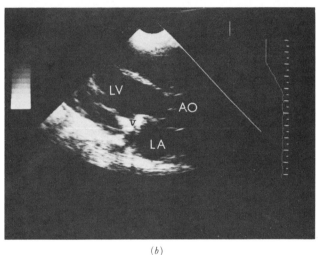

(b)

FIG. 7.50. Two dimensional echocardiogram long axis views in diastole (a) and systole (b) showing a large vegetation (v) on the anterior cusp of the mitral valve. (Left ventricle (LV), left atrium (LA) and aorta (AO) are labelled in b).

Radionuclide Studies

Measurement of left heart valvar regurgitation from gated cardiac blood pool studies has been referred to in the section on aortic regurgitation; the technique does not differentiate aortic from mitral leak but is of use in either if the other valve is competent.

Cardiac Catheterisation: Angiocardiography

The information on cardiac output and pressures obtained at catheterisation is of importance in overall assessment but quantitation of mitral regurgitation is by left ventriculography which, despite considerable limitations, is the generally accepted standard.

Left ventriculography allows assessment of the amount and cause of mitral regurgitation and gives a measure of left ventricular function. Cinefilming is necessary for such dynamic study and the right anterior oblique is the preferred single projection for the reasons given in the section on mitral stenosis; if there is biplane facility, the left anterior oblique can be usefully added for the additional information it gives on the anterior mitral cusp and left ventricular posterior and septal wall motion.

It is usual to make a subjective grading of mitral regurgitation from the extent of observed left atrial opacification, for example grades 1 to 4 indicating mild, moderate, severe and gross regurgitation respectively, but the implied accuracy has little justification (Honey et al., 1969) despite its wide acceptance. Variation in catheter placement and contrast delivery, ectopic beats with artefactual mitral leak, atrial opacification by insignificant diastolic regurgitation, variations in left atrial and ventricular size and contractility all make for difficulty in assessment, even for experienced observers. Measurement of the regurgitant volume by subtracting left ventricular stroke volume, obtained by quantitative analysis of the ventriculogram, from forward stroke volume, derived from some other measure of cardiac output (Dodge, 1971), overcomes some of these difficulties but is not widely used in routine clinical practice.

Features which point to the cause of mitral regurgitation are ventricular size and contraction pattern, the appearances of the valve itself, the nature of the regurgitant stream (Wexler et al., 1971) and the configuration of the left atrium.

In chronic rheumatic disease, the left ventricular volume at end diastole is increased but end systolic volume and ejection fraction are normal until the stage of left ventricular failure; the valve cusps often show some calcification and, when outlined by contrast medium on their atrial and ventricular surfaces, are seen to be thick; the regurgitant stream is typically central or diffuse and, if sufficient, will show a large atrium and large appendage (Fig. 7.51).

In non-rheumatic diseases the cusps are thin and often difficult to see except as the interface between differing ventricular and atrial opacification. Mitral valve prolapse is most commonly confined to the posterior cusp and is often localised to just one of the three scallops of this structure (Fig. 7.52), usually the posteromedial scallop. Posterior cusp prolapse is diagnosed from the right anterior oblique ventriculogram when one or more scallops bulge into the left atrium in systole (Ranaganathan et al., 1973) (Fig. 7.53a); anterior cusp prolapse is poorly shown in this projection and a left anterior oblique view is helpful for its diagnosis (Fig. 7.53b) (Ranaganathan et al., 1974) though it is rarely seen without posterior cusp prolapse. Slight normal systolic bulging of the valve cusps and anatomical variation in the adjacent inferior wall of the left

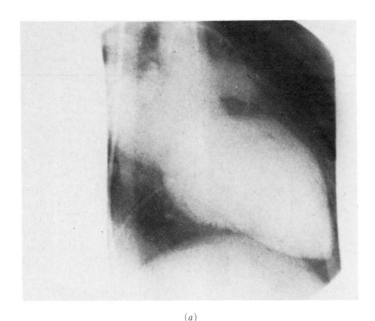

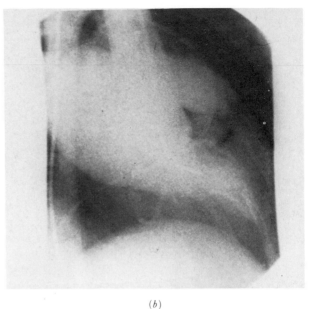

(a)   (b)

Fig. 7.51. Right anterior oblique left ventriculogram in diastole and systole showing a large left ventricle, mitral regurgitation and a large left atrium and appendage.

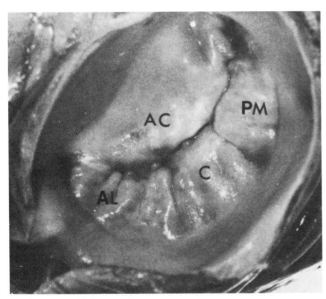

Fig. 7.52. The anterior (AC) and posterior cusps of the mitral valve as seen from the left atrium. Note the three scallops of the posterior cusp, the anterolateral (AL), central or middle (C) and the postero-medial (PM) scallops. (Reproduced with permission from Davies, M. J. (1980) *Pathology of Cardiac Valves*. London: Butterworths.)

ventricle simulating prolapse have lead to mistaken angiographic reports of the condition which can be avoided if strict diagnostic criteria are followed (Spindola-Franco *et al.*, 1980). Mitral regurgitation is not invariable in prolapse but when present the regurgitant stream is usually eccentric. Torn chordae tendineae or the much rarer papillary muscle rupture also show eccentric regurgitation and in such cases the involved flail cusp can usually be seen everting completely into the atrium; left ventricular contraction is normal or hyperdynamic in ruptured chordae but papillary muscle rupture is a complication of myocardial infarction, evident as a regional contraction abnormality. Papillary muscle dysfunction does not give the torrential mitral leak of acute rupture but is also characterised by left ventricular dysfunction and eccentric regurgitation; the valve cusps may show slight prolapse. When mitral regurgitation is functional, the ventriculographic appearances are dominated by the causative ventricular dilation and generalised contraction abnormality, the leak is diffuse rather than localised, the valve cusps, if seen, appear normal and the left atrium is only slightly enlarged; in practice it can occasionally be difficult to distinguish an organic valve fault with secondary ventricular changes from ventricular abnormality with functional regurgitation (and they can of course be additive).

Aortography is usually included if the mitral lesion is rheumatic because of the frequent association with aortic regurgitation.

Coronary arteriography is indicated as part of the catheter assessment if the patient has any feature suggestive of causative or coexistent coronary disease. It is unusual for chest pain in mitral valve prolapse to be typically cardiac but it may necessitate coronary

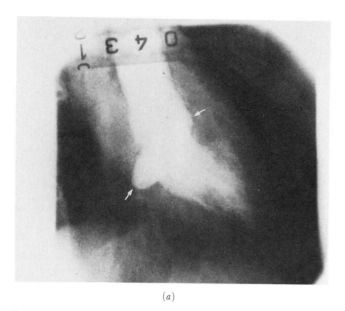
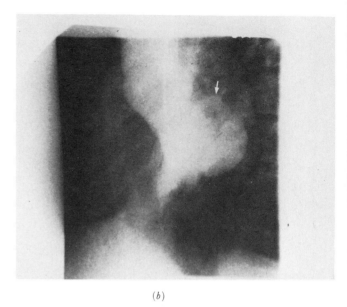

(a)

(b)

FIG. 7.53. (a) Right anterior oblique left ventriculugram in mitral valve prolapse. The bulge of the prolapsing posteromedial scallop of the posterior cusp is indicated by the inferior arrow and that of the anterolateral scallop by the superior arrow (the middle scallop is overshadowed by contrast medium in the left ventricular outflow tract and aortic root). There is no mitral regurgitation in this case despite the total prolapse. (b) Left anterior oblique projection of the same ventriculogram showing prolapse of the anterior cusp (arrow) in addition to the posterior cusp.

arteriography and an association with coronary spasm has already been mentioned.

TRICUSPID AND PULMONARY VALVE DISEASE

The tricuspid and pulmonary valves show many similarities to the mitral and aortic valves respectively but are rarely affected by acquired organic disease and when there is a lesion it is usually the least important feature of multiple valve disease.

Tricuspid stenosis can occur in rheumatic disease and the carcinoid syndrome and the valve can be obstructed by a right atrial myxoma. These conditions, together with infective endocarditis (notably in 'mainlining' drug addicts), tricuspid valve prolapse (similar to and often associated with mitral prolapse), ischaemic heart disease and trauma, can all give acquired **tricuspid regurgitation**, though the only common cause is not an intrinsic valve fault but 'functional' regurgitation due to annular stretching in right ventricular dilation and failure. The radiological hallmark of tricuspid disease is right atrial enlargement with dilation of the superior vena cava and azygos vein on the posteroanterior chest radiograph (Fig. 7.54a) and often posterior displacement and posterior convexity of the inferior vena caval shadow on the lateral (Toombes & Miller, 1979) (Fig. 7.54b). Echocardiographic features are very similar to those seen in analagous mitral valve lesions (but more difficult to obtain); abdominal ultrasound examination will detect not only the hepatic enlarge-

ment of high central venous pressure but also dilation of hepatic veins and the inferior vena cava. Angiography is seldom performed; tricuspid stenosis is better assessed by the transvalvar pressure gradient and the general problems of angiographic assessment of valve leak are added to by the necessarily transvalvar placement of a right ventricular catheter.

Pulmonary stenosis is nearly always congenital but

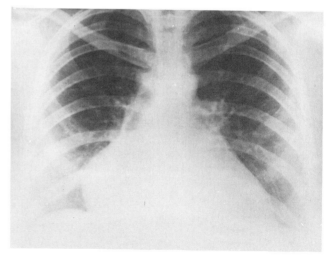

FIG. 7.54. (a) Posteroanterior chest radiograph of a patient with moderate mitral stenosis and severe tricuspid stenosis and regurgitation.

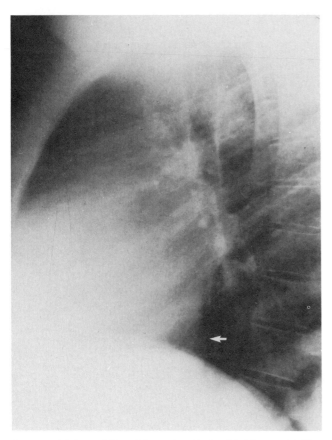

FIG. 7.54. (b) Lateral film of the patient depicted in Fig. 7.54(a). Note the posterior displacement and convexity of the inferior vena cava (arrowed).

acquired obstruction to right ventricular outflow can occur in the carcinoid syndrome or when there is obstruction by intracavitary tumour or even massive thromboembolism.

Pulmonary regurgitation is usually due to the annular dilation which accompanies pulmonary artery enlargement in pulmonary hypertension. Infective endocarditis can involve the pulmonary valve with consequent regurgitation. Rheumatic valvulitis can be virtually ignored as a cause of pulmonary stenosis or regurgitation except in conditions of high altitude living (Vela *et al.*, 1969).

Pulmonary valve disease is not only rare but also of little haemodynamic importance unless there is acute obstruction; there are no specific radiographic features and echocardiographic signs can be predicted from the causes described.

MIXED STENOSIS AND REGURGITATION: MULTIPLE VALVE DISEASE

There is some artificiality in detailed discussion of

isolated single valve faults, the least common worldwide form of acquired valvar disease, but this approach has been used in the above sections to emphasize their effects and radiological signs which are seen in various combinations in mixed and multiple valve disease. In general, acquired stenosis of heart valves occurs in relatively few diseases, often associated with some degree of regurgitation (which can predominate or can be seen in isolation in many of these same diseases); in contrast, solely regurgitant valves occur in a long list of diseases where stenosis is unknown. Mixed stenosis and regurgitation in a single valve is almost certain to be due to chronic rheumatic valvulitis or dystrophic calcification, though myxomas should be remembered amongst the rarities. Multiple valve disease suggests a rheumatic cause but functional regurgitation of an upstream (proximal) valve can add confusion to organic single valve disease.

Chest radiograph signs in mixed and multiple valve disease can be completely misleading if taken out of clinical context, for example the common combination of rheumatic mitral stenosis and aortic regurgitation will have plain film features suggesting mitral regurgitation. There are certain signs worth emphasising in reports even if in disagreement with initial clinical findings; left atrial enlargement evidenced by more than just a double shadow of the heart to the right of the spine suggests mitral valve disease and this is highly likely (and usually rheumatic) if the appendage is disproportionately large; enlargement of the ascending aorta suggests aortic valve disease; enlargement of the right atrium, admittedly a tenuous plain film diagnosis, in the absence of signs of pulmonary arterial hypertension suggests organic tricuspid disease (such right atrial enlargement is usually seen in the presence of the much more obvious left atrial enlargement of coexistent mitral disease); the presence of valve calcification (which can only be excluded by fluoroscopy) indicates disease of that valve, though not necessarily its significance.

CARDIAC TUMOURS

Cardiac tumours can be radiologically 'silent' but include among their manifestations chest radiograph appearances so like acquired valvar disease that they warrant brief description here.

Secondary tumour involvement of the heart by direct extension or distant metastasis is far more common than primary neoplasia but is usually an incidental autopsy finding or just one feature in widespread malignancy; lung cancer, breast cancer, malignant melanoma, malignant lymphoma and leukaemia are the commonest sources. Most primary cardiac tumours are benign and their importance as surgically correctable mimics of virtually any form of heart disease far outweighs their rarity. Myxomas, which constitute about half of all primary tumours (Heath, 1968), are pedunculated, intracavitary, friable masses most commonly found in the left atrium; they are benign and there is even suggestion that they represent organised thrombus not true neoplasm (Salyer *et al.*, 1975) though both familial and multiple occurrence is known and there is a recurrence rate after surgery of about 5% (Sutton *et al.*, 1980). Other benign tumours include rhabdomyomas which are often associated with tuberous sclerosis. Malignant primary tumours are almost invariably sarcomas derived from the various mesenchymal elements of the heart.

Sarcomas and, of the benign lesions, myxomas typically occur in middle age; rhabdomyomas, fibromas and teratomas are seen particularly in children. Clinical presentation of benign tumours depends on site and size: intramural lesions can cause arrhythmia, obstruction to chamber inflow or outflow or ventricular failure; intracavitary lesions can obstruct valves or make them regurgitant and can be a source of emboli. Cardiac sarcomas can produce any of these features, usually in the right heart, but are highly malignant and associated with rapid progression, pericardial effusion and metastases. Systemic effects of primary cardiac tumours (apart from their embolic and metastatic consequences) include the malaise, weight loss, fever, arthralgia, clubbing, haematological and plasma protein abnormalities which can occur with myxomas (Goodwin, 1968).

Chest Radiographs: Fluoroscopy

Plain film features of cardiac tumours depend on cell types and tumour position; they include non-specific cardiomegaly (Fig. 7.55), signs of pericardial effusion, bizarre heart shape (Fig. 7.56) and frankly misleading signs suggesting valve (usually mitral) disease. In disseminated malignancy, the primary tumour (particularly lung cancer) dominates radiological appearances. Non-cardiac thoracic metastasis and an abnormal heart shadow can be due to a cardiac primary (Fig. 7.56) but there are obviously commoner causes for such a combination. Tumour calcification is seen in 10% of myxomas (Davis *et al.*, 1969) and can be gross enough for plain film diagnosis (Fig. 7.57), but like all cardiac calcification, is best assessed by fluoroscopy. The intracavitary position of a calcified myxoma allows virtually

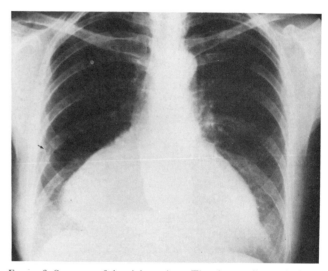

FIG. 7.56. Sarcoma of the right atrium. The chest radiograph shows a bizarre heart shadow and a pathological fracture of a rib (arrow). Multiple skeletal metastases were shown by radionuclide bone scan.

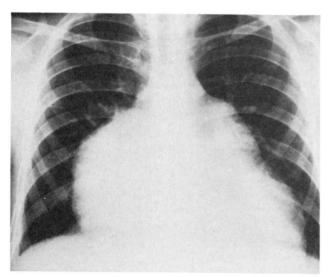

FIG. 7.55. Cardiac enlargement due to a primary sarcoma of the heart in a child.

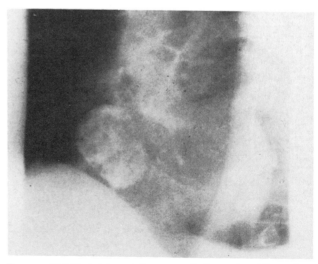

FIG. 7.57. Calcified right atrial myxoma. Left anterior oblique view.

no other differential diagnosis except calcified thrombus; if the calcification moves with blood flow as if on a stalk, myxoma is almost certain.

Tumour obstruction of the right heart can give generalised reduction in pulmonary vascularity and intracavitary right heart tumours can present with signs of acute pulmonary embolus or pulmonary arterial hypertension due to repeated small tumour emboli (Heath & Mackinnon, 1964). Diastolic prolapse of left atrial myxoma into (often through) the mitral valve causes mitral obstruction and sometimes, by repeated impact damage to the valve apparatus, mitral regurgitation. This can be indistinguishable from rheumatic mitral valve disease and similarly associated with radiographic signs of pulmonary venous and arterial hypertension.

Despite these numerous possible signs it must be emphasised that the plain film and fluoroscopic examination is often normal in the presence of cardiac tumour and even when there are clinically significant metastases to the heart the majority of cases show no plain film cardiac abnormality (Abrams *et al.*, 1971).

Echocardiography

Intracavitary tumours are so well demonstrated by this technique that it is an essential examination whenever such a tumour is suspected or is a possible cause of a patient's initial diagnosis (e.g. unexplained systemic or pulmonary embolus or 'mitral valve disease'). This may be considered an overstatement but even the author's limited experience of cardiac tumours includes three left atrial myxomas which presented with systemic emboli, two cerebral and one femoropopliteal (all with normal chest X-rays), two left atrial myxomas diagnosed at cardiac catheterisation for 'mitral valve disease' (no echocardiography before the catheters), one left atrial myxoma diagnosed at surgery for 'rheumatic mitral valve disease' (no echocardiography, missed at catheter) and one right atrial myxoma diagnosed echocardiographically months after an initial presentation with pulmonary infarction.

The echocardiographic features of intracavitary tumours are typified by the commonest example, left atrial myxoma: M-mode examination shows a mass of echoes in the left atrial cavity (Fig. 7.58a) which move to an atrioventricular position behind the anterior mitral cusp if there is diastolic prolapse (Fig. 7.58b). A frozen frame from the two-dimensional echocardiographic demonstration of such a tumour (Fig. 7.59) does little justice to the dramatic real time display of the tumour mass and its motion. The general applications of echocardiography have obvious relevance to cardiac tumour diagnosis, particularly the demonstration of pericardial effusion.

Other Examinations

Cardiac catheterisation and angiocardiography have been virtually replaced by the recent advances in echocardiography unless coexistent disease (e.g. coronary disease) requires preoperative documentation; it is nevertheless interesting to compare an angiographic demonstration of left atrial myxoma (Fig. 7.60) with the echocardiographic picture (Fig. 7.59). If for some reason angiocardiography is required, the general rule is that the angiographic catheter must be kept away from the suspected tumour site to avoid tumour embolus: left atrial myxomas are shown by pulmonary artery injections of contrast medium followed through to the left

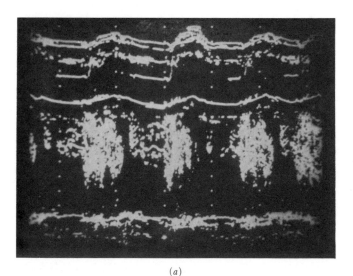

(a)

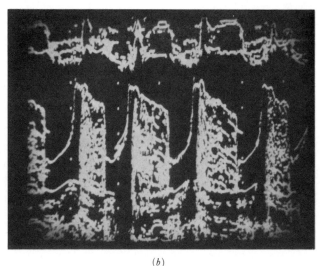

(b)

FIG. 7.58. (a) and (b). M-mode echocardiogram of left atrial myxoma. The mass of echoes from the tumour is seen in the left atrium in systole (a) and behind the anterior mitral cusp in diastole (b).

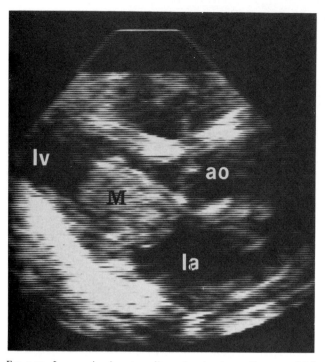

FIG. 7.59. Long axis view two dimensional echocardiogram of left atrial myxoma. The echoes from the myxoma (M) are seen prolapsing through the mitral valve in this diastolic frame (left ventricle (v), left atrium (la) and aorta (ao) are labelled).

heart and right atrial myxomas are best demonstrated by simultaneous inferior and superior vena caval injections (to avoid streaming artefact). Coronary arteriography can demonstrate tumour neovascularity but does not distinguish benign from malignant tumours or even tumours from the more commonly seen neovascularity of organised thrombus (Soulen *et al.*, 1977).

Radionuclide angiocardiography is less sensitive than echocardiography in the diagnosis of myxomas but it can detect them and its increasing use in the screening of cardiac disease must give it some importance.

Peripheral arteriography may be required when there is systemic embolus from a cardiac tumour and the arteriographer must be alert to the possible diagnosis of myxoma in the event of unexplained embolus.

REFERENCES

ABRAMS, H. L., ADAMS, D. F. & GRANT, H. A. (1971) The radiology of tumours of the heart. *Radiol. Clin. N. Amer.*, **9**, 299–326.

AKINS, C. W., KIRKLIN, J. K., BLOCK, P. C., BUCKLEY, M. J. & AUSTEN, W. G. (1979) Preoperative evaluation of subvalvular fibrosis in mitral stenosis. A predictive factor in conservative vs replacement surgical therapy. *Circulation*, **60**, 1.71–1.76.

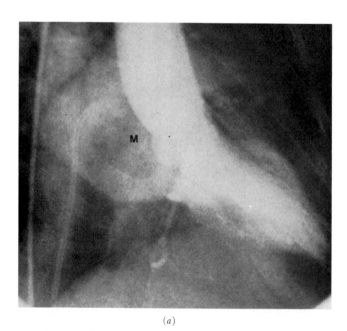

(a)

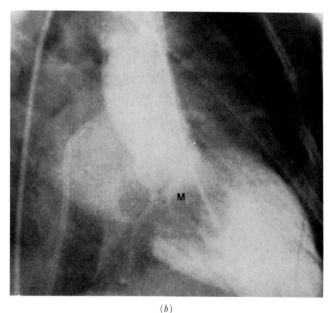

(b)

FIG. 7.60. (a) and (b). Left anterior oblique left ventriculogram of a patient catheterised with presumptive diagnosis of rheumatic mixed mitral valve disease (no preliminary echocardiography). In systole the myxoma (M) is seen in left atrium as a filling defect (there was mitral regurgitation) (a) and in diastole the myxoma is seen prolapsing into and partly through the mitral valve (b).

Armstrong, P. W., Dinsmore, R. E., Harthorne, I. W. & Sanders, C. A. (1973) Hemodynamic clues to the discrepancy between the angiographic and intraoperative assessment of aortic regurgitation. *J. Thoracic Cardiovascular Surg.*, **66**, 265–270.

Baron, M. G. (1971) The angiocardiographic diagnosis of valvular stenosis. *Circulation*, **44**, 143–154.

Beppu, S., Kawazoe, K., Nimura, Y., Park, Y. D., Sakakibara, H. & Fujita, T. (1982) Echocardiographic study of abnormal position and motion of the posterobasal wall of the left ventricle in cases of giant left atrium. *Amer. J. Cardiol.*, **49**, 467–472.

Bon Tempo, C. P., Ronan, J. A., De Leon, A. C. & Twigg, H. L. (1975) Radiographic appearance of the thorax in systolic click-late systolic murmur syndrome. *Amer. J. Cardiol.*, **36**, 27–31.

Braunwald, E. (1969) Mitral regurgitation. Physiologic, clinical and surgical considerations. *New England J. Med.*, **281**, 425–433.

Braunwald, E. & Awe, W. C. (1963) Syndrome of severe mitral regurgitation with normal left atrial pressure. *Circulation*, **27**, 29–35.

Burch, G. E., DePasquale, N. P. & Phillips, J. H. (1968) The syndrome of papillary muscle dysfunction. *Amer. Heart J.*, **73**, 399–415.

Camishion, R. C., Gibbon, J. H., Pierucci, L. & Iida, J. (1966) Paralysis of the left recurrent laryngeal nerve secondary to mitral valvular disease: report of two cases and literature review. *Annals Surg.*, **163**, 818–827.

Chen, J. T. T., Behar, V. S., Morris, J. J., McIntosh, H. D. & Lester, R. G. (1968) Correlation of roentgen findings with hemodynamic data in pure mitral stenosis. *Amer. J. Roentgenol.*, **102**, 280–290.

Child, J. S., Skorton, D. J., Taylor, R. D., Krivokapich, J., Abbasi, A. S., Wong, M. & Shah, P. D. (1979) M-mode and cross-sectional echocardiographic features of flail posterior mitral leaflets. *Amer. J. Cardiol.*, **44**, 1383–1390.

Cohen, M. V. (1978) Real-time sector scan study of the mitral valve prolapse syndrome. *Brit. Heart J.*, **40**, 964–971.

Cohen, M. V. & Gorlin, R. (1972) Modified orifice equation for the calculation of mitral valve area. *Amer. Heart J.*, **84**, 839–840.

Cope, G. D., Kisslo, J. A., Johnson, M. L. & Behar, V. S. (1975) A reassessment of the echocardiogram in mitral stenosis. *Circulation*, **52**, 664–670.

Curry, G. C., Elliott, L. P. & Ramsey, H. W. (1972) Quantitative left ventricular angiocardiographic findings in mitral stenosis. Detailed analysis of the anterolateral wall of the left ventricle. *Amer. J. Cardiol.*, **29**, 621–627.

Darsee, J. R., Mikolich, J. R., Nicoloff, N. B. & Lesser, L. E. (1979) Prevalence of mitral valve prolapse in presumably healthy young men. *Circulation*, **59**, 619–622.

Davies, M. J. (1980) *Pathology of Cardiac Valves*. London: Butterworths.

Davis, G., Kincaid, O. & Hallermann, F. (1969) Roentgen aspects of cardiac tumours. Seminars in Roentgenology, **4**, 384–394.

Demany, M. A., Kay, E. B. & Zimmerman, H. A. (1966) An angiocardiographic sign for the evaluation of the stenotic mitral valve. *Amer. J. Cardiol.*, **18**, 843–846.

Dodge, H. T. (1971) Determination of left ventricular volume and mass. *Radiol. Clin. N. Amer.*, **9**, 459–467.

Edler, I. & Gustafson, A. (1957) Ultrasonic cardiogram in mitral stenosis. *Acta Med. Scand.*, **159**, 85–90.

Edwards, J. E. (1961) Editorial: The congenital bicuspid aortic valve. *Circulation*, **23**, 485–488.

Ellis, P. R., Cooley, D. A. & De Bakey, M. E. (1961) Clinical considerations and surgical treatment of annulo-aortic ectasia: report of successful operation. *J. Thoracic Cardiovascular Surg.*, **42**, 363–370.

Galloway, R. W., Epstein, E. J. & Coulshed, N. (1961) Pulmonary ossific nodules in mitral valve disease. *Brit. Heart J.*, **23**, 297–307.

Gelfand, M. L., Cohen, T., Ackert, J. J., Ambos, M. & Mayadag, M. (1979) Gastrointestinal bleeding in aortic stenosis. *Amer. J. Gastroenterol.*, **71**, 30–38.

Glancy, D. L., Freed, T. A., O'Brien, K. P. & Epstein, S. E. (1969) Calcium in the aortic valve. Roentgenologic and hemodynamic correlations in 149 patients. *Annals Int. Med.*, **71**, 245–250.

Godley, R. W., Green, D., Dillon, J. C., Rogers, E. W., Feigenbaum, H. & Weyman, A. E. (1981) Reliability of two-dimensional echocardiography in assessing the severity of valvular aortic stenosis. *Chest*, **79**, 657–662.

Goodwin, J. F. (1968) The spectrum of cardiac tumours. *Amer. J. Cardiol.*, **21**, 307–314.

Gorlin, R. & Gorlin, S. G. (1951) Hydraulic formula for calculation of the area of the stenotic mitral valve, other cardiac valves, and central circulatory shunts. *Amer. Heart J.*, **41**, 1–29.

Gould, L., Reddy, C. V. R., De Palma, D., De Martino, A. & Kalish, P. E. (1976) Cardiac manifestations of ochronosis. *J. Thoracic Cardiovascular Surg.*, **72**, 788–791.

Graboys, T. B. & Cohn, P. F. (1977) The prevalence of angina pectoris and abnormal coronary arteriograms in severe aortic valvular disease. *Amer. Heart J.*, **93**, 683–686.

Green, C. E., Kelley, M. J. & Higgins, C. B. (1982) Etiologic significance of enlargement of the left atrial appendage in adults. *Radiology*, **142**, 21–27.

Hatle, L. Angelsen, B. A. & Tromsdal, A. (1980) Non-invasive assessment of aortic stenosis by Doppler ultrasound. *Brit. Heart J.*, **43**, 284–292.

Heath, D. (1968) Pathology of cardiac tumours. *Amer. J. Cardiol.*, **21**, 315–317.

Heath, D. & Mackinnon, J. (1964) Pulmonary hypertension due to myxoma of the right atrium with special reference to the behaviour of emboli of myxoma in the lung. *Amer. Heart J.*, **68**, 227–235.

Heller, S. J. & Carleton, R. A. (1970) Abnormal left ventricular contraction in patients with mitral stenosis. *Circulation*, **42**, 1099–1110.

Higgins, C. B. & Wexler, L. (1975) Reversal of dominance of the coronary arterial system in isolated aortic stenosis and bicuspid aortic valve. *Circulation*, **52**, 292–296.

Honey, M., Gough, J. H., Katsaros, S., Miller, G. A. H. & Thuraisingham, V. (1969) Left ventricular cine-angiocardiography in the assessment of mitral regurgitation. *Brit. Heart J.*, **31**, 596–602.

Jefferson, K. & Rees, S. (1980) *Clinical Cardiac Radiology*. Second Edition. London: Butterworth.

Karnegis, J. N. & Heinz, J. (1979) The risk of diagnostic cardiovascular catheterisation. *Amer. Heart J.*, **97**, 291–297.

Kimbiris, D., Iskandrian, A. S., Segal, B. L. & Bemis, C. E. (1978) Anomalous aortic origin of coronary arteries. *Circulation*, **58**, 606–615.

King, M., Huang, J. & Glassman, E. (1969) Paget's disease with cardiac calcification and complete heart block. *Amer. J. Med.*, **46**, 302–304.

Kirklin, J. W. & Kouchoukos, N. T. (1981) Editorial: Aortic valve replacement without myocardial revascularization. *Circulation*, **63**, 252–253.

Klatte, E. C., Yune, H. & Burney, B. (1979) Radiographic manifestations of aortic stenosis and aortic valvular insufficiency. *Sem. Roentgenol.*, **14**, 122–130.

Kostuk, W. J., Boughner, D. R., Barnett, H. J. M. & Silver, M. D. (1977) Strokes: A complication of mitral-leaflet prolapse? *Lancet*, ii, 313–316.

Layton, C., Gent, G., Pride, R., McDonald, A. & Brigden, W. (1973) Diastolic closure rate of normal mitral valve. *Brit. Heart J.*, **35**, 1066–1074.

Lendrum, A. C., Scott, L. D. W. & Park, S. D. S. (1950) Pulmonary changes due to cardiac disease with special reference to haemosiderosis. *Qu. J. Med.*, **19**, 249–262.

Levisman, J. A., Abbasi, A. S. & Pearce, M. L. (1975) Posterior mitral leaflet motion in mitral stenosis. *Circulation*, **51**, 511–514.

Lewis, R. P., Bristow, J. D. & Griswold, H. E. (1971) Radiographic heart size and left ventricular volume in aortic valve disease. *Amer. J. Cardiol.*, **27**, 250–253.

McLAURIN, L. P., GIBSON, T. C., WAIDER, W., GROSSMAN, W. & CRAIGE, E. (1973) An appraisal of mitral valve echocardiograms mimicking mitral stenosis in conditions with right ventricular pressure overload. *Circulation*, **48**, 801–809.

MARTIN, R. P., RAKOWSKI, H., KLEIMAN, J. H., BEAVER, W., LONDON, E. & POPP, R. L. (1979) Reliability and reproducibility of two-dimensional echocardiographic measurement of the stenotic mitral valve orifice area. *Amer. J. Cardiol.*, **43**, 560–568.

MAUTNER, R. K., KATZ, G. E., ITELD, B. J. & PHILLIPS, J. H. (1981) Coronary artery spasm. A mechanism for chest pain in selected patients with the mitral valve prolapse syndrome. *Chest*, **79**, 449–453.

MILLS, P., ROSE, J., HOLLINGSWORTH, J., AMARA, I. & CRAIGE, E. (1977) Long-term prognosis of mitral-valve prolapse. *New England J. Med.*, **297**, 13–18.

MORGAN, D. J. R. & HALL, R. J. C. (1979) Occult aortic stenosis as cause of intractable heart failure. *Brit. Heart J.*, **1**, 784–787.

MORROW, A. G., ROBERTS, W. C., ROSS, J., FISHER, R. D., BEHRENDT, D. M., MASON, D. T. & BRAUNWALD, E. (1968) Obstruction to left ventricular outflow. Current concepts of management and operative treatment. *Annals Int. Med.*, **69**, 1255–1286.

OBEYESEKERE, H. I., DULAKE, M., DEMERDASH, H. & HOLLISTER, R. (1965) Systemic hypertension and mitral valve disease. *Brit. Med. J.*, **2**, 441–445.

POMERANCE, A. (1972) Pathogenesis of aortic stenosis and its relation to age. *Brit. Heart J.*, **34**, 569–574.

POMERANCE, A. (1974) Pathology of heart disease in the elderly. *Brit. J. Hosp. Med.*, **11**, 245–252.

PROCACCI, P. M., SAVRAN, S. V., SCHREITER, S. L. & BRYSON, A. L. (1976) Prevalence of clinical mitral-valve prolapse in 1169 young women. *New England J. Med.*, **294**, 1086–1088.

QUINONES, M. A., YOUNG, J. B., WAGGONER, A. D., OSTOJIC, M. C., RIBEIRO, L. G. T. & MILLER, R. R. (1980) Assessment of pulsed Doppler echocardiography in detection and quantification of aortic and mitral regurgitation. *Brit. Heart J.*, **44**, 612–620.

RAHIMTOOLA, S. H., DUFFEY, J. P. & SWAN, H. J. C. (1966) Hemodynamic changes associated with injection of angiocardiographic contrast medium in assessment of valvular lesions. *Circulation*, **33**, 52–57.

RAMSDALE, D. R., FARAGHER, E. B., BENNETT, D. H., BRAY, C. L., WARD, C. & BETON, D. C. (1982) Preoperative prediction of significant coronary artery disease in patients with valvular heart disease. *Brit. Med. J.*, **284**, 223–226.

RANGANATHAN, N., SILVER, M. D., ROBINSON, T. I., KOSTUK, W. J., FIELDERHOF, C. H., PATT, N. L., WILSON, J. K. & WIGLE, E. D. (1973) Angiographic-morphologic correlation in patients with severe mitral regurgitation due to prolapse of the posterior mitral valve leaflet. *Circulation*, **48**, 514–518.

RANGANATHAN, N., SILVER, M. D. & WIGLE, E. D. (1974) Mitral valve prolapse. *Circulation*, **49**, 1268–1269.

RIGO, P., ALDERSON, P. O., ROBERTSON, R. M., BECKER, L. C. &

WAGNER, H. N. (1979) Measurement of aortic and mitral regurgitation by gated blood scans. *Circulation*, **60**, 306–312.

ROBERTS, W. C., MORROW, A. G., McINTOSH, C. L., JONES, M. & EPSTEIN, S. E. (1981) Congenitally bicuspid aortic valve causing severe, pure aortic regurgitation without superimposed infective endocarditis. *Amer. J. Cardiol.*, **47**, 206–209.

SAHN, D. J., WOOD, J., ALLEN, H. D., PEOPLES, W. & GOLDBERG, S. J. (1977) Echocardiographic spectrum of mitral valve motion in children with and without mitral valve prolapse: The nature of false positive diagnosis. *Amer. J. Cardiol.*, **39**, 422–431.

SALYER, W. R., PAGE, D. L. & HUTCHINS, G. M. (1975) The development of cardiac myxomas and papillary endocardial lesions from mural thrombus. *Amer. Heart J.*, **89**, 4–17.

SELTZER, R. A., HARTHRONE, J. W. & AUSTEN, W. G. (1967) The appearance and significance of left atrial calcification. *Amer. J. Roentgenol.*, **100**, 307–311.

SIMON, G. (1972) The value of radiology in critical mitral stenosis—an amendment. *Clin. Radiol.*, **23**, 145–146.

SOULEN, R. L., GROLLMAN, J. H., PAGLIA, D. & KREULEN, T. (1977) Coronary neovascularity and fistula formation. A sign of mural thrombus. *Circulation*, **56**, 663–666.

SPINDOLA-FRANCO, H., BJORK, L., ADAMS, D. F. & ABRAMS, H. L. (1980) Classification of the radiological morphology of the mitral valve. Differentiation between true and pseudoprolapse. *Brit. Heart J.*, **44**, 30–36.

SUTTON, M. G., ST. J., MERCIER, L. A., GIULIANI, E. R. & LIE, J. T. (1980) Atrial myxomas. A review of clinical experience in 40 patients. *Mayo Clin. Proc.*, **55**, 371–376.

THUILLEZ, C., THEROUX, P., BOURASSA, M. G., BLANCHARD, D., PERONNEAU, P., GUERMONPREZ, J. L., DIEBOLD, B., WATERS, D. D. & MAURICE, P. (1980) Pulsed Doppler echocardiographic study of mitral stenosis. *Circulation*, **61**, 381–387.

TOOMBES, B. D. & MILLER, S. W. (1979) Clinical implications of the convex supradiaphragmatic inferior vena cava. *Radiology*, **132**, 577–581.

VELA, J. E., CONTRERAS, R. & SOSA, F. R. (1969) Rheumatic pulmonary valve disease. *Amer. J. Cardiol.*, **23**, 12–18.

WALLER, B. F., CARTER, J. B., WILLIAMS, H. J., WANG, K. & EDWARDS, J. E. (1973) Bicuspid aortic valve. Comparison of congenital and acquired types. *Circulation*, **48**, 1140–1151.

WALLER, B. F., MORROW, A. G., MARON, B. J., DEL NEGRO, A. A., KENT, K. M., McGRATH, F. J., WALLACE, R. B., McINTOSH, C. L. & ROBERTS, W. C. (1982) Etiology of clinically isolated, severe, chronic, pure mitral regurgitation: Analysis of 97 patients over 30 years of age having mitral valve replacement. *Amer. Heart J.*, **104**, 276–288.

WEXLER, L., SILVERMAN, J. F., DeBUSK, R. F. & HARRISON, D. C. (1971) Angiographic features of rheumatic and nonrheumatic mitral regurgitation. *Circulation*, **44**, 1080–1086.

WHITNEY, B. & CROXON, R. (1972) Dysphagia caused by cardiac enlargement. *Clin. Radiol.*, **23**, 147–152.

WILSON, L. A., KEELING, P. W. N., MALCOLM, A. D., RUSSELL, R. W. R. & WEBB-PEPLOE, M. M. (1977) Visual complications of mitral leaflet prolapse. *Brit. Med. J.*, ii, 86–88.

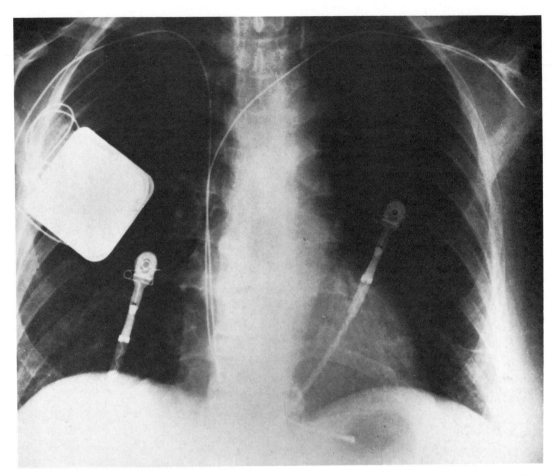

FIG. 8.08. Functioning transvenous pacing system inserted on the right after failure of previous system inserted from the left. The latter electrode could not be removed and was cut proximally and anchored with subcutaneous sutures.

outdated before publication in this rapidly changing field; cross reference should be made to specialist publications (e.g. 'Pace') when required.

REPLACED HEART VALVES

During the 1950s techniques of cardiopulmonary bypass progressed to a stage where open heart valve surgery under direct vision became practicable and this lead to development of a wide variety of firstly mechanical and then biological prostheses in the next decade. The earliest mechanical valves were caged balls and the Starr-Edwards caged ball prosthesis (Figs. 7.01, 7.02) is still widely used. Low profile valves were then developed to lessen the obstruction at and beyond the valve inherent in the large caged ball models; caged discs (Figs. 7.01, 7.02) had short-lived popularity and were abandoned because of high complication rates but tilting or pivoting discs have been shown to be effective and reliable; the Bjork-Shiley, Hall-Kaster and St. Jude

Medical disc prostheses are notable examples in use today. Valve replacement with a mechanical prosthesis entails anticoagulation against thrombotic complications and the low incidence of thrombosis on biological valves has been one of the factors stimulating their development. Homologous (cadaveric!) and autologous (transposed pulmonary valve) heart valves and valves constructed from dura mater or fascia lata have been successfully employed but commercially produced heterografts (the Hancock and the Carpentier-Edwards porcine aortic valves, the Ionescu-Shiley bovine pericardial valve) are now most frequently used when an alternative to a mechanical valve is required.

Open heart surgery is performed through a median sternotomy and the wire sutures frequently used for closure remain as a chest radiograph sign of the operation (Fig. 8.10); in cases of rheumatic mitral disease there may also be evidence of a previous left thoracotomy (rib and pleural changes, Fig. 8.11) for an earlier closed mitral valvotomy.

Mechanical valves have radiopaque housings, later

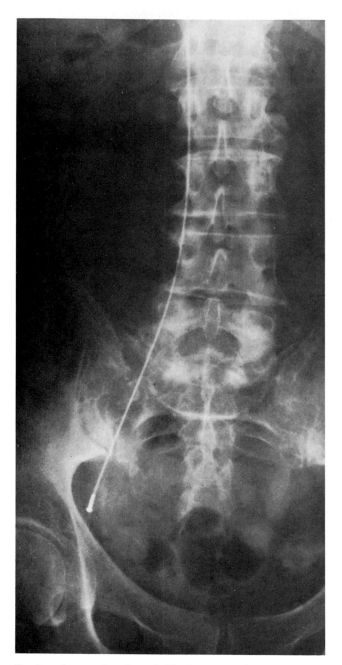

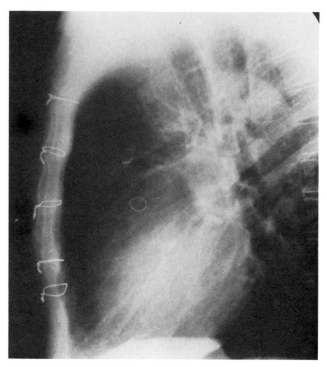

FIG. 8.10. Lateral projection to show sternal wire sutures after open heart surgery (in this case for coronary artery bypass grafts; note the metallic markers sutured to the ascending aorta to indicate the graft insertions to facilitate follow-up graft arteriography).

FIG. 8.09. Same patient shown in Fig. 8.08 one week later after check chest radiograph revealed migration of the cut electrode despite its previous anchorage points; it was removed by Dotter's basket technique of catheter retrieval via the right femoral vein (Dotter *et al.*, 1971).

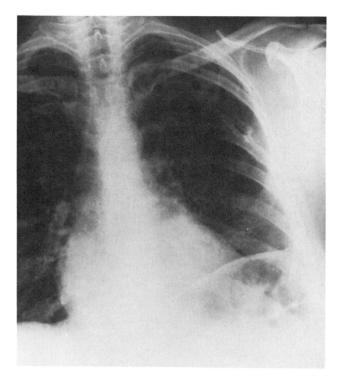

FIG. 8.11. PA projection, previous lateral thoracotomy for mitral valvotomy. The rib and pleural changes and elevation of the left hemidiaphragm shown are so gross as to be a caricature of the more usual subtle signs of trace periosteal new bone formation and blunt costophrenic angle. Note absence of an atrial appendage bulge; the appendage was amputated.

generation Starr-Edwards valves have opaque balls (Figs. 7.01 and 7.02) and several disc valves have semiopaque discs (Fig. 8.13) or incorporated opaque ring markers (post 1975 Bjork-Shiley valves). Biological valves are only recognisable on plain films if mounted on metal frames or stents (Fig. 8.12) though they can also calcify to a considerable degree. Radiographically visible prostheses can be identified as aortic, mitral or tricuspid by the criteria applied to valve calcification in Chapter 7. The cage of an aortic Starr-Edwards valve has three struts, a mitral has four. Caged valves are additionally localised by their alignment; aortic cages are directed cephalad, mitral and tricuspid are directed anteriorly (Figs. 7.01 and 7.02). The direction of opening of an opaque disc gives similar information.

Successful treatment of a haemodynamic fault by valve replacement can remove signs of ventricular failure when this is reversible and can dramatically reduce heart size when there has been volume overload

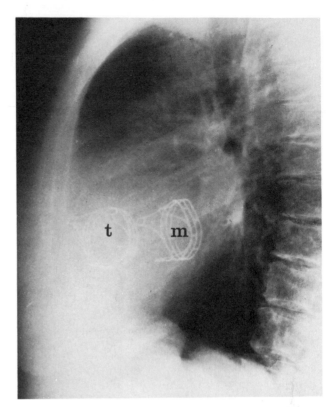

FIG. 8.12. Frame mounted mitral (m) and tricuspid (t) homograft valves. An unframed aortic homograft is also in place but undetectable. Note that the sternal suture material is nonopaque in this case.

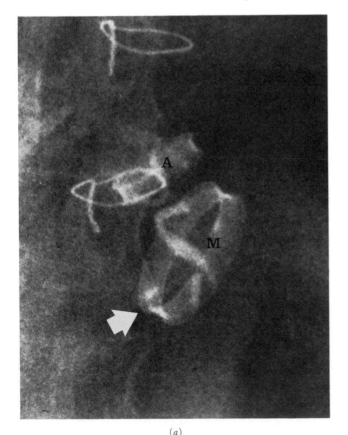

(a)

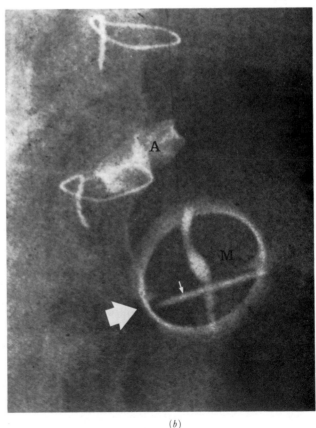

(b)

FIG. 8.13. Right anterior oblique projection, systolic (a) and diastolic (b) cine frames of aortic (A) and mitral (M) Hall-Kaster disc valves. The mitral valve ring flaps about an anchoring point (large arrow) indicating partial detachment; its semiopaque and centrally pivoted disc opens fully and is clearly seen when profiled in diastole (small arrow).

but it is rare for the heart and pulmonary vascular signs of rheumatic mitral valve disease to regress completely and they can remain unaltered despite considerable symptomatic improvement.

Prosthetic valve dysfunction is, in general, investigated in like manner to native valve disease and the various imaging techniques described in Chapter 7 are similarly applied. Fluoroscopy, preferably with cinerecording, deserves particular mention as important information can be quickly and simply obtained by this technique when the valve in question is radiopaque. Paravalvar leak due to ring dehiscence (inadequate or detached sutures) can be diagnosed by excessive rocking or flapping of the valve ring (Fig. 8.13) which, according to the observations of Gimenez et al. (1968) on aortic and mitral Starr-Edwards prostheses, should not normally exceed 9°; 'normal' motion does not, however, exclude regurgitation or partial detachment. Incomplete motion of a valve disc or ball (movements so rapid that cinefluoroscopy is essential for analysis) suggests stenosis when there is failure of opening and regurgitation if there is failure of closure. Disc valves have known opening amplitudes, for example 60° for the Bjork-Shiley (Bjork et al., 1977), which can be measured by cinefluoroscopy if an appropriate projection can be obtained; impaired motility can result from obstruction by thrombus, adjacent tissue or sutures. Echocardiography can give similar but less exact information but is of course also applicable to radiolucent valves; echocardiography also allows a much wider cardiac assessment and has particular use in assessing stenosis (as judged by left ventricular filling characteristics) of prosthetic mitral valves (St. J. Sutton et al., 1981). The value of echocardiography in the noninvasive study of prosthetic valves has been one factor leading to neglect of the complementary and often more direct role of cinefluoroscopy and the latter has received welcome reemphasis in a recent report (Sands et al., 1982).

REFERENCES

Bjork, V. O., Henze, A. & Hindmarsh, T. (1977) Radiopaque marker in the tilting disc of the Bjork-Shiley heart valve. *J. Thoracic Cardiovasc. Surg.*, **73**, 563–569.

Dotter, C. T., Rosch, J. & Bilbao, M. K. (1971) Transluminal extraction of catheter and guide fragments from the heart and great vessels: 29 collected cases. *Amer. J. Roentgenol.*, **111**, 467–471.

Gimenez, J. L., Soulen, R. L. & Davila, J. (1968) Prosthetic valve detachment: its roentgenological recognition. *Amer. J. Roentgenol.* **103**, 595–600.

Gondi, B. & Nanda, N. C. (1981) Real-time, two dimensional echocardiographic features of pacemaker perforation. *Circulation*, **64**, 97–106.

Hewitt, M. J., Chen, J. T. T., Ravin, C. E. & Gallagher, J. J. (1981) Coronary sinus atrial pacing: radiographic considerations. *Amer. J. Roentgenol.*, **136**, 323–328.

Krug, H. & Zerbe, F. (1980) Major venous thrombosis: a complication of transvenous pacemaker electrodes. *Brit. Heart J.*, **44**, 158–161.

Sands, M. J., Lachman, A. S., O'Reilly, D. J., Leach, C. N., Sappington, J. B. & Katz, A. M. (1982) Diagnostic value of cinefluoroscopy in the evaluation of prosthetic heart valve dysfunction. *Amer. Heart J.*, **104**, 622–627.

Sorkin, R. P., Schurrmann, B. J. & Simon, A. B. (1976) Radiographic aspects of permanent cardiac pacemakers. *Radiology*, **119**, 281–286.

St. J. Sutton, M., Roudaut, R., Oldershaw, P. & Bricaud, H. (1981) Echocardiographic assessment of left ventricular filling characteristics after mitral valve replacement with the St. Jude medical prosthesis. *Brit. Heart J.*, **45**, 365–368.

Steiner, R. M., Morse, D. P. & Tegtmeyer, C. J. (1982) Pacemaker lead pseudo-fracture. *Radiology*, **143**, 793.

Zoll, P. M. (1952) Resuscitation of the heart in ventricular standstill by external electric stimulation. *New England J. Med.*, **247**, 768–771.

CHAPTER 9

DISEASES OF HEART MUSCLE

Maurice Raphael

INTRODUCTION

Heart failure is usually due to obvious mechanical factors leading to a pressure or volume overload on the heart, as in valvular or hypertensive heart disease, or to the destruction of muscle as in ischaemic heart disease. When cardiac failure occurs in the absence of these factors it is attributed to disease of heart muscle. The term 'cardiomyopathy' is defined as a disease of heart muscle of unknown cause or association. When a cause or association is known the condition is so described, e.g. haemochromotosis heart disease. Ischaemic necrosis of heart muscle, the commonest cause of cardiac failure from heart muscle disease, is dealt with in Chapter 6.

CONGESTIVE OR DILATED CARDIOMYOPATHY

This is the commonest form of cardiomyopathy. The condition is usually asymptomatic until cardiac failure develops, often suddenly, producing an influenza-like illness which may be thought to have initiated the illness. In addition to the clinical evidence of congestive cardiac failure there is always evidence of serious cardiac dysfunction with an atrial tachycardia and a third sound gallop. A systolic murmur of mitral regurgitation may be present. About 10% of patients may have cardiac pain and some patients may present with peripheral emboli.

At necropsy the heart is enlarged with a large and rather globular left ventricle with effacement of the trabecula, and there may be clot in the interstices. Pathologically there is interstitial fibrosis and fibre hypertrophy, appearances which are entirely non-specific and may also be seen in patients with mechanical cardiac failure.

At presentation all patients will have an abnormal chest radiograph showing cardiomegaly. The heart may be globular in shape (Fig. 9.01) if all chambers are involved, or show a pronounced left ventricular configuration if enlargement is confined to the left ventricle (Fig. 9.02). Rarely the heart may not be grossly enlarged overall but left ventricular enlargement may be seen, more rarely only on the lateral view. The aorta is normal in size and shape. A pericardial effusion may be present. In untreated patients lung changes will be seen varying from upper lobe blood diversion to gross alveolar pulmonary oedema.

The response to treatment varies from complete radiological remission when the heart reduces to normal and the lungs clear (Fig. 9.03), to only minor improvement. The general course is downhill with each relapse into cardiac failure responding less well to treatment.

There are two treatable conditions which may be confused with congestive cardiomyopathy; silent aortic stenosis may only be recognised if calcification in the region of the aortic valve is seen on the lateral chest radiograph, or during echocardiography. Left ventricular aneurysm may be indistinguishable clinically from congestive cardiomyopathy, as may cardiac failure from diffuse ischaemic destruction of myocardium.

All patients with congestive cardiomyopathy should be investigated first by echocardiography and then by left ventriculography and coronary arteriography. The characteristic angiographic appearance in congestive cardiomyopathy is of a large smooth and often globular left ventricle with only a small concentric excursion of its wall between diastole and systole, and often with a variable amount of mitral regurgitation (Fig. 9.04). The other conditions which may lead to clinical confusion should all be immediately recognisable at coronary arteriography. The distinction between mitral regurgitation due to congestive cardiomyopathy and mitral regurgitation causing congestive cardiac failure may be difficult even after angiocardiography.

HEART MUSCLE DISEASE OF KNOWN CAUSE OR ASSOCIATION

Infections

Coxackie B virus. Sudden onset of a febrile illness and a high or rising titre of antibody, associated with the syndrome of congestive cardiac failure, suggests this diagnosis. When myocarditis is clinically likely an endocardial biopsy should be done. The demonstration of inflammatory cells eroding the myocardial muscle fibres confirms the diagnosis which is important to the management and prognosis.

Diphtheria. Cardiac failure 10–14 days after the

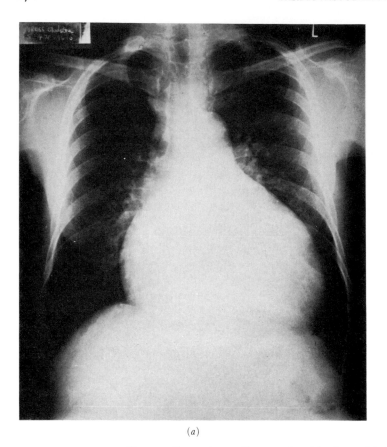
(a)

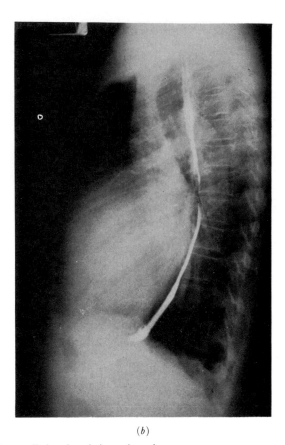
(b)

FIG. 9.01. Congestive cardiomyopathy with a large globular heart, all chambers being enlarged.

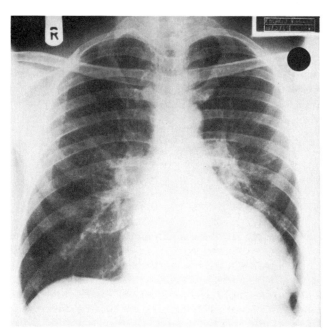

FIG. 9.02. Congestive cardiomyopathy with primarily left ventricular enlargement.

onset of infection may develop as the bacterium releases its specific toxin.

Chagas disease. This condition, occurring mainly in Latin America, is due to a T Cruzi infection which produces a patchy destruction of the heart, after a long latent period. It also produces appearances similar to achalasia of the cardia in the oesophagus at barium swallow.

Collagen Diseases

Rheumatic fever may itself lead to congestive cardiac failure in the acute phase before organic valve damage has developed. The other collagen diseases may also involve the heart leading to arrhythmias or to congestive cardiac failure.

Systemic lupus erythematosus, while usually producing a pericardial effusion when it involves the heart, rarely produces curious vegetations (Libman-Sacks) on the mitral and aortic valves which may lead to incompetence.

Infiltrations

Haemochromatosis. About one-third of patients die

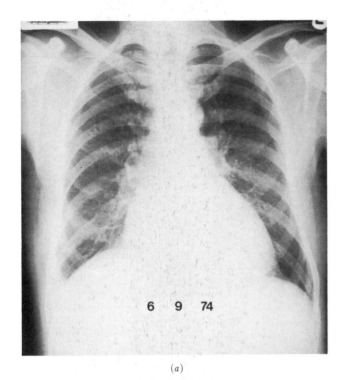
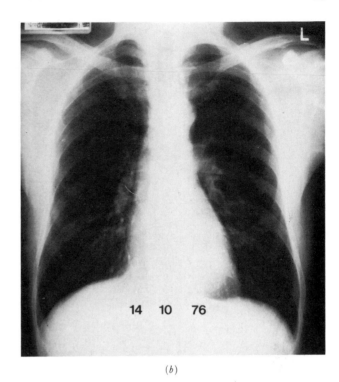

(a) (b)

Fig. 9.03. Congestive cardiomyopathy. 6.9.74 at first presentation the heart is enlarged and there is upper lobe blood diversion. 14.10.76 following good clinical remission the heart has returned to a normal size and the lungs are clear.

from congestive cardiac failure due to iron deposition in the heart.

Sarcoidosis. Sarcoid involvement of the heart usually presents with arrhythmias but congestive cardiac failure or malfunction of a cardiac valve, usually the mitral from papillary muscle involvement, may occur. The condition may present with sudden death. Sarcoid involvement of the heart may precede other manifestations of the disease in other parts of the body by several years.

Amyloid heart disease. Amyloid may involve the heart alone or as part of a generalised disorder. Cardiac involvement is manifest as a very severe and intractable low output cardiac failure with low volume pulse and low blood pressure, often murmur free. The ECG shows a relatively low voltage. Plain film appearances are variable. The heart shadow will be large if there is a pericardial effusion, which is common, but may be only slightly large in its absence. A variable degree of pulmonary venous hypertension and oedema may be seen. The findings of cardiac catheterisation and angiocardiography are suggestive of the diagnosis. Within the left ventricle diastolic pressures are high, both in early- and end-diastole. The ventricle however is usually only slightly enlarged and with a moderately reduced ejection fraction. The appearances are distinctive from congestive cardiomyopathy where the elevation in the

end-stolic pressure in the left ventricle is usually commensurate with the left ventricular dilatation.

Glycogen storage disease. This condition may rarely present as heart failure before the characteristic muscle weakness becomes obvious. Gross cardiomegaly with either a left ventricular or a non-specific shape will be seen. The liver may be seen to be enlarged. The condition is immediately recognisable at left ventriculography by the enormously increased thickness and irregularity of the left ventricular wall, associated with a moderate cavity dilatation.

Metabolic Disorders

Thyroid disease. *Myxoedema* characteristically produces a pericardial effusion but the heart muscle itself may be involved with some cardiac dilatation. *Thyrotoxicosis* produces atrial fibrillation and if this leads to cardiac failure the heart will be dilated. Cardiac dilatation may also occur in association with the high cardiac output and this may lead to high output failure.

Acromegaly. This may be associated with the syndrome of congestive cardiomyopathy but, as there is a high incidence of both hypertension and coronary artery disease, the exact basis of acromegalic heart disease is uncertain.

Beriberi. Deficiency of thiamine leads to high, or rarely a low, output cardiac failure, with a large heart

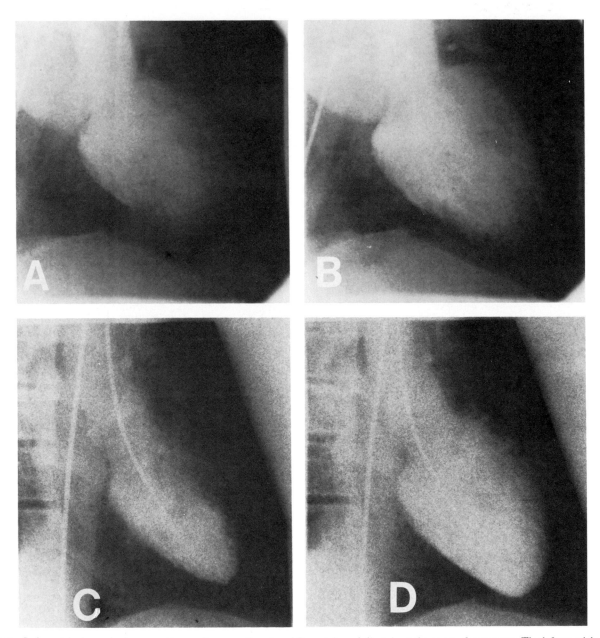

FIG. 9.04. Left ventriculography in congestive cardiomyopathy. A and B, systole and diastole at the onset of symptoms. The left ventricle is large and its trabecula effaced. The change in size from diastole to systole is small. There is mitral regurgitation. C and D, systole and diastole after successful treatment. The ventricle is smaller though still enlarged. Wall excursion has increased. There is no mitral regurgitation. This is the same case as in Fig. 9.03 showing that quite significant left ventricular enlargement can be present in the presence of an apparently normal chest X-ray.

and pulmonary congestion. The response to thiamine is usually dramatic.

Drugs and Poisons

Alcoholic heart disease. Excessive consumption of alcohol may lead to cardiac failure and the syndrome of congestive cardiomyopathy. The specific diagnosis may be made by eliciting the history of excessive alcohol consumption. The condition usually improves if alcohol is forsaken.

Beta blocking drugs. Large doses of beta blocking drugs may lead to cardiac dilatation and cardiac failure, and this is reversible if the drug is discontinued. Almost always underlying heart disease is present.

Cytotoxic drugs. *Daunorubicin* is a well recognised cause of congestive cardiac failure in patients treated for malignant disease.

Other Conditions

Postpartum cardiomyopathy. Congestive cardiac failure developing after pregnancy, in an otherwise healthy patient, is a well recognised condition. It usually responds to treatment but often relapses with subsequent pregnancies.

Neuromuscular disorders. A syndrome of congestive cardiomyopathy is associated with a variety of heredofamilial neuromuscular disorders, and may be the cause of death in a number of patients. The radiological appearances are those of non-specific congestive cardiomyopathy.

Anaemias. Any severe anaemia may lead to high-output cardiac failure. There may be cardiomegaly with a non-specific cardiac outline in mild anaemia. As the heart becomes less able to support the high output, the lung fields develop signs of pulmonary venous hypertension and there may also be enlargement of the azygos vein and superior vena cava due to systemic venous hypertension. There is seldom any recognisable sign of pulmonary plethora.

HYPERTROPHIC CARDIOMYOPATHY

This condition is characterised by an inappropriate hypertrophy of the myocardium, usually of the left ventricle but occasionally involving both ventricles. In the typical case the involvement is asymmetrical and predominantly in the septum, but uniform hypertrophy may rarely be seen. The histological appearances are of fibre hypertrophy and fibrosis. The excessive muscle apparently contracts well as systolic function, evidenced by ventricular emptying, is good, though a few patients enter a congestive terminal phase. The major functional abnormality is that the increased muscle bulk prevents the left ventricle from filling properly in diastole. Mitral regurgitation is frequent though rarely severe and may be due to abnormal muscle action reopening the mitral valve in systole. This reopening may be responsible for the intracavitary gradient which was at one time considered to be the hallmark of the condition. The condition is frequently familial with the history of sudden death in older members of the family. A cardiac abnormality pathologically identical to hypertrophic cardiomyopathy is seen in patients with Friedreich's ataxia and in Noonan's syndrome.

The presentation of the disorder is variable. Arrhythmias or even sudden death may occur. Dyspnoea may initially be due to a high venous pressure from difficulty in filling the stiff left ventricle. Anginal pain, presumably from the demands of the large amount of muscle, is common. The diagnosis may be made clinically in the typical case. The pulses are jerky, as opposed to the plateau pulse of aortic stenosis. The left ventricular impulse is sustained and an atrial beat is frequently palpable, indicating left ventricular hypertrophy. A mid-systolic murmur may be heard, resembling the murmur of aortic stenosis, this may be due to intracavitary obstruction or to mitral regurgitation and the murmur may also resemble the murmur of non-rheumatic mitral regurgitation. The ECG usually shows left ventricular hypertrophy and may resemble ischaemia. M-mode echocardiography, competently performed, will show the small left ventricular cavity, the septum disproportionately thick compared with the free wall of the left ventricle, and the systolic anterior movement of the anterior leaflet of the mitral valve, though not all features are present in every case.

The appearances of plain film radiography will depend on the stage of the illness. Initially, appearances may vary from virtually normal (Fig. 9.05) to those of gross left ventricular enlargement (Fig. 9.06), often with a rather chunky rounding of the apex, slightly resembling the appearances of a left ventricular aneurysm. The aorta is usually normal. Congestive changes may be seen in the lungs. A few patients may show a surprisingly large left atrium, even in the absence of mitral regurgitation, strongly resembling mitral valve disease radiologically.

The appearances usually remain stable for several years but deterioration is heralded by the onset of atrial fibrillation. The heart shadow increases in size and takes on a globular shape (Fig. 9.05). This is almost always due to enlargement of chambers other than the left ventricle, which only rarely goes into a dilated terminal phase. The left atrium may be large at this stage, and rarely a prominent atrial appendage may be seen.

The range of findings of cardiac catheterisation and angiocardiography is considerable, and depends on the degree of septal involvement. Filling pressure in the left ventricle is usually increased. An intracavitary gradient may be present at rest or may be induced by a variety of manoeuvres. The left ventricle (Fig. 9.07) may be near normal in shape and size in diastole but empties excessively in systole with a small amount of contrast only remaining under the aortic valve, and rarely contrast may be trapped at the apex of the ventricle. The axis of the left ventricle is usually curved downwards and may be grossly so. The papillary muscles are prominent and in systole may often be seen bulging into the cavity. The free wall is often thickened with an increase in trabeculation and the bulge of the thickened upper septum may be seen on the right anterior oblique angiogram. In some cases the appearances may be extremely bizarre due to the indentation of numerous methods of muscle, in others the appearances are indistinguishable from normal.

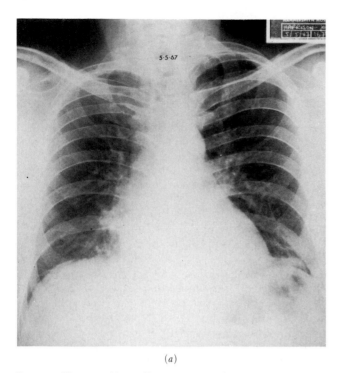 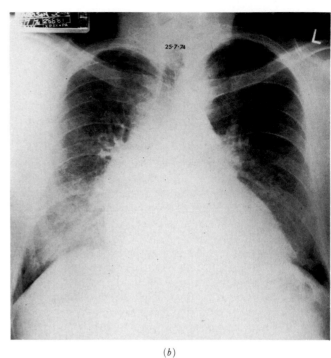

(a)   (b)

FIG. 9.05. Hypertrophic cardiomyopathy. 5.5.67. Apart from slight non-specific cardiac enlargement the appearances are normal. 25.7.74 after marked clinical deterioration the heart shadow is much larger, all chambers being involved. There is perihilar pulmonary oedema. Serial angiography showed that the left ventricle had not changed in size or shape between the two dates.

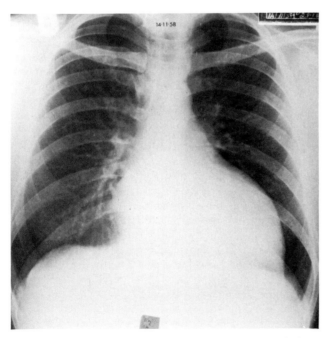

FIG. 9.06. Hypertrophic cardiomyopathy. The plain radiograph shows gross left ventricular enlargement with a slightly chunky left border.

Differential Diagnosis

A combination of left ventricular hypertrophy, systolic murmur and abnormal ECG leads to consideration of aortic stenosis at either valvar or subvalvar level, non-rheumatic mitral regurgitation, or hypertrophic cardiomyopathy. The echogram and cardiac catheterisation will usually serve to distinguish these three conditions. A murmur is not necessary for the diagnosis which hinges on the evidence of inappropriate left ventricular hypertrophy.

Right Ventricular Hypertrophic Cardiomyopathy

If asymmetrical involvement of the septum causes the hypertrophic myocardium to bulge to the right it will encroach on the outflow tract of the right ventricle leading to a syndrome of infundibular obstruction. The angiographic appearances of the right ventricle may resemble those of congenital infundibular stenosis but the clinical and angiographic evidence of left ventricular disease will point to the diagnosis.

RESTRICTIVE CARDIOMYOPATHY

Involvement of the endocardial layer of the right or the left (or both) ventricles by fibrosis leads to the syndrome

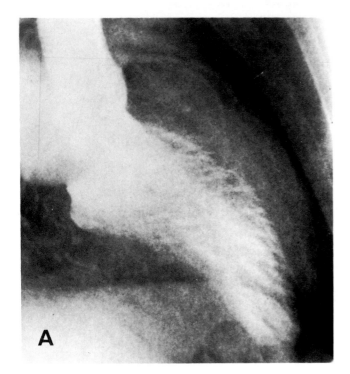
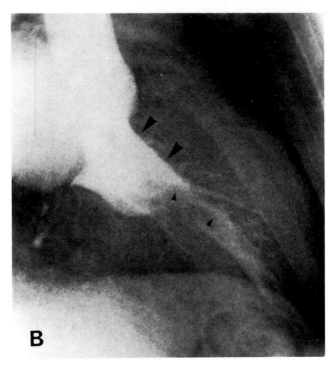

FIG. 9.07. Left ventriculography in hypertrophic cardiomyopathy. Same case as Fig. 9.05. A, diastole. The cavity is a normal size but shows a typical curved axis. Trabeculation is coarse, the left ventricular wall is thickened. B, systole. The cavity is almost completely empty apart from some contrast under the aortic valve. The posterior papillary muscle is very prominent (small arrows). Asymmetric septal hypertrophy indents the upper cavity (large arrows).

of restrictive cardiomyopathy which is characterised by normal contraction but abnormal relaxation. There are two pathological causes recognised for the condition, endomyocardial fibrosis which is largely confined to Africans, and Loeffler's endocarditis which is basically the name given to the same condition when it occurs in Europeans. The role of eosinophilia in the causation of these conditions is gradually becoming clear with evidence that sustained eosinophilia can damage the heart and produce endomyocardial fibrosis, and this may progress even after the eosinophilia has died down. In Europeans the condition commonly involves the left ventricle more than the right, with fibrosis effacing the apex of the ventricle and spreading round to involve the mitral valve producing mitral incompetence. In Africans the condition tends to involve more the right ventricle, again with effacement of the right ventricular apex and a reduction in cavity size. It spreads on to the tricuspid valve leading to tricuspid regurgitation.

The condition may be suspected when an African patient presents with gross right heart failure with incompetence of the tricuspid valve and with a third heart sound. In Europeans right- or left-sided failure may be associated with incompetence of the appropriate atrioventricular valve and a third heart sound.

The plain film appearances are again variable. When the left ventricle alone is involved the heart is usually not enlarged unless mitral regurgitation is gross. The involvement of the right ventricle in African patients leads to a large heart with evidence of marked right heart chamber enlargement and often with a pericardial effusion in addition. Curvilinear calcification of the apical endocardium of either ventricle may rarely be seen and may be suggestive of the diagnosis.

CHAPTER 10

ACQUIRED DISEASES OF THE AORTA

Maurice Raphael

THORACIC AORTA

Normal Appearances

The normal thoracic aorta is divided for descriptive purposes into three parts. Rising from the aortic valve on the right side of the anterior part of the superior mediastinum is the ascending aorta. The arch turns backwards, crossing the mediastinum from right to left to pass to the left of the trachea and oesophagus at the level of D4, then becoming the descending thoracic aorta which turns down in the posterior part of the left superior mediastinum to pass through the aortic hiatus of the diaphragm at the T12 level. On the right side the superior vena cava conceals the outer aspect of the normal ascending aorta. The posterior part of the arch casts a shadow on the chest radiograph, known as the aortic knob, and the left border of the descending aorta can usually be identified as a faint straight line shadow to the left of the vertebral column, where its left border is in contact with the left lung.

Age Related Changes

The neonate. In the neonate, particularly when the thymus is large, the arch of the aorta cannot be identified as a discrete shadow, the ascending aorta is concealed within the mediastinum, and unless radiographic technique is first class the descending aorta cannot be identified.

The older child and adult. With regression of the thymus the arch of the aorta becomes recognisable as the aortic knob at the level of the manubrium and the left border of the descending aorta becomes recognisable as a slightly oblique straight edge descending in the thorax slightly to the left of the vertebral column and its pleural reflection. The ascending aorta remains concealed by the superior vena cava.

Elderly patients. With advancing age the aorta both elongates and becomes dilated. These changes result in the ascending aorta bulging beyond the right border of the superior mediastinum (Fig. 10.01). The knob shadow of the aortic arch becomes larger and higher and the descending aorta follows an undulating course; this may become so pronounced as to kink the vessel giving an appearance resembling a mass lesion or an aneurysm (Fig. 10.2). Difficulty in diagnosis will be avoided if the possibility is kept in mind. A penetrated

view will usually outline the descending aorta and demonstrate the relationship of any shadows to it and a lateral view, supplemented if necessary by fluoroscopy, will usually show that the aortic walls retain their parallelism making an aneurysm unlikely. In the elderly calcification commonly develops in the wall of the aortic arch and is of no particular pathological significance.

Pseudoachalasia. Extreme kinking of the lower end of the thoracic aorta may cause pressure on the lower end of the oesophagus producing dysphagia, and this is known as pseudoachalasia because its radiological appearances on barium swallow may closely resemble those of achalasia, with a tapered narrowing of the oesophagus allowing occasional release of held up

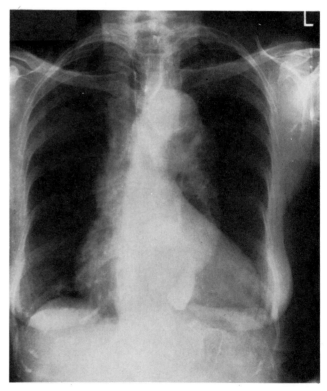

FIG. 10.01. Elongation of the aorta. Slightly penetrated chest X-ray of an elderly patient with barium in the oesophagus. The aorta is dilated and elongated, its ascending part bulges to the right, its knob is enlarged and elevated and its descending thoracic part bulges to the left of the spine and is also slightly irregular.

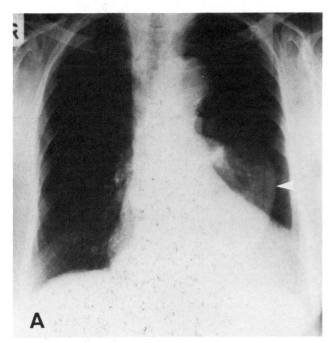

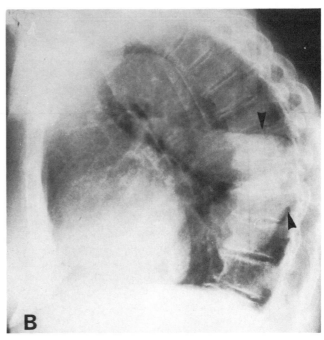

FIG. 10.02. Kinked aorta. (A) and (B) frontal and lateral chest X-ray. The apparent mass lesion of the left chest seen on the frontal view (arrow) may be seen in the lateral view to be a kinked descending thoracic aorta (arrows). There is no loss of parallelism of the aortic walls so this is simple elongation, an age change.

FIG. 10.03. Pseudoachalasia. There is hold-up of barium at the lower end of the oesophagus. The lower end is tapered and compressed by the elongated and dilated aorta.

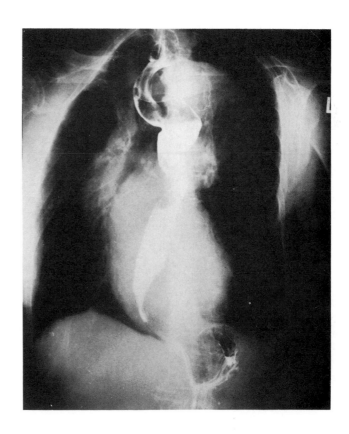

barium (Fig. 10.03). As achalasia is rare in the elderly the possibility of aortic compression should be considered when the relationship of the dilated and tortuous descending aorta to the oesophageal abnormality will become obvious.

AORTITIS

A number of conditions which have as their common factor a characteristic ridged appearance of the inner aspects of the aorta (resembling the bark of a tree) are grouped together under the term aortitis. They may be distinguished from each other histologically. All may be associated with dilatation of the involved part of the aorta, involvement of the aortic valve ring and rarely the cusps, and aortic incompetence. All may be associated with dystrophic calcification in the scarred media. Secondary atheroma is frequent and may obscure the underlying abnormality. All may progress to aneurysm formation.

Aortitis is characterised radiologically by the fine,

linear calcification occurring in the wall of the aorta, usually in the aortic root of the ascending aorta (Fig. 10.04). If extensive it will give an indication of the size of the aorta and may indicate the formation of aneurysm. This fine calcification must be distinguished from the thicker irregular calcification of atheroma, though aortitis may predispose to a severe secondary atheroma. Occasionally, an aorta may be recognised as being dilated by aortitis in the absence of calcification. In the presence of aortic incompetence commensurate left ventricular enlargement will be noted. Valve calcification is not a feature of aortitis though all types of aortitis may affect the valve.

Syphilis is now a rare cause of aortitis, which is only recognised when aortic incompetence develops. Coronary ostial stenosis may cause ischaemic cardiac pain in syphilitic aortitis. Involvement of the aorta by *rheumatoid arthritis* and *ankylosing spondylitis* is characterised by aortic incompetence which increases with the duration of the disease. Dilatation of the aortic root and occa-

sional aneurysm formation may occur. *Giant cell arteritis* is complicated by aortitis and aortic incompetence in a small proportion of cases. In *relapsing polychondritis* about 10% of patients show aortitis with dilatation of the aortic ring. In *Reiter's Syndrome* ascending aortitis is complicated by aortic incompetence in 2–5% of patients. In non-specific *aorto-arteritis* of Asians (Takayasu disease) (see p. 315) up to 2% of patients have aortic incompetence from dilatation of the aortic ring, and ostial stenosis of the coronary arteries may occur. Enlargement of the aorta may be recognised by plain radiography. Localised dilatations and narrowings of any part of the intrathoracic aorta may also occur and calcification may vary from fine line to grossly irregular.

ANEURYSMS OF THE AORTA

Aneurysms of the aorta are localised dilatations. True aneurysms where remnants of the aortic wall structures are recognised histologically in the wall of the aneurysms

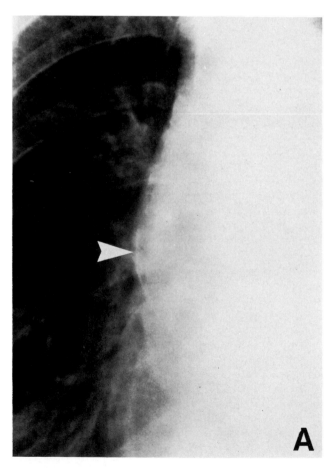
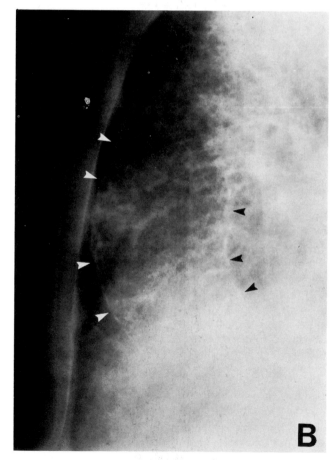

FIG. 10.04. Aortitis. Close up view of the aorta, (A) frontal view, (B) lateral view. In (A) fine curvilinear calcification may be seen in the right wall only (arrow). In (B) calcification may be seen in both walls (arrows) demonstrating that parallelism is retained and no aneurysm has yet developed.

are distinguished from dissecting aneurysms (p. 183) and false aneurysms (p. 192) where the sac is formed by adventitia only. All forms of aortitis may lead to aneurysm formation, as may atheroma (now probably the commonest cause), Marfan's disease and mucopolysaccharidosis. Mycotic aneurysms may result from infection. Congenital aneurysms of the aorta are rare, and often associated with other abnormalities, such as coarctation.

Aneurysms may present clinically in a variety of ways. They may be asymptomatic, being detected on plain radiography for some unrelated reason. Such aneurysms may expand slowly for many years. Symptomatic aneurysms may present as mass lesions in the thorax, pressing on the structures of the mediastinum such as the trachea or bronchi, the superior vena cava, or pulmonary artery. They may even erode vertebrae, characteristically leaving the discs intact. Pain and haemoptysis may mimic a carcinoma of the lung. If an aneurysm involves the aortic root, aortic incompetence may be the presenting feature. Rupture of an aneurysm usually leads to sudden death.

Aneurysms may be saccular or fusiform. In both, plain radiography is virtually always abnormal if the aneurysm develops beyond the pericardial reflection. *Saccular* aneurysms develop as masses of soft tissue density (Fig. 10.05), and may have calcification in the wall. Their outline is commonly sharp though it may be blurred by an inflammatory pleural reaction. They may be round or an irregular shape and may be lobulated. They may appear as a mass lesion apparently unrelated to the aorta, but careful radiography, if necessary with fluoroscopic positioning, will demonstrate that they are continuous at the edge with the aorta. They may resemble a carcinoma of the lung, both clinically and radiologically and any mass lesion which cannot be separated from the aorta, by appropriate radiography, should be investigated for aneurysm before needle biopsy.

Fusiform aneurysms (Fig. 10.06) are usually gross and the involved part of the aorta is obviously enlarged in a fusiform manner; appropriate radiography demonstrates loss of parallelism of the aortic walls, the hallmark of aneurysm development. Difficulty may be encountered in a dilated, elongated and kinked aorta of the type seen in the elderly, but careful radiography in this situation usually shows that a parallelism of the aortic wall is retained. Fluoroscopy to study the type of pulsation of mediastinal masses on the assumption that expansile pulsation may be recognised in aneurysms and be diagnostically useful, is now no longer carried out as the majority of such aneurysms do not show expansile pulsation.

Intrapericardial Aneurysms

Aneurysms of the low aortic root developing within the pericardium are much more difficult to recognise as they do not present radiologically with a local bulge; loss of parallelism of the aortic wall is difficult to detect, as both walls of the aorta are not well seen in any one view in this situation.

Quite large aneurysms may be entirely concealed in the pericardium and in the frontal chest radiograph the aorta may appear normal (Fig. 10.07). More usually the superior mediastinum bulges to the right, and appears to contain simply a prominent ascending aorta, and indeed a very marked prominence may be present. There is rarely a localised bulge. This prominent ascending aorta may rise smoothly from the cardiac shadow, or there may be a notch between it and the right atrium (Fig. 10.08). In the lateral view the enlarged aortic root can usually be seen though the aortic root, not being in contact with the lung, is not well outlined. Occasionally aortic root aneurysms may displace the pulmonary trunk to the left, making it appear prominent. These appearances may be puzzling if no aorta is prominent on the right side of the mediastinum (Fig. 10.09). Intrapericardial aneurysms are usually of the Marfan type or more rarely due to aortitis. Rarely, Marfan type aneurysms may also show curvilinear calcification.

Mycotic Aneurysms

Arterial aneurysms may be caused by infection weakening the arterial wall, either by embolisation, as in bacterial endocarditis, or by direct extension of infection, as by a tuberculous gland. Such aneurysms are rare in the aorta but may occur at sites of wall abnormality, either with minor degrees of coarctation, or at the site of duct origin from the aorta. Any abnormal shadow contiguous with the aorta, developing in the course of bacterial endocarditis must be suspected to be a mycotic aneurysm (Fig. 10.10). The only characteristic feature that may show is their tendency to expand rapidly, and they may also rupture early.

Special Investigations

Aneurysms beyond the pericardium are almost invariably visible as abnormal shadows related to the aorta, and only their nature is in doubt. Contrast CT scanning, where a third generation scanner is available, will demonstrate the connection of the mass to the aorta and the presence of contrast-containing blood within it (Fig. 10.05). A reconstruction of the longitudinal extent of the abnormality is also possible. In the absence of modern CT, if the distinction between a fusiform aneurysm and simple aortic dilatation is to be made, or prior to surgery, aortography is indicated. The lumen of the aneurysm connecting with the aorta is usually obvious providing that care is taken to select a projection which profiles the abnormal shadow. In aneurysms near the arch it is important to recognise the involve-

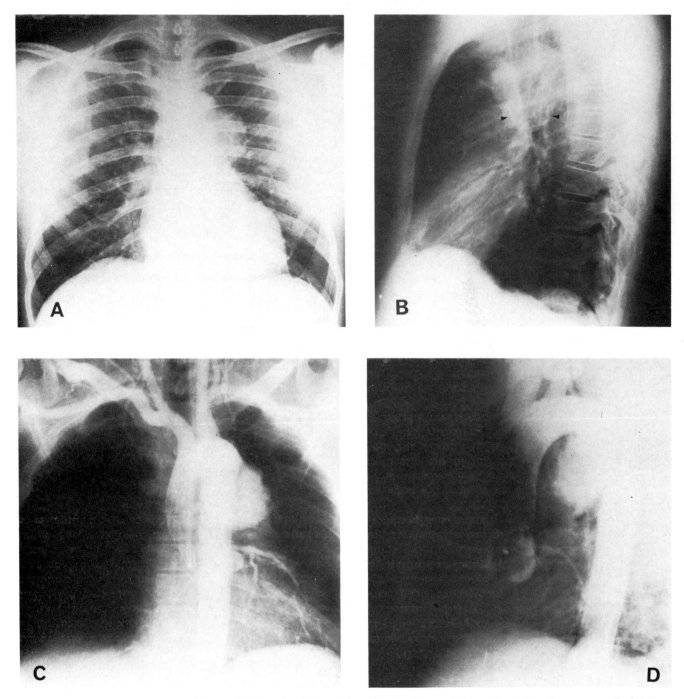

FIG. 10.05. Saccular aortic aneurysm. (A) and (B) frontal and lateral chest X-rays. (C) and (D) frontal and lateral aortograms. In (A) there appears to be a mass lesion in the upper part of the left hilum which is seen (arrows) to overlap the aorta in (B). In (C) and (D) it is seen to fill with contrast from the aorta. (E) CT scan of a similar patient; (F) with contrast enhancement (*Courtesy Dr G. Verney*).

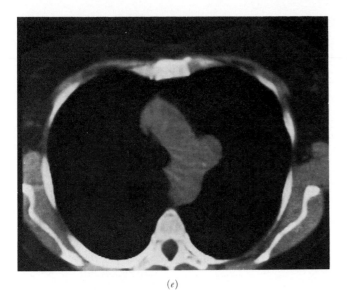

(e)

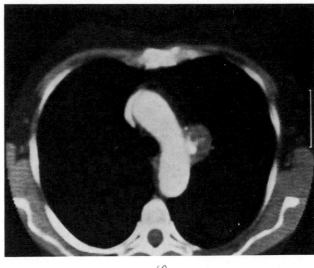

(f)

ment of the great arteries. Aneurysms are commonly lined with a variable amount of clot so that the opacified lumen may be smaller, and quite markedly so, than the soft tissue mass visualised at plain radiography. Only rarely an aneurysm may be completely full of clot leading to considerable difficulty in diagnosis. Almost invariably in this situation some abnormality of the opacified aorta is visible to suggest the nature of the lesion (Fig. 10.11).

Intrapericardial aneurysm may be suspected when an abnormal shadow is recognised at the root of the aorta in a patient with aortic incompetence or may be suspected with an abnormal root shadow in a patient with Marfan's disease. CT should in theory be helpful in recognising an aneurysm as should 2D echocardiographs, but usually aortography, combined with cardiac catheterisation, is required to demonstrate the presence and extent of an aneurysm and the degree of aortic regurgitation. The characteristic appearance is of a globular or fusiform dilatation of the aortic root involving the aortic valve ring, and the sinuses of Valsalva, the so called triple sinus aneurysm (Fig. 10.09). The abnormal dilatation extends up the ascending aorta, but almost invariably stops short of the origin of the innominate artery. When Marfan's disease is the cause, echocardiography or left ventriculography should also be performed to detect the characteristic prolapse of the mitral valve.

DISSECTING ANEURYSM OR DISSECTING HAEMATOMA

In this condition blood tracks in the aortic media dissecting the intima away from the adventitia. The media is abnormal, usually showing pathological appearances of Erdheim's cystic medial necrosis or Marfan's syndrome. The dissection is initiated by a split in the intima and the dissecting blood may re-enter the true aortic lumen from the false lumen created, at a distal re-entry point. Three types of aortic dissection have been defined by De Bakey et al. (1955). In type 1 a dissection initiates in the ascending aorta and spreads round the arch into the descending aorta and often beyond, into the abdomen. Type 2 begins in the ascending aorta but stops short of the great arteries of the arch. Type 3 begins with a split in the intima in the upper descending aorta just distal to the left subclavian artery and descends distally, again often into the abdominal aorta. In all three groups the dissection tends to follow a pattern. It lies on the right aspect of the ascending aorta, spirals on to the superior aspect of the arch and then into the left posterior aspect of the descending aorta descending on the left and tending to turn more posteriorly as it reaches the abdominal aorta (the left renal artery is frequently included).

At any stage of its formation the spreading haematoma may rupture through the aortic adventitia either in the pericardium from the ascending aorta or into the left pleural cavity from the descending aorta. As the dissection spreads it involves the branches of the aorta and may occlude them, often intermittently. If the patient survives the acute phase the adventitial sac created by the dissection progressively enlarges over a period of months or years until death results either from rupture or a fresh spread of dissection. The clinical features mirror the pathology. The majority of patients are hypertensive males, though pregnancy, coarctation of the aorta, Turner's syndrome or Marfan's disease are

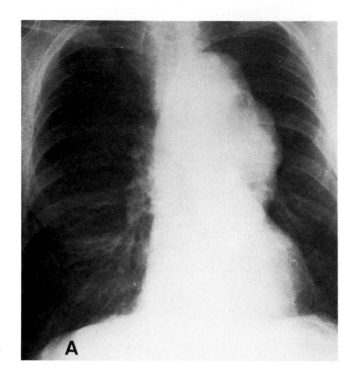

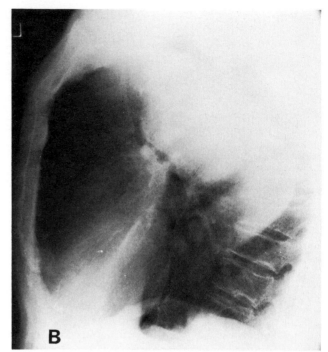

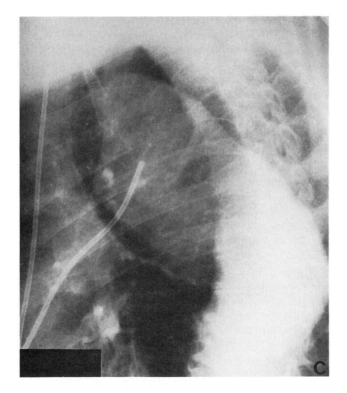

FIG. 10.06. Fusiform aortic aneurysm. (A) and (B) frontal and lateral chest X-rays. (C) lateral venous aortogram. The aneurysm involves the arch and thoracic aorta. Note the tracheal compression.

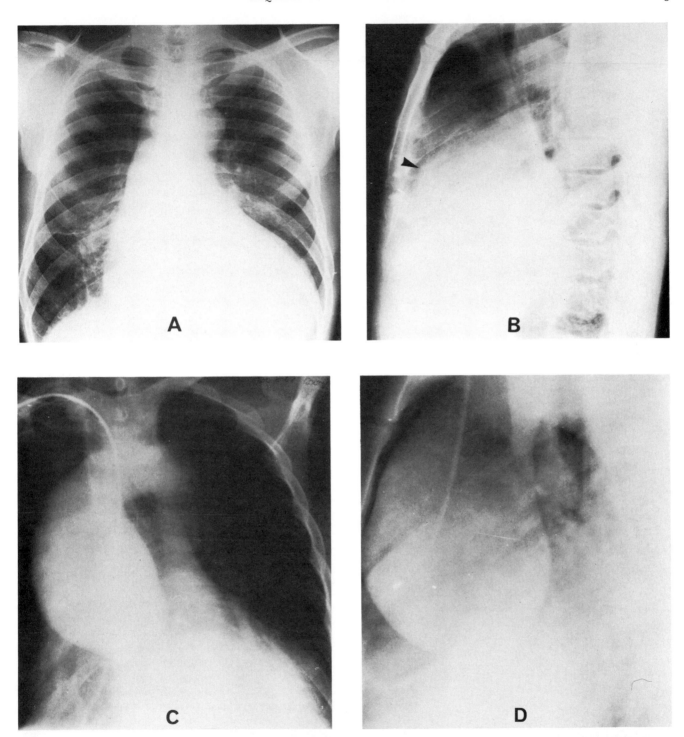

FIG. 10.07. Concealed intrapericardial aneurysm. A patient with syphilitic aortic incompetence. (A) frontal chest X-ray. The left ventricle is large, commensurate with severe aortic incompetence, but the aorta is only slightly large and does not appear aneurysmal. (B) lateral chest X-ray. This shows the large heart. The anterior wall of the aorta (arrow) appears to bulge anteriorly. Its posterior wall cannot be seen. (C) and (D) frontal and lateral root aortograms. These reveal an intrapericardial aneurysm of the aortic root with opacification of the left ventricle through the leaking aortic valve.

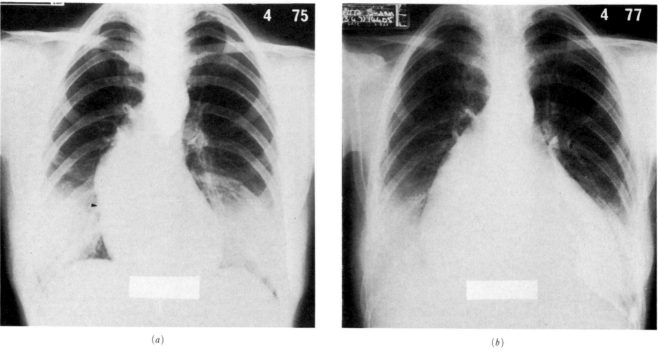

(a)

(b)

FIG. 10.08. Marfan aneurysm of the aortic root. In 1975 (A) there is localised prominence of the ascending aorta, separated by a notch (arrow) from the right heart border. The heart is not enlarged but already has a left ventricular configuration from aortic incompetence. By 1977 (B) the aneurysm of the aortic root is larger but blends with the now very much larger heart shadow which has dilated from increasing aortic incompetence.

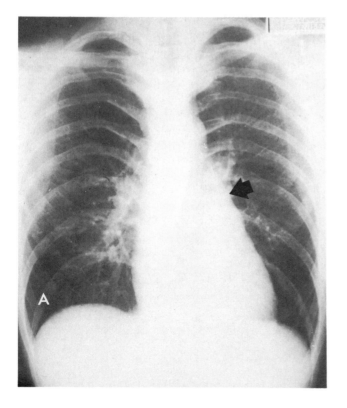

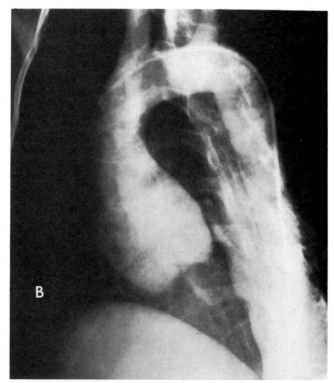

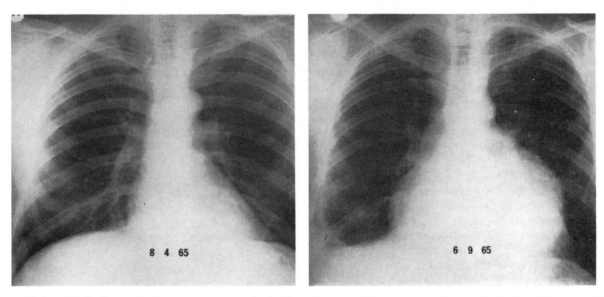

FIG. 11.01. Pericardial effusion. 8.4.65 Normal appearances. 6.9.65 There is a gross globular apparent increase in the size of the heart with a left upper border bulge. The lungs are clear; there is a right pleural effusion. These appearances are typical of a pericardial effusion, particularly when the increase in heart size has been as rapid and as marked as this.

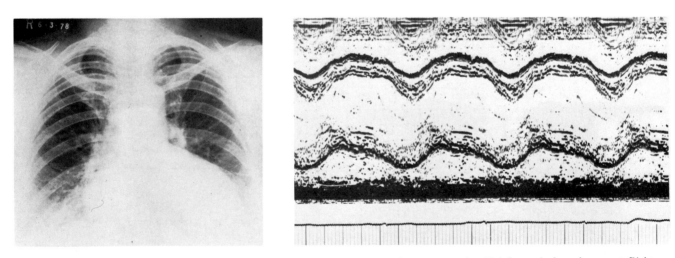

FIG. 11.02. Pericardial effusion due to myxoedema. Left.—The chest X-ray shows the heart apparently with left ventricular enlargement. Right.— Echogram shows a posterior pericardial effusion. In this case pericardial effusion mimicked left ventricular enlargement.

free) space behind the left ventricle and in front of the right ventricle (Fig. 11.02). This method only fails when it is technically impossible to obtain an adequate echocardiogram or when fluid collects in an unusual place, as it rarely does over the left ventricle.

Angiocardiography may be required if echocardiography is not successful or the clinical syndrome of tamponade is produced by a solid pericardial tumour. The normal thickness of tissue over the right atrium (right atrial wall and pericardium) is 3 mm and any

increase above 4 mm indicates a pericardial abnormality. The combination of ultrasound and angiocardiography can usually determine whether the pericardial abnormality is fluid or solid, or a combination of both.

Once a pericardial effusion has been diagnosed its nature must be determined. In many instances the pericardial effusion may occur in the course of, or complicate, a number of conditions, and lead to tamponade.

Secondary malignant disease, often breast.

Infections, bacterial, tuberculous, or viral.

Heart disease, cardiac failure, myocardial infarction with Dressler's syndrome.

Endocrine diseases, myxoedema.

Collagen diseases, systemic lupus erythematosus, rheumatic fever, rheumatoid arthritis, scleroderma, polyarteritis nodosa.

Uraemia.

Haemopericardium, trauma, rupture of the heart, dissecting aneurysm.

When the aetiology of the pericardial effusion is unclear, or a tamponade is present, it may be necessary to aspirate the effusion, usually under fluoroscopic control. Once the pericardium has been aspirated carbon dioxide may be injected into the pericardium to outline the inner aspect of the pericardium. Tumour masses may be identified and the thickness of the pericardium demonstrated.

A large globular heart and clear lungs may be seen in treated congestive cardiomyopathy, triple valve rheumatic heart disease, Ebstein's malformation of the tricuspid valve, critical pulmonary valve stenosis with right heart dilatation, and pulmonary atresia with intact ventricular septum and tricuspid regurgitation. Whereas these may resemble each other radiologically on the plain film there is no difficulty in distinguishing them on the basis of the clinical findings.

CONSTRICTIVE PERICARDITIS

This is a syndrome in which thickening and rigidity of the pericardium impede the filling of the cardiac chambers. Usually filling of the right heart is more affected than the left. The common causes are viral or tuberculous pericarditis or more rarely haemopericardium; collagen diseases may also lead to constriction. The clinical findings are those of oedema, hepatomegaly and ascites though without dyspnoea. The heart is murmur free and the diagnosis may be missed and oedema attributed to other causes if the neck veins are so distended that pulsation in them is not seen.

Plain Film Appearances

The heart may be normal in size or show a variable degree of enlargement (Fig. 11.03). There may be straightening of either or both borders of the heart with loss of outline of individual structures so that the heart and mediastinal structures are bounded by a continuous curved edge. An ill-defined shaggy outline of the heart suggests the presence of pleuropericardial fibrosis which may be associated with constriction. Constriction usually affects the right heart predominantly and in this situation the lungs are relatively clear. If the pulmonary veins are constricted or if the constriction involves the

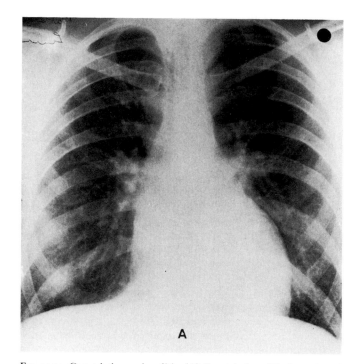
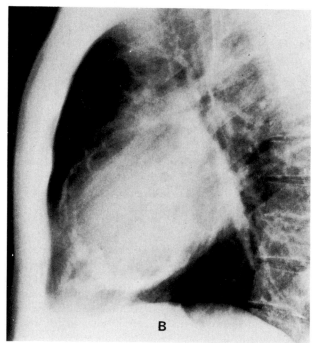

FIG. 11.03. Constrictive pericarditis. (A) Frontal view. The heart is only slightly large but the right border is represented by a continuous curve. (B) Lateral view. Pericardial calcification is present over the right ventricle.

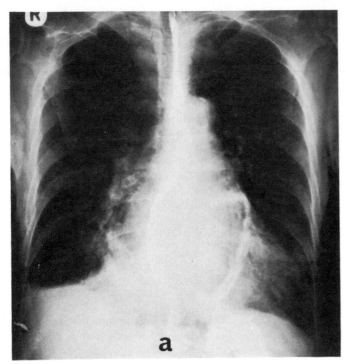 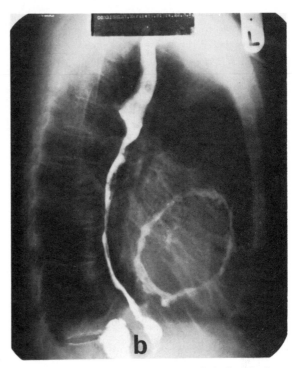

FIG. 11.04. Calcification in the atrioventricular groove. (*a*) Frontal view. (*b*) Lateral view. Note the continuous ring of calcium in both projections.

atrioventricular ring obstructing the left atrium then pulmonary oedema may be seen.

Pericardial calcification occurs in about half the patients with constriction, though it may be seen in the absence of constriction. It develops where pericardial effusions collect, inferiorly, anteriorly and laterally, but not posteriorly. It often collects specifically in the atrioventricular groove, outlining it on plain films and fluoroscopy (Fig. 11.04). While pericardial calcification is not invariably indicative of constriction, its presence is strongly suggestive of it.

Even gross constriction may be difficult to distinguish clinically from heart muscle disease. Cardiac catheterisation will demonstrate equal diastolic pressures in the two ventricles and right atrial angiography will show pericardial thickening (Fig. 11.05) and if this is gross suggests fluid as well. Angiography is also useful in demonstrating a normally functioning left ventricle. Constrictive pericarditis is a very difficult condition to recognise clinically as the evidence pointing to heart disease as the cause of oedema may be difficult to recognise. Even if heart disease has been recognised the distinction between constrictive pericarditis and disease of heart muscle may be impossible on clinical grounds or even after investigation. In any case of doubt the pericardium must be explored surgically.

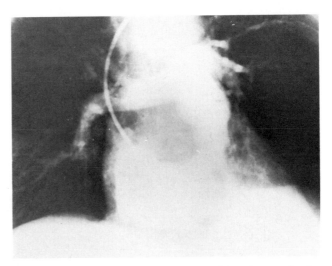

FIG. 11.05. Constrictive pericarditis. Right atrial angiogram showing the increase in thickness of the tissue over the right atrium.

PNEUMOPERICARDIUM

Gas within the pericardium is most commonly introduced by doctors either intentionally or inadvertently during the aspirations of the pericardial sac or as a result of surgery. Other forms of trauma may lead to gas in the pericardium and it is possible that suppurative infections could produce gas.

Appearances will depend on the amount of gas and also on any associated fluid present in the pericardium. The thin gas density may be seen at the edge of the

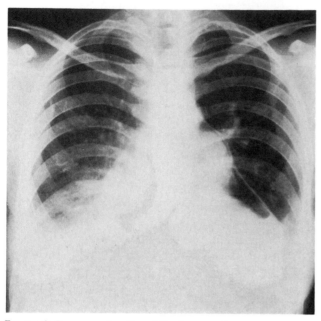

FIG. 11.06. Pneumopericardium following open heart surgery. Note the thinness of the normal pericardium. Beneath it the main pulmonary artery and left atrial appendage are outlined by air. The air rises only to the reflection of the pericardium.

heart on either side of the frontal view or in front in the lateral view. With larger amounts of gas the pericardium will be outlined on its inner aspect, and its thickness can be evaluated (Fig. 11.06). The heart may be seen within the pericardium and structures such as the left atrial appendage may be outlined. A gas–fluid level may be seen in the erect position.

When the gas is extensive there is usually little doubt about the diagnosis though intestinal hernias may cause difficulty. The chief difficulty lies in distinguishing between pneumopericardium and a pneumomediastinum. The presence of a fluid level points to a pneumopericardium but in its absence the lateral view is helpful as gas within the pericardium cannot rise above the superior extent of the pericardium whereas mediastinal gas is not limited in that way.

TUMOURS OF THE PERICARDIUM

The only common pericardial tumour is the springwater cyst (synonym pleuro-pericardial cyst, pericardial coelomic cyst). These are unilocular thin walled cysts attached either intimately or by pedicle to the pericardium. They are similar to pericardial diverticula, which communicate with the pericardial cavity. These tumours occur in the pericardiophrenic angle, much more commonly on the right. Small cysts may be teardrop in shape and lie in the lower end of the oblique fissure (Fig. 11.07). The larger ones are spherical

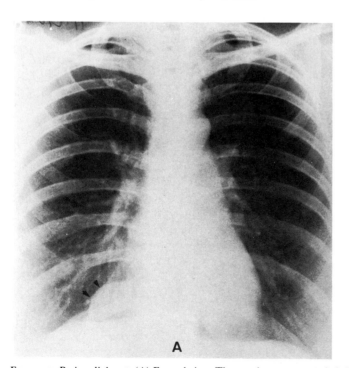

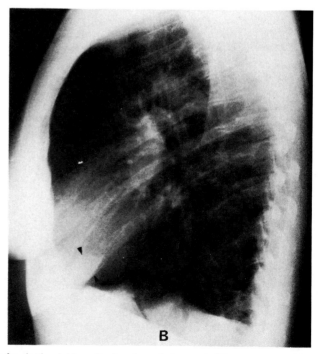

FIG. 11.07. Pericardial cyst. (A) Frontal view. The cyst is seen as rounded shadow in the right cardiophrenic angle (arrows). (B) Lateral view. The cyst lies in the lower end of the oblique fissure (arrows).

(Fig. 11.08). They may change shape with respiration. The diagnosis is immediately suggested by their characteristic position in the right cardiophrenic angle anteriorly, though rarely Morgani hernias, which in the elderly are filled with omentum, may cause confusion. A barium study will demonstrate the elevation of the transverse colon in a Morgani hernia. Primary malignant tumours of the pericardium are rare and may

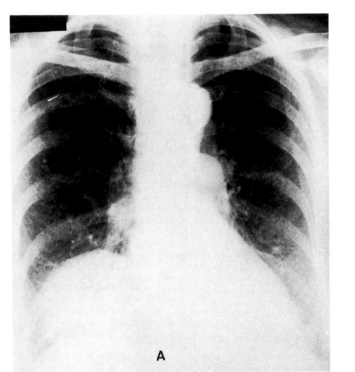
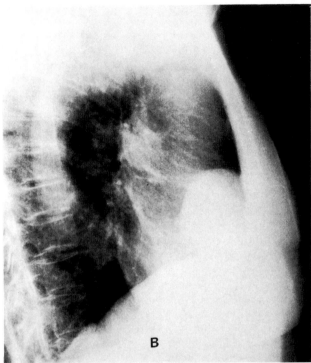

FIG. 11.08. Large pericardial cyst. (A) Frontal view. There is a very large rounded density in the right cardiophrenic angle. (B) Lateral view. The large round shadow lies anteriorly.

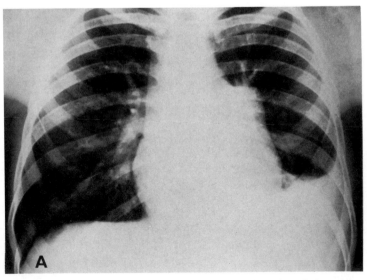
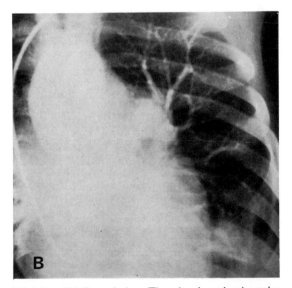

FIG. 11.09. Herniation of the atrial appendage through a congenital partial pericardial defect. (A) Frontal view. There is a large but irregular bulge in the position of the left atrial appendage. There is also a left pleural effusion. The appendage was partly strangulated. (B) Venous angiogram, frontal projection. This shows that the bulge consists of a left atrial appendage. The body of the left atrium is of normal size.

appear as a mass or a pericardial effusion or both. Secondary malignant involvement of the pericardium is common producing a pericardial effusion and often tamponade.

CONGENITAL PERICARDIAL DEFECTS

Partial defects of the left pericardium may lead to herniation of the structures of the left heart border, the pulmonary artery or left atrial appendage, producing a prominence on the plain radiograph. They may be associated with a slightly odd murmur causing a mis-diagnosis of either rheumatic mitral valve disease or of pulmonary stenosis. The lack of other evidence of heart disease on clinical grounds and the otherwise normal left atrium on radiological grounds will raise the possi-bility of a pericardial defect (Fig. 11.09). Torsion of the atrial appendage has been recorded through a pericar-dial defect; this may be fatal.

Complete absence of the left pericardium (Fig. 11.10) leads to displacement of the heart to the left, prominence of the main pulmonary artery and often a bulge in the position of the left atrial appendage. The translucency of interposed lung between the heart and the diaphragm will suggest the absence of the left pericardium as the normal pericardium is bound down to the diaphragm beneath the heart. Apart from the abnormalities of the left heart border there will be no other features either clinically or radiologically to suggest that there is heart disease. Gas can be made to enter the pericardium if a left pneumothorax is induced, and this will confirm the

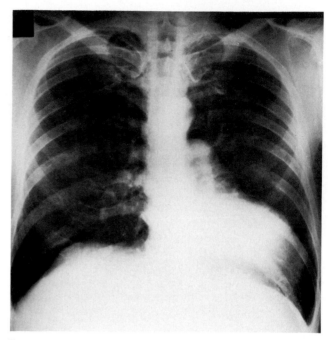

FIG. 11.10. Complete absence of the left pericardium. The heart is displaced to the left with a prominent main pulmonary artery. A radiolucent area can be seen between the heart and the left diaphragm (*Courtesy Dr J. B. Partridge*).

diagnosis. The appearances of the plain radiograph are usually sufficiently distinctive for a confident diagnosis to be made. Absence of the right pericardium is very much rarer, as is that of the whole pericardium.

CHAPTER 12

CONGENITAL HEART DISEASE
BASIC PRINCIPLES

John Partridge and Leon Gerlis

INTRODUCTION

Congenital heart disease is an infrequent problem in routine radiological practice and consists of a large number of pathologies which may be in combination. The aim of these chapters is to present firstly an outline of the basic principles of morphology and haemodynamics, and then a systematic review of pathologies. The emphasis will be on the plain chest radiograph and other non-invasive techniques; angiocardiograms will be used to illustrate the conditions rather than to instruct the reader in present day angiographic techniques. The reader is urged not to disregard this chapter; a proper understanding of disordered cardiac physiology is essential to the correct radiological interpretation of all imaging techniques.

The plain chest radiograph is often non-specific on congenital heart disease and is only moderately accurate in reflecting its severity. This is particularly so in the neonate, in valvar stenoses and in left to right shunts. Yet the plain film is essential in the clinical evaluation of the patient and, taken with the clinical signs and an electrocardiogram, it is quite surprising how accurate an experienced diagnostician can be. Throughout these chapters the reader should relate the signs described to this general pattern in which the plain film contributes in all cases:

(a) The detection of abnormal situs or cardiac position.

(b) Cardiac size.

(c) Cardiac configuration and the inferences of individual chamber size and position that it may make.

(d) The position of the aortic arch.

(e) The state of the pulmonary circulation.

(f) Chest wall signs such as notching or evidence of surgery. Some of these signs have been discussed in previous chapters, and it is assumed that the reader has covered them before beginning this section.

DEVELOPMENT OF THE HEART

The first appearance of the heart is heralded by the development of a cardiogenic plate of mesodermal tissue which lies below a coelomic cleft at the extreme head end of the embryonic disc and projects backwards on each side in a horse-shoe shape. Rapid development and flexion of the head cause this cardiac anlage to come to lie below the head and mouth, in front of the foregut, and behind the coelomic cleft. Meanwhile the two lateral extensions of cardiac tissue become hollowed out to form a pair of endothelial tubes, and at the same time the infolding and fusion of the lateral portions of the embryonic plate bring together these two cardiac tubes which come to lie side by side, and in turn fuse to form the primitive cardiac tube. Paired veins from the trunk, liver, yolk sac and placenta enter the heart tube from below and a series of arterial arches emerge from the upper end.

The endothelial heart tube becomes invested in a loose mantle of cells which is destined to form the myocardium and it expands, elongates and loops upon itself and projects into, and becomes invested by, the coelomic cleft which becomes the pericardial cavity. During the expansion and looping of the single heart tube four different portions become recognisable (Fig. 12.01); from below upwards these are, the sinus venosus, the primitive atrium, the primitive ventricle and the truncus arteriosus. These regions later become separated by three sets of valves. The ventricular chamber becomes further divided by looping which separates an inlet chamber, into which the atrium opens from above, and an outlet chamber, sometimes called the bulbus cordis, which opens distally into the truncus arteriosus.

This ventricular looping is normally associated with a right-handed or dextral (d) twist, such as if the free portion of the loop, that is the apex of the heart, is rotated anticlockwise. At this stage of development the inlet portion is, therefore, on the left side and the outlet portion or bulbus is on the right side. The segmentation, dilatation and looping of the heart result in the loss of the early tubular form, and functional maturity is brought about by valved separation of the chambers and longitudinal septation.

The sinus venosus comes to open into the right side of the atrium and the opening is guarded by two venous valve folds which are originally prominent (Fig. 12.02). Regression of these valves results in the sinus venosus becoming absorbed into the (right) atrium as the 'smooth' lateral portion and the three main venous

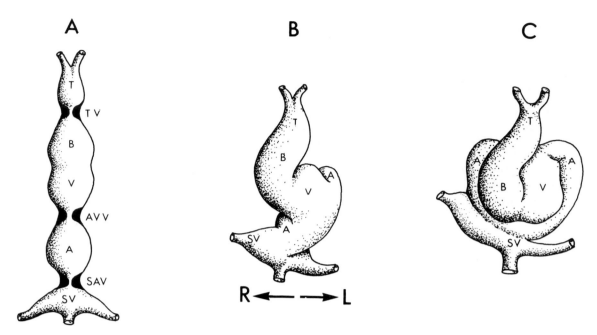

FIG. 12.01. The development of the heart tube. (A) Simple tubular heart. (B) Early looping. (C) Established looping and early definition of unseptated cardiac chambers.

A.	Atrium	R.	Right.	T.	Truncus arteriosus.
AVV.	Atrio ventricular valve site.	SAV.	Sinuatrial valve site.	TV.	Truncal Valve site.
B.	Bulbus cordis	SV.	Sinus venosus.	V.	Ventricle.
L.	Left.				

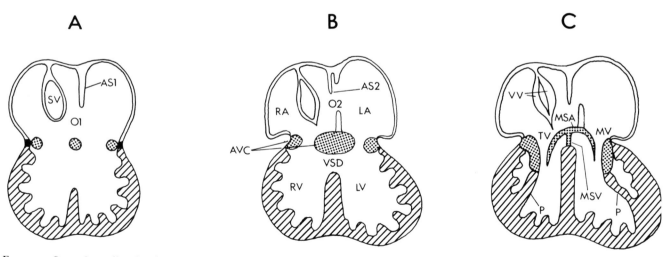

FIG. 12.02. Stages in cardiac chamber septation; the diagrams represent coronal sections of the heart. (A) Primary intra-atrial and intraventricular openings still widely patent. (B) Atrial ostium primum closed and ostium secundum and septum secundum forming. Ventricular septation is incomplete. (C) Septation complete and membraneous septum formed. The atrioventricular valves have been defined by growth of the cushion tissue and excavation of the myocardium.

AS1.	Atrial septum primum.	MSV.	Membraneous septum;	RV.	Right ventricle.
AS2.	Atrial septum secundum.		interventricular portion.	SV.	Sinus venosus orifice.
AVC.	Atrioventricular cushions.	MV.	Mitral valve.	TV.	Tricuspid valve.
LA.	Left atrium.	O1.	Ostium primum.	VS.	Ventricular septum.
LV.	Left ventricle.	O2.	Ostium secundum.	VSD.	Ventricular septal defect.
MSA.	Membraneous septum;	P.	Papillary muscle.	VV.	Venous valves.
	atrioventricular portion.	RA.	Right atrium.		

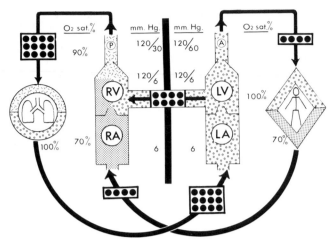

FIG. 12.04(D). Large ventricular septal defect with hyperkinetic pulmonary hypertension.

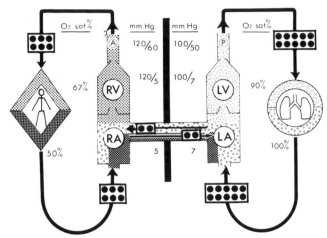

FIG. 12.04(G). Transposition of the great vessels.

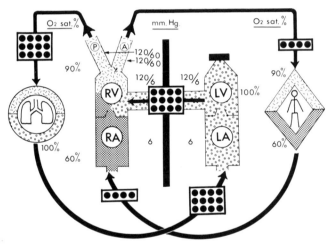

FIG. 12.04(E). Double outlet right ventricle with no pulmonary stenosis.

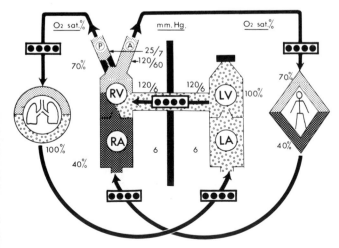

FIG. 12.04(F). Double outlet right ventricle with pulmonary stenosis.

those malformations listed above as left to right shunts when pulmonary vascular occlusive disease has risen to a level that causes the shunt to reverse (Fig. 12.04C). Other situations include severe pulmonary stenosis with right to left shunt at atrial level, Ebstein's malformation of the tricuspid valve with the same, VSD with severe pulmonary stenosis (with or without 'corrected transposition'), transitional circulation, and pulmonary artery to pulmonary vein fistula.

(d) Common Mixing Situations. Some complex cardiac malformations have traditionally been described as involving 'bidirectional shunting'. This confusing concept can be simplified by appreciating that most of them involve, at some point in the circulation, the mixing of all pulmonary and systemic blood streams. The malformations include:

Totally anomalous pulmonary venous drainage.
Univentricular heart.
Double outlet right or left ventricle.
All valve atresias.
Truncus arteriosus.

In all these malformations the common stream of blood provides an identical oxygen saturation in both pulmonary and systemic circuits. It follows that some degree of systemic desaturation will be present. The degree of cyanosis is dictated by the ratio of pulmonary to systemic flow, and this ratio in turn is dictated by the ease of access of the common flow to the pulmonary circuit. Double outlet right ventricle is a good example of the haemodynamic variability of this group. Figure 12.04E shows the circulation in a case where there is a large ventricular septal defect, no pulmonary stenosis and no significant rise in the pulmonary vascular resistance. Pulmonary blood flow is elevated and the radiograph will show plethora. The high ratio between pulmonary and systemic venous return means that the saturation of the mixed flow, and therefore of the aortic blood, is 90%, which is barely detectable clinically as cyanosis. Figure 12.04F shows the effect of valvar pulmonary stenosis on the same pathology. Equalised systemic and pulmonary flows lower the systemic saturation to 70% producing moderate clinical cyanosis. More severe pulmonary stenosis would further depress pulmonary flow and therefore systemic saturation. The various malformations each have a number of possible physical restrictions to pulmonary blood flow; these will be enumerated later. All those which have a high pulmonary flow initially will probably, if untreated, develop a low pulmonary flow due to the onset of pulmonary vascular occlusive disease.

(e) Parallel Circulations. In practical terms, the only malformation here is transposition of the great vessels. Figure 12.04G shows how the pulmonary and systemic circuits are essentially independent; life is sustained only by partial mixing at atrial level, ventricular level or across a patent ductus. It is the only cause of *severe* cyanosis with obviously plethoric lung fields. Systemic saturation is usually higher when pulmonary flow is high as this encourages atrial mixing; pulmonary flow is higher in those cases with a VSD or PDA. These relationships are not invariable, however, and the exact mechanisms in play are not fully understood. Pulmonary vascular occlusive disease can develop before six months of age.

(f) Left to Left Shunts. These rare malformations return fully oxygenated blood to the left side of the heart. The commonest cause is a fistula in the lungs between an abnormal aortic collateral vessel and a pulmonary vein, usually as part of a broncho-pulmonary sequestration.

(g) Right to Right Shunt. This is mentioned for completion. It exists as pre-capillary pulmonary artery to bronchial vein anastomoses and is a minor feature of some complex defects.

(h) 'Obstructive' Pathologies. Defects which hinder blood flow include the valvar stenoses and regurgitations, the causes of myocardial failure, aortic and pulmonary coarctation, constrictive pericarditis and pulmonary venous stenosis. The group is divided between those in which there is no other defect, in which the haemodynamic response is hypertension of the chamber proximal to lesion, and those in which a septal defect or other malformation allows the proximal chamber to decompress. In the former group signs of pulmonary or systemic venous hypertension predominate; in the latter, the effects of a septal defect are accentuated (e.g. coarctation with ventricular septal defect) or diminished (e.g. ventricular septal defect with pulmonary stenosis) or even reversed (tetralogy of Fallot).

SUBACUTE BACTERIAL ENDOCARDITIS (S.B.E.)

The general aspects of S.B.E. in children are no different from those mentioned in the section on adult disease. All congenital pathologies which can produce turbulent blood flow are susceptible to S.B.E. In general, the risk increases with the degree of turbulence, and this in turn depends on the pressure drop that is causing the turbulence. The pathologies at particular risk are:

Small ventricular septal defects
Gerbode defects
Mitral and aortic regurgitation
Small PDA
Coarctation, and coarctation repair
Aortic stenosis.

For some reason, pulmonary valvar stenosis is not particularly susceptible.

Cerebral Abscess

Any pathology that allows systemic venous blood into the systemic arteries without passage through the lungs can produce a cerebral abscess. In other words, any cyanotic lesion can do this, and the greater the degree of cyanosis, the greater the risk.

PULMONARY VASCULAR PATTERNS IN CONGENITAL HEART DISEASE

This section is complementary to an understanding of the haemodynamics of the pulmonary circuit as elegantly demonstrated by Professor Milne in Chapter 3.

(a) Plethora. This term describes the visible changes of the pulmonary vessels secondary to an increased flow in them. The pulmonary arteries are enlarged, they are more numerous, they extend further towards the periphery of the lung than normal, and there is equalisation of the relative flows in the upper and lower zones. These structural changes are usually absent in conditions where the increase in flow is of recent onset, and may regress slowly or not at all in established cases when the cause is removed.

FIG. 12.05. Pulmonary vascular patterns. (a) Mild plethora. ASD with 1.4:1 shunt. Borderline enlargement of the pulmonary arteries. (b) Moderate plethora. PDA with 2:1 shunt. Equalised flow in the upper and lower zones. (c) Severe plethora. VSD with 4:1 shunt. Note the vessel blurring due to 'shunt failure'. (d) Mild oligaemia. Tetralogy of Fallot. (e) Severe oligaemia. Tetralogy of Fallot. Note that the artery seen end on, just lateral to the hilum, is much smaller than its attendant bronchus. (f) Pulmonary venous hypertension. Six year old girl with congenital mitral stenosis. Upper lobe blood diversion (note the small lower lobe artery despite hilar enlargement), perivascular oedema and bronchial cuffing, but no septal lines.

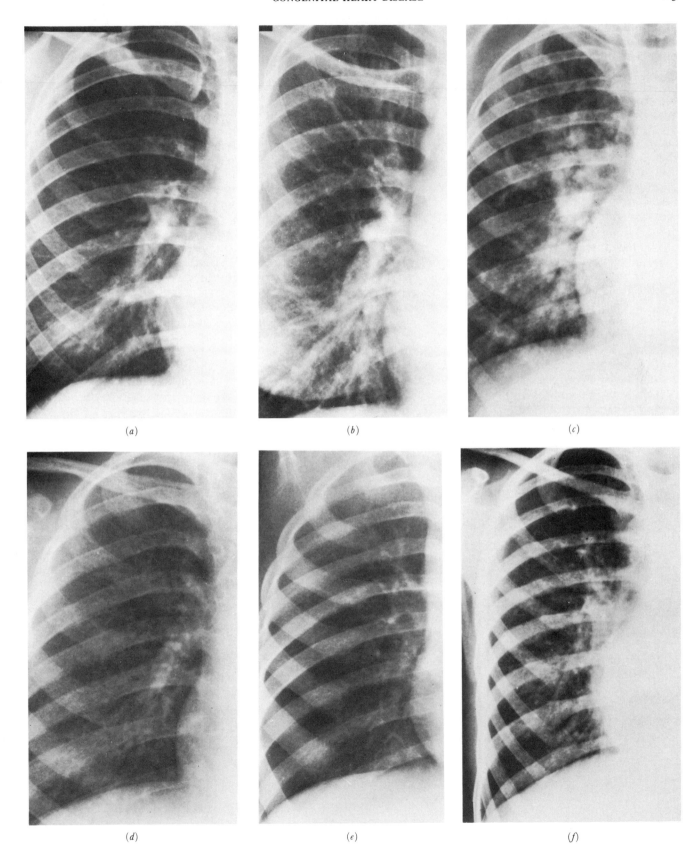

(a)　　　　　　　(b)　　　　　　　(c)

(d)　　　　　　　(e)　　　　　　　(f)

Plethora does not automatically mean that there is a simple left to right shunt as other pathologies (e.g. anaemia, transposition of the great arteries) may produce it. In the infant, a large shunt may generate a high left atrial pressure and cause superadded signs of pulmonary venous hypertension ('shunt failure'). Plethora can usually be detected if the pulmonary blood flow is twice normal or more, i.e. if there is a simple shunt, a ratio of 2:1 or more. Borderline changes are difficult to assess. Enlargement of the pulmonary arteries, which is best judged by the comparison of an 'end on' arterial shadow with its bronchus, is a moderately reliable sign; recruitment of the upper zone arteries is an early sign but very subjective and liable to confusion with pulmonary venous hypertension.

(b) Oligaemia. This in turn is the appearance of chronically reduced pulmonary blood flow; the pulmonary arteries are small, less numerous than normal and do not extend as far as normal into the lung fields. These features are usual in the first day or two of life. Mild oligaemia is extremely difficult to be sure of. The decrease in arterial size is quite a constant feature of moderate oligaemia. I suspect that the subjective 'emptyness' of the lungs in severe oligaemia is due also to collapse of the pulmonary veins.

(c) Pulmonary venous hypertension. This is an unusual situation in congenital heart disease, and so easily missed. Several pathologies, e.g. totally anomalous pulmonary venous drainage, may present in the neonate without murmurs and with widespread pulmonary consolidation and be taken for pulmonary disease. Such infants usually show air space consolidation with a tendency to perihilar distribution. Older children with milder hypertension show features more typical of adult disease, save that septal B lines are often absent.

(d) Secondary pulmonary arterial hypertension. As previously described, pulmonary arterial hypertension may be hyperdynamic due to a shunt, or secondary due to pulmonary vascular occlusive disease. When it is secondary to a shunt it is characterised by progressive dilatation of the main pulmonary artery and the lungs often retain a plethoric appearance even if the shunt is neutralised. In those occasional cases where there has been no plethoric phase, the pulmonary vasculature may have normal appearances.

(e) 'Bronchial' circulation. Some patients with Fallot pulmonary atresia show a nodular pattern in the lungs due to abnormal systemic arteries. Signs of oligaemia at the hila are invariable, but the peripheral pattern can sometimes mimic plethora.

All these patterns are to be seen in the following chapters. Figure 12.05 serves to give a convenient comparison of some of the common types.

For this and the following three chapters, we thank the Department of Medical Illustration at St James's University Hospital, Leeds, and the secretarial assistance of Miss J. Cooney, Miss S. Tyrell and Mrs D. M. Partridge.

FURTHER READING

VEREL, D. & GRAINGER, R. G. (1979) *Cardiac Catheterisation and Angiocardiography*. 3rd Edn. London: Churchill Livingstone.

CHAPTER 13

SIMPLE CONGENITAL HEART DISEASE

John Partridge and Leon Gerlis

INTRODUCTION

This chapter includes malformations that usually occur in isolation and without any situs or connection abnormality. This does not preclude the occasional case in situs inversus atria. Combinations of them do occur but will only be mentioned when they are particularly relevant.

ATRIAL SEPTAL DEFECT (ASD)

Morphology

Most ASDs are of the *ostium secundum* type in which the defect lies in the middle portion of the atrial septum between septum primum and septum secundum, where normally the fossa ovalis is found. It may exist alone or complicate virtually any other defect. *Ostium primum* ASDs are part of the spectrum of atrioventricular defects which will be described later in this chapter. When uncomplicated by a ventricular septal defect they are haemodynamically and radiologically identical to other ASDs. The *sinus venosus* type of ASD is the least common and lies high in the septum, between the septum secundum and the orifice of the superior vena cava. It is frequently (if not always, according to some authors) complicated by anomalous drainage of the right upper pulmonary vein to the superior vena cava. Combinations of these three types of ASD are uncommon.

Haemodynamics

Shunting across an uncomplicated defect is from left to right and happens during ventricular diastole, not because of any pressure gradient between the atria but because the right ventricle relaxes more easily (i.e. has greater compliance) than the left ventricle because of its thinner myocardium. There will be no shunting at birth as the right ventricle is then as thick as the left. Right ventricular involution to a normal wall thickness takes several months during which the shunt slowly develops. Despite quite a large shunt, the pulmonary artery pressure is only mildly raised in childhood and dyspnoea is slight or absent. The defect is typically discovered at routine school medical examination because of a systolic flow murmur across the pulmonary valve. Pulmonary vascular obstructive disease may never develop and cases may present late in adult life without any pulmonary hypertension. Usually, however, there is a slow rise in pulmonary arterial pressure reaching significant levels around the age of thirty and reversing the shunt in the fifties. The pulmonary hypertension may exceed systemic pressure before the consequent right ventricular hypertrophy becomes severe enough to cause right ventricular compliance to fall below left. As the shunt diminishes so does dyspnoea but it is replaced by fatigue and cyanosis. Eventually the right ventricle fails and death ensues. An occasional presentation is with atrial fibrillation, usually late in life and when the shunt is still large; this may precipitate heart failure.

Radiology

The plain chest film shows cardiomegaly and plethora which parallel the size of the shunt. Since the shunt develops well after birth, the pulmonary arteries have thin walls and dilate readily with the increased flow; shunts of 2:1 or more usually appear plethoric. The main pulmonary artery is enlarged and the aortic knuckle often appears small. The cardiac shape is non-specific; the apex tends to have a rounded contour and there may be a mild right atrial prominence (Fig. 13.01). The superior vena cava is often shallow in secundum and venosus defects, and may not form the right upper mediastinal border at all, leaving it quite bare (Fig. 13.02a). This sign is said by some to be suggestive of complicating anomalous right upper pulmonary venous drainage, but it is far from a reliable sign. Indeed, some sinus venosus defects have a prominent superior vena cava (Fig. 13.02b). Occasionally an anomalous pulmonary vein can be seen as an unusually horizontal vessel in the right upper hilum, sometimes it simply increases the number of vessels in the hilum. More often than not, however, the plethora disguises the presence of the vein and so the plain film is a poor diagnostic test for it. With increasing pulmonary hypertension, the thin walled pulmonary arteries dilate readily and when the pressure reaches systemic they may be truly enormous (Fig. 13.03). Nevertheless, even when the pressure exceeds systemic, the peripheral arteries retain a plethoric appearance; embolic or other obliterative causes of pulmonary hypertension of late onset usually have obvious peripheral oligaemia.

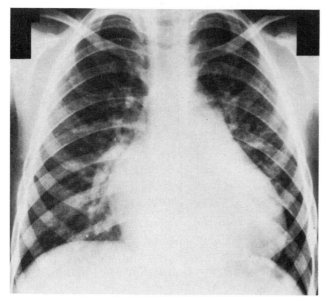

FIG. 13.01. Typical large atrial septal defect.
(*Courtesy Dr D. P. Montgomery.*)

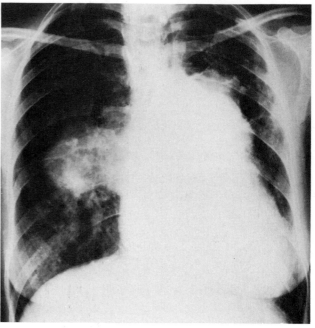

FIG. 13.03. Eisenmenger atrial septal defect. Gross main and hilar
pulmonary artery dilatation.

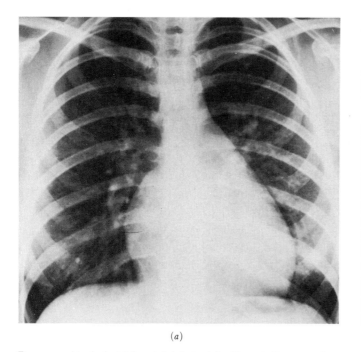

(*a*)

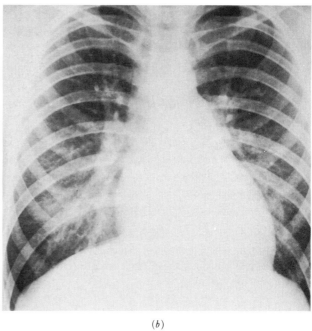

(*b*)

FIG. 13.02. Atypical atrial septal defects: (*a*) with a shallow superior vena caval shadow, (*b*) with a dilated superior vena cava (sinus venosus
defect). (*Courtesy Dr D. P. Montgomery.*)

Echocardiography

Real-time two-dimensional imaging can detect atrial septal defects of significant size with considerable reliability. The defect must have consistent and sharply defined edges and be seen in more than one view to avoid mis-diagnosing septal dropout as a defect (Fig. 13.04). The apical or subcostal four chamber views are best; ostium primum defects abut the atrioventricular valves; secundum defects are seen in the mid-part of the septum and so have a rim of septum on both sides in all views. Venosus defects lie at the upper rim of the septum, completely opposite the valves. M-mode recordings do not identify the defect directly and show only the secondary and non-specific features of increased right ventricular stroke volume. Contrast echocardiography can be useful; despite a large left to right shunt some bubbles delivered to the right atrium will cross to the left atrium, often enough to be identified on real time imaging.

Isotope studies are only helpful in the detection and quantification of the shunt.

Management

Surgical closure is undertaken in all defects but the very smallest. The risks of the operation are very low.

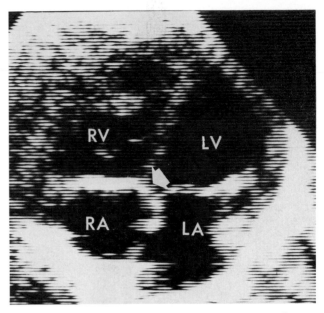

FIG. 13.04. Ostium secundum atrial septal defect; echocardiogram, four chamber view. The defect is bounded on both sides by atrial septum. The atrioventricular septum is arrowed; note the discontinuity of the lines of the tricuspid and mitral valves.

VENTRICULAR SEPTAL DEFECT (VSD)

Morphology

In isolation or with other defects, holes in the ventricular septum are the commonest congenital cardiac defect. There are several different types and it is not the brief of this text to describe them in great detail. They fall into three broad categories (Fig. 13.05):

(1) **Perimembraneous defects.** Any defect that involves the membraneous interventricular septum is included in this group. The defect lies below the aortic valve on the left ventricular side but is distant from the pulmonary valve on the right ventricular side. The group includes the common *subcristal defects* (which are illustrated in Fig. 13.05 and 13.06) and *inflow defects* which extend inferiorly alongside the tricuspid valve (these are found in the atrioventricular defects which are described below). The septal defects of many complex conditions (e.g. tetralogy of Fallot) are also essentially perimembraneous.

(2) **Infundibular defects,** also known as supracristal or doubly committed defects, are also subaortic but are higher than the perimembraneous type and enter the right ventricle immediately below the pulmonary valve.

(3) **Muscular defects.** Single (Fig. 13.07) or multiple, these are found anywhere in the muscular septum. Sometimes the septum is riddled with small defects and is graphically described as a 'Swiss-cheese' septum.

(4) **Combinations.** Combinations of two of the three

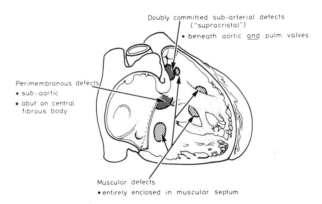

FIG. 13.05. Diagram of the three types of ventricular septal defect; perimembraneous, which may be subcristal (as shown) or inflow (extending downwards to abut on the central fibrous body); infundibular ('supracristal'); and muscular. The defects are shown as if viewed from the right ventricular side of the septum.
(*Courtesy Professor R. H. Anderson.*)

types are occasionally found. Some very large defects are a confluence of two types.

Haemodynamics

The shunt through a VSD occurs during ventricular systole. The size of the shunt is determined in small defects by the size of the defect itself, and in large defects by the resistance of the pulmonary circuit relative to systemic resistance. As a general rule, the defect has to

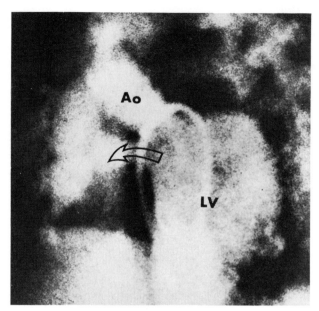

FIG. 13.06. Perimembraneous ventricular septal defect in the subcristal position. The defect is close to the aortic valve. Left ventricular angiogram, left anterior oblique view. LV = left ventricle; Ao = aorta.

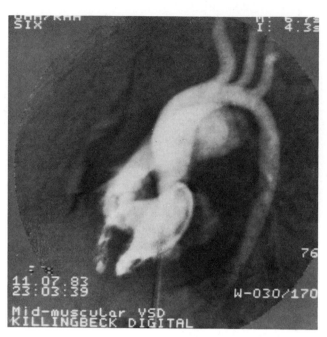

FIG. 13.07. Muscular ventricular septal defect. Left ventricular angiogram, left anterior oblique view. The defect is well below the aortic valve and is single.

be as large as the aortic valve before pulmonary resistance limits the size of the shunt. The haemodynamic spectrum varies from negligible shunts through to large shunts presenting with heart failure and pulmonary hypertension in neonatal life, as described in Chapter 12. Untreated, a large defect will cause pulmonary vascular occlusive disease which seldom becomes established before two years of age but which progresses inexorably towards shunt reversal. Cyanosis will then increase and death ensues usually before thirty.

Smaller defects can produce a shunt large enough for, in time, pulmonary hypertension to develop, but this seems to be an unusual course. Small defects usually give a small, asymptomatic shunt that is detected on routine medical examination. Adults with small defects are quite rare; this is because most small defects close spontaneously in teenage life or earlier (Fig. 13.08); perimembraneous defects are closed by membraneous tissue growing across the defect; muscular defects close by muscular encroachment. Large defects (other than inflow) can also close spontaneously, sometimes within two years from birth. Adults with large, pulmonary hypertensive defects are documented but are quite rare.

Radiology

The plain chest radiograph shows non-specific cardiomegaly in those cases with a large shunt (Fig. 13.09). Plethora is usual in large shunts, but can be surprisingly slight; as the large shunt began early in life, the

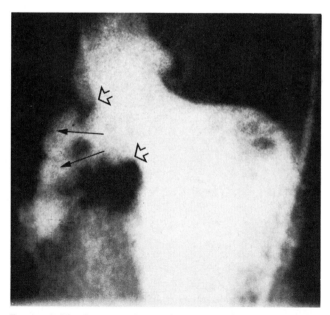

FIG. 13.08. Membraneous closure of a subcristal defect. Left ventricular angiogram, left anterior oblique view. The limits of the septal defect are shown by the open arrows. The membrane on the right ventricular side of the defect limits the flow to two small channels (solid arrows).

pulmonary arteries retain a thick wall and do not readily dilate. The main pulmonary artery is usually prominent in large shunts, only mildly so when pulmonary artery pressure is low and more so when pressure is high; even so, many neonates with large shunts do not show any prominence despite angiographic evidence of pulmonary arterial dilatation. When the defect closes spontaneously, the signs regress. When

the defect is small the chest radiograph is frequently normal.

In cases where pulmonary vascular occlusive disease reduces the shunt, the main pulmonary artery is usually clearly prominent and slowly becomes more so (Fig. 13.10). The peripheral pulmonary arteries usually retain a mildly plethoric appearance but can look quite normal. Occasionally the chest film can look virtually normal (Fig. 13.11). Whenever the shunt is large and there is no atrial septal defect, the left atrium is enlarged and this can be seen as prominence of its rightward border on the chest film. It is often hardly apparent because of generalised cardiomegaly but is quite a frequent sign if looked for. Large shunts presenting in the neonate may also have signs of interstitial pulmonary oedema as the left heart fails to cope with torrential pulmonary venous return. In contrast, and rarely, some cases with large defects never drop their pulmonary resistance after birth and go straight into the Eisenmenger situation.

Echocardiography

At the time of writing echocardiography has advanced to the point where many investigators can reliably demonstrate any large single defect. This requires a thorough approach, visualising the ventricular septum from as many aspects as possible. Membraneous closure can often be detected but its extent across the defect may not be accurately assessed. Figure 13.12 is an example of a muscular defect; see also Fig. 14.13.

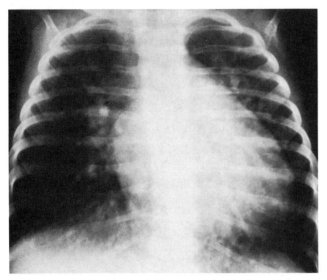

FIG. 13.09. Typical large ventricular septal defect in an infant.

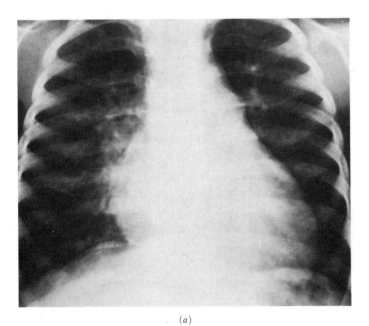

(a)

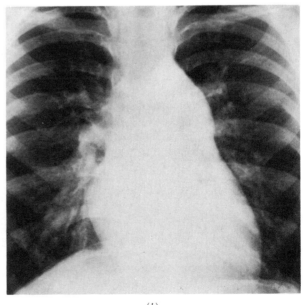

(b)

FIG. 13.10. Progression of a ventricular septal defect. (a) Age four years; clinically a moderate shunt, with no electrocardiographic evidence of pulmonary hypertension. (b) Age nine years, having been lost to follow-up in the interval. Severe pulmonary hypertension with shunt reversal.

Contrast echocardiography using a wedged pulmonary artery injection will improve shunt detection but is unlikely to improve placement of the defect. Left atrial enlargement is more easily judged than on the plain film. Angiocardiography will probably remain the arbiter in cases where multiple or muscular defects are involved; compound angular views are required and will not be described here.

Isotope techniques are confined to the detection and quantification of the shunt.

Management

A pulmonary hypertensive ventricular septal defect without PVOD needs surgical closure sooner or later. Early closure before two years of age is preferable (if the expertise is available) to avoid pulmonary vascular occlusive disease. If not, pulmonary artery banding can delay the need for closure until the child grows. A non-hypertensive defect can be closed at a later date, providing it shows no sign of impending spontaneous closure or is not so small that PVOD is not a risk.

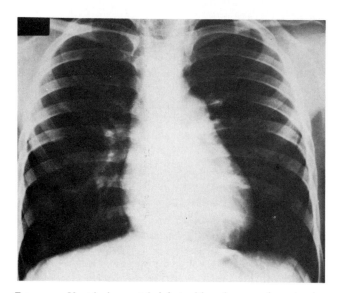

FIG. 13.11. Ventricular septal defect with pulmonary hypertension and reversed shunt. There is only mild prominence of the main pulmonary artery and hilar vessels. This is probably an example of severe pulmonary hypertension persisting from birth.

VENTRICULAR SEPTAL DEFECT WITH AORTIC REGURGITATION

Morphology

In most perimembraneous and in all infundibular defects, part of the aortic valve ring is unsupported by ventricular myocardium. Consequently there may be diastolic prolapse of part or whole of an aortic leaflet. The prolapsed part falls into the septal defect and may partly or completely occlude it. The prolapse allows aortic regurgitation which can be severe.

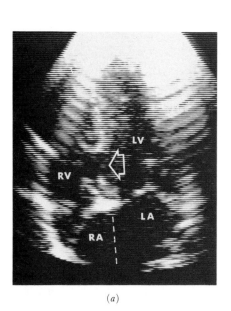

(a)

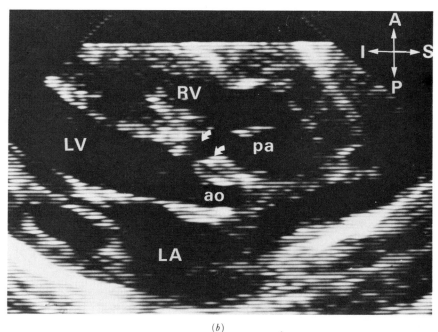

(b)

FIG. 13.12. Echocardiograms of ventricular septal defects. (a) Four chamber view showing a mid-muscular defect (arrow). (b) Long axial view showing a perimembraneous defect (arrows). (*Courtesy Dr G. R. Sutherland.*)

Haemodynamics

The effective size of the septal defect and the degree of regurgitation affect the haemodynamic state. Combinations of the two tend to be more symptomatic than cases of a comparable uncomplicated septal defect.

Radiology

This will not be different from ordinary defects unless the aortic regurgitation is severe, when the signs of regurgitation will predominate.

Echocardiography

This is similarly a variable combination of the two. Prolapse of the aortic leaflet is presently not a consistently recognised feature but this situation may well change as the quality of real time equipment improves.

Management

This is a serious pathology. The VSD might be easily closed but the aortic valve may well require repair (with variable success) or replacement (with the prospect of replacement as the patient grows). It is often prudent to settle for some residual regurgitation rather than to interfere too much with the aortic valve.

GERBODE DEFECT

Morphology

The true Gerbode defect is very rare indeed and is a defect in the atrioventricular septum between the left ventricle and the right atrium. The term is often used more loosely to describe a subcristal defect in which the tricupsid valve has become adherent to the defect and allows the shunt to stream through its commissures (or through a cleft in its valves) into the right atrium.

Haemodynamics

There is nothing to hinder a shunt from the high pressure left ventricle to the low pressure atrium save the size of the defect—a situation described as an 'obligatory shunt'. These defects, if large, do not have to wait for pulmonary vascular resistance to fall to become clinically obvious.

Radiology

Most of these defects show no plain film distinction from ordinary VSDs. Right atrial prominence is an occasional feature. Left ventricular angiocardiography is the definite test.

Echocardiography

A lack of consistent data on these defects reflects their rarity. As in the angiogram, echo contrast has to be delivered to the left ventricle to clearly establish the pattern of shunting.

ATRIOVENTRICULAR DEFECTS

Also known as atrioventricular canal defects or endocardial cushion defects.

Morphology

This important group has a common anatomical defect in that the embryonic common atrioventricular valve fails to develop into separate mitral and tricuspid valves. This is always accompanied by, and possibly is due to, shortness of the inlet portion of the ventricular septum. It is virtually unknown for the common atrioventricular valve to be correctly attached to the atrial septum primum above it, and so a low and usually large atrial septal defect is present (an 'ostium primum ASD'). The group is sub-categorized according to the relationship of the valve to the ventricular septum. The valve may be unattached to the ventricular septum, so allowing a large inlet ventricular septal defect to exist beneath it (a 'complete' defect, Fig. 13.13), or may be

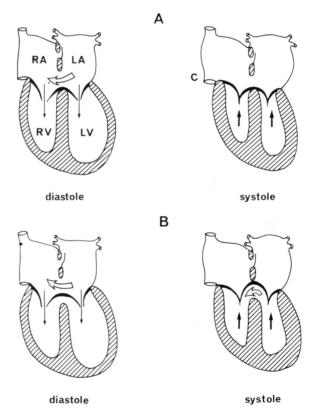

Fig. 13.13. Atrioventricular defects.
(A) With no ventricular septal defect. The central portion of the common valve is attached to the ventricular septal crest. The shunt through the low atrial septal defect occurs during diastole. (B) With a ventricular septal defect, which is present because the valve is unattached to the septal crest. Note that in both cases the atrioventricular portion of the membranous septum (MSA in Fig. 12.02) has not developed.

irregularly attached to the septal crest leaving small inlet VSDs (an 'intermediate' defect), or firmly attached leaving no VSD (a 'partial' defect, Fig. 13.13, 13.14). The atrioventricular valve leaflets show a variety of configurations and in complete defects the chordae may straddle the septum and seriously complicate surgical repair. 'The 'mitral' valve is tricuspid, since the two components which normally fuse to form the anterior leaflet remain separated by a cleft. Both 'mitral' and 'tricuspid' valves may be incompetent.

Haemodynamics

An ostium primum atrial defect alone has the same haemodynamics as an ordinary atrial defect. Added 'mitral' incompetence, unless truly gross, simply increases the shunt across the defect. Although the regurgitation may be directed into the right atrium because of the low atrial septal defect, the shunt is not obligatory as the atria are in communication. When there is a ventricular septal defect of significant size the haemodynamic picture is principally affected by it, but as a rule the complete defects present a cumulative picture of the two septal defects and 'mitral' incompet-

ence. It is typically more severe and earlier in presentation than a large ventricular septal defect alone. Secondary left ventricular failure in infancy is quite common.

Radiology

Partial and intermediate forms appear as atrial septal defects on the plain film, complete defects as a large VSD, and there is nothing to suggest an underlying atrioventricular defect. Angiocardiography is required for a radiological diagnosis; a full discussion is beyond the scope of this volume, but the shortness of the inlet septum gives rise to a striking appearance first described by Baron in 1964 (*Am. J. Cardiol.*, **13**, 162) and since dubbed the 'goose neck' deformity, which has become a popular term (Fig. 13.15).

Echocardiography

Real time studies are consistently diagnostic of the basic defect and reliably demonstrate the atrial defect and any large ventricular septal defect. The view of choice is the apical four chamber followed closely by the subcostal four chamber. The continuity of the common

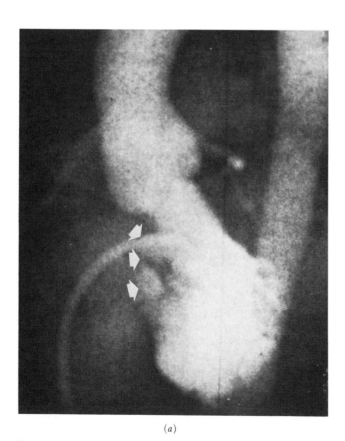

(a)

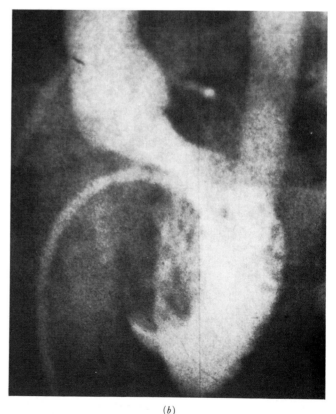

(b)

FIG. 13.14. Atrioventricular defect with no ventricular septal defect. Left ventricular angiogram, left anterior oblique view. (a) In systole. (b) In diastole. The irregular attachment of the abnormal atrioventricular valve to the septum is seen in systole (arrows). In diastole, the 'mitral' orifice is 'D' shaped and abuts the septum. There is no atrioventricular septum.

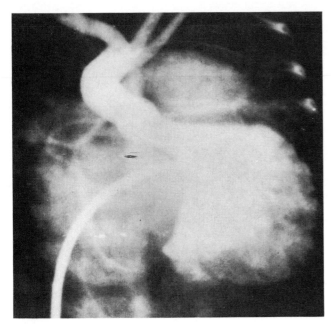

FIG. 13.15. Atrioventricular defect. Left ventricular angiogram, frontal view. The typically excavated appearance of the outflow tract is called the 'goose neck' deformity.

valve across the ventricular septum is a cardinal feature and is easily appreciated in the moving image (Fig. 13.16, 13.17). The M-mode trace is usually diagnostic when the transducer angles slightly more medially than for the normal mitral valve and sweeps through on to the 'tricuspid' valve (Fig. 13.18). Right ventricular overload is usual and, if a significant VSD can be excluded on other grounds, left ventricular overload suggests a significant degree of 'mitral' regurgitation.

Associations

Atrioventricular defects are usually isolated and there is a strong relationship between complete defects and Down's syndrome and may co-exist with Tetralogy of Fallot in this group. Single ventricle is often complicated by an atrioventricular defect, as are the atrial isomerisms.

Management

Closure of the ASD of a partial defect is not of itself a difficulty but runs the risk of inducing or worsening any 'mitral' regurgitation. Asymptomatic defects are, therefore, managed medically for a longer period than secundum defects. The 'mitral' regurgitation may itself demand operative intervention; usually repair of the cleft or occasionally valve replacement is required. Complete defects have a poor prognosis untreated but surgical repair is difficult and the greater expertise is found in units where patients with Downs' syndrome

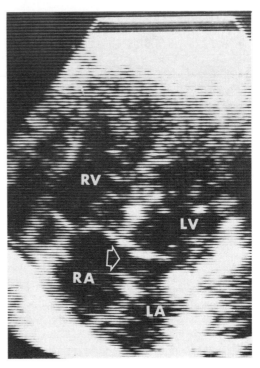

FIG. 13.16. Atrioventricular defect with no ventricular septal defect (ostium primum ASD). Echocardiogram, four chamber view. The atrial septal defect (arrow) is only bounded on one side by atrial septum (c.f. Fig. 13.04). There is no atrioventricular septum and the 'mitral' and 'tricuspid' valves are continuous across the septum.

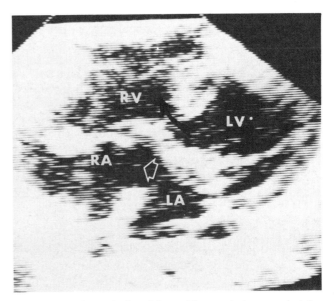

FIG. 13.17. Atrioventricular defect with ventricular septal defect ('complete canal' defect). The atrial defect is similar to that of Fig. 13.16 (open arrow). The VSD lies just below the common atrioventricular valve (black arrow).

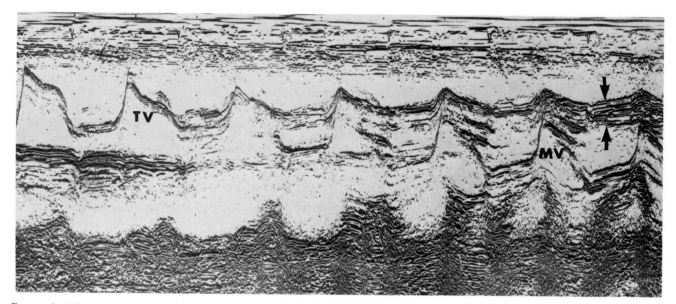

FIG. 13.18. Atrioventricular defect. M-mode echocardiographic trace swept from the 'tricuspid' valve (TV) to the 'mitral' valve (MV) shows how they merge across the septal echo (arrowed).

are regularly accepted for surgery. Pulmonary artery banding is a poor substitute for intracardiac repair as the atrial shunt is relatively unaffected by it.

TRICUSPID ATRESIA

Morphology

In tricuspid atresia proper the tricuspid 'valve' is an imperforate sheet of fibrous tissue between the right atrium and right ventricle (Fig. 13.19B). Clinically it is indistinguishable from absence of the right atrioventricular connection (Fig. 13.19A) which is more properly considered to be a variety of univentricular heart. Indeed, most cases of 'clinical' tricuspid atresia are probably the absent connection type. In both instances a ventricular septal defect is present, but it may be quite small. The right ventricle is hypoplastic. Pulmonary stenosis is usual. Transposition of the great vessels is occasionally associated with it. If there is no ventricular septal defect the entire right heart may be absent. An atrial communication is essential for life, so that systemic venous return may pass through to the left atrium.

Haemodynamics

Essentially a common mixing situation as the mitral valve is a common pathway for total venous return. The degree of pulmonary stenosis will usually determine the degree of cyanosis but occasionally the VSD restricts pulmonary blood flow more than the pulmonary valve. The typical case has severe pulmonary stenosis and severe desaturation. Complicating transposition has no intrinsic effect, unless the VSD is small and obstructs

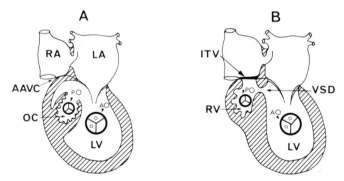

FIG. 13.19. Types of tricuspid atresia. (A) Absent atrioventricular connection (AAVC), in which there is an outflow chamber (OC) which usually leads to the pulmonary orifice (PO), the aortic orifice (AO) remaining with the left ventricle. (B) Imperforate tricuspid valve (ITV), with a small but correctly connected right ventricle beneath it.

aortic outflow which is a serious situation with a poor prognosis.

Radiology

The typical case with severe cyanosis presents in neonatal life with pulmonary oligaemia. There is a very hollow pulmonary bay below which the left ventricle forms a very rounded left heart border; the junction between the two is often shelf-like (Fig. 13.20). Cardiac enlargement is rare. Atypical cases with little or no pulmonary stenosis show pulmonary plethora, the main pulmonary artery is normal or prominent and the appearances, therefore, mimic a large VSD. Cases with

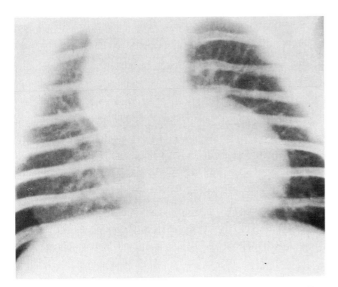

FIG. 13.20. Tricuspid atresia. The rounded left heart border and the hollow pulmonary bay join in a typically 'shelf' like fashion.

transposition look like uncomplicated transpositions. Those with coarctation will usually demand operative intervention before notching can become a visible feature.

Echocardiography

This will easily demonstrate, in the four chamber views, a single atrioventricular valve and the large left ventricle into which it opens. Closer analysis should allow the mitral valve to be distinguished from a common atrioventricular valve. The small right ventricle may or may not be identified; if not then the distinction from a single ventricle cannot be made. Mitral atresia can give a similar ventricular formation but the remaining atrioventricular (tricuspid) valve is usually clearly related to the right atrium and the aorta will not be hypoplastic in tricuspid atresia. The position and the connections of the great vessels should be apparent if high quality images are obtained; the pulmonary artery may be very small.

Management

Early in life palliative procedures to either increase pulmonary blood flow by a shunt or decrease it by pulmonary artery banding may be required. More corrective surgery entails the diversion of systemic venous flow to the pulmonary arteries either by the Glenn, Fontan or similar procedures.

TRICUSPID STENOSIS

Tricuspid stenosis is an occasional complication of other pathologies; it is virtually unknown as an isolated lesion.

It can be seen in chronic rheumatic valvar disease in children.

TRICUSPID REGURGITATION

This also is virtually unknown as a primary disorder but is frequently seen as a complication of any pathology that results in right ventricular failure, when it is as a result of dilatation of the valve ring. There is no diagnostic radiological feature but severe right atrial enlargement is always suggestive of it. At echocardiography increased pulsation of the right atrium and the inferior vena cava may be seen but, when it is, the liver is usually clinically pulsatile anyway.

EBSTEIN'S ANOMALY

Morphology

This is a moderately rare malformation of the tricuspid valve in which the leaflets of the valve are stuck down on to the right ventricular myocardium, starting at the tricuspid annulus and extending, in a sheet-like manner, a variable distance towards the ventricular apex. The effective valve ring is, therefore, displaced towards the apex. Despite its tetherings, the leaflets are enlarged and so can still appose, but the result is a severely incompetent valve. The ventricular chamber proximal to it is 'atrialised' and cannot contribute to ventricular performance. The remaining distal right ventricle is usually quite small (Fig. 13.21). The anomaly may complicate other malformations, particularly 'corrected transposition'.

Haemodynamics

At birth, when pulmonary vascular resistance is high, the feeble right ventricle, compounded by the incompetence of the tricuspid valve, cannot sustain an adequate forward flow and many cases present in neonatal life with right heart failure with secondary right to left shunting at atrial level. As pulmonary resistance falls the patient can improve, sometimes quite dramatically, and in quite a few cases a normal right heart output can be attained and the patient is asymptomatic at rest. Exercise tolerance is usually impaired, however. This period of relative well-being ends at about ten years of age when the right ventricle begins to fail to respond to the increasing demands of growth, and cyanosis returns. Many patients cannot survive the neonatal period without assistance.

Radiology

(Fig. 13.22.) There is nearly always a typical appearance on the chest film of a large, globular heart, due to considerable enlargement of the right heart without any hypertrophy. The lung fields are either normal, or, if

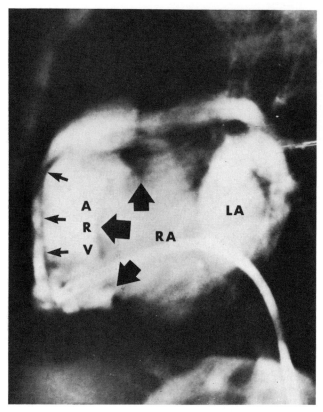

Fig. 13.21. Ebstein's anomaly. Right ventricular angiogram, lateral view. The abnormal tricuspid valve (small arrows) is displaced anteriorly away from the true tricuspid annulus (large arrows); between the two is the atrialised portion of the right ventricle (ARV). The hepatic veins are opacified because of severe tricuspid incompetence. RA = right atrium; LA = left atrium.

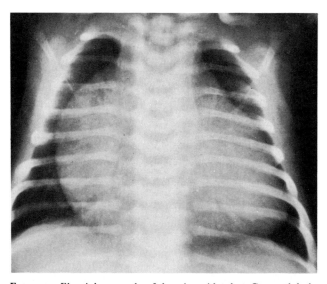

Fig. 13.22. Ebstein's anomaly of the tricuspid valve. Gross, globular cardiomegaly and pulmonary oligaemia.

cyanosis is evident, oligaemic. The differential diagnosis from the film is of a pericardial effusion, congestive cardiomyopathy, critical pulmonary or aortic stenosis, or Uhl's disease. Less severe cases show mild, non-specific cardiomegaly.

Echocardiography

On the four chamber or long axial views the apical displacement of the unattached part of the tricuspid valve is quite easily seen (Fig. 13.23). Minor degrees of displacement may be difficult to detect, but the lesion is usually gross. The right atrium is usually very large. On the M-mode trace the diagnosis is not so easy, but again depends on detecting the anterior displacement; suspicion is usually aroused by the ease with which the valve is identified.

Management

The severely cyanosed infant may require a shunt procedure but there is hope that pharmacological pulmonary vascular dilatation may be a reasonable alternative (some of the prostaglandins have this effect). Valve replacement is a logical procedure in the larger child but has not in practice proved satisfactory. Semi-corrective surgery, e.g. the Fontan procedure, is presently the treatment of choice, but for it pulmonary resistance must be low and this is not always the case if the child has previously had a shunt.

PULMONARY ATRESIA

Morphology

This section is not concerned with pulmonary atresia with VSD, which is a severe form of tetralogy of Fallot (see Chapter 14). Pulmonary atresia with an intact septum does not involve any obstruction at infundibular

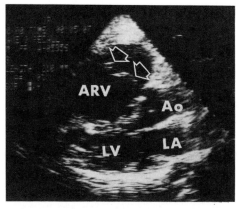

Fig. 13.23. Ebstein's anomaly. Echocardiogram, long axial view. The right heart is greatly dilated and the tricuspid valve (arrows) is anteriorly displaced. ARV = atrialised right ventricle.

level, the valve leaflets alone being atretic. Below it, the right ventricle is minuscule and heavily trabeculated; what little blood enters the ventricle leaves either by tricuspid regurgitation or via sinusoidal venous channels through the right ventricular myocardium to the cardiac veins (Fig. 13.24). The tricuspid valve is also severely hypoplastic. The left ventricle is enlarged; the pulmonary arteries are supplied by a patent ductus arteriosus and are small (Fig. 13.25). The main pulmonary artery extends back to the atretic valve leaflets and so is separated from the right ventricular cavity by only the thickness of the valve. Aorto-pulmonary collaterals are hardly ever seen.

Haemodynamics

Common mixing occurs at the mitral valve. Since the ductus is usually small, cyanosis is severe and these patients usually present as neonates. Furthermore, the ductus will try to close and so the cyanosis will rapidly worsen.

Radiology

(Fig. 13.26.) Pulmonary oligaemia is the rule and the pulmonary bay is hollow. Cardiomegaly is absent, slight or occasionally moderate. Despite sharing, with tricuspid atresia, a large left ventricle and small right ventri-

cle, the cardiac apex is either non-specific or mildly suggestive of right ventricular hypertrophy.

Echocardiography

Echocardiography will initially reveal only one obvious ventricle (the left), one large atrioventricular valve (mitral) and a normally positioned and connected aorta. The diagnosis rests on the demonstration of the

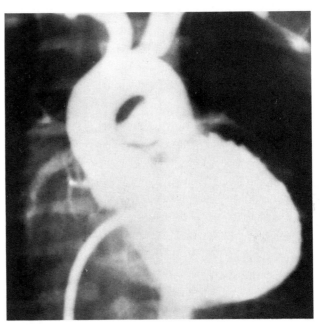

FIG. 13.25. Pulmonary atresia. Left ventricular angiogram, frontal view. The left heart outline is formed by the enlarged left ventricle. Small pulmonary arteries fill via a patent ductus arteriosus.

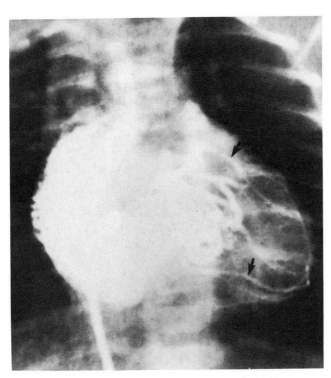

FIG. 13.24. Pulmonary atresia with intact ventricular septum. Right ventricular angiogram, frontal view. The right ventricle is tiny and is heavily trabeculated and some contrast is forced retrogradely into the coronary arteries (arrows). There is moderate tricuspid incompetence.

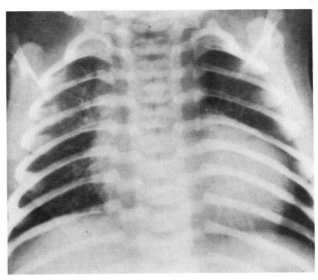

FIG. 13.26. Pulmonary atresia. Hollow pulmonary bay and oligaemia.

small, squat, thickened right ventricle and the hypo-plastic but patent tricuspid valve which is normally related to the right ventricle. The small pulmonary artery may not be identified.

Management

Untreated, this condition is fatal within one year, and is usually so before a few weeks have passed. The atretic valve can be perforated and dilated, but this is only palliative since the valve ring is small and flow through it is limited. Many centres combine this procedure with a shunt as a regular policy. In time, the right ventricle will sometimes increase in volume and de-hypertrophy. Eventually the child may grow large enough to have a proper valved conduit from the right ventricle to the pulmonary artery, or some form of right heart bypass.

PULMONARY STENOSIS

Morphology

Stenosis at valvar level is by far the commonest form (Fig. 13.27). The leaflets are thickened and the commissures fused to a varying degree. The valve ring is of a normal size unless the stenosis is severe, when it may be small. The main pulmonary artery shows post-stenotic dilatation when the degree of stenosis is mild, moderate or tending towards severe. Truly trivial stenosis may not show any post-stenotic dilatation, nor will many severe or critical cases, since there may be insufficient turbulence when the cardiac output falls. Also with increasing severity and/or chronicity, right ventricular hypertrophy will be manifest and at the level of the crista this may lead to end-systolic muscular infundibular stenosis which can be quite severe.

Sub-pulmonary stenosis without valvar stenosis is uncommon. It takes the form of an infundibular obstruction usually due to irregular bundles of muscle (Fig. 13.28) or occasionally to a more fixed fibrous subvalvar ring. It may co-exist with valvar stenosis, with only its irregular appearances to differentiate it from secondary infundibular hypertrophy. Post-stenotic dilatation of the main pulmonary artery is less striking than in the valvar stenoses, but is still usual.

Post-stenotic dilatation may extend into the proximal left branch pulmonary artery since it is more in line with the main trunk than is the right pulmonary artery. Valvar and infundibular pulmonary stenosis are very common complications of more complex malformations and will be mentioned many times again in subsequent sections.

Haemodynamics

With all but severe or critical stenosis, right ventricular hypertrophy enables a normal cardiac output to be maintained across the valve. Right ventricular pressure

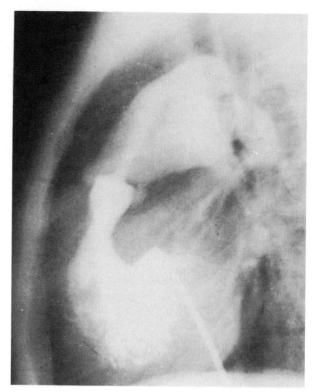

Fig. 13.27. Valvar pulmonary stenosis. Right ventricular angiogram, lateral view. The valve leaflets form a dome, and contrast passing through them forms a jet. Note the post-stenotic dilatation of the main pulmonary artery. (*Courtesy Dr J. K. Walker.*)

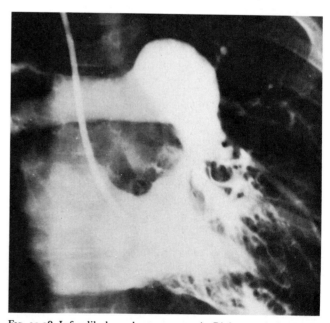

Fig. 13.28. Infundibular pulmonary stenosis. Right ventricular angiogram, frontal view. Multiple irregular bands of muscle obstruct the subvalvar outflow tract. Note the post-stenotic dilatation of the main pulmonary artery.

may exceed left ventricular, occasionally twofold. With severe stenosis right atrial pressure rises as the ventricular compliance decreases due to hypertrophy. If the foramen ovale is not sealed shut a mild to moderate right to left shunt may occur and the patient can become clinically cyanosed. Also, as right ventricular pressure increases, the tricuspid valve may become incompetent.

Critical pulmonary stenosis usually presents in the neonate as gross right ventricular failure with a low cardiac output. Right ventricular pressure may not be very high as there has not been sufficient time for hypertrophy to develop. In older children, since the valve orifice does not grow with the child, the effective stenosis will increase and in most cases, sooner or later, will become critical and right ventricular failure will ensue. Witness to this is the rarity of pulmonary stenosis presenting in adult life.

Radiology

Heart size is normal in all but severe or critical cases. The classic features of right ventricular hypertrophy are strangely infrequent; severe cases show a rather squat cardiac shape and critical stenosis in the newborn can mimic the globular heart of Ebstein's malformation (Fig. 13.29). Turbulence in the main pulmonary artery leads to post-stenotic dilatation of it in most cases (Fig. 13.30, 13.31); exceptions are those cases with very mild stenosis, or with very severe stenosis and a reduced cardiac output. Most cases of infundibular stenosis also demonstrate post-stenotic dilatation. Post-stenotic dilatation may also extend into the left main pulmonary artery and so cause enlargement of the left hilum. The combination of an enlarged main and left pulmonary

artery and a normal or small right pulmonary artery is virtually diagnostic of pulmonary stenosis (Fig. 13.31). When the cardiac output is normal, which is in 80% of cases, the peripheral pulmonary vasculature is *normal*.

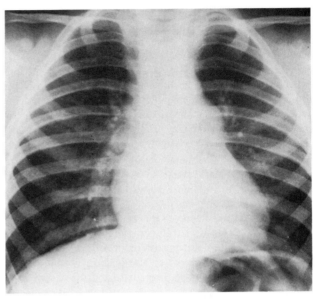

FIG. 13.30. Mild valvar pulmonary stenosis. Normal intra-pulmonary vessels.

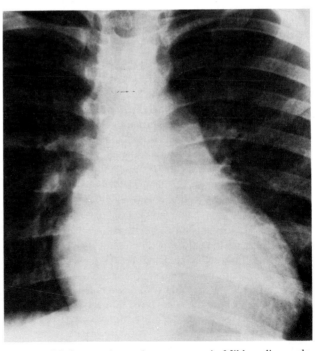

FIG. 13.31. Moderate valvar pulmonary stenosis. Mild cardiomegaly. Left pulmonary artery is mildly prominent due to post-stenotic dilatation; right pulmonary artery is small.

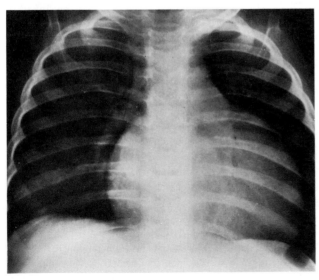

FIG. 13.29. Severe valvar pulmonary stenosis. The large heart has a squared outline and there is no post-stenotic dilatation of the pulmonary artery. The lungs are oligaemic.

Severe cases may show moderate oligaemia and sometimes severe oligaemia. Moderate oligaemia can coexist with central post-stenotic dilatation.

Echocardiography

The pulmonary valve has a typical M-mode echo appearance in pulmonary stenosis, and real time images from the xiphisternal notch may demonstrate the dome of the stenosed valve as seen on the angiogram. In general, the normally placed pulmonary valve is not easy to demonstrate, particularly in the older child, nor is the thickness of the trabeculated right ventricle or the dimensions of its outflow tract. For these reasons the echo is not very accurate in the assessment of the severity of pulmonary stenosis.

Management

Relief by open pulmonary valvotomy is required for any significant degree of stenosis, which is generally taken as a gradient across the valve of 60 mm Hg or more. Relief is required before severe ventricular hypertrophy, oligaemia or right ventricular failure are evident. Infundibular resection of secondary subvalvar stenosis is often required, or the post operative period may be complicated by intractable right ventricular failure.

DYSPLASTIC PULMONARY VALVE

There are two types of dysplastic pulmonary valve, the 'absent' type which is discussed in the section on tetralogy of Fallot, and the thicker, principally stenotic sort, associated with Noonan's syndrome. Patients with Noonan's syndrome have an external appearance very similar to Turner's syndrome but are of either sex and the chromosomes are normal. Pulmonary stenosis is the most frequent cardiac abnormality; aortic stenosis, coarctation and hypertrophic cardiomyopathy have also been reported. Radiologically, apart from the angiographic and echocardiographic appearances of a very thick and immobile pulmonary valve, there are no diagnostic cardiovascular features.

PULMONARY REGURGITATION

This virtually is unknown as a primary congenital defect. In childhood it is most usually the result of chronic pulmonary arterial hypertension. It is a particular feature of the 'absent' pulmonary valve, which seldom exists in isolation. Radiologically there is dilatation of the main pulmonary artery and, when severe, non-specific cardiac enlargement.

MITRAL STENOSIS

Morphology

Congenital mitral stenosis is a rare condition, nearly always due to one particular deformity, the *parachute mitral valve*. The valve leaflets themselves are not primarily stenosed, but all the chordae are attached to one papillary muscle and this limits valve opening. It usually occurs in association with coarctation.

Haemodynamics

When the atrial septum is intact there is pulmonary venous hypertension, which may be severe. Secondary pulmonary arterial hypertension may be found, usually in severe cases which tend to present soon after birth. If there is an associated atrial septal defect, the venous hypertension is less severe since the left atrium can drain freely to the right atrium. With mild stenosis the picture will, therefore, be of a large ASD; with severe stenosis, the child may present as a large ASD but in infancy, much earlier than an uncomplicated ASD.

Radiology

Mild cases with an ASD show plain film changes of an ASD. Those with an intact atrial septum and mild to moderate mitral stenosis show the same features as adults with mitral stenosis; left atrial enlargement, pulmonary venous congestion, variable interstitial oedema and, sometimes, pulmonary arterial hypertension and cardiomegaly. Severe cases presenting in the first months of life have not had time for these chronic changes to become established and show severe interstitial alveolar pulmonary oedema and mild non-specific cardiomegaly, features common to coarctation, cor triatriatum, hypoplastic left heart syndrome and some cases of totally anomalous pulmonary venous drainage.

Echocardiography

The mitral valve echogram has the same basic pattern of movement as adult mitral stenosis, without any significant thickening of the leaflets or calcification. Nevertheless, it can be a difficult diagnosis to make as the leaflets are quite mobile and in the infant with a fast heart rate the E–F slope can be too short for easy analysis of its gradient. Real-time visualisation of the dome of the stenosed valve is rather more reliable, but experience of this rare condition is limited.

Management

Cases presenting early demand valvotomy, but the risks are high. The indications for surgery in older cases mirror the adult cases, except that simple valvotomy is often not possible when the valve is structurally abnormal.

SUPRAVALVAR MITRAL RING

This very rare condition consists of a thin membrane across the mitral orifice, just above the valve and below any atrial septal defect; it is not to be confused with cor triatriatum. The haemodynamics and radiology are identical to severe neonatal mitral stenosis. Echocardiography is diagnostic if the membrane can be visualised as being separate from the mitral leaflets; otherwise the pattern mimics mitral stenosis. Resection of the membrane is indicated and, if successful, the prognosis can be very good.

MITRAL REGURGITATION

Morphology

When it occurs as a truly congenital and isolated lesion of the valve itself, this is a rare pathology and usually the valve shows a parachute deformity. Many of the non-rheumatic causes of acquired mitral regurgitation can occur in childhood, not forgetting the transient regurgitation of acute rheumatic fever. Regurgitation secondary to true congenital disease includes causes of left ventricular failure such as endocardial fibro-elastosis, mucopolysaccharidoses and anomalous left coronary artery. Myxomatous, 'floppy' mitral valve can present in childhood and may be silently present at birth; mitral prolapse in childhood is usually gross.

Regurgitation of the 'mitral' component of the common atrioventricular valve in atrioventricular defects is common but tends to be overshadowed by the septal defect(s).

Haemodynamics

Pulmonary venous hypertension increases with severity of incompetence and secondary pulmonary arterial hypertension may ensue. The clinical picture of a dyspnoeic child with a pansystolic murmur is so much like a VSD that it is occasionally the chest radiograph that gives the clue to the true diagnosis. In general, mitral incompetence in childhood is better tolerated and usually presents later than mitral stenosis.

Radiology

Since few of these patients have a rheumatic aetiology, obvious prominence of the left atrial appendage is an unusual feature, but generalised left atrial enlargement is the rule (Fig. 13.32). Cardiomegaly is present in those with significant regurgitation. Older children often show the chronic signs of pulmonary venous hypertension described in the section on acquired mitral disease, including upper lobe blood diversion.

Echocardiography

This shows the non-specific features of mitral regurgitation, with or without prolapse.

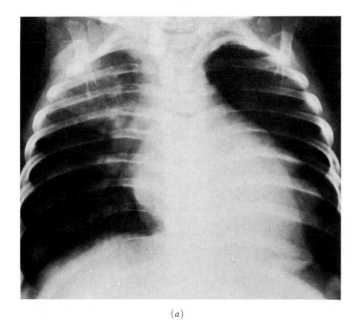

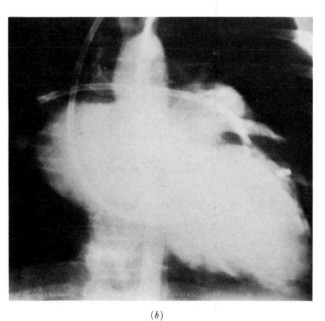

(a)   (b)

FIG. 13.32. Mitral regurgitation: (a) plain film (b) left ventricular angiogram, frontal view. The left atrium is considerably enlarged, and the left lower lobe is collapsed.

HYPOPLASTIC LEFT HEART SYNDROME

Morphology

This syndrome embraces the separate or combined atresias of the mitral and aortic valves (Fig. 13.33). Of the two lone atresias, aortic atresia is the commonest. Aortic atresia leads to marked hypoplasia of the ascending aorta, since it exists only to perfuse the coronary arteries (Fig. 13.34). Systemic perfusion depends upon the ductus arteriosus, which closes shortly after birth leading to acute distress and neonatal death. When, as is usually the case, the ventricular septum is intact the left ventricle and mitral valve are miniscule. If there is a VSD the ventricle may show only moderate hypoplasia. Mitral atresia with no VSD also leads to left ventricular, aortic valve and arch hypoplasia, sometimes so extreme that the aortic valve is also atretic and the left ventricle reduced to a microscopic slit in the myocardium. Mitral atresia with a VSD is the one member of this group where the aortic valve and ascending aorta are reasonably normal, provided the VSD is of reasonable size and allows a good flow into the left ventricle.

Haemodynamics

The aortic atresias, combined atresias and mitral atresia with intact ventricular septum all have initially a common mixing situation with the aorta perfused by the patent ductus. As the ductus closes, they present as neonatal emergencies with circulatory collapse and poor peripheral pulses. Life is measured in days. Only mitral atresia with a VSD may escape, but even then the left atrium often has to empty through a restrictive ASD (unlike tricuspid atresia when the flap of the foramen ovale can open towards the left atrium) with secondary pulmonary venous hypertension. All the other members of the group can be similarly affected by a restrictive ASD.

Radiology

There is a variable picture with cardiomegaly, usually significant but occasionally only slight; there may be pulmonary oedema (Fig. 13.35), a mixture of oedema and plethora or, occasionally, plethora alone. In general the smaller hearts are associated with the purer signs of pulmonary oedema, probably reflecting the importance of the role of the restrictive ASD. The heart shape is non-specific so the diagnosis cannot be made from chest radiography.

Echocardiography

This has proved to be most helpful and cardiac catheterisation can usually be avoided. The crux of the diagnosis is the detection or visualisation of the hypoplastic ascending aorta. This can be easy to do with real-time imaging as the vertically oriented aorta is

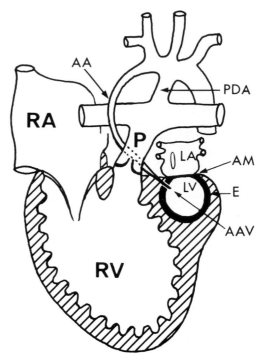

FIG. 13.33. The hypoplastic left heart syndrome, which consists of various combinations of aortic valve atresia (AAV), atretic mitral valve (AM), atresia or hypoplasia of the ascending aorta (AA), left ventricular hypoplasia with endocardial fibroelastosis (E) and patent ductus arteriosus (PDA).

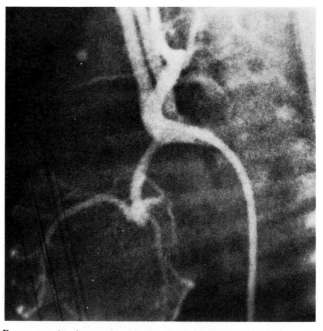

FIG. 13.34. Aortic atresia. Aortogram, lateral view. The ascending aorta is severely hypoplastic.

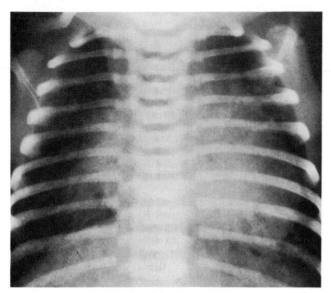

FIG. 13.35. Aortic atresia. Moderate cardiomegaly with mild pulmonary oedema.

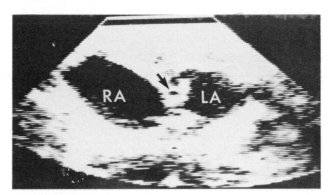

FIG. 13.36. Aortic atresia. Echocardiogram, high short axial view. The minuscule aorta is seen in cross section (arrow).

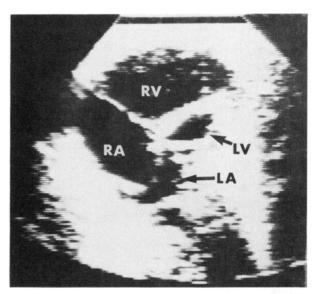

FIG. 13.37. Hypoplastic left heart syndrome (aortic atresia). Echocardiogram, four chamber view. The left ventricle and mitral valve are hypoplastic.

quite reliably shown as a small, tubular structure posterior to the pulmonary artery or right ventricular outflow tract (Fig. 13.36). The only possible differential would be a transposed, hypoplastic pulmonary artery, but the clinical presentation here would be of severe cyanosis with oligaemic lung fields. The other features are predictable; a small left ventricle in many cases (Fig. 13.37); sometimes only one ventricle and a solitary tricuspid valve are seen. Mitral atresia with a large VSD is the one instance where the aorta is of more normal size; the mitral valve often exists as an imperforate membrane which moves like a severely stenosed valve and confirmatory catheterisation and angiocardiography is necessary.

Management

This is generally held to be a hopeless condition. Efforts to palliate the condition centre around shunt procedures from the pulmonary arteries to the systemic to improve systemic flow, and balloon atrial septostomy to relieve any left atrial hypertension. These may succeed, but pulmonary blood flow will be excessive unless there is distal pulmonary artery banding, which will entail subsequent, and very risky, refashioning as the child grows.

AORTIC STENOSIS

Morphology

(a) Valvar aortic stenosis is nearly always the result of a bicuspid aortic valve, in turn usually due to fusion of the right and left coronary leaflets. The other commissures may occasionally fuse, and rarely there may be no commissures at all (the 'unicuspid' aortic valve). Occasionally stenosis of a tricuspid valve is seen, due either to myxomatous valve dysplasia or to a congenitally small aortic valve ring. In all these cases the valve leaflets fail to open to the aortic wall in systole but form a dome around the stenosed orifice (Fig. 13.38). The leaflets are nevertheless quite mobile and calcification in childhood is very rare. As had been noted in Chapter 7, congenital aortic stenosis often presents in the adult.

Bicuspid aortic valve frequently complicates coarctation of the aorta but is seldom the dominant pathology. Left dominant coronary artery anatomy is much more frequent with bicuspid aortic valves.

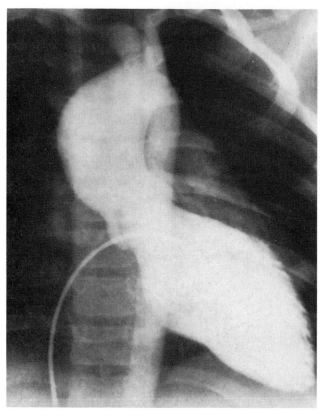

FIG. 13.38. Aortic stenosis. Angiogram, frontal view, showing aortic valve doming and post stenotic dilatation of the ascending aorta.

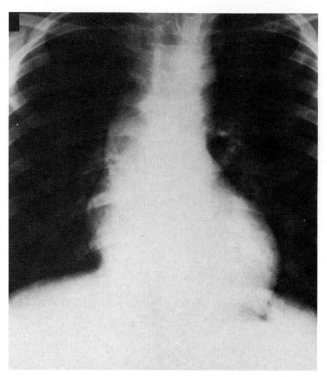

FIG. 13.39. Typical aortic stenosis. Prominent ascending aorta; left ventricular hypertrophy.

(b) Subvalvar aortic stenosis, or subaortic stenosis, is an uncommon pathology with a varied morphology. Usually it is of the *membraneous* variety in which a thin obstructing membrane lies quite close to the aortic valve, so close at times that it may be overlooked at angiography. At the other end of the spectrum is a long, fixed and concentric fibromuscular stenosis – 'subaortic tunnel'. In between are various combinations of the two. All types may extend on to the anterior mitral valve leaflet and cause some mitral incompetence. Turbulence above the stenosis can damage the aortic valve and render it incompetent.

Rarely, subaortic stenosis may be due to redundant mitral valve tissue, usually in the atrioventricular defects.

(c) Hypertrophic obstructive cardiomyopathy (HOCM) is not at all unknown in children and occasionally can present in infancy. It has been fully discussed in Chapter 10.

(d) Supra-aortic stenosis is a disease of the aortic wall and will be considered in Chapter 15.

Haemodynamics

Left ventricular hypertension increases with the severity of the stenosis, so maintaining a normal cardiac output in most cases. With severe stenosis there may be signs of an impaired response to exercise with effort-induced angina or syncope or frank left ventricular failure with pulmonary oedema, which is associated with a very poor prognosis if left untreated.

Radiology

Heart size is usually normal, even in quite severe cases, or may be moderately enlarged. The cardiac outline is usually typical for left ventricular enlargement. Post-stenotic dilatation of the ascending aortic arch is usually seen in cases of valvar or sub-valvar stenosis (Fig. 13.39). The dilatation can reach the apex of the aortic arch but never affects the aortic knuckle. When left ventricular failure is present there are the usual signs of pulmonary venous hypertension or oedema but the failure is hardly ever chronic enough to lead to radiological signs of left atrial enlargement.

Two variations merit a mention. Critical aortic stenosis in the neonate usually presents as left ventricular failure with considerable cardiac enlargement of non-specific shape with no post-stenotic dilatation of the aorta; occasionally the cardiomegaly is gross and globular, and mimics a severe cardiomyopathy or coarctation (Fig. 13.40). Secondly, in some cases of moderate stenosis and for no clear reason, pure aortic stenosis

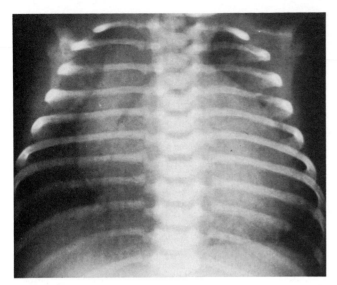

FIG. 13.40. Critical aortic stenosis. Neonate with gross non-specific cardiomegaly and interstitial oedema.

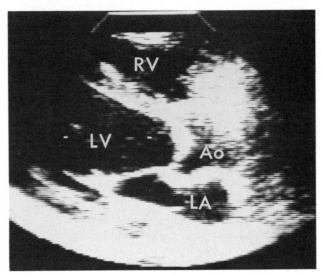

FIG. 13.42. Aortic stenosis, echocardiogram, long axial view, shows doming of the valve.

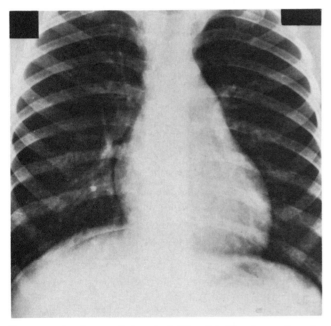

FIG. 13.41. Aortic stenosis (atypical). The plain film shows a 'pseudo-shunt'; the main pulmonary artery is mildly prominent. Catheter confirmed that aortic stenosis was the lone pathology.

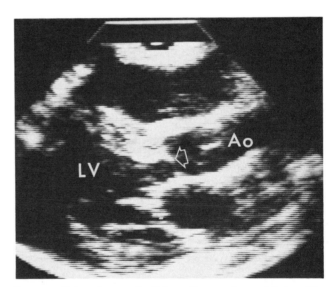

FIG. 13.43. Subaortic stenosis. Echocardiogram, long axial view. The subvalvar region is narrowed by septal hypertrophy and a thin membrane (arrowed).

may produce a radiograph that looks like a left to right shunt with no aortic prominence, a large main pulmonary artery and mild dilatation of the hilar vessels (Fig. 13.41). It may be that post-stenotic dilatation affecting the leftward wall of the aorta leads to secondary displacement of the main pulmonary artery, but the 'pseudo shunt' plethora is inexplicable.

Echocardiography

(a) **Valvar stenosis.** Fig. 13.42). The features are in general the same as in the adult, but the valve usually is only mildly thickened and the leaflets are mobile; if an M-mode trace is taken low in the sinuses, valve opening may seem deceptively good. Real-time images are more sensitive and can identify the pattern of leaflet fusion.

(b) **Subaortic stenosis.** (Fig. 13.43). Both echo modalities can clearly and easily demonstrate the diffuse narrowing of the left ventricular outflow tract of the subaortic tunnels. As the obstruction tends towards the membraneous variety, so the diagnosis becomes less obvious. Thin membranes close to the aortic valve may escape notice on all but the best real-time images; on the M-mode it may still be seen as a thin echo between the mitral and aortic valves. An important clue to the diagnosis is, in the presence of a clinical suspicion of aortic stenosis, a normally opening but fluttering aortic valve trace.

(c) **Hypertrophic cardiomyopathy,** has been previously considered.

Management

(a) **Valvar.** Surgical relief by valvotomy, or occasionally valve replacement, is indicated in all symptomatic cases since symptoms mean that severe stenosis is present and the risk of syncopal death is significant. Asymptomatic cases may also demand relief if the stenosis is significant, but the decision to operate is very difficult to make. Nearly always the valve is made incompetent by the valvotomy and the likelihood of subsequent reoperation for valve replacement is high. Various parameters are used to judge the severity, mainly the pressure gradient across it as measured at cardiac catheterisation, but any clear electro or echo cardiographic evidence of severe left ventricular hypertrophy may also prompt surgical intervention. The child should never be allowed to progress to the stage of chronic left ventricular failure.

(b) **Subvalvar.** Thin membranes can be excised with a good result, provided the aortic valve itself is undamaged by jet turbulence. Fibromuscular or tunnel stenoses are virtually impossible to resect and a number of drastic procedures, aimed at either dilating the outflow tract by using a patch or bypassing it entirely, have been described. Perhaps the most unusual is the insertion of a valved conduit from the left ventricular apex to the abdominal aorta.

AORTIC REGURGITATION

Morphology

Aortic regurgitation due to congenital aortic valve disease usually occurs as a complication of a bicuspid valve, with or without stenosis. As a rule it is less severe than any stenosis unless the valve has been damaged by infective endocarditis or surgical valvotomy. It may complicate a subaortic VSD or subaortic stenosis, as previously described, and tetralogy of Fallot. Some acquired causes may present in childhood; by far the most important is Marfan's syndrome (see Chapter 10).

Haemodynamics

Left ventricular stroke volume increases to maintain a normal net forward cardiac output in most cases. In severe cases the left ventricle fails to compensate; the features of left ventricular failure indicate a poor prognosis.

Radiology and echocardiography

On the plain film the general cardiac outline is similar to aortic stenosis. Cardiac enlargement due to the dilated left ventricle is common in moderate or severe incompetence and the echocardiogram shows a hyperdynamic ventricle. More advanced cases show considerable cardiac enlargement, with or without pulmonary oedema, and their echoes reveal reduced left ventricular contractility.

NEONATAL MYOCARDIAL FAILURE

This section deals with congenital 'heart failure' when there is no gross anatomical malformation. Acquired cardiomyopathies have been discussed in Chapter 9 and it must be remembered that any cardiomyopathy or myocarditis, including acute rheumatic fever, may present in childhood or even in the neonatal period (including the hypertrophic group).

(a) **Endocardial fibro-elastosis** is the commonest cause of primary ventricular failure in childhood. It is not a cardiomyopathy proper, since it does not directly affect the myocardium. It consists of thickening of the left ventricular endocardium by stiff, non-contractile tissue. The left ventricle is splinted by it; there is often hypertrophy of the myocardium in response, but this only adds to a concomitant loss of diastolic compliance. The ventricular cavity is dilated and contractility is severely depressed. The papillary muscles are often abnormally sited and shortened and mitral incompetence is usual and often severe. Presentation in the neonatal period is not uncommon; in the first year of life it is usual and later in childhood unusual. There is, of course, the possibility that the late presenters do not have truly congenital disease.

A very similar if somewhat patchy situation can severely complicate severe infantile or neonatal aortic stenosis and/or coarctation.

The chest radiograph reveals non-specific cardiac enlargement with or without pulmonary signs of left ventricular failure (Fig. 13.44). Echocardiography shows diffuse left ventricular hypokinesia and not infrequently mild left atrial enlargement. The prognosis is not necessarily poor or brief. Admittedly the diagnosis is often one of exclusion as endocardial biopsy is seldom employed in small children, but cases with this diagnosis have been known to spontaneously improve.

(b) **Glycogen storage disease,** usually Pompe's disease, affects both ventricles. Hepatomegaly is a constant feature of the disease itself, so this otherwise reliable sign of congestive heart failure in this age group

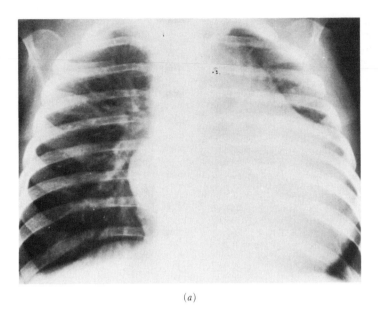

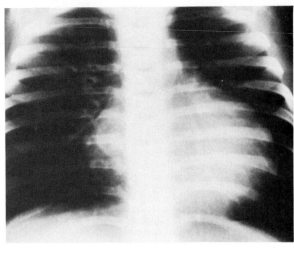

(a)   (b)

FIG. 13.44. Endocardial fibroelastosis. (a) In infancy and in heart failure. (b) Age two years, clinically much improved.

is not available. Any degree of left ventricular failure may be present, reflected in the lung fields on the plain film. Cardiomegaly is usual but may be relatively mild. Echocardiography reveals greatly the thickened myocardium, mimicking a hypertrophic cardiomyopathy, but in contrast contractility is very poor. Angiography is confirmatory.

(c) Uhls disease is the replacement of the right ventricular myocardium by thin, fibrous tissue. The ventricle is grossly dilated and non-contractile. The haemodynamic consequences are very similar to Ebstein's malformation, as is also the plain radiograph. Echocardiography and angiocardiography show a large, non-contractile right ventricle with a normally positioned tricuspid valve. The condition is extremely rare.

(d) Dysrhythmias can cause non-specific cardiomegaly due to congestive heart failure. Isolated tachycardias are usually of atrial origin. Congenital heart block is surprisingly well tolerated; the idioventricular rate is higher than in the adult type and asystole is unusual. The heart block is present *in utero* and, unless it has been recognised earlier in the pregnancy, the delivery may be induced early because the intra partum foetal bradycardia may be erroneously taken to indicate foetal distress. There is a high incidence of clinical or sub-clinical systemic lupus erythematosus in the mothers of children with complete heart block. The 'sick sinus syndrome' may feature episodes of both tachy or brady-cardia. Accessory atrioventricular pathways, of which the Wolf-Parkinson-White syndrome is the commonest example, lead to a variety of tachycardias.

(f) Transient heart failure of the newborn is a

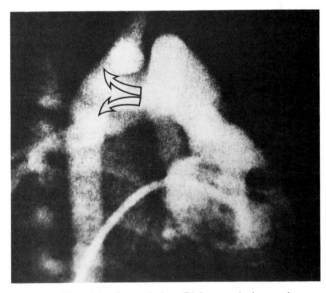

FIG. 13.45. Transitional circulation. Right ventricular angiogram, right anterior oblique view. The systemic arteries fill from the pulmonary artery via a large patent ductus arteriosus.

period of mild to moderate left ventricular failure, present from birth, usually resolving spontaneously in a few days. It is presumed to be due to myocardial ischaemia secondary to birth anoxia; most cases have a history of a difficult delivery. The pyrophosphate cardiac scintigram is strongly positive in this condition.

(g) Transitional circulation. This condition is proving to be quite common. In it, the ductus arteriosus

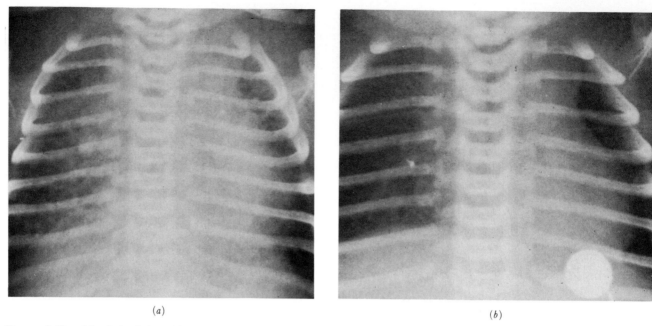

(a)   (b)

FIG. 13.46. Transitional circulation with left ventricular failure. (a) Cardiomegaly and pulmonary oedema on the first day of life. (b) One day later after antifailure treatment and dopamine.

remains patent and pulmonary vascular resistance is only a little lower than the foetal level. There is consequently a large right to left shunt across the PDA (Fig. 13.45). The infant is usually at term, cyanosed and ill; the condition carries a 20% risk of death. There is usually a history of a complicated birth. Radiologically there is a spectrum of appearances from a small heart with pulmonary oligaemia to a large heart with pulmonary oedema (Fig. 13.46). The latter group has ischaemic left ventricular failure; there is an overlap with 'transient heart failure of the newborn'. Echocardiography is helpful in demonstrating normal intracardiac anatomy.

(h) Hypertension occasionally is a problem in the neonatal period and can occur as a withdrawal response if the mother had been on antihypertensive drugs.

(i) Anomalous left coronary artery will be discussed in Chapter 15.

FURTHER READING

JEFFERSON, L. & REES, S. (1980) *Clinical Cardiac Radiology.* London: Butterworth.

ELLIOT, L. P. & SCHIEBLER, G. L. (1979) *The X-ray Diagnosis of Congenital Heart Disease in Infants, Children and Adults.* Springfield, Illinois: Charles C. Thomas.

CHAPTER 14

COMPLEX CONGENITAL HEART DISEASE

John Partridge and Leon Gerlis

INTRODUCTION

Malformations which involve an abnormality of chamber connection or position are in this group. The aim of this chapter is to give most space to those pathologies which are common in clinical practice. The segmental approach will be used in the description of them but there will not be any attempt to illustrate fully some of the rarer combinations of situs, atrioventricular connection and ventriculo-arterial connections.

SITUS, SEGMENTS AND POSITIONS

Complex congenital heart disease includes those cases which have one or more malformations which fall into any of these three categories:
(*a*) Disorders of body situs.
(*b*) Disorders of chamber connection.
(*c*) Cardiac malposition.
Before the discussion one important convention of nomenclature must be fully understood. The atria and ventricles all have a typical morphology, but are regrettably named after their position in the normal. Throughout this book, the terms right or left atrium and right or left ventricle refer to their morphology and *not* to their position. The chambers may also be described as 'sided', e.g. the right-sided atrium, but this in turn does not indicate its morphology. Hence the phrase 'right-sided left atrium' means that the morphologically left atrium is on the right side of the other atrium.

(A) Situs

A number of organs of the body show a particular asymmetry in the horizontal plane, i.e. right and left sidedness. They are the abdominal viscera, the lungs and the atria (Fig. 14.01). The cardiac ventricles and the great vessels are not included, for reasons that will become apparent, nor is dextrocardia. Atrial situs is naturally the one which affects our nomenclature of a complex cardiac malformation; it cannot be identified directly by plain radiography and can still be indeterminate after angiocardiography, so it is useful to try to predict it from one of the other two compartments. Abdominal situs can be judged from the position of the liver density and stomach bubble on the plain film (with barium if needed); unfortunately, this can be misleading

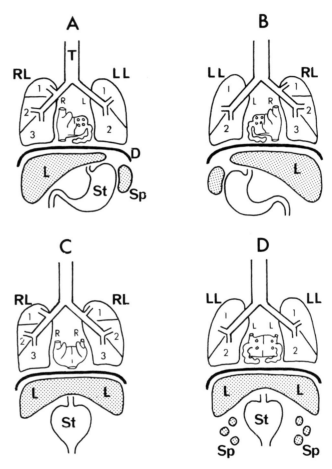

Fig. 14.01. Viscero-atrial situs variations. (A) Situs solitus. (B) Situs inversus. (C) Situs ambiguous and asplenia with bilateral morphologically 'right' lungs and right atrial isomerism. (D) Situs ambiguous and polysplenia with bilateral morphologically 'left' lungs and left atrial isomerism. L, R=Left and right atria; RL=right (trilobed) lung; LL=left (bilobed) lung; T=trachea; D=diaphragm; L=liver; St=stomach; Sp=spleen or multiple splenunculi.

and in addition the abdominal situs can be different from atrial situs (Fig. 14.02). Lung situs is much more reliable; it requires the bronchi to be seen either by tomography or by high kilovoltage radiography and interpretation is based on the fact that the left main bronchus is at least twice as long as the right.

Situs solitus is the term that describes the usual situation of the right atrium, trilobed lung and liver all being on the right side, with the left atrium a bilobed lung, the stomach and the spleen on the left side.

Situs inversus means the reversal of usual anatomy; it nearly always includes all three compartments. Situs inversus *totalis* is used when there is no complicating cardiac abnormality and the individual is a complete mirror image of the normal. Usually there is added heart disease, which can be of any sort but which tends to be a major connection problem. In solitus or inversus atria, the *connections* of the systemic and pulmonary veins are reasonably straightforward; usually the systemic veins drain into the right atrium and the pulmonary veins into the left; abnormalities of both can occur but are quite rare apart from totally anomalous pulmonary venous drainage. More complex are the *isomerisms*, in which both sides of the body try to assume the same morphology. They are also described as situs ambiguous, or visceroatrial heterotaxy.

Right isomerism is also known as the asplenia syndrome since the spleen (a morphologically left structure) is absent; this is associated with the presence of Howell-Jolly bodies in the peripheral blood. The liver and stomach tend to lie in the mid-line, the lungs are both trilobed and both bronchi are short with the branching pattern of a right lung. The atria both show right morphology; abnormalities of systemic venous drainage are frequent, each atrium tending to take hepatic veins directly from the nearest lobe of the liver, and two superior vena cavae may drain directly to their ipselateral atrium. The IVC is present but may be on either side. With no morphologically left atrium, it is no surprise that totally anomalous pulmonary venous drainage is common. Multiple pathologies are common, and pulmonary atresia is particularly frequent.

Left isomerism is the polysplenia syndrome; small multiple spleens are found on both sides of the abdomen. The liver and stomach, as in right isomerism, tend to be midline and so the two isomerisms cannot be differentiated on the abdominal film. Moreover, particularly in left isomerism, the liver and stomach can be laterallised and appear to be in situs solitus or inversus (Fig. 14.03). The lungs are both bilobed and the bronchi are both long (Fig. 14.04). Both atria have left morphology; each may receive the ipselateral pulmonary veins. Because the atria differentiate partly from the sinus venosus, systemic venous drainage abnormalities are common and again include bilateral superior vena cavae. Unlike right isomerism the inferior vena cava often fails to connect to either atrium and systemic venous return from the lower half of the body passes through dilated azygous systems. These anomalies are discussed further in the section on venous abnormalities.

In theory, splenic isotope scanning should differentiate between the isomerisms, but erratic hepatic uptake

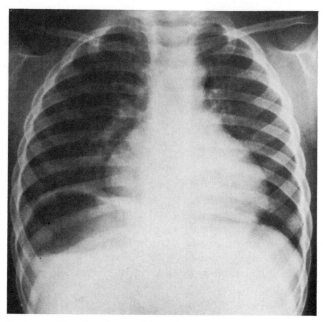

FIG. 14.02. Complex situs problem. The stomach is right-sided and the blood film suggested asplenia syndrome. However, the lungs and atria were in situs solitus. (*Reproduced by permission of the Editor*, Clinical Radiology.)

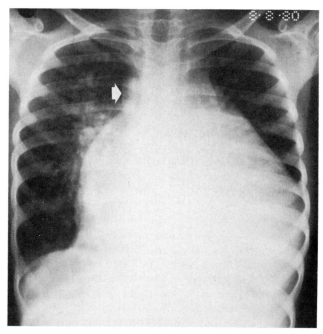

FIG. 14.03. The large heart is on the left, the stomach on the right. The bulge on the right upper mediastinum (arrowed) is a large azygous vein. (*Courtesy Dr J. Reidy.*)

usually renders it equivocal. Cholecystography is of no value as the position of the gall bladder is of no consequence.

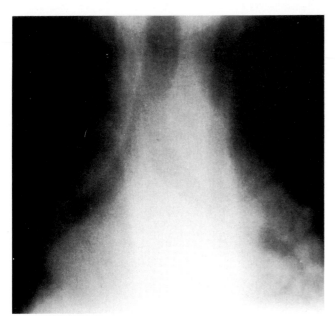

FIG. 14.04. Tomogram of a similar case as in Fig. 14.03. Both bronchi are long and have left morphology. Polysplenia syndrome.

(B) Chamber Connections (Fig. 14.05)

(1) **Atrioventricular connections** are *normal* when the right ventricle is connected to the right atrium and the left ventricle to the left atrium. The tricuspid or mitral valves do not have to be patent to satisfy this definition nor is it invalid if there is a common atrioventricular valve; the important point is that the inflow portions of the ventricles are each attached to the correct atrium. It follows that in solitus atria the normally connected right ventricle is right sided and in inversus atria it is left sided. *Atrioventricular concordance* is the term used when the ventricles are normally connected. *Atrioventricular discordance* means that the left ventricle is connected to the right atrium and the right ventricle is connected to the left atrium. *Double inlet ventricle* describes the situation where both atria are connected to only one ventricle.

When there is an atrial isomerism there is neither a normal way of connecting the ventricles nor a truly discordant way. The embryology section (Chapter 12) described how normally the right ventricle comes to lie to the right and so become connected to the right sided atrium because of rightward looping of the primitive heart tube (d-loop). If the loop is leftward (l-loop) then the right ventricle connects to the left sided atrium (this would be normal for atrial inversus). The terms 'd-loop' and 'l-loop' are therefore used to describe the atrioventricular connection when there is atrial isomerism. *Ventricular inversion* is a phrase which is not part of this particular system of nomenclature but which is still in popular usage. It simply means that the right ventricle

is on the left and the left ventricle is on the right, irrespective of the status of atrial situs or the atrioventricular connections.

(2) **Ventriculo-arterial connections** are *normal* when the aorta arises from the left ventricle and the pulmonary artery from the right. The definition is unaffected by the atrioventricular connection or the spatial position of any of the chambers or great vessels; the connection is the only inference. A great vessel is *transposed* when it arises from the wrong ventricle; 'transposition of the great arteries' therefore means that both are transposed. When both arise from one ventricle (which is usually the right) there is a *double outlet ventricle*. Lastly there may be a *single outlet heart* due to a persistent truncus arteriosus or to pulmonary or aortic atresia.

(C) Malpositions

Whether there is a disorder of atrial situs or cardiac connection or not, a number of positional abnormalities require a terminology and form this heterogenous group. Abnormal positions of the cardiac apex are the commonest. Normally the ventricular mass points leftwards so that the heart seems left sided on the frontal chest radiograph; this is *laevocardia*. Sometimes it points to the right (*dextrocardia*, Fig. 14.06) and occasionally it is midline (*mesocardia*). Mesocardia is usually associated with a connection disorder. The other two positions are mainly related to ventricular looping. Laevocardia is usual when the left ventricle is on the left and dextrocardia when the left ventricle is right-sided, *irrespective* of atrial situs. Therefore, laevocardia is usual in atrial solitus with normally connected ventricles, and dextrocardia is expected in atrial inversus with normally connected ventricles (i.e. right sided left atrium drains to the right sided left ventricle). A classic situation is when abdominal situs suggests atrial inversus but there is laevocardia (so called 'isolated laevocardia'); in this case atrioventricular discordance is quite likely (Fig. 14.07). Exceptions, needless to say, do occur.

'*Two-tier*' and '*criss cross*' hearts are very rare positional anomalies; they are not apparent on the plain film. They come about by twisting of the ventricles along their long axis, so that they wrap around each other. Thus, a right ventricle draining from a right sided atrium may come to lie on top or underneath the left ventricle, the septum being horizontal ('two-tier'). It may even lie mostly on the left, despite retaining its connection to the right atrium, with the left ventricle passing to the right ('criss cross'). Neither is considered to be a disorder of connection since the inlet portion of each ventricles remains related to the correct atrium.

The *great vessels* can also show positional abnormalities. Normally the aortic valve lies posterior and rightward of the pulmonary valve. In transposition of the great arteries the aorta is usually anterior and rightward to the pulmonary artery, but may be directly anterior or

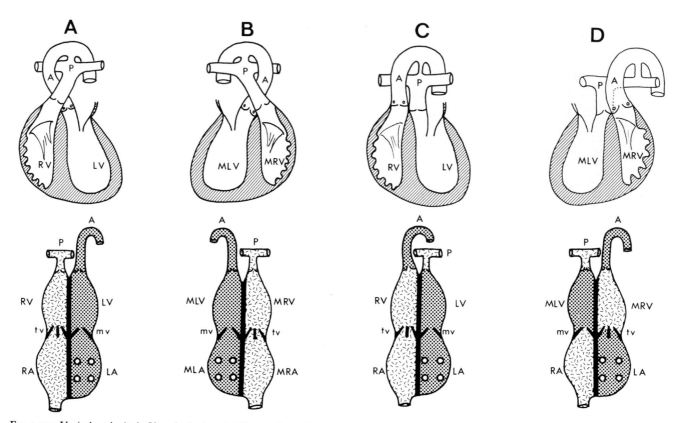

FIG. 14.05. Variations in Atrio-Ventriculo-Arterial Connections. Top Row: Anatomical forms. Bottom Row: Morphological connections. The dark hatching represents morphologically left-sided structures; the light hatching represents morphologically right-sided structures. (A) Normal conditions. Solitus atria, atrio-ventricular concordance; ventriculo-arterial concordance. ('D' loop ventricles). (B) Mirror-image dextrocardia. With apex lying to the right (as in situs inversus totalis). Inverted atria; atrio-ventricular concordance; ventriculo-arterial concordance. ('L' loop ventricles). (C) Complete transposition of the great arteries. Solitus atria; atrioventricular concordance; ventriculo-arterial *dis*cordance ('D' loop ventricles). (D) Congenitally corrected transposition of the great arteries. Solitus atria; atrio-ventricular *dis*cordance; ventriculo-arterial *dis*cordance. ('L' loop ventricles). In this instance the apex is lying to the right (dextrocardia). MLA, MRA = Morphologically left and right atria. MLV, MRV = Morphologically left and right ventricles. A = Aorta. P = Pulmonary artery.

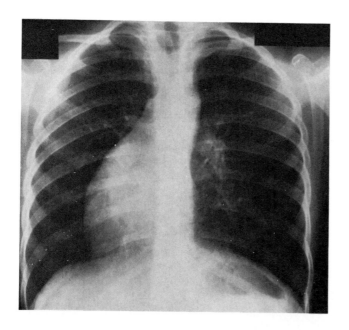

FIG. 14.06. Dextrocardia with visceroatrial situs solitus. Transposition with atrioventricular discordance.

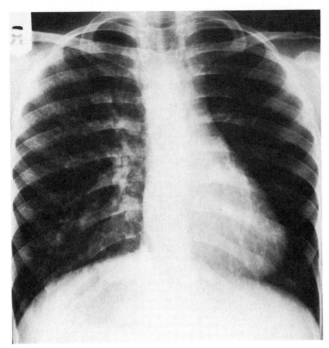

FIG. 14.07. 'Isolated laevocardia'. The stomach is on the right. Transposition with atrioventricular discordance.

anterior and leftward. These anterior positions have a shorthand: d—(dextro), o—(zero) or l—(laevo) respectively. Thus, d—transposition (dextro-transposition) describes the usual situation. In double outlet right ventricle and very occasionally with normally connected great vessels, these positional abnormalities can again occur. Since they are not transpositions, the aortic position is termed malposition. For example, double outlet right ventricle with l-malposition means that both great vessels arise from the right ventricle with the aorta anterior and leftward of the pulmonary artery.

THE SEGMENTAL APPROACH

This is the description given to a currently popular system of describing complex heart disease. In it the initial description is of atrial situs, followed by the atrioventricular connection and ventriculoarterial connection. Other intra cardiac abnormalities are then listed, and finally any arterial malformation. Malpositions are appended to any relevant statement. When any of these facets is normal it is left unsaid, but care must be taken to employ the definitions of normal as outlined above, particularly atrioventricular connections. For example; solitus atria, normally connected ventricles and transposition with the aorta anterior and rightward of the pulmonary artery and a VSD is shortened to 'd-transposition of the great arteries with VSD'.

In the following chapters, all the pathologies described will be in atrial situs solitus. There will not be any deeper discussion of the isomerisms. All the reader will have to remember is that, in theory, all the pathologies can exist in atrial situs inversus, and can be reproduced by viewing the illustrations in a mirror.

TETRALOGY OF FALLOT

Morphology

This is a disorder of the ventriculo-arterial junction due to unequal division of the truncus arteriosus with displacement of the truncal and infundibular septa towards the pulmonary arterial side. This single basic abnormality is responsible for the four classical features of tetralogy.

(1) **Narrowing of the pulmonary valve ring and its subvalvar infundibulum** (Fig. 14.08). This usually includes stenosis of the valve itself, which is often bicuspid. There is nearly always secondary hypertrophy of the infundibular muscle leading to labile subpulmonary stenosis which is generally more severe than the valvar stenosis above it. Hypoplasia usually also affects the proximal part of the main pulmonary artery and may extend upwards as far as the origins of the right and left pulmonary arteries, though never as far as the hilar vessels.

(2) **A ventricular septal defect** (Fig. 14.09). Since the truncoinfundibular septum is displaced it cannot fuse in a normal way with the ventricular septal crest. A high subaortic ventricular septal defect in the perimembranous area results. It is always large but may be partly occluded by membraneous tissue.

(3) **Aortic overriding** of the septum (Fig. 14.09). This is not due to displacement of the aorta as a whole, but to the displacement of the infundibular septum. Since the pulmonary outflow is reduced in size, the aorta is correspondingly larger, and as the infundibular septum is thus over the right ventricular cavity it follows that the aorta, which is on the other side of the septum, must arise partly from the right ventricle, i.e. it overrides the ventricular septal crest. There is a normal relationship between the leftward margin of aorta and the left ventricular outflow tract and mitral valve.

(4) **Right ventricular hypertrophy** is present because of the pulmonary stenosis. It is seldom gross as the VSD ensures that right ventricular pressure does not exceed systemic unless the VSD is obstructed.

It is most unusual for tetralogy of Fallot to be present with atrial situs inversus or with atrioventricular discordance. Other major associated pathologies are also rare; the most notable is an atrioventricular defect with Down's syndrome.

Right aortic arch is present in 13%; it usually has

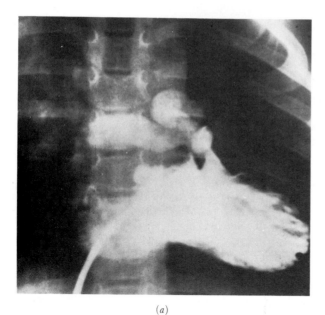

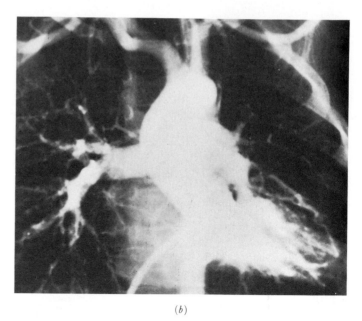

(a)   (b)

Fig. 14.08. Tetralogy of Fallot. Right ventricular angiogram, frontal view. (a) An early frame shows the stenosed right ventricular outflow tract and pulmonary valve. (b) A later frame shows filling of the left aortic arch via the VSD.

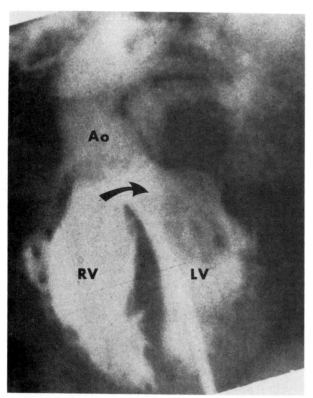

Fig. 14.09. Tetralogy of Fallot. Right ventricular cineangiogram, left anterior oblique with caudocephalic angulation, showing the aorta overriding the septum above the ventricular septal defect (arrow). (*Reproduced by permission of the Editor*, British Heart Journal.)

mirror image branching: occasionally there is an aberrant left subclavian artery.

The picture is sometimes complicated by atresia of one of the branch pulmonary arteries, usually the right. The affected lung may then be perfused by a major aortopulmonary collateral artery. These collaterals are more fully discussed in the section on Fallot pulmonary atresia. They may also be present in tetralogy of Fallot when all the pulmonary arteries are present.

Haemodynamics

Cyanosis is usual and is due to right to left shunting "across the VSD", or to be more exact, to part of the right ventricular stroke volume exiting via the over-riding aorta. In young children and infants the pulmonary stenosis may not be so severe and the haemodynamics may be those of a left to right shunt at ventricular level (the 'pink Fallot' syndrome). The muscular infundibular element of the pulmonary stenosis can at times become transiently more severe, producing a 'spell' of increased cyanosis, even when the child is a 'pink Fallot'. The cyanosis may be profound, with circulatory collapse and sometimes death.

Radiology

Cardiomegaly is rare. The cardiac apex often shows the uptilted apex of right ventricular hypertrophy (Fig. 14.10). The pulmonary artery bay is concave, usually frankly hollow. These two features lead to an overall cardiac shape that has been likened to a boot (the 'coeur en sabot' heart). The aortic arch may be right sided (Fig. 14, 11). The pulmonary arteries may be normal but some degree of oligaemia is usual. It is not uncommon for the chest radiograph, when viewed without any clinical information, to be considered normal. With atresia of one of the branch pulmonary arteries the affected lung is obviously oligaemic and smaller than its opposite number, with mild secondary mediastinal shift (Fig. 14.12).

In the 'pink Fallot' group, the lung fields are usually plethoric but the main pulmonary artery is not significantly enlarged and the pulmonary artery bay therefore remains hollow. Cardiomegaly is usual. The picture is very similar to that of a truncus arteriosus.

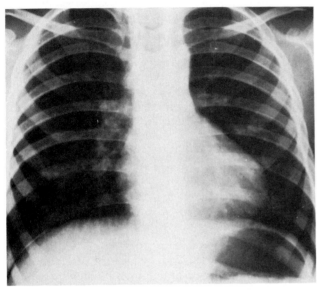

FIG. 14.10. Tetralogy of Fallot. Hollow pulmonary bay, uptilted cardiac apex.

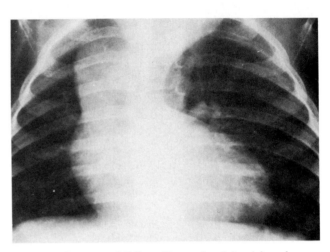

FIG. 14.12. Tetralogy of Fallot with atresia of the right pulmonary artery. The right lung is small and the mediastinum is shifted towards it.

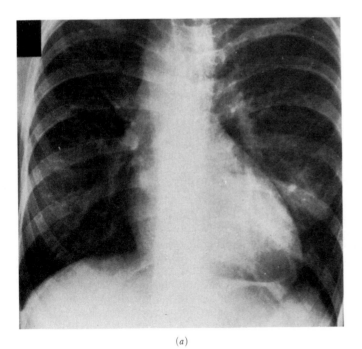

(a)

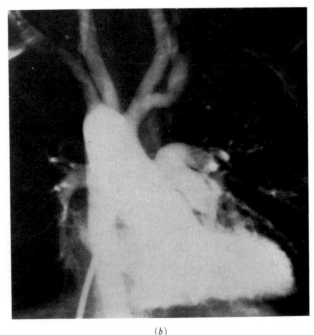

(b)

FIG. 14.11. Tetralogy of Fallot with right aortic arch. (a) Plain film. Note deviation of the trachea to the left. (b) Angiogram. Mirror image brachiocephalic branching.

Echocardiography

Two ventricles with separate atrioventricular valves are present but the left ventricle may be small. One large great vessel (the aorta) is easily identified and it lies in continuity with the mitral valve: the anterior margin is discontinuous with the septum, lying anterior to it (Fig. 14.13); real time images more clearly show that the discontinuity is due to the aortic override. The

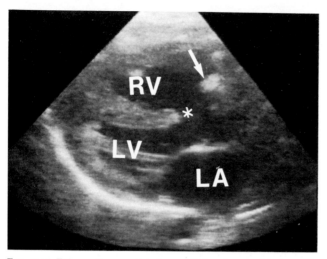

Fig. 14.13. Echocardiogram, tetralogy of Fallot. Long axial view. The anterior wall of the aorta (arrowed) overrides the crest of the septum, above the VSD (star).

right ventricular outflow tract is in the usual position but is hypoplastic. Not infrequently it cannot be identified and the appearances mimic Fallot pulmonary atresia or truncus arteriosus.

Management

Total repair entails closure of the VSD, enlargement of the pulmonary valve ring by a patch and resection of the infundibular stenosis. This usually results in a moderate degree of pulmonary regurgitation, which is well tolerated provided that there is no residual pulmonary stenosis. Total correction can be performed at any age but only a few centres do so in children under 10 kg body weight. In these small children a shunt procedure defers total correction. The decision to intervene surgically depends on the degree of cyanosis or the frequency and severity of cyanotic spells.

TETRALOGY OF FALLOT WITH ABSENT PULMONARY VALVE

Morphology

This rare but interesting group have a typical VSD and mild aortic overriding. The pulmonary valve ring is small causing a moderate degree of stenosis. The pulmonary valve leaflets are thickened, deformed and incompetent. The main and branch pulmonary arteries show gross dilatation and deform the left atrium and the bronchial tree (Fig. 14.14).

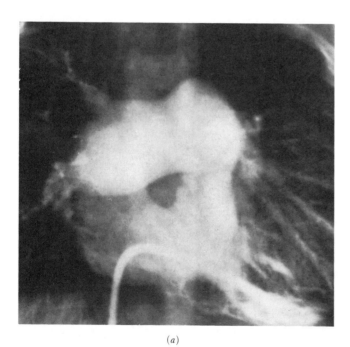

(a)

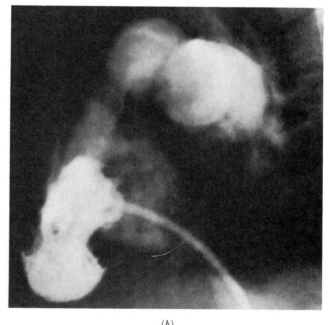

(b)

Fig. 14.14. Tetralogy of Fallot with absent pulmonary valve. Angiogram (a) Frontal view (b) Lateral view. The central pulmonary arteries are massively enlarged.

Haemodynamics

Many of these children present as neonates in severe respiratory difficulty due to the bronchial compression; cardiac signs may be unimpressive, but it is said to be the only cardiac pathology to have a pan-systolic murmur in the first day of life. Those without early respiratory problems present later with the signs of tetralogy of Fallot and the murmur of pulmonary regurgitation.

Radiology

The heart may be mildly enlarged and the ventricular outline is as in uncomplicated tetralogy. In contrast, the pulmonary artery is enlarged and there may be visible enlargement of the hilar pulmonary arteries (Fig. 14.15). Oligaemia is seldom more than mild.

Echocardiography

This seldom shows more than the usual features of an uncomplicated tetralogy. Real time imaging may reveal the dilated pulmonary arteries just above the left atrium.

Management

The respiratory problems are very difficult to treat. The compression is so low that even intubation can be of little benefit. Neonatal cyanosis is likely to be respiratory more than cardiac and shunt procedures are not required. The older child can be repaired in the usual way.

FALLOT PULMONARY ATRESIA

Morphology

This is also known as pulmonary atresia with ventricular septal defect; the pathology is a tetralogy of Fallot with pulmonary atresia rather than stenosis: indeed, some cases are known originally to have been very severe tetralogies which have advanced to pulmonary atresia after shunt procedures. The malformation is quite unlike pulmonary atresia with intact septum (Chap. 13) not only in the intracardiac malformation but also in the way that the lungs are eventually perfused. A patent ductus arteriosus, usual when the ventricular septum is intact, is rare in the Fallot type; instead the lungs are perfused by collateral branches of the aorta. These are of two sorts:

(A) Bronchial and other mediastinal collaterals. Also known as 'secondary bronchial collaterals'. These are anatomically normal vessels, enlarged because they carry extra blood flow that will perfuse the pulmonary arteries via a pre-alveolar capillary network (Fig. 14.16). Pulmonary arteries fed in this way are at low pressure as the systemic pressure in the bronchial arteries is dissipated in the capillary anastomoses. These collaterals are not exclusive to Fallot pulmonary atresia; they can occur to a lesser degree in any cyanotic disease including transposition, even if pulmonary blood flow is high.

(B) Major aortopulmonary collateral arteries (MAPCAs). These are large arteries which are addi-

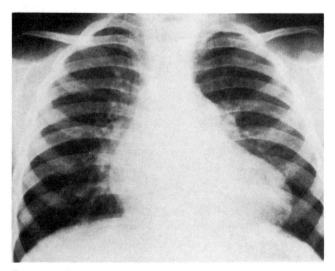

FIG. 14.15. Tetralogy of Fallot with absent pulmonary valve. This is the only situation in which a tetralogy shows a prominent main pulmonary artery.

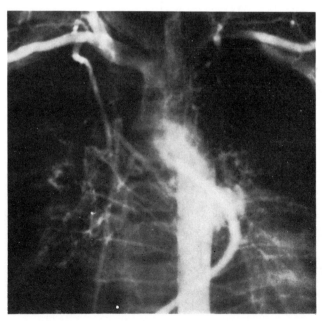

FIG. 14.16. Bronchial collaterals in Fallot pulmonary atresia. Multiple small arteries arise from the descending aorta and form a peribronchial network.

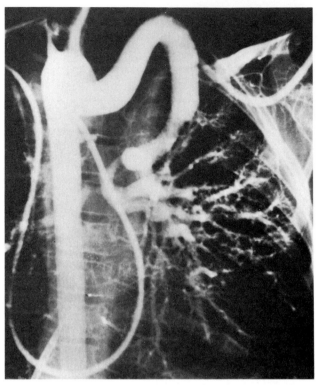

FIG. 14.17. A large major aorta-pulmonary collateral artery (MAPCA) from the left subclavian artery (right aortic arch) supplies most of the left lung. The distal pulmonary arteries have the 'pruned' appearance of severe pulmonary hypertension.

tional to the normal branches of the aorta. Usually between one and four in number, they may arise from the descending aorta, the brachiocephalic arteries (Fig. 14.17) or from the coronary tree. Those from the descending aorta are sometimes erroneously known as 'primary bronchial collaterals' (Fig. 14.18). They are attached directly to the pulmonary arteries, usually to a lobar branch, and may supply additional territory through capillary networks, as with bronchial collaterals. The direct anastomosis between the MAPCA and its pulmonary artery negates the pulmonary artery any central connection to the main pulmonary artery. In effect, it replaces the embryonic anastomosis between the parenchymal pulmonary artery and the sixth arch branches (main pulmonary arteries). In extreme cases, all the lung fields are supplied by MAPCAs and the sixth arch derivatives are absent. Such cases usually have multiple MAPCAs from the descending aorta, and are incorrectly called by some 'type 4 truncus arteriosus'. Generally the main pulmonary artery is present but is small and has a limited distal distribution. There may be stenoses at the junction of the MAPCA and its pulmonary artery.

Pulmonary atresia of the Fallot type can complicate other major defects, notably transposition of the great arteries and double outlet right ventricle.

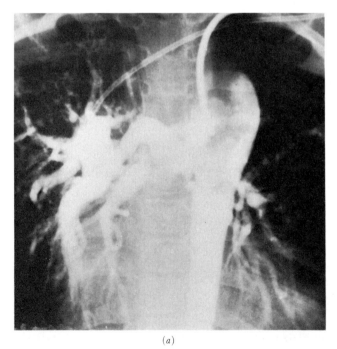

(a)

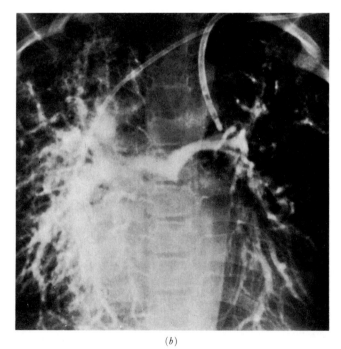

(b)

FIG. 14.18. Multiple MAPCAs from the descending aorta; descending aortogram. (a) Early frame showing their widespread distribution. (b) Late frame showing delayed filling of the central pulmonary arteries which have a limited distal distribution. The main pulmonary artery is just a stump.

Haemodynamics

There is a common mixing at the aortic valve. Pulmonary blood flow is very variable; it can be high in areas supplied by unstenosed MAPCAs, and these areas run the risk of pulmonary vascular occlusive disease. In areas supplied by stenosed MAPCAs or secondary bronchial collaterals, pulmonary blood flow is low. Some patients with high flow in most zones are barely cyanosed; in most cases, however, there is moderate to severe cyanosis.

Radiology

The heart size and shape are similar to tetralogy of Fallot except that a normal shape is quite rare and often the changes are florid (Fig. 14.19). The apex may be very high. MAPCAs can produce unusual mediastinal contours as they emerge from the brachiocephalic vessels and penetrate the lungs (Fig. 14.20). The rare cases with only collaterals and an absent main pulmonary artery can show a diffuse pulmonary nodularity due to the many randomly spaced vessels (Fig. 14.20). Pulmonary vascularity can be anything from moderately plethoric to severely oligaemic, and variations in perfusion from zone to zone are common. The main pulmonary artery is never enlarged.

Echocardiography

Intracardiac appearances are similar to tetralogy of Fallot, except that no pulmonary outflow tract is seen.

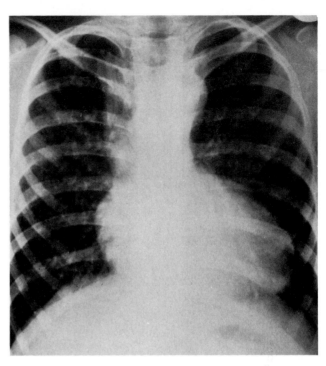

FIG. 14.20. Fallot pulmonary atresia with multiple collaterals to the right lung giving a nodular pattern.

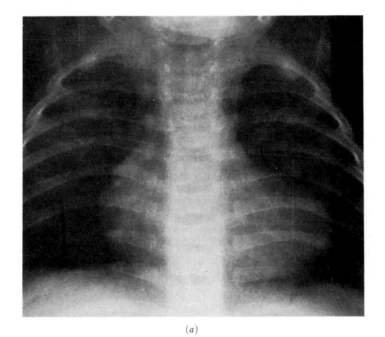

(a)

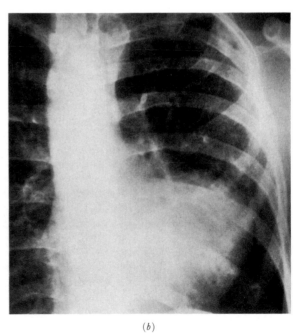

(b)

FIG. 14.19. Fallot pulmonary atresia. (a) Neonate, looking similar to tetralogy of Fallot. (b) In an older child; the apex is very high. Notching of the left ribs is due to a previous left Blalock-Taussig shunt.

There are no reports yet of collaterals being identified. *Isotope perfusion lung imaging* can be helpful in quantitating regional pulmonary blood flow; taken with the angiogram, the contribution of each collateral pathway can be assessed.

Management

This is complicated; there are three main situations:

(A) When there are no central pulmonary arteries and the lungs are supplied by MAPCAs with pulmonary vascular occlusive disease, or by bronchial collaterals alone, nothing can be done.

(B) When there are central pulmonary arteries of reasonable size and distribution, they can be shunted from a systemic artery or attached by a conduit to the right ventricle (together with closure of the VSD). Coexisting MAPCAs can be ligated or embolised.

(C) Occasionally a single, large MAPCA which is at low pressure can be treated as a normal pulmonary artery as in B.

In general, the long term prognosis of a case presenting with severe cyanosis is not much altered by these procedures, but good palliative results are quite common.

TRANSPOSITION OF THE GREAT ARTERIES

Morphology

This term describes the situation when the aorta arises from the morphologically right ventricle and the pulmonary artery from the left, and where the atrioventricular connections are normal (Fig. 14.21). It may be found when the atria are in situs inversus, but solitus is usual. The relationship of the great vessels to their connected chambers are reversed also; the aorta arises from a muscular outflow tract above the crista supraventricularis and the pulmonary valve lies in continuity with the mitral valve. Complicating atrial and ventricular septal defects, and patent ductus arteriosus are very common; almost always one of them is present. The left ventricular outflow tract is frequently narrowed by the septum, which is convex into the left ventricle since the right ventricle is at systemic pressure. This narrowing may produce a significant stenosis, either by itself or by provoking subaortic stenosis of the same sort as is found in hypertrophic obstructive cardiomyopathy. Valvar pulmonary stenosis is also frequent.

The aorta, arising from the right ventricle, is usually anterior and rightward of the pulmonary artery (d-transposition). Occasionally it is anterior and left, or directly anterior, as earlier described in this chapter. Very rarely it lies posterior to the pulmonary artery.

Haemodynamics

Transposition is the usual cause of parallel circulations as described in Chapter 12. There is an inconstant relationship between the degree of cyanosis and the degree of pulmonary plethora; the larger any septal defects are, the greater (usually) is pulmonary blood flow and also greater is the degree of mixing between the two circuits. Occasionally a child will present after two weeks of age with mild cyanosis and torrential pulmonary blood flow, and may be thought to have truncus arteriosus. Transpositions usually present with severe cyanosis in the first week of life. In cases with pulmonary stenosis severe enough to cause oligaemia, cyanosis is severe or profound.

Radiology

Like tetralogy of Fallot, it is not unusual for transpositions to present with a reasonably normal cardiac outline on the plain chest radiograph (Fig. 14.22). There is a typical appearance of moderately severe cases presenting three to ten days after birth. The arch of the aorta runs in an anteroposterior plane rather than in the normal oblique plane and the pulmonary artery sits in the midline (Fig. 14.21); if, as is usually the case, the infant is so ill that the thymus is shrunken, the superior mediastinum (known by cardiologists as the 'pedicle') will be narrow. The heart is normal in size or mildly enlarged and has an ovoid shape. The combination of the two has been dubbed the 'egg on a stick' appearance (Fig. 14.23). The lungs are usually moderately plethoric but, as noted above, extremes do occur. When the child presents in the first two days of life plethora is seldom obvious as the pulmonary arterial resistance is still high, but the cardiac configuration is the same as described. After treatment by septostomy or surgery, the thymus usually regenerates and the typical appearances are lost.

Echocardiography

The atria, atrioventricular valves and ventricles appear normal. The pulmonary valve lies in the same position as a normal aortic valve. A ventricular septal defect, usually perimembraneous, may be visualised. The diagnosis rests on a careful appraisal of the position of the great vessels; the aorta, arising anteriorly, arches over the pulmonary artery. This cannot be visualised in its entirety but the clue lies in the reasonably vertical orientation of the ascending aorta when compared to the more horizontal disposition of the normal pulmonary artery. The result is that the aorta is more readily identified as a tubular structure both on M-mode and real time studies (Fig. 14.24). The M-mode may record *both* semilunar valves at the same time, both showing the box configuration of a normal aortic valve. Real time images may yield a more specific feature in that the anterior wall of posterior great vessel (the pulmonary artery arising from the posterior ventricle) is seen to pass posteriorly just above the heart (so marking the

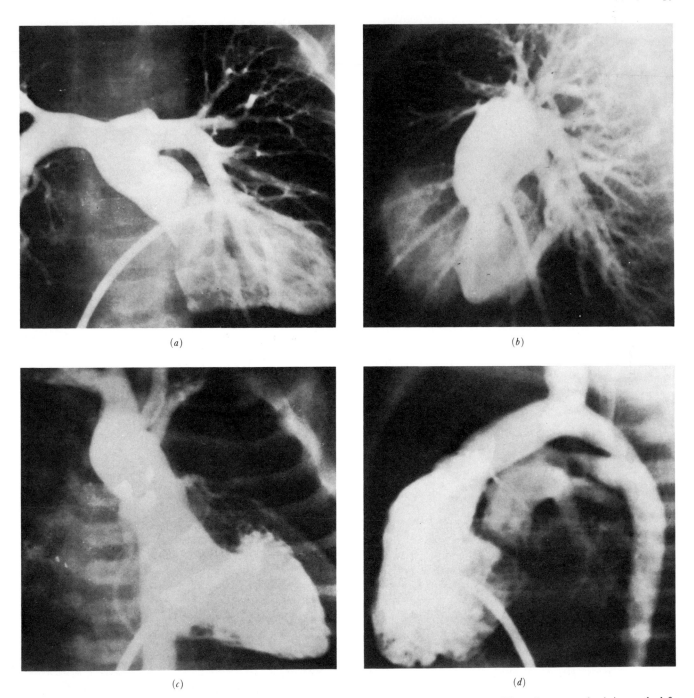

(a)

(b)

(c)

(d)

FIG. 14.21. Transposition of the great arteries. (a, b) frontal and lateral views, left ventricular angiogram. The pulmonary valve is just to the left of the midline. (c, d) frontal and lateral views, right ventricular angiogram. The pulmonary artery fills via a small patent ductus arteriosus; note that it lies almost directly behind the ascending aorta.

bifurcation of the main pulmonary artery), in contrast to a normal aorta which passes without uninterruption out of view (Fig. 14.25).

These signs are, strictly speaking, those of abnormally positioned great vessels but, taken in the clinical context of a cyanosed neonate, are unlikely to be due to other pathologies. In any event, identification of some abnormality of the great vessels should be cause enough for the patient's referral to a specialist centre.

Contrast echocardiography is useful in transposition,

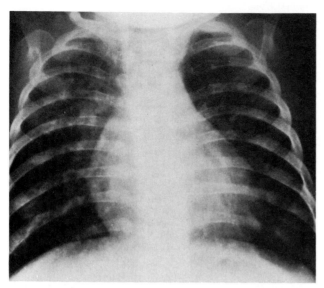

FIG. 14.22. Transposition of the great arteries; a typical chest radiograph. The heart shape is non-specific. Moderate pulmonary plethora.

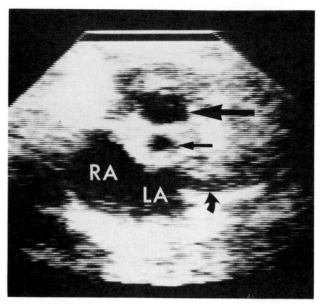

FIG. 14.24. Transposition of the great arteries. Echocardiogram, short axis view at great vessel level; both vessels show as circular echoes (straight arrows) indicating an abnormal configuration. The curved arrow indicates a pulmonary vein.

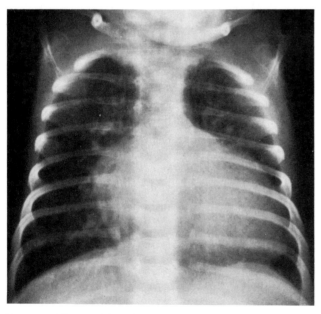

FIG. 14.23. Transposition of the great arteries. 'Egg shaped' heart with a narrow superior mediastinum.

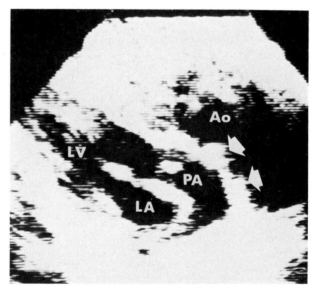

FIG. 14.25. Transposition of the great arteries, high long axial echocardiogram. Note the posterior swing of the anterior wall of the main pulmonary artery (arrows). PA = pulmonary artery, Ao = aorta, LA & LV = left atrium and ventricle.

but will be only briefly described here as it is a technique that is more suited to an investigative centre. It relies upon the ascending aorta being consistently anterior to the pulmonary artery when viewed high up from the suprasternal notch, no matter what position the aortic valve is in. In transposition, contrast bubbles injected into a vein will appear in the aorta before the pulmonary artery. The pulmonary artery will opacify

as bubbles pass through the sites of mixing, but it will clear before the aorta clears. Care is needed to distinguish this pattern from pulmonary atresia and patent ductus arteriosus, when the pulmonary artery will opacify well after the aorta and clear later too.

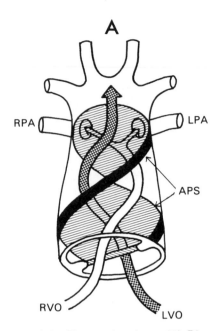
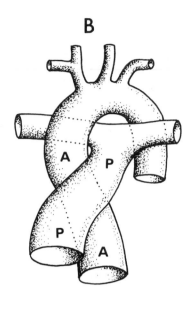

FIG. 15.02. Septation of the Truncus Arteriosus. (A) Diagram showing the spiral septum within the primitive truncus arteriosus which is continuous with the bulbar septum below and which separates the outflow streams from the two ventricles. The distal attachment of this septum to the posterior wall distal to the origin of the 6th aortic arches directs the flow from the right ventricle into the lungs. (B) The aorta and pulmonary arteries defined after septation and separation are completed showing the persisting spiral relationship.

A.	Aorta.	LPA. RPA.	Left and right pulmonary arteries.
P.	Pulmonary artery trunk.	LVO. RVO.	Left and right ventricular outflows.
APS.	Aortico-pulmonary septum.		

to the aorta, then passes to the left side of it and then posteriorly. The upper extremity of the truncal (now aortico-pulmonary) septum joins the posterior wall of the aortic sac above the outlet of the sixth or most proximal pair of aortic arches which then become continuous with the pulmonary artery trunk and supply blood to the lungs. The distal portion of the right sixth arch, connecting with the right paired descending aorta, disappears; the corresponding arterial segment on the left side persists throughout foetal life as the ductus arteriosus.

A useful aid to the understanding of normal aortic arch development and of most of the common arch malformations is the 'embryonic double arch' (Fig. 15.03). It consists of the paired fourth aortic arches; it has the same configuration as an actual double aortic arch (see below). Various segments of it are indicated by letters; the various arch configurations are mostly explained by disappearance of one or two of these segments. The normal left aortic arch (Fig. 15.04) is the result of disappearance of segment A. The aorta passes upwards, first behind and then to the right side of the pulmonary trunk. It continues into the left fourth aortic arch, which passes over the left bronchus to join the left paired descending aorta and continues into the posterior descending aorta ('dorsal aorta' in Fig. 15.01

etc). The fifth aortic arches on each side and the right paired descending aorta disappear; in this way the left fourth arch becomes the definitive aorta and the right fourth arch becomes the innominate artery. The first and second pairs of aortic arches contribute towards the formation of the internal maxillary and stapedial arteries respectively. The upper portions of the ventral aorta and paired dorsal aortas with the third aortic arches form the carotid arteries. The subclavian arteries develop from the seventh cervical inter-segmental branches of the paired dorsal aortas. Different rates of growth in the constituent portions of the foetal arterial system enable the primitive pattern to be moulded into the final anatomical form. At the junction of the primitive truncus arteriosus and the bulbus four endocardial cushions develop; two of these, in opposing position, are continuous with the lower extremities of the spiral endocardial truncal ridges and are divided with the development of the truncal or aortico-pulmonary septum and the ingrowth of the muscular walls of the separated arteries. A hollowing-out process completes the transformation of the original four truncal cushions into six semilunar cusps which form the two tricuspid valves of the pulmonary artery and aorta (Fig. 15.05). The two coronary arteries take exit from behind the two aortic valve sinuses which are adjacent

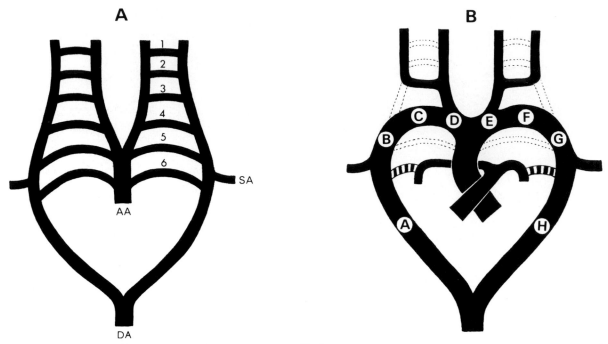

FIG. 15.03. (A) The basic primitive arch pattern in two dimensions. (B) The 'embryonic double arch' system. Atresia of the various lettered segments yields all the common arch configurations (see text).

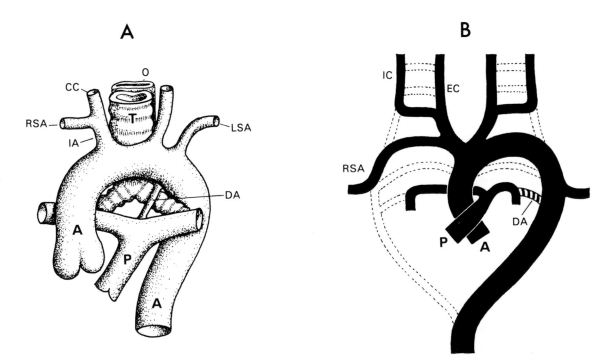

FIG. 15.04. The great arteries—normal pattern. (A) Anatomical arrangement. (B) Embryological diagram. This results from disappearance of segment A of the embryonic double arch.

A.	Aorta.	IA.	Innominate artery.
CC.	Common carotid artery.	LSA. RSA.	Left and right subclavian arteries.
EC.	External carotid artery	P.	Pulmonary artery trunk.
IC.	Internal carotid artery.	O.	Oesophagus.
DA.	Ductus arteriosus.	T.	Trachea.

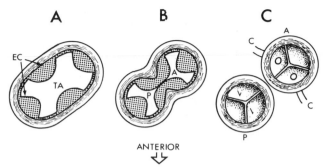

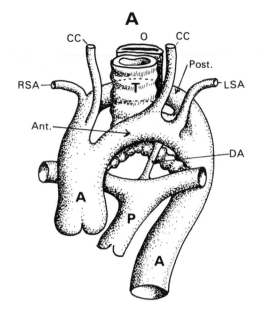

FIG. 15.05. Septation of the truncus arteriosus and formation of the arterial valves. (A) Early stage showing the truncus arteriosus origin with four endocardial cushions. (B) Early septation by confluence of an opposing pair of endocardial cushions which are themselves undergoing division and which are continuous with the aortico-pulmonary septum. There is commencing ingrowth of the vessel wall. (C) Septation completed with modelling of the resultant six endocardial cushions to form the two tricuspid arterial valves.

A.	Aorta.	P.	Pulmonary artery trunk.
C.	Coronary artery.	TA.	Truncus arteriosus.
EC.	Endocardial cushions.	V.	Semi-lunar valves.
Ant.	Anterior.		

to the pulmonary artery. There are two umbilical arteries, one arising from each internal iliac artery; these carry deoxygenated blood from the foetus to the placenta.

MALFORMATIONS OF THE AORTIC ARCH

Double aortic arch. Persistence of the embryonic 'double arch' system (Fig. 15.06, 15.07) is a rare pathology. The plain film may suggest right or left aortic arch as one limb is often larger than the other. Dysphagia is the rule and the barium swallow is always abnormal (Fig. 15.08).

Aberrant right subclavian artery is the consequence of interruption of the embryonic ring at sections B and C in Fig. 15.03 (Fig. 15.09). Dysphagia occurs in only a few cases. The barium swallow shows a shallow posterior indentation a short distance above the carina which is only clearly seen when the oesophagus is well distended (Fig. 15.10).

Right aortic arch occurs when the embryonic ring divides on the left side. When it is unassociated with intracardiac disease the atretic segment is usually at point F/G in Fig. 15.03, producing a right aortic arch with aberrant left subclavian artery, or at point E, yielding a right arch with aberrant left innominate artery (see Fig. 15.12, 15.13). Both these aberrant systems produce a posterior indentation on the barium swallow. Right aortic arch with mirror image branching is the result of atresia at point H (Fig. 15.11), and frequently complicates the conotruncal malformations, particularly tetralogy of Fallot (Fig. 14.11). In the adult

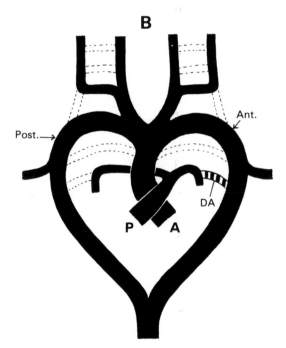

FIG. 15.06. Double aortic arch. (A) Anatomical arrangement. (B) Embryological diagram. The aorta descends on the left side which is the same side as the ductus arteriosus. There is no 'innominate artery' as such. Ant. A. Anterior or left arch. Post A. Posterior or right arch. Other abbreviations as for Fig. 15.04.

or older child, right arch of any sort is quite easily diagnosed as the aortic knuckle is clearly to the right (Fig. 15.12). It may be mistaken for mediastinal lymphadenopathy. In children, where the knuckle is obscured by thymic tissue, the diagnosis is made from

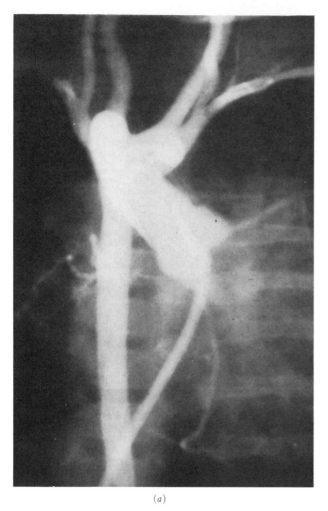

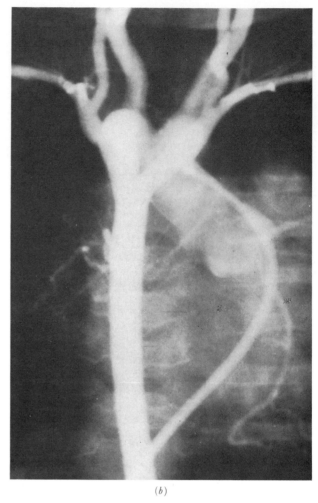

(a)   (b)

FIG. 15.07. Double aortic arch, angiogram. (A) Early phase. (B) Late film; as the ascending aorta clears, the joining of the two arches posteriorly is revealed.

the tracheal shadow. The normal left aorta deviates the trachea mildly to the right in the upper mediastinum; in right arch it is deviated to the left (see also Fig. 15.62b).

Cervical aortic arch covers a variety of rare malformations in which the arch is the persistence of the third (Fig. 15.13, 15.14) or second branchial arches rather than the fourth. Usually it is a right arch as well. The patient may present with a pulsatile mass in the neck or with dysphagia because of a complicating branching abnormality. The plain film may show a high, shallow or absent aortic knuckle, with or without a right aortic arch.

The Management of Vascular Rings

This text has deliberately made no effort to describe each and every one of the many sub-types of arch anomaly. It is enough to remember that, because the embryonic double arch surrounds the oesophagus and trachea, any arch configuration may produce a compressive vascular ring since the encirclement may partly consist of fibrous remnants ('ligaments') of the ring, still attached to the vessels proper (e.g. the ductus ligament). For an arch anomaly to produce compression, some part of it must lie posterior to the oesophagus. The management of *any* patient with unexplained stridor or dysphagia must therefore include a barium swallow. Any *symptomatic* ring will certainly show an oesophageal impression; it can be argued that a normal swallow excludes any vascular ring. Efforts to diagnose the exact type of ring from the swallow serve no purpose; the final diagnosis and the operative approach rely entirely upon an arch aortogram.

Pulmonary Artery Sling

This is the one cause of a symptomatic vascular ring

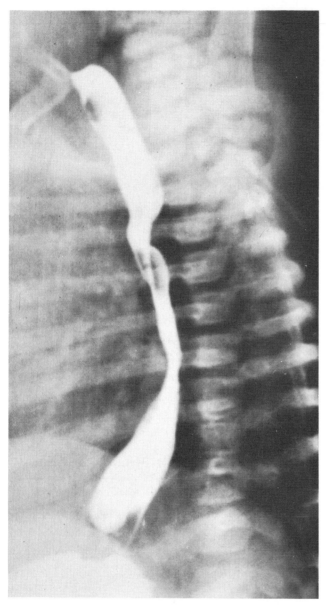

Fig. 15.08. Double aortic arch; barium swallow shows a large posterior indentation which is due to the posterior arch.

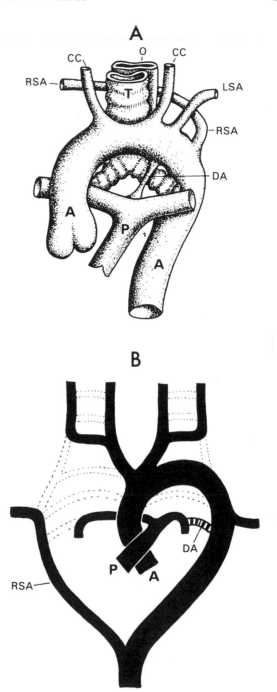

Fig. 15.09. Aberrant right subclavian artery. (A) Anatomical arrangement. (B) Embryological diagram. This arrangement is due to disappearance of segments B and C (Fig. 15.03). Abbreviations as in Fig. 15.04.

where the aortic arch is not involved. The left pulmonary artery fails to develop anterior to the trachea; instead it passes to the right and backwards before turning to the left to go towards the left lung, passing between the trachea and oesophagus (Fig. 15.15). The artery is not stenosed by this abnormal path, and pulmonary vascularity is normal. Nor is the oesophagus significantly affected, although a carefully performed barium swallow will demonstrate an *anterior* indentation just above the level of the carina (Fig. 15.16). The trachea is posteriorly

indented at the same level, and this usually leads to stridor which is often severe and which requires surgical relief. The frontal chest film is normal; the tracheal indentation can sometimes be seen on the lateral view.

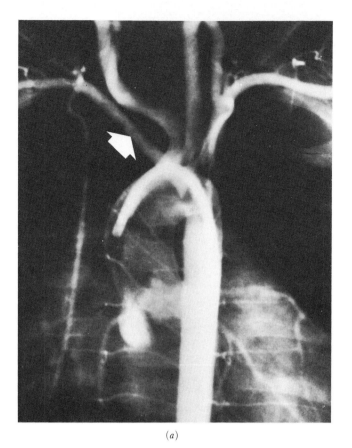

(a)

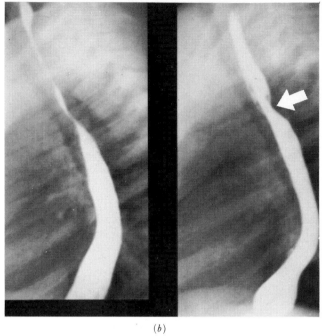

(b)

FIG. 15.10. Aberrant right subclavian artery. (a) Angiogram. The artery is arrowed. (b) Barium swallow. The posterior indentation (arrow) is only seen when the oesophagus is distended with contrast.

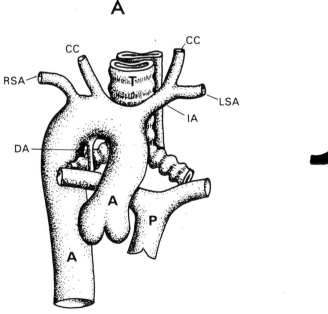

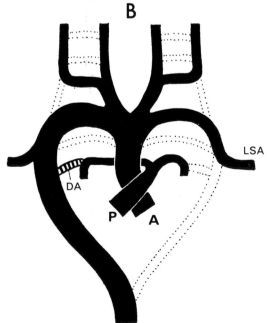

FIG. 15.11. Right sided aortic arch. (A) Anatomical arrangement. (B) Embryological diagram. This is a mirror image of the normal and is due to disappearances of segment H in Fig. 15.03. Abbreviations as for Fig. 15.04. See also Fig. 14.11b.

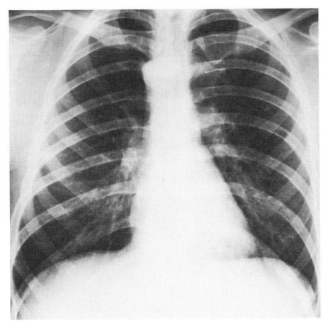

FIG. 15.12. Right aortic arch. The aortic knuckle is clearly visible on the right upper mediastinal border. No associated intracardiac disease.

FIG. 15.13. Cervical right aortic arch with aberrant left subclavian artery and left descending aorta. The descending aortic position is not always on the same side as the arch.

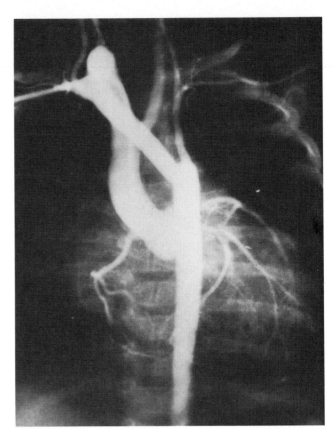

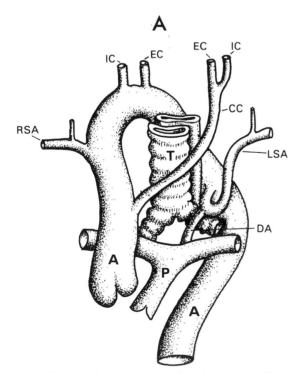

A

B

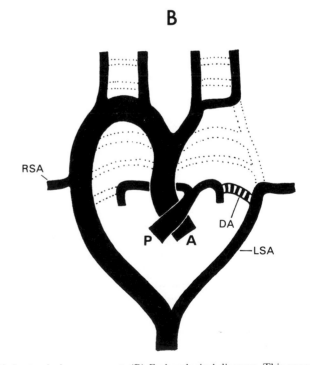

FIG. 15.14. Diagram of the same cervical aortic arch as in Fig. 15.13. (A) Anatomical arrangement. (B) Embryological diagram. This anomaly results from non-development of the fourth aortic arches on both sides with persistence of the whole of the right posterior descending artery. The left sided position of the ductus arteriosus determines the anatomical side of the descending aorta and this is responsible for the aortic arch passing behind the oesophagus and not the left subclavian artery. Note that there is no right common carotid artery as such and the right internal and external carotid arteries each arise directly from the abnormally high aortic arch. Abbreviations as for Fig. 15.04.

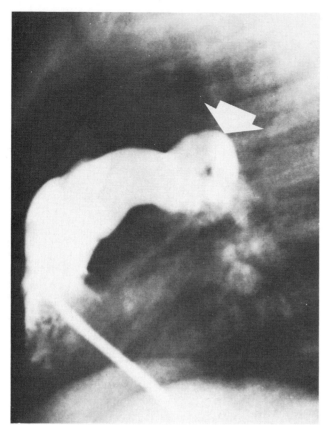

FIG. 15.15. Aberrant left pulmonary artery ('pulmonary artery sling'). Pulmonary angiogram, lateral view. The left pulmonary artery (arrow) shows as an abnormally high structure as it passes above the right pulmonary artery before turning posteriorly and leftward to cross the midline between oesophagus and trachea.

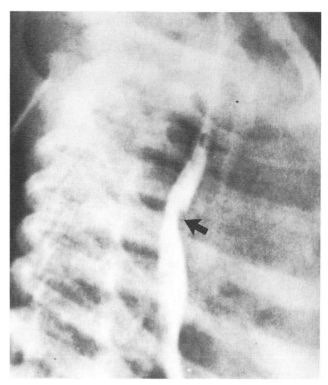

FIG. 15.16. Barium swallow, aberrant left pulmonary artery, lateral view. There is a high, anterior impression (arrow).

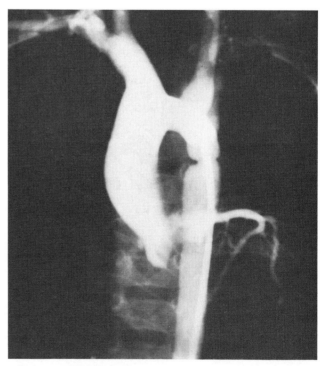

FIG. 15.17. Mild, shelf-like, coarctation of the aorta. Aortogram.

COARCTATION OF THE AORTA

Morphology

This is a common malformation and is found frequently in association with other conditions such as patent ductus arteriosus, bicuspid aortic stenosis, other causes of left ventricular outflow obstruction, and perimembraneous ventricular septal defect. The condition covers any narrowing of the aorta at the isthmus, which is defined as that segment between a normally arising left sub-clavian artery and the ductus arteriosus or its ligamentous remnant. The narrowing may be a short shelf-life stenosis (Fig. 15.17), an hour glass stenosis (Fig. 15.18), or a long segment of narrowing ending in a more severe localised stenosis (Fig. 15.19). Theories on its pathogenesis are varied; two strong contenders are, firstly, that exuberant ductal tissue (which is histologically distinct from aortic endothelium) invades the aortic lumen and, secondly, that in utero the isthmus may be a point of zero blood flow if the ductus is large,

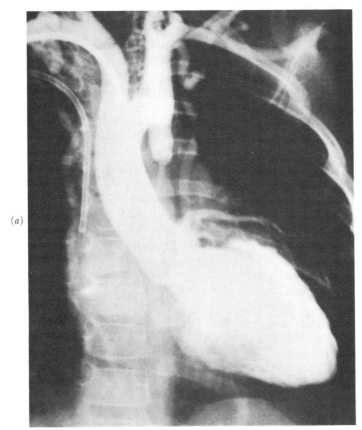

(a)

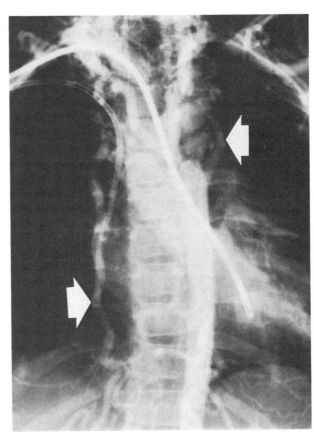

FIG. 15.18. Moderate coarctation; aortogram. (a) Early frame. There is a jet of contrast passing through the coarcted segment. (b) Late frame. Sustained opacification of the descending aorta due to collateral flow. The enlarged internal mammary arteries are arrowed.

FIG. 15.19. Severe coarctation. The isthmus (small arrows) is hypoplastic and ends as a severe coarctation (large arrow).

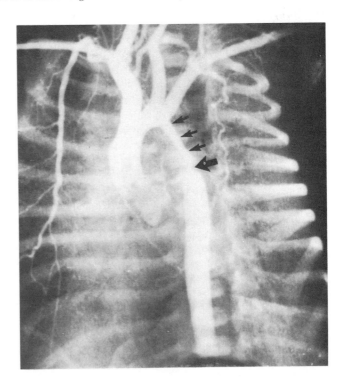

and therefore does not grow. Whatever the cause the coarctation is adjacent to the ductus (see Fig. 15.33). In the infant the ductus is usually patent and opens below the coarctation ('preductal coarctation'). In some infants, and in the majority of later presentations, the ductus is shut. The minority of cases left are those in which a patent ductus opens into the aorta at or above the coarctation ('post ductal coarctation'). It is inaccurate to think of all infantile cases as preductal. The coarctation may lie close to the origin of the left subclavian artery, and in a few cases that artery is involved in the process and is stenosed at its origin; when this happens it cannot participate in the collateral circulation. There is occasionally an aberrant right subclavian artery, whose origin is always distal to the coarctation (Fig. 15.20).

Coarctation presenting in the older child or adult can be associated with berry aneurysm of the intracerebral vessels. There is a small but definite risk of bacterial

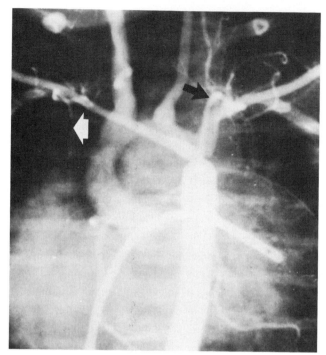

FIG. 15.20. Moderate coarctation with an aberrant right subclavian artery whose origin is posterior, just below the coarctation. The right internal mammary artery (white arrow) is not part of the collateral circulation and is small; the left internal mammary is enlarged (black arrow).

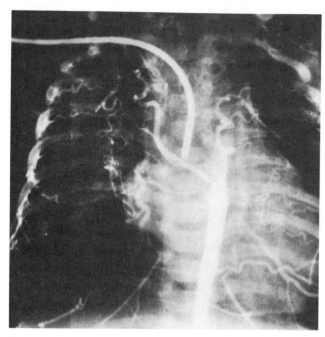

FIG. 15.21. Severe coarctation. Aortogram, late phase, showing tortuous subcostal arteries.

infection on the coarctation which, despite being strictly an endarteritis tends still to be called endocarditis. There is a high incidence of coarctation in Turner's syndrome.

Collateral Circulation

Any significant coarctation will quite quickly cause the opening up of collateral channels to bypass the obstruction. There are two main sets. In one, anastomoses between anterior and posterior intercostal arteries develop, reversing normal flow in the latter and so perfusing the descending aorta (Fig. 15.18). The anterior intercostals are fed mainly by the internal mammary arteries, which also dilate (Fig. 15.18b). The upper two intercostal arteries do not contribute to this circuit as both anterior and posterior branches originate from the brachiocephalic arteries; notching of the first or second ribs therefore suggest causes other than coarctation (which include neurofibromatosis, Blalock-Taussig shunts and vena caval obstructions).

Notching of the underside of the ribs in coarctation is due to tortuosity of the intercostal arteries (Fig. 15.21). The cortical margin may be indistinct but is intact (Fig. 15.22). Irregular indentation of the inferior border of the posterior medial third of a rib is not unusual in the normal, and so a diagnosis of notching must be

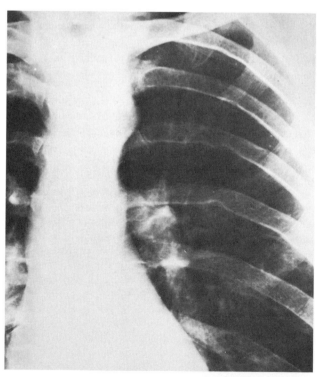

FIG. 15.22. Coarctation with notching. Note the medial displacement of the upper descending aorta.

made on abnormalities more laterally placed. The internal mammary arteries which feed the intercostals are also enlarged and may notch the posterior border of the sternum. Unilateral notching can be due to stenosis of one of the subclavian arteries or to a subclavian artery arising anomalously from below the coarctation; the possibilities are complex when combinations with right aortic arch are included.

The second group of collaterals is found in the mediastinum, usually quite small but often as haemodynamically important as the intercostal set. There is often one large vessel running from the right subclavian artery to the descending aorta, the *arteria aberans*.

Haemodynamics

Systemic hypertension develops above the coarctation as the circulation strives to maintain renal perfusion, but no amount of collateral enlargement can properly overcome the stenosis. In the infant, the ductus often perfuses the lower half of the body, necessarily at high pressure, but with desaturated blood giving differential cyanosis of the lower extremities. In the neonate the electrocardiogram usually shows right ventricular strain which changes slowly to the more expected left ventricular pattern. Left ventricular failure is the usual presentation for a neonate with severe coarctation. Lesser degrees usually escape detection until the effects of hypertension become manifest in later life, which can be at almost any time, or until either notching or absent femoral pulses are detected at routine medical examination.

Radiology

Neonates in heart failure (Fig. 15.23) present with moderate to gross cardiomegaly of non-specific shape. The lung fields often show interstitial oedema, with plethora if there is a complicating VSD. The older patient has a normal or mildly enlarged heart, with or without left ventricular hypertrophy, depending upon the severity of the lesion. Notching is unusual below the age of seven but can occur from the age of three. It always indicates that the coarctation is severe enough to require repair. Notching generally regresses slowly after repair of the defect but may persist, especially in the adult. Provided that it is unobscured by thymus, the aortic knuckle is usually abnormal. The coarctation lies just below the knuckle, and displaces the line of the descending aorta medially (Fig. 15.22). This displacement may extend over a considerable length, flattening the knuckle and sometimes elevating its position. Alternatively, the distal arch above and the descending aorta below may be dilated around a short coarctation, producing a 'figure three' sign (Fig. 15.24).

Echocardiography is presently unable to visualise a coarctation reliably, though convincing images can be produced in the neonate.

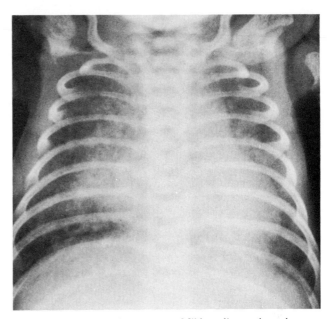

FIG. 15.23. Coarctation in a neonate. Mild cardiomegaly, pulmonary oedema.

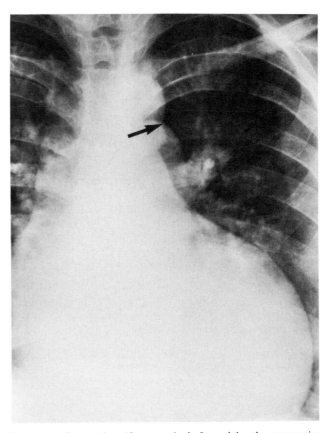

FIG. 15.24. Coarctation: 'figure 3 sign', formed by the coarctation indenting (arrow) the otherwise prominent descending aorta.

Management

Repair is usually indicated in the neonate and at present the left subclavian artery is sacrificed to provide a flap of autologous tissue for a patch repair. End-to-end anastomosis in this age group usually leads to restenosis. In the older patient who is not in failure, any coarctation severe enough to have caused either hypertension or notching merits repair. Some, however, will not respond by normalising the blood pressure. There is conflict in the two to ten year old group between the need for early operation to avoid irreversible hypertension and the desirability of allowing the aorta to grow to adult proportions before repair.

AORTIC INTERRUPTION

This pathology is at the severest end of the spectrum of coarctation, when the affected segment is atretic rather than simply stenosed. These cases present in neonatal life and a PDA usually supplies the descending aorta. Heart failure is severe. The atretic segment, if short, can be repaired like a coarctation, but usually the length of the defect precludes adequate surgery.

PSEUDO COARCTATION

Occasionally an otherwise normal aorta shows mild tortuosity of the distal arch (Fig. 15.25) which deforms the knuckle on the plain film, mimicking a coarctation. There is never any notching as there is no more than trivial stenosis.

SUPRA AORTIC STENOSIS

Morphology. This uncommon condition is a diffuse narrowing of the ascending aorta, beginning at the top of the coronary sinuses and extending upwards often to the brachiocephalic vessels or sometimes beyond (Fig. 15.26). If measured, the entire aorta is often found to be smaller than normal, and rarely there may be other localised stenoses. Similar stenoses of the pulmonary arteries frequently complicate the situation. There is a strong association with idiopathic hypercalcaemia of infancy; mental subnormality is common but the hypercalcaemia has usually resolved by the time the aortic disease is identified.

Haemodynamics. Because of its length, the effective severity of the narrowing is usually severe; the haemodynamic consequences are the same as those of valvar aortic stenosis.

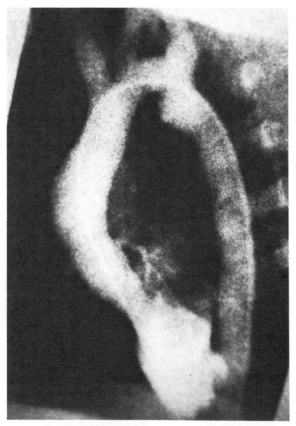

FIG. 15.25. Pseudocoarctation. LV angiogram, left anterior oblique view. The distal arch is tortuous but not stenosed.

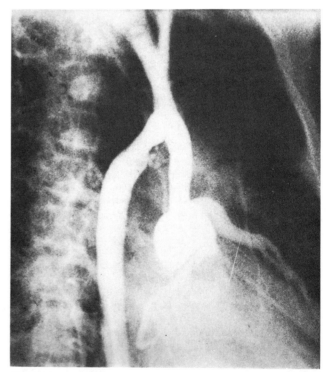

FIG. 15.26. Supraaortic stenosis. Aortogram, right anterior oblique view. The ascending aorta and the arch are narrowed. The aortic sinuses are normal but the coronary arteries are proximally dilated.

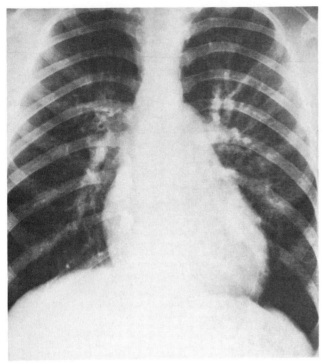

FIG. 15.27. Supraaortic stenosis. Same patient as Fig. 15.26. The aortic knuckle is shallow. Dilatation of the left upper pulmonary arteries due to associated peripheral stenoses.

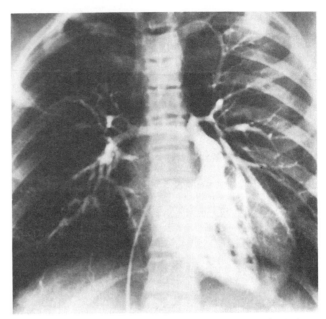

FIG. 15.28. Severe pulmonary artery stenoses. The central vessels are most severely affected.

Radiology (Fig. 15.27). Since the ascending aorta is the seat of the pathology, there is no post stenotic dilatation in this condition. The combination of clinically severe aortic stenosis and no visible ascending aorta on the frontal chest film is therefore quite suggestive of this disease. Patchy dilatations of the peripheral pulmonary arteries, secondary to stenoses, may provide another clue.

Management. Replacement of the ascending aorta is sometimes attempted.

COARCTATION OF THE PULMONARY ARTERIES

Morphology. This is also known as 'peripheral pulmonary artery stenosis'. There are diffuse narrowings of the pulmonary arteries, sometimes with patchy post stenotic dilatation. Mild forms often complicate supra aortic stenosis. Severe, isolated cases usually affect the arteries diffusely, the main pulmonary artery being mainly affected (Fig. 15.28).

Haemodynamics are essentially those of valvar pulmonary stenosis. Surprisingly, it may not progress appreciably as the patient grows.

Radiology. There is no post stenotic dilatation of the main pulmonary artery. Patchy dilatations of the peripheral pulmonary arteries may be seen. In severe cases

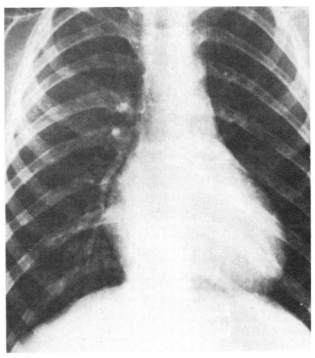

FIG. 15.29. Severe pulmonary artery stenoses. Same patient as Fig. 15.28. The hilar pulmonary arteries are tiny and there is peripheral oligaemia.

the hilar pulmonary arteries are small (Fig. 15.29) and the heart may be enlarged.

Management is non-surgical.

BRANCH PULMONARY ARTERY ATRESIA

Morphology. This is an occasional malformation. Usually the right pulmonary artery is affected (Fig. 15.30). The ipselateral lung is small. It may be perfused by an aorto pulmonary collateral (MAPCA, Chap. 14) when there is associated intracardiac pathology (typically tetralogy of Fallot); otherwise it is supplied by enlarged bronchial arteries.

Haemodynamics. There is evidence to suggest that when only one lung takes all the cardiac output in early childhood, pulmonary vascular occlusive disease may develop. This is not too surprising as the perfusion, as far as that lung is concerned, is the same as a 2:1 shunt. This situation also holds true for pneumonectomy in childhood.

Radiology (Fig. 15.31). The affected lung is small and hyperlucent, but unlike McCleod's syndrome shows no air trapping. The mediastinum is shifted towards the small lung. The other lung is plethoric.

Management. Since there are no distal pulmonary arteries, there is no satisfactory treatment.

PATENT DUCTUS ARTERIOSUS (PDA)

Morphology

The ductus arteriosus is the distal half of the left sixth aortic arch and is patent throughout foetal life. It may remain patent after birth to give a left to right shunt (Fig. 15.32), to be part of a coarctation complex (Fig. 15.33), to perfuse the lungs in cases of cyanotic heart disease or the body in hypoplastic left heart syndrome. It frequently complicates hyaline membrane disease; either it gives a complicating left to right shunt for which surgery is required or, in severe cases, allows pressure relief of the pulmonary arteries with a right to left shunt, in which case closure is of dubious value. Its patency can be pharmacologically altered. Some prosta-

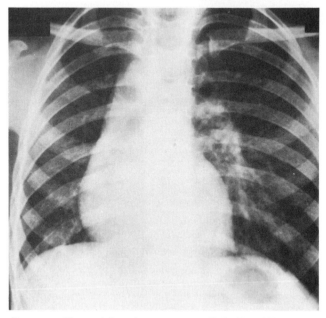

Fig. 15.31. Absent right pulmonary artery. Plain film of Fig. 15.30.

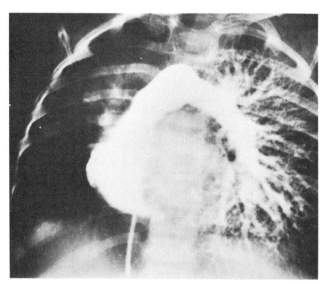

Fig. 15.30. Absent right pulmonary artery. Right ventricular angiogram. The left lung is plethoric.

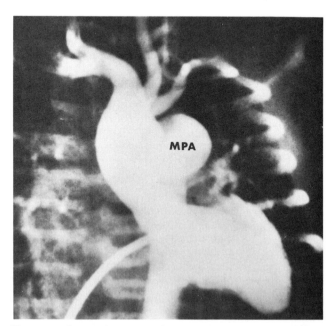

Fig. 15.32. Patent ductus arteriosus. Left ventricular angiogram, frontal view. The enlarged main pulmonary artery (MPA) has opacified. Note that the aortic knuckle is not prominent.

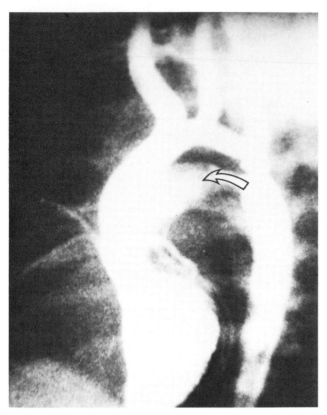

FIG. 15.33. Patent ductus arteriosus; left ventricular angiogram, left anterior oblique. The ductus (arrow) lies just below a shallow coarctation.

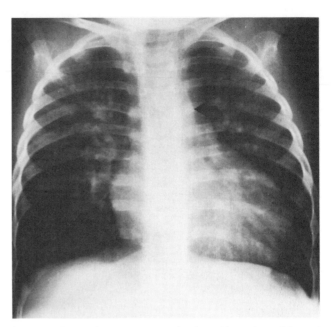

FIG. 15.34. Patent ductus arteriosus, showing a 'ductus bump' (arrow) on the upper descending aorta. Moderate cardiomegaly and plethora.

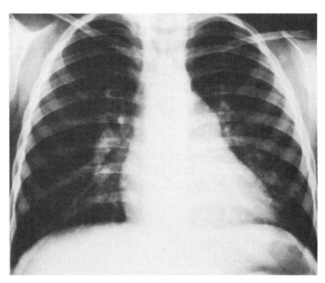

FIG. 15.35. Small patent ductus arteriosus; mild plethora with a prominent main pulmonary artery.

glandins are very affective in opening it; others, and phenylbutazone, can sometimes close it.

Haemodynamics

Alone, or with a VSD, there is a left to right shunt which develops in neonatal life as the pulmonary resistance falls. Pulmonary vascular occlusive disease usually develops but its incidence is less and its presentation later than with a large VSD. Presentation may well be delayed until adulthood. When in combination with other defects its effects are varied, depending upon the exact pathology.

Radiology

Only isolated PDA will be considered. In the neonate or infant there may be cardiomegaly, plethora or heart failure depending upon the size of the shunt. The heart shape is seldom specific but on occasions there is a bulge on the line of the upper descending aorta, visible on the frontal film (the 'ductus bump', Fig. 15.34). The older child will show varying degrees of plethora and cardiomegaly. The main pulmonary artery is usually prominent; more so than might be expected from the

size of the shunt. This is ascribed to turbulence in it from the ductal stream (Fig. 15.35). The aortic knuckle tends to be normal or large, in contrast to the intracardiac shunts, but this is an unreliable sign. Pulmonary hypertension brings increasing enlargement of the main pulmonary artery. Occasionally an adult will present with severe pulmonary hypertension, pulmonary artery calcification and, sometimes, calcification of the duct

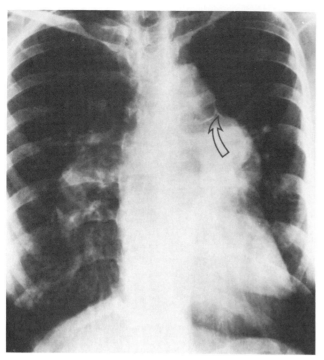

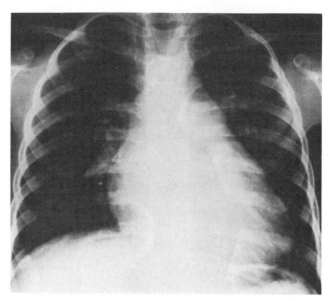

Fig. 15.37. Patent ductus arteriosus with severe pulmonary hypertension. Atypical appearances; the pulmonary arteries are not enlarged. Cardiomegaly is due to right ventricular failure.

Fig. 15.36. Adult patent ductus arteriosus with severe pulmonary hypertension and shunt reversal. The pulmonary arteries are greatly enlarged and show fine linear calcification secondary to atheromatous disease. The wall of the ductus itself is calcified (arrow).

itself (Fig. 15.36). Sometimes the pulmonary vessels retain their foetal thickness so well that Eisenmenger shunt reversal does not lead to obvious enlargement of the main or branch pulmonary arteries (Fig. 15.37).

Echocardiography can sometimes visualise the ductus but is not presently a reliable method. Left atrial size increases with the size of the shunt and this can be used as a monitor of ductal patency in the neonate.

Management

Surgical closure is virtually free from serious risk unless it is associated with neonatal respiratory distress and is advocated for all cases with a left to right shunt who have no pulmonary vascular occlusive disease.

AORTOPULMONARY WINDOW

Morphology. This defect is due to non-fusion of part of the truncal septum above the semilunar valves; the result is a long, slit-like communication which often runs from the valves up to the distal arch. The pulmonary and aortic valves are normally formed (Fig. 15.38). The defect is usually large and severe heart failure is common. Patent ductus arteriosus may complicate it.

Haemodynamics are the same as for a large patent ductus.

Radiology. There is nothing on the plain film to distinguish a window from other large left to right shunts (Fig. 15.39).

Echocardiography has been shown to be able to visualise the defect, but it is so rare that it is difficult to know how sensitive the technique is.

TRUNCUS ARTERIOSUS

Morphology

In this malformation the truncal septum fails to develop in the region of the intended aortic and pulmonary valves. The embryonic truncal valve therefore persists. Since the cono-truncal septum contributes to the mature interventricular septum there is invariably a high ventricular septal defect and the truncal valve usually straddles the ventricular septum. Above the valve the great vessels are usually separate; the pulmonary artery usually takes origin from the leftward anterior face of the trunk. There may be a long main pulmonary artery (type I) or a short one (type II) (Fig. 15.40). More rarely the right and left pulmonary arteries take separate origins from the ascending aorta (type III). There is a type IV in some systems of nomenclature, in which the pulmonary arteries are said to arise from the descending aorta; however, these cases are in fact Fallot pulmonary atresia with absent central pulmonary arteries and MAPCAs from the descending aorta.

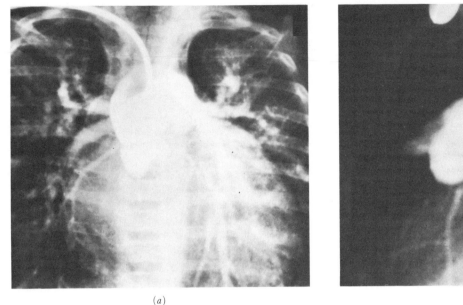

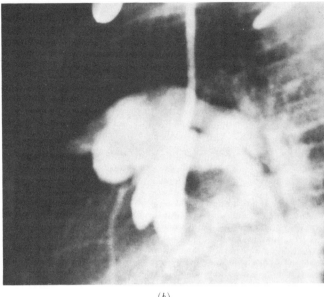

(a)   (b)

FIG. 15.38. Aortopulmonary window. Aortogram. (a) Frontal view shows simultaneous filling of aorta and pulmonary arteries. (b) Lateral view shows that separate pulmonary and aortic valves exist (compare with Fig. 15.40).

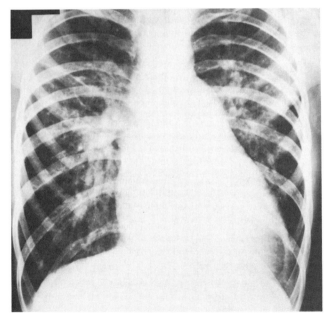

FIG. 15.39. Aortopulmonary window. Moderate plethora.

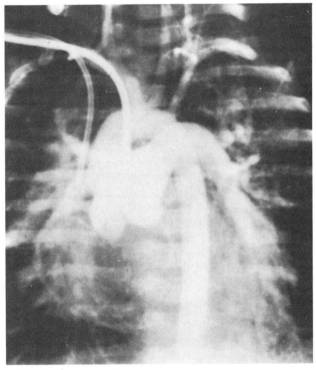

FIG. 15.40. Truncus arteriosus (type II). There is only one semilunar valve (compare with Fig. 15.38).

Haemodynamics

This is a common mixing situation, usually with no restriction to pulmonary blood flow (pulmonary artery stenosis is occasionally seen). Pulmonary blood flow is therefore high and cyanosis is minimal. The picture may be complicated by stenosis or incompetence of the truncal valve.

Radiology

(Fig. 15.41). There is typically plethora and cardiomegaly. As only the type I cases have anything like a normally pulmonary artery, the pulmonary bay is usually hollow, in contrast to a typical PDA or VSD. The heart shape is otherwise non-specific. Right aortic arch is occasionally seen.

Echocardiography

Two ventricles, the VSD and a single overriding great vessel are seen. Similar appearances are present in Fallot pulmonary atresia or sometimes in acyanotic Tretralogy when the right ventricular outflow tract is not apparent. Truncal stenosis may also be visualised.

Management

Surgical repair is feasible but regular success is unusual. Pulmonary vascular occlusive disease usually develops quite quickly in untreated cases.

MISCELLANEOUS GREAT VESSEL SHUNTS

A number of systemic and pulmonary arteriovenous malformations may present as 'heart disease'. Some of the more common are presented here.

Sinus of Valsalva Fistula

These begin as aneurysms, presumably congenital, of one of the coronary sinuses; as such they are clinically silent and may be sometimes detected as an incidental finding at aortography (Fig. 15.42(a)). The right coronary sinus is most frequently affected. They present if and when they rupture into the heart, usually into the right ventricle but sometimes into the right atrium or left ventricle. The rupture is classically precipitated by minor trauma or acute but strenuous exertion. The shunt can be quite large and being acute is poorly tolerated. The chest radiograph usually shows mild cardiomegaly and borderline plethora. Unusually, a large aneurysm may show as a bulge on the right heart border (Fig. 15.42(b)).

Coronary Artery Fistula

Either coronary artery may form a fistulous connection with any of the cardiac chambers or with the pulmonary artery. Most commonly the right atrium is the receiving chamber (Fig. 15.43). The shunt is seldom severe. Clinically they can be mistaken for a small

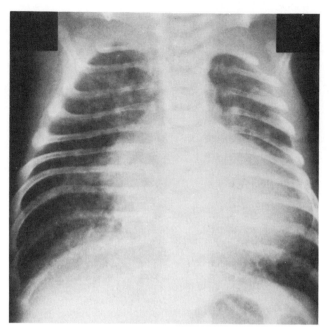

FIG. 15.41. Truncus arteriosus. Infant, severe plethora and cardiomegaly. Shallow pulmonary bay.

patent ductus arteriosus or for aortic regurgitation. The chest radiograph shows, if anything, non-specific signs of a left to right shunt.

Systemic Arteriovenous Malformations

These are uncommon. Small, asymptomatic fistulae can occur in the brachiocephalic vessels and in the spine. Some cerebral and hepatic malformations, particularly the 'aneurysm' of the vein of Galen (Fig. 15.44) may be so large as to cause heart failure in the infant (Fig. 15.45). The haemodynamics are the same as for a left ventricular to right atrial shunt. Less common are malformations between anomalous aortic vessels and the pulmonary veins; these are part of the spectrum of pulmonary sequestration but there is usually no visible lung lesion on the plain chest radiograph. The shunt is often missed at catheterisation as it returns saturated blood to the left atrium and this does not give any step-up in the saturations recorded. Aortography is required for definitive diagnosis.

Pulmonary Arteriovenous Malformations

Pulmonary artery to left atrium shunts are due to either large, single or multiple arteriovenous malformations which are easily seen on the plain chest film (Fig. 15.46), or to widespread small fistulae that can only be seen on pulmonary angiography (Fig. 15.47). Both types produce a pure right to left shunt that may be large enough to give clinical cyanosis. Both may also be associated with familial telangectasia.

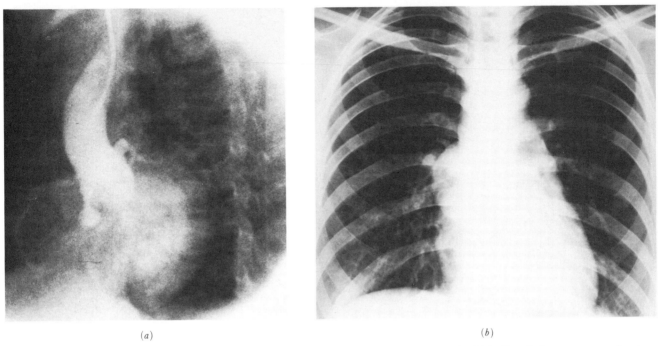

(a)   (b)

FIG. 15.42. Aneurysm of the sinus of Valsalva. (a) Aortogram, showing the flask-shaped aneurysm. (b) Plain film of a large aneurysm, forming a bulge above the right atrium.

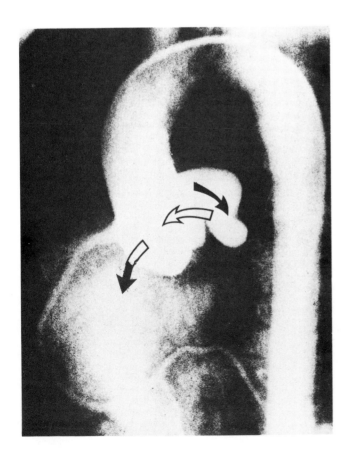

FIG. 15.43. Fistula, left coronary artery to right atrium. The greatly enlarged left coronary artery (arrowed) doubles back behind the aortic root to opacify the right heart. The normal left coronary artery branches filled later.

ANOMALOUS LEFT CORONARY ARTERY

In this condition the left coronary artery arises from the main pulmonary artery trunk (Fig. 15.48). After birth, this leads to perfusion of most of the left ventricular myocardium with desaturated blood. Later, as pulmonary vascular resistance falls, collaterals between the right and left coronary systems open up and allow a left to right shunt. This leads to a 'steal' of blood from the myocardium. At either stage the myocardium at risk is likely to infarct; the electrocardiogram typically shows the pattern of an antero-septal infarction. Reversible ventricular dysfunction is present in those in whom infarction has not yet taken place and it is in this small group that a coronary artery bypass graft holds some hope. The plain chest film shows non-specific cardiomegaly, with or without pulmonary venous congestion. Echocardiography may reveal a segmental pattern of myocardial dysfunction as the antero-septal zone of the left ventricle is principally affected.

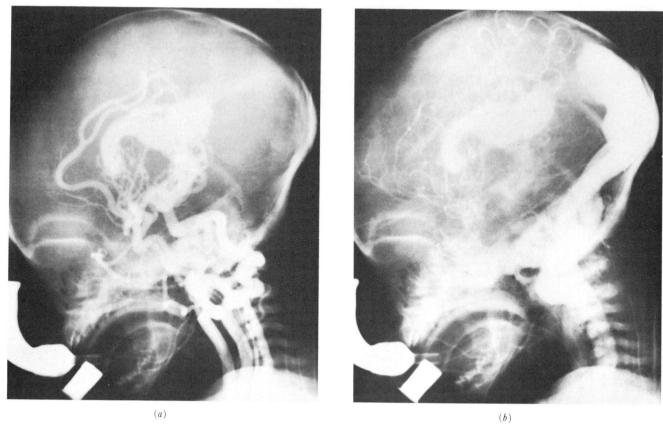

(a)   (b)

FIG. 15.44. Aneurysm of the vein of Galen. (a) Arterial phase. All four cerebral arteries feed the malformation. (b) Venous phase.

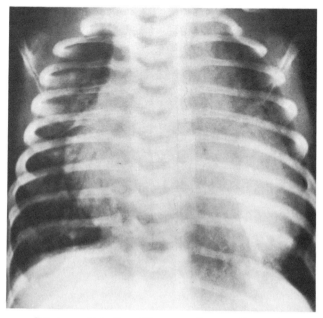

FIG. 15.45. Plain film of Fig. 15.44. Gross cardiomegaly.

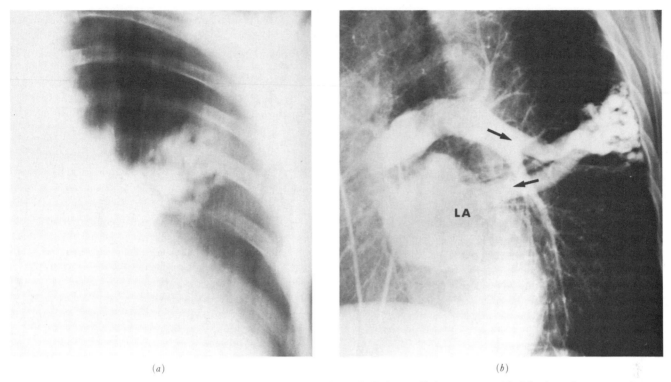

(a)   (b)

FIG. 15.46. Pulmonary arteriovenous fistula. (a) Tomogram showing the typically 'worm-like' appearance. (b) Selective pulmonary angiogram, showing drainage to the left atrium (LA) (*Courtesy Dr M. Sidaway*).

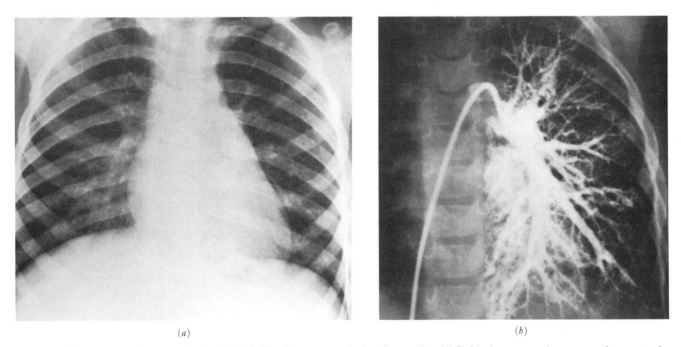

(a)   (b)

FIG. 15.47. Pulmonary arteriovenous fistula. (a) Plain film shows no convincing abnormality. (b) Left pulmonary angiogram reveals an extensive capillary blush in the whole of the left lower lobe due to widespread fistulae.

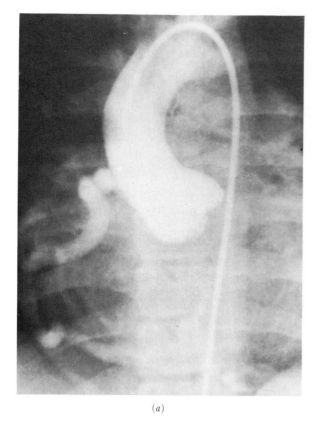 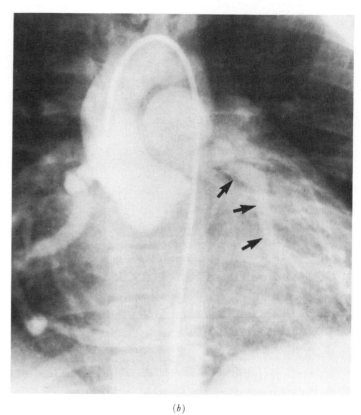

(a)   (b)

FIG. 15.48. Anomalous left coronary artery. Aortogram. (a) Early film shows filling of a right coronary artery only. (b) Late film shows the left coronary artery (arrows) filled retrogradely by collaterals from the right coronary artery and draining back to the pulmonary artery (*Courtesy Dr J. Walker*).

THE NORMAL DEVELOPMENT OF THE VEINS

(Fig. 15.49). The early foetal sinus venosus has two lateral extensions or horns, each of which receives three veins. The medial pair of veins are the vitelline veins which pass upward from the primitive yolk sac. They become united by a plexus around the upper part of the intestine, and between this region and the sinus venosus they become incorporated into the developing hepatic vasculature. The upper part of the right vitelline vein becomes the upper portion of the definitive inferior vena cava whilst the periduodenal plexus condenses into the portal vein and receives vessels from the spleen and intestinal tract. The two umbilical veins bring oxygenated blood from the placenta to the foetus. These too become incorporated into the developing liver; they lose direct connection with the sinus venosus but communicate freely with the intra-hepatic vitelline vein sinusoids. The right umbilical vein becomes atrophic and the total return blood flow from the placenta passes through the left umbilical vein, along the lower margin of the falciform ligament, into the liver where a new channel develops to take it directly into the upper portion of the right vitelline vein, which has become the hepatic vein. This channel is the ductus venosus; it closes shortly after birth when the placental circulation ceases. The lateral horns of the sinus venosus are each continuous with a common cardinal vein, or Cuvierian duct, which receives two vessels, an anterior cardinal vein which drains the head and arms, and a posterior cardinal vein which drains the trunk and legs.

The two anterior cardinal veins become connected by a transverse cervical anastomosis which evolves into the innominate vein. The upper part of the left common cardinal vein becomes atrophic, the lower part persists as the coronary sinus, and the intermediate portion remains represented as the oblique vein of the left atrium and the ligament of Marshall. The right anterior and common cardinal veins become the superior vena cava. With the descent of the heart from a subpharyngeal to a thoracic position, the anterior and common cardinal veins become elongated and the junctions with the posterior cardinal veins come to lie above the heart. The venous drainage of the lower half of the body

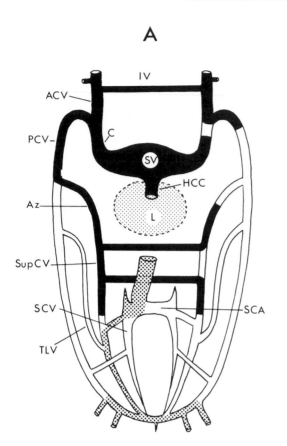

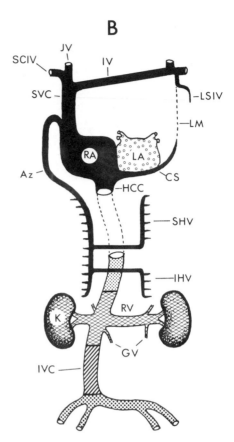

FIG. 15.49. Development of the systemic veins. (A) The constituent embryonic elements of the venous system. The vessels which persist and drain into the superior vena cava are shown in black; those which form the inferior vena cava are shaded. (B) The mature systemic venous pattern; the constituent portions of the inferior vena cava are indicated.

ACV.	Anterior cardinal vein.		LA.	Left atrium.
AZ.	Azygos vein.		LM.	Ligament of Marshall.
C.	Cuvierian duct.		LSIV.	Left superior intercostal vein.
CS.	Coronary sinus.		PCV.	Posterior cardinal vein.
GV.	Gonadal vein.		RA.	Right atrium.
HCC.	Hepato cardiac channel.		RV.	Renal vein.
IHV.	Inferior hemiazygos vein.		SCA.	Subcardinal anastomosis.
IV.	Innominate vein.		SCV.	Subcardinal vein.
IVC.	Inferior vena cava.		SCIV.	Subclavian vein.
JV.	Jugular vein.		SHV.	Superior hemiazygos vein.
K.	Kidney.		SV.	Sinus venosus.
L.	Liver.		SVC.	Superior vena cava.
			Sup. CV.	Supracardinal vein.

becomes taken over by the development of various other longitudinal veins including the azygos system. The proximal portions of the posterior cardinal veins remain as the superior intercostal veins and the terminal portion of the (right) azygos vein. The distal extremity of the right posterior cardinal vein also persists and forms the lower extremity of inferior vena cava. The remainder of the inferior vena cava has a complex origin and is derived from segments of several veins of distinct embryological origin.

The lungs originate as outgrowths from the anterior aspect of the pharynx with which, initially, they share a common venous plexus draining into the systemic venous system. As the lungs develop they acquire a secondary pulmonary venous plexus which condenses into a common inter pulmonary vein (Fig. 15.50). At the same time an outgrowth from the left side of the primitive atrial chamber, the primary pulmonary vein, grows towards the inter pulmonary vein and makes connection with it. The main pulmonary venous drainage thus comes to enter the left side of the atrium; the original splanchnic venous elements persist as the

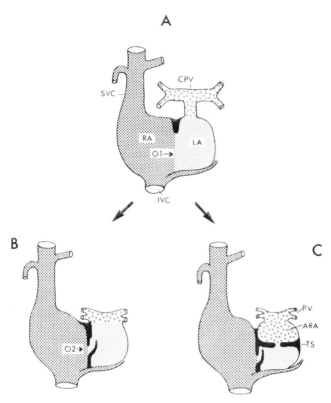

FIG. 15.50. Development of the pulmonary veins. (A) Normal stage of connection of the common pulmonary vein to the left atrium. (B) Normal absorption of the common pulmonary vein into the left atrium. (C) Abnormal incorporation of a dilated common pulmonary vein *without* absorption into the primitive left atrial chamber, and with a small aperture between them, to give cor triatriatum.

ARA.	Accessory left atrial chamber.	O2.	Ostium secundum.
CPV.	Common pulmonary vein.	PV.	Pulmonary veins.
IVC.	Inferior vena cava.	RA.	Right atrium.
LA.	Left atrium.	SVC.	Superior vena cava.
O1.	Ostium primum.	TS.	Transverse septum.

bronchial veins which drain into the systemic system through the azygos veins.

Meanwhile, the sinus venosus has been absorbed into the right side of the primitive atrium, the primary and inter pulmonary veins are absorbed into the left side and subsequent atrial septation completes the separation of the systemic venous blood from the main pulmonary return flow.

COR TRIATRIATUM

This exceedingly rare malformation is due to the persistence of a flange between the common pulmonary vein and the left atrium. The result is an obstructing membrane, leading to usually severe pulmonary venous hypertension (Fig. 15.50). The clinical picture is the same as for severe congenital mitral stenosis, and neonatal presentation is typical. The plain film shows

non-specific cardiomegaly, which may be severe, and pulmonary oedema. Echocardiography can detect the membrane if it is not too close to the mitral valve. Surgical resection is hazardous but is the only hope.

ANOMALOUS PULMONARY VENOUS DRAINAGE

Morphology

The lungs originate as outgrowths of the pharynx, and their venous plexus initially drains into the systemic splanchnic circulation. The definitive pulmonary venous flow is brought about by condensation of a secondary plexus to form a transverse common pulmonary vein which joins an outgrowth from the left atrium and eventually becomes absorbed into the left atrial chamber. If this condensation and conjunction fails to occur normally, some or all of the pulmonary veins will open into one or more of the systemic veins, and so drain to the right atrium. Anomalous pulmonary venous drainage may be total or partial, and may be described as supracardiac, cardiac or infracardiac according to the level at which the pulmonary flow joins the systemic.

Supracardiac drainage enters the primary cardinal venous system, represented by the superior vena cava. Usually the lungs drain into a transverse common pulmonary vein from which an anomalous vertical vein ascends to open into the left extremity of the innominate vein at the confluence of the left subclavian and jugular veins (Fig. 15.51). The ascending vein generally passes in front of the left pulmonary artery but it may pass behind it and become liable to compression. Supracardiac drainage may also be into the superior vena cava directly, a persistent left superior vena cava or to an azygos vein.

Anomalous drainage at cardiac level may be into the right atrium directly or into the coronary sinus, which is the terminal portion of the left cardinal vein.

In infracardiac pulmonary venous drainage, an anomalous vertical vein passes downwards from the common pulmonary vein and pierces the diaphragm to join the portal vein (Fig. 15.52); the flow is generally obstructed by postnatal closure of the ductus venosus. In the mixed type the pulmonary venous flow enters the systemic system by more than one of the above mentioned routes in a variety of combinations.

Associated cardiac malformations are present in many cases and the foramen ovale always remains open. Visceral heterotaxy and splenic abnormalities are frequently present with the infracardiac type.

In partial anomalous pulmonary venous drainage the veins from one lung, part of a lung, or parts of both lungs, enter the systemic veins (Fig. 15.53) or the right atrium directly. The right lung is more frequently affected than the left. When drainage from the whole of one lung is involved the term *hemianomalous pulmonary*

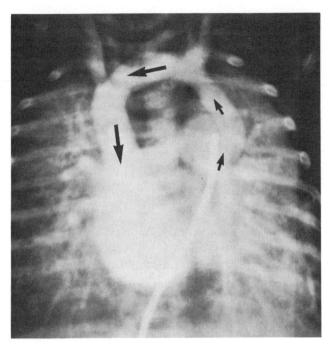

FIG. 15.51. Supracardiac totally anomalous pulmonary venous drainage. Pulmonary angiogram, venous phase. The pulmonary veins drain to an anomalous common vein (short arrow) and thence to the left innominate vein and superior vena cava (long arrows).

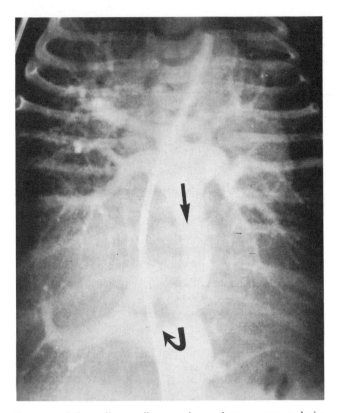

FIG. 15.52. Infracardiac totally anomalous pulmonary venous drainage. Pulmonary angiogram, venous phase. Pulmonary venous blood flows down to a common vein (straight arrow) to drain into the portal venous system (curved arrow).

venous drainage is appropriate. Partial anomalous drainage of the right upper lobe is frequently a complication of sinus venosus atrial septal defect.

Haemodynamics

In totally anomalous pulmonary venous drainage (TAPVD) all pulmonary and systemic venous return passes to the right atrium and so there is a common mixing situation. However, it is complicated by pulmonary venous hypertension in all cases of infradiaphragmatic drainage as the portal venous bed is moderately obstructive to flow. Some cases of supracardiac drainage also are obstructed by stenosis of the anomalous vein. The obstructed varieties present in neonatal or early infant life; unobstructed presentation may be delayed until adult life.

Partial anomalous drainage acts as a moderate but obligatory left to right shunt at atrial level, which is seldom large; these cases present clinically like an uncomplicated atrial septal defect.

Radiology

Those cases of totally anomalous drainage with obstructed return show either a normal heart size or mild cardiomegaly of non-specific shape. The lungs will usually show considerable evidence of pulmonary venous hypertension (Fig. 15.54).

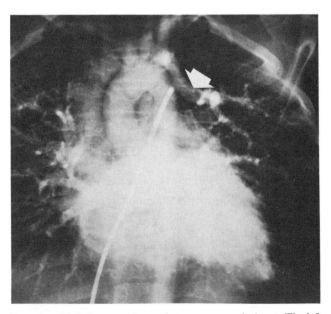

FIG. 15.53. Partially anomalous pulmonary venous drainage. The left upper pulmonary vein (arrow) drains to the left innominate vein.

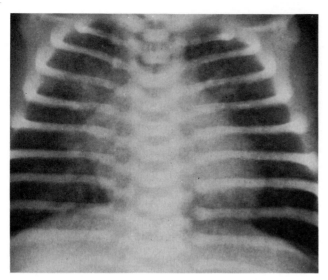

FIG. 15.54. Infracardiac TAPVD. Mild cardiomegaly; alveolar pulmonary oedema due to pulmonary venous obstruction.

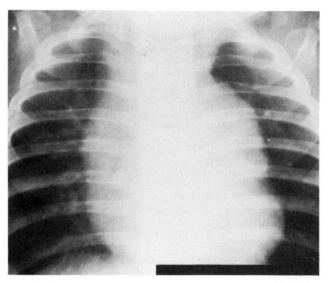

FIG. 15.55. Supracardiac TAPVD. 'Cottage loaf' shape.

The unobstructed varieties show plethora and cardiomegaly which are more severe in less cyanosed patients. The cardiac shape is often non-specific but the supracardiac types usually have a broad upper mediastinum which is due to the dilated anomalous vein on the left and a dilated superior vena cava on the right. The appearance is likened to a 'cottage loaf' or 'snowman' (Fig. 15.55).

Partial anomalous drainage also causes cardiomegaly and plethora but usually these signs are partly or mainly due to an associated atrial septal defect. The anomalous vein can not be reliably identified on the plain film.

Echocardiography

A two-dimensional 'real time' scanner of reasonable quality can usually identify pulmonary veins as they enter the left atrium. It is not possible to identify the absence of a solitary vein; in any event the number of orifices is not constant in the normal. There are claims, however, that totally anomalous drainage can be reliably identified; apart from the total lack of any pulmonary vein orifice, the left atrium and ventricle are small, the right ventricle is volume overloaded and not infrequently the anomalous common pulmonary vein can be identified as a chamber as large as the left atrium and lying just posterior to it (Fig. 15.56).

Management

Direct anastomosis of the anomalous vein to the posterior wall of the left atrium is advocated for all cases of totally anomalous drainage; this carries a reasonable

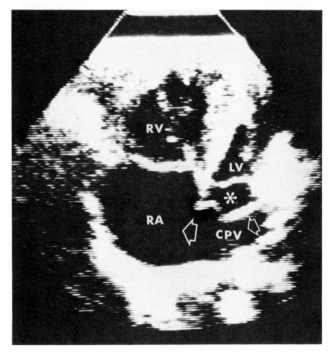

FIG. 15.56. TAPVD. Echocardiogram, apical four chamber view. The left atrium (star) and ventricle are small. Posterior to the left atrium is the common pulmonary vein (CPV) which in this case drains directly, as the coronary sinus, to the right atrium.

chance of success. Partial anomalous drainage associated with an atrial septal defect is repaired when the ASD is closed. Uncomplicated cases of partial anomalous drainage are probably best left alone.

HYPOGENETIC RIGHT LUNG SYNDROME

Morphology. This is a particular form of hemianomalous pulmonary venous drainage and is also known as the 'Scimitar syndrome'. All the veins of the right lung join to form a vertical vein which passes parallel to the right heart border to drain to the inferior vena cava at the level of the diaphragm (Fig. 15.57a). The right lung is hypogenetic and the mediastinum is displaced to the right. The lung architecture is not as abnormal as a dysplastic lung, but often it has no external fissures. The right pulmonary artery is reasonably normal but a variable amount of the lung is supplied by one or more aortic collateral vessels from the abdominal aorta; these vessels can be quite large (Fig. 15.57b). There is often an atrial septal defect.

Haemodynamics. An effective left to right shunt of 2:1 might be anticipated. In fact it is often greater because of the high pressure flow from the aortic collaterals.

Radiology (Fig.15.58). The mediastinum is displaced to the right and the right lung is small. The vascularity of both the affected and unaffected lungs is usually increased. The heart may be enlarged. In many cases the common pulmonary vein on the right is seen as a vertical vascular marking passing from mid lung down to the right diaphragm, and its shape gives rise to the condition being known as 'scimitar syndrome'.

Management. The large shunt usually results in pulmonary hypertension and demands relief. Total

correction is far from easy but is sometimes achieved. A useful palliation can often be achieved when the aortic collaterals are large, by ligating them at right thoracotomy or by catheter embolisation of them.

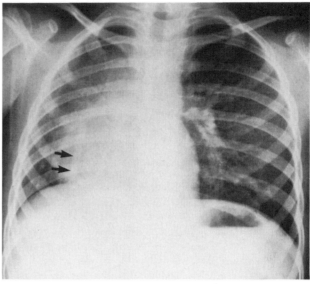

FIG. 15.58. Scimitar syndrome. Same case as in 15.57. One of the vertical veins (arrows) forms the 'scimitar' shadow. The right lung is hypogenetic.

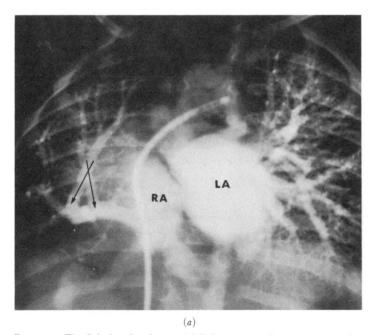

(a)

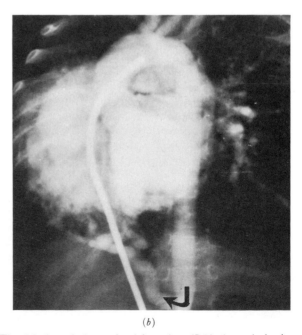

(b)

FIG. 15.57. The Scimitar Syndrome. (a) Pulmonary angiogram, venous phase. The right lung drains to the right atrium (RA) via vertical veins (arrows). The left lung drains normally to the left atrium (LA). (b) A later frame shows a large aortic collateral from the abdominal aorta perfusing the right lower lung field.

INTERRUPTION OF THE INFERIOR VENA CAVA

This is usually associated with left atrial isomerism and is due to failure of development of the hepatic portion of the inferior vena cava. Venous flow from the lower half of the body, apart from the hepatic veins, passes mainly via an enlarged azygos vein to the superior vena cava (Fig. 15.59). Dilation of the azygos is often visible on the plain chest film in the older child or adult (Fig. 15.60, also Fig. 14.3). Echocardiography is quite reliable for the diagnosis as there is no sign of the intrahepatic segment of the inferior vena cava; care has to be taken not to confuse a large hepatic vein (which will drain directly into the right atrium) with the inferior vena cava.

LEFT SUPERIOR VENA CAVA

This is a frequent anomaly which may complicate any other cardiac malformation. It is due to persistence of the left anterior cardinal vein which otherwise would have become the coronary sinus. It drains usually to the right atrium, entering in the same position as the coronary sinus in the normal (Fig. 15.61). Occasionally it may drain to the left-sided atrium; this usually means that there is atrial isomerism. On the plain film it may be seen as a straight border slightly laterally up the left upper mediastinal border (Fig. 15.62), but it is often lost within the shadow of the thymus. There is no distinctive echocardiographic feature.

CARDIAC SURGERY FOR CONGENITAL DISEASE

Corrective Procedures

These are the operations which return the heart to a reasonably normal morphology and function. They include the simple closures of atrial and ventricular septal defects, valvotomies, coarctation repair and correction of tetralogy of Fallot. Also in this group is the *switch* operation for transposition, where the aorta and pulmonary artery trunks are detached and replaced in their correct position. Many of these procedures involve a ventriculotomy, usually through the right ventricle. The scar that results can form a fibrous aneurysm (Fig. 15.63) which may calcify (Fig. 15.64).

Physiological Correction

Some operations correct the physiology of the malformation but not the gross morphology.

Atrial redirection (Mustard or Senning procedures).This involves the removal of the atrial septum and the insertion of a patch of synthetic material or pericardium in such a way that the pattern of atrio-

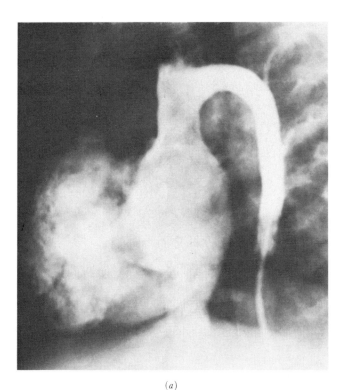

(a)

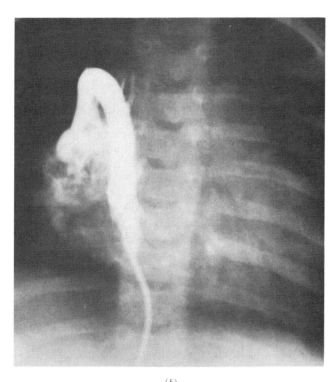

(b)

FIG. 15.59. Interrupted inferior vena cava. The azygos vein is enlarged as it is the main route of venous return from the lower half of the body. Selective angiogram, (a) lateral and (b) frontal views.

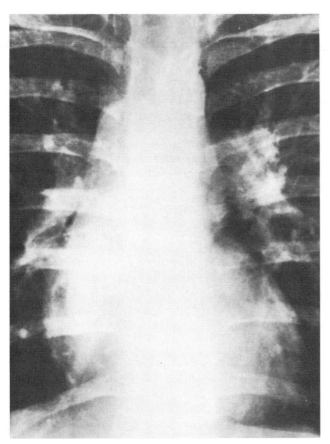

FIG. 15.60. Interrupted IVC. Plain film showing enlargement of the azygos vein.

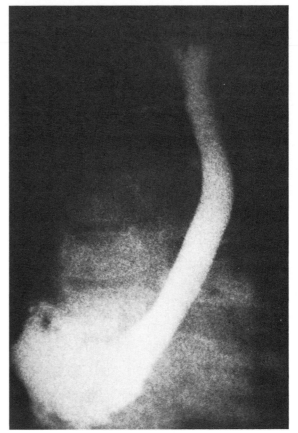

FIG. 15.61. Left superior vena cava. Selective angiogram shows it draining to the right atrium.

ventricular drainage is reversed (Fig. 15.65). It is mostly used for transposition of the great arteries; systemic venous return is led over to the left ventricle and then to the pulmonary artery; pulmonary venous flow is taken to the right ventricle and thence to the aorta. The results in the short term can be dramatically good but there is concern that the right ventricle, which remains as the systemic ventricle, may fail early in adult life. One of the three venous channels (superior systemic, inferior systemic or pulmonary venous) may develop obstruction or stenosis.

The Rastelli procedure. Some cases of severe tetralogy of Fallot, transposition with ventricular septal defect, and double outlet right ventricle with VSD are repaired by this operation. The VSD is closed with a patch that angles across to include the aortic orifice in the left ventricle, but in so doing it compromises the pulmonary orifice. The right ventricle is therefore connected to the pulmonary arteries by a prosthetic conduit (Fig. 15.66). The procedure can also be used to correct malformations that are complicated by unrelievable pulmonary stenosis. The conduit usually undergoes

slow fibrosis and distortion, and may calcify (Fig. 15.67).

The Fontan Procedure involves the connection of the pulmonary arteries with the right atrium either directly or by a conduit; it is used to overcome situations where there is only one functioning ventricle. To be successful, pulmonary resistance must be low.

Valve Replacement

In the paediatric age group this is complicated firstly by the patients growth, which may quickly make a prosthetic valve relatively too small, and secondly by a high rate of calcification of tissue valves.

Palliative Shunts

Systemic artery to pulmonary artery shunts are designed to improve pulmonary blood flow in cyanotic disease by perfusing the lungs with desaturated systemic blood. They may be complicated by secondary pulmonary hypertension or by surgical stenosis of the implanted pulmonary artery.

The Blalock-Taussig shunt is an end to side anas-

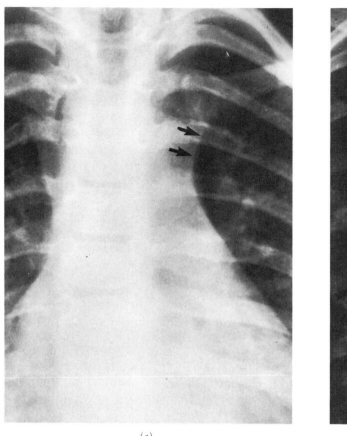

(a)

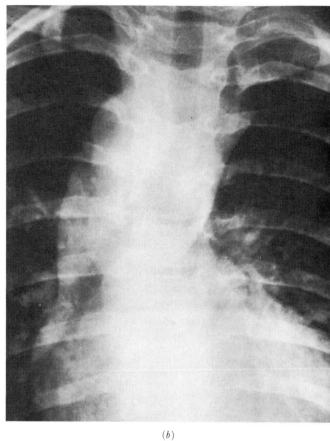

(b)

FIG. 15.62. Left superior vena cava. The vessel shows as a straight left upper mediastinal border which does not extend above the clavicle. (a) The vein is arrowed on this typical film. (b) The vein is more prominent in this case where there is a right aortic arch.

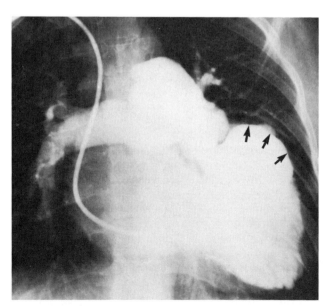

FIG. 15.63. Right ventricular aneurysm (arrows) at the site of a previous right ventriculotomy.

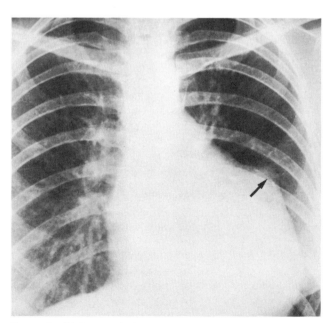

FIG. 15.64. Right ventricular aneurysm (same case as Fig. 15.63). Plain film shows linear calcification of the aneurysm.

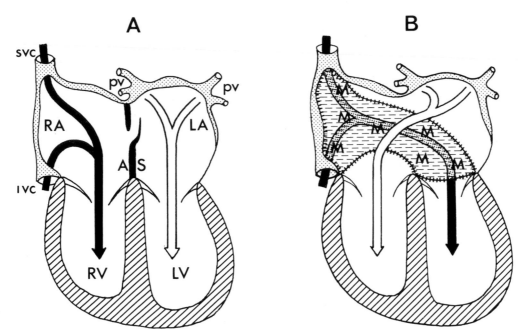

FIG. 16.65. Atrial redirection. (A) Pre-operative state; systemic blood from the superior (SVC) and inferior (IVC) vena cavae passes via the right atrium (RA) to the right ventricle (RV), whilst pulmonary return goes via left atrium (LA) to left ventricle (LV). The atrial septum (AS) is intact. (B) After a Mustard type of redirection; the atrial septum is removed and the Mustard baffle (M) switches the atrial flows.

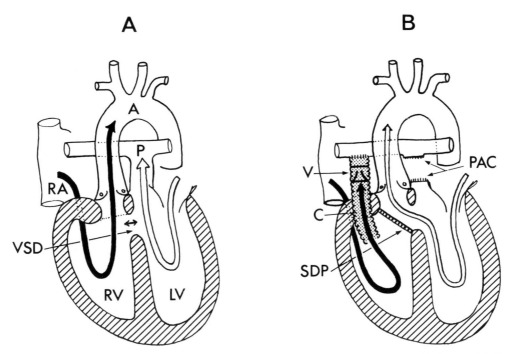

FIG. 15.66. The Rastelli procedure. Here shown as a repair for transposition of the great arteries with ventricular septal defect (VSD). (A) pre-operative anatomy. (B) Post-operative result. The VSD is closed with a septal defect patch (SDP) so as to include the aorta in the effective left ventricle, the main pulmonary artery is closed (PAC) and the right ventricle is connected to the pulmonary arteries by a prosthetic conduit (C) which may contain a tissue valve (V).

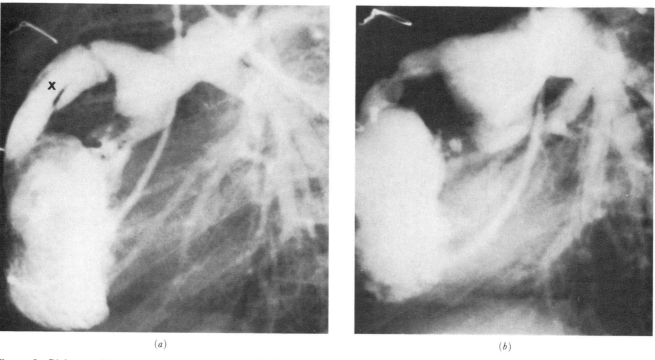

(a)   (b)

FIG. 15.67. Right ventricle to pulmonary artery conduit. (a) Soon after surgery. This particular type contains a valve (X). (b) Some years later, the conduit has fibrosed and stenosed.

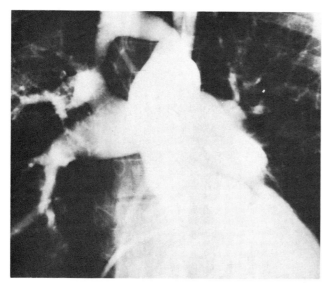

FIG. 15.68. Right Blalock-Taussig shunt (here into the right upper lobar pulmonary artery).

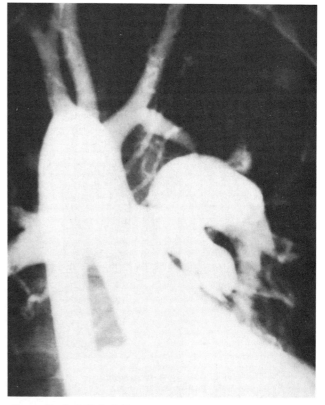

FIG. 15.69. Left Blalock-Taussig shunt. Note the right aortic arch.

tomosis of either subclavian artery to the ipselateral pulmonary artery (Fig. 15.68, 15.69). There is the risk of over perfusion of the lung on the same side as the shunt (Fig. 15.70). Blood supply to the ipselateral arm is interrupted but this has surprisingly little effect.

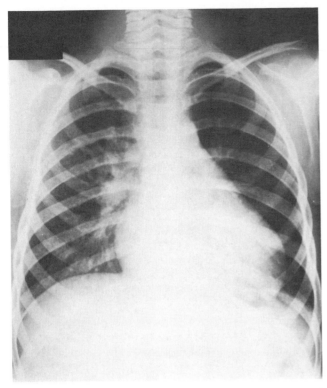

Fig. 15.70. Right Blalock-Taussig shunt. Plain film shows preferential flow to the right lung.

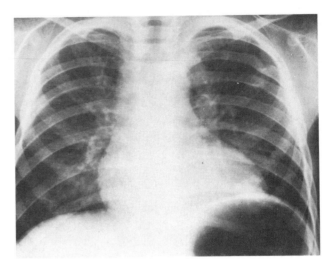

Fig. 15.71. Left Blalock-Taussig shunt. The displaced left subclavian artery forms a shadow just lateral to the upper left heart border. Note the notched left fifth rib.

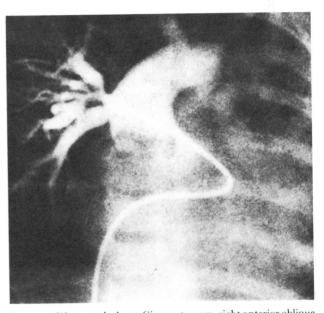

Fig. 15.72. Waterston's shunt. Cine aortogram, right anterior oblique. There is no retrograde filling of the pulmonary arteries to the left of the anastomosis.

Collaterals to the arm develop and can notch the upper ribs on the affected side (Fig. 15.71).

Waterston's procedure is a side to side anastomosis of the ascending aorta and the right pulmonary artery (Fig. 15.72); this can severely stenose the pulmonary artery and sometimes lead to acquired atresia of it.

Potts' operation is a side to side anastomosis of the descending aorta with the left pulmonary artery.

Anterior shunts between the ascending aorta and main pulmonary artery may be direct (Davidson's) or via a short prosthetic conduit.

Systemic vein to pulmonary artery shunts are more physiological in their action but need a very low pulmonary artery pressure to be effective.

The Glenn procedure is an end to side anastomosis of the superior vena cava and the right pulmonary artery with ligation of the proximal pulmonary artery to encourage flow. Abrams' procedure is a side to side anastomosis of the two, without ligation of the pulmonary artery.

Pulmonary Artery Banding

Large shunts, and common mixing situations with high pulmonary flow, may be palliated by narrowing the main pulmonary artery with a band of nylon tape (Fig. 15.73). The effect is to simulate pulmonary stenosis, reduce pulmonary blood flow and protect the lungs from pulmonary vascular occlusive disease. Unfortunately, the debanding procedure ultimately required carries a significant mortality. Many centres have found that early total correction often carries less risk than early banding and late repair with debanding.

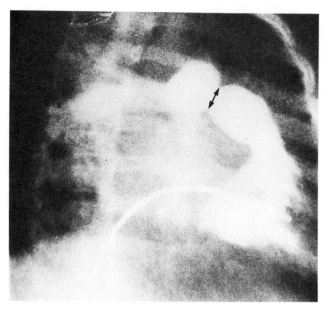

FIG. 15.73. Pulmonary artery band (arrow). Right ventricular cine angiogram, right anterior oblique.

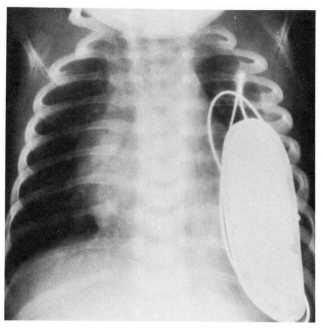

FIG. 15.74. Pacemaker in the left pleural cavity of a neonate. Congenital heart block.

Pacemakers

Artificial pacemakers are occasionally required in childhood, generally for complete heart block after VSD closure, but also for the 'sick sinus syndrome' ('bradytachycardia syndrome'), and very occasionally for congenital heart block (Fig. 15.74).

FURTHER READING

SHUFORD, W. H. & SYBERS, G. (1974) *The Aortic Arch and its Malformations*. Illinois: Charles C. Thomas.

CHAPTER 16

DISEASES OF THE PERIPHERAL ARTERIES

Alan Hugh

PLAIN FILM

Although plain films are frequently requested in suspected arterial disease, they are of very limited clinical value, since arterial calcification is a very frequent radiological finding. The reason for this is that most arterial calcification is not accompanied by a corresponding luminal obliteration. In older people, calcification of the media of the vessel is more likely to be a sign of longstanding hypertension. This type of calcification is termed dystrophic calcification and, when widespread (which is most common in the arteries of the lower limbs) is termed Monckeberg's sclerosis.

Calcification is of importance to the radiologist in the plain film detection of aortic and other aneurysms. A lateral film of the abdomen taken with low kV may well show patchy calcific plaques in a vessel clearly of a diameter greater than that of a normal abdominal aorta. Most aneurysms contain layered clot, so that an indication of the vessel lumen cannot be derived, but serial films are of some value in assessing the progress of an otherwise untreated aneurysm.

Calcification in arm arteries is very much less common than in the leg vessels, as is the incidence of atheroma. Although atheroma may become calcified there is a poor correlation between the dystrophic calcification of the media of an artery already mentioned and the amount of atheroma within its lumen, slightly surprising because in both atheroma and arteriosclerosis, hypertension is a common predisposing condition. Possibly, more attention will be paid to atheromatous calcification following a report that calcification can be detected in the internal carotid origin using C.T. Using soft tissue techniques normally used for mammography, Hugh and Eggleton (unpublished) have demonstrated flecks of calcification in the internal carotid origin undetectable using normal radiographic factors. Again, in this situation, there appears to be little correlation between wall calcification and the deposition of atheroma.

There is an increased incidence of arterial calcification in peripheral arteries in diabetic patients, and in other conditions where there may be hyperlipaemia. This is probably a variety of dystrophic calcification, where a mixture of hypertension and abnormal blood content are also relevant, together with local infection (Fig. 16.01).

The alternative type of arterial calcification is less common than dystrophic calcification and is termed 'metastatic' calcification. It is usually a manifestation of a metabolic disease with an elevated serum calcium-phosphate product, e.g. hyperparathyroidism, and is not accompanied by clinical evidence of arterial insufficiency even though on occasion there may be sufficient calcium deposited for the radiographic appearances to resemble an angiogram. Unlike dystrophic calcification, metastatic calcification can regress if the underlying condition is treated or alters, and is seen equally in both upper and lower limbs, particularly in the smaller arteries of the hands and feet. Why metastatic calcification is seen in the walls of arteries but not veins is conjectural. Pressure must be of importance in relation to dystrophic calcification because pulmonary artery calcification is only seen in pulmonary hypertension.

TRANSVENOUS ARTERIOGRAPHY

Digital Subtraction Imaging. The transvenous approach to the arterial system, at one time the only one available, is enjoying a resurgence of interest because of the introduction of computer techniques to the well established principle of 'image subtraction'. 'Subtraction' consists of taking two films of the region of interest, one directly before or after, and one during the presence of contrast medium. If the control film is reversed photographically and superimposed upon the film with contrast agent, provided the reversal density is appropriate, the black and white images of the bones cancel out, leaving a clear image of the contrasted vessel (Fig. 16.02). This technique is simple and can be done by dark room staff, and is considered to be a standard requirement by some radiologists, particularly for studies of the aortic arch and its major branches in the neck and head.

The introduction of computers has allowed venous injections to produce adequate pictures of arteries; the technique is also described as 'digital vascular arteriography (DVA)' or 'digital vascular imaging (DVI)'. Instead of using X-ray films, the X-ray information emerging from the patient is captured by a fluoroscopic image intensifier as in conventional fluoroscopy. The

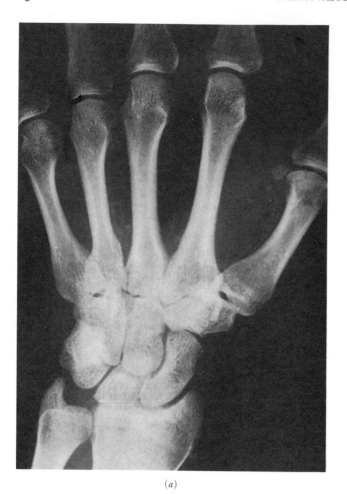

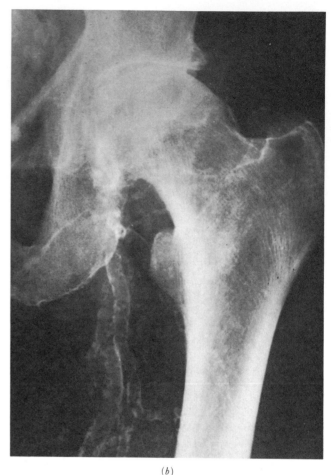

(a)   (b)

FIG. 16.01. Arterial calcification in a diabetic patient.

resulting intensified light image is scanned by a TV camera and is fed to an 'analogue-to-digital' converter, which transposes the image into a digital form. This is stored in a computer which is equipped with a double memory. One (or a number) of control images are stored in one memory, and 'reversed' by the computer to form a 'mask' image; further images are stored on the second memory at the appropriate time following a bolus injection of contrast medium given intravenously. The computer subtracts the mask image from the contrasted ones, enhances the contrast of the residual image, i.e. the opacified vessels, and displays the resulting image on a video display unit from which a photographic image can be taken. Provided that there has been little or no patient movement between the control and opacified images, the resulting arterial image can be of excellent diagnostic quality, allowing a display of atheromatous lesions in the neck and head, and other peripheral vessels (Fig. 16.03).

Movement artefacts, limited field size and cost are the major drawbacks preventing this out-patient technique supplanting conventional angiography, where contrast has to be introduced directly into the arterial system with the attendant problems of an in-patient procedure and possible complications.

Conventional radiographic venous angiography can be supplemented with xeroradiography, tomography or photographic subtraction, and can be used to distinguish between aortic aneurysms and other abdominal masses when more sophisticated techniques are not available or advisable.

Enhanced computer tomography. Soon after the introduction of computer tomography it became obvious that an intravenous injection of contrast would 'enhance' the visibility of certain intracerebral tumours and other vascular abnormalities. The development of scanners with much shorter scanning times has resulted in vascular abnormalities being detected and demonstrated in other parts of the body (dynamic scanning), using either venous (Fig. 16.04) or, sometimes, selective

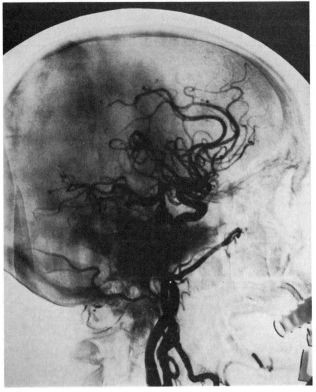

FIG. 16.02. Photographic subtraction (persistent trigeminal artery).

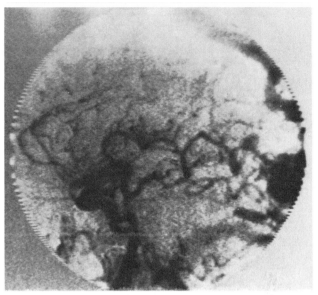

FIG. 16.03. Digital (computed) subtraction of carotid angiogram.

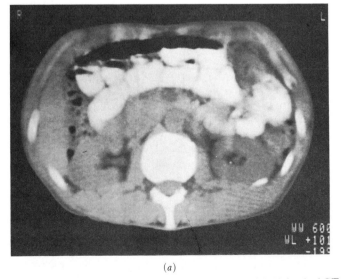
(a)

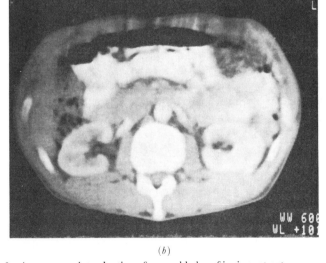
(b)

FIG. 16.04. (a) Abdominal CT before contrast. (b) Abdominal CT after intravenous introduction of a 50 ml bolus of ionic contrast.

arterial contrast injection (Fig. 16.05) to opacify larger arteries and veins. The 'hot flush' experienced by the patient shortly after the intravenous introduction of a bolus of conventional (ionic) contrast medium signifies that the contrast has reached the arterial side of the circulation and may be used to time the scan for arterial imaging. Dynamic scanning, using high and low kV pulses, allows flow studies through a particular organ to be carried out, i.e. build-up and clearance factors, in the same way as computer-connected gamma cameras.

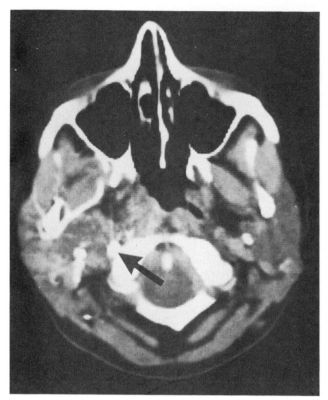

FIG. 16.05. CT of neck with selective introduction of contrast into the right common carotid artery. Recurrent tonsillar tumour.

ARTERIAL INTRODUCTION OF CONTRAST MEDIUM

Arteriography has been practised in various ways for over half a century. During this time, many techniques have been used and every named vessel has been demonstrated radiographically for some purpose or other. The first record of angiography is by a Frenchman named Moniz who, in 1927, described the localisation of cerebral tumours radiographically. Following this, direct arterial needle puncture was supplemented by a number of important advances. The advent of catheters, the ability to introduce catheters into arteries without directly opening the artery, and radio-opaque and steerable catheters, malleable for selective insertion into branch vessels, have resulted in arteriography becoming a highly sophisticated technique. Simultaneously, improvements in contrast media, injection pumps, X-ray tubes, generators, image intensifiers and film changers have brought about a situation where arteriography can be easily and safely practised in any hospital or clinic possessing a reasonable X-ray set. The reduction in demand for arteriography due to the introduction of other imaging techniques and alternative diagnostic tools will probably result in less purpose-built angiographic suites in the future than has been fashionable in recent years.

There are two possible major approaches to arterial injection; direct puncture by needle with injection of contrast locally, and catheter techniques where the contrast medium is injected some distance from where the catheter enters the artery.

Direct Needle Injection

This technique has been extensively employed in the past, no major vessel being safe from puncture at the hands of an enthusiastic operator. Currently, the common carotid artery in the neck, the lumbar aorta and the femoral artery are the ones commonly examined by this technique, and an increasingly used refinement is one where the metal needle is covered by a Teflon sheath, so that once the vessel is successfully entered, the needle can be withdrawn leaving a blunt flexible plastic tube within the artery rather than a sharp bevelled needle tip, whose movement during injection might cause trauma to the arterial media. The use of a sheath in this way has a drawback, namely that on withdrawal of the needle there is a free flow of blood before a syringe or extension tube is attached; this also means that there is a possibility of the connection blowing apart when a forceful injection is made unless a 'lock' connection is used, and even so, the free arterial flow might panic the inexperienced into a faulty connection. In all direct puncture examinations, where the operator has an assistant, he should ensure that the assistant realises that owing to the obliquity of the needle entry, the puncture in the skin does not lie directly over the puncture in the artery, and that if arterial compression were needed in the absence of the operator, e.g. while films were being viewed, pressure should be applied upstream rather than downstream of the puncture in the artery. This is particularly important in retrograde femoral puncture, both for needle and catheter examinations.

Carotid Arteriography. The common carotid artery is a very accessible vessel. In experienced hands it can be easily and safely punctured, as it can be localised and immobilised by two fingers of one hand, and the needle inserted with the other hand. Disposable combinations of prejoined 18 gauge needle with 35 cm of plastic connection to attach to a Luer fitting syringe are available, very suitable for direct puncture carotid angiography. The needle and connector are filled with saline and the plastic connector clamped with forceps to retain the saline within the syringe until the needle tip has pierced the skin, but released before the artery is punctured. This prevents air being sucked into a negative pressure jugular vein and allows a clean, blood-free surface from which the operator and assistant can work. If the vessel is transfixed and the needle withdrawn at a lower angle than it was introduced, a distinct 'click' is felt and the operator will know that the tip of the needle is safely within the lumen of the vessel. If this is not felt, or if the flow-back of blood is not clearly of the arterial spurting variety, it is wise to remove the needle, compress the vessel at the puncture point, and repeat the procedure after a few minutes. The artery should be entered as low in the neck as is reasonably possible, as the carotid bifurcation is quite variable in position and can be surprisingly low; however, too low an entry produces the possibility of a pneumothorax as the apex of the lung lies appreciably above the clavicle.

Another hazard of carotid puncture is entry into the jugular vein, which lies adjacent to the carotid artery. The negative pressure here tends to suck saline from the needle and syringe connection and air embolisation could occur if this possibility was not realised. A further complication of direct carotid puncture is haematoma, either into the carotid sheath or into the neck tissues. Before proceeding to a bilateral examination, the operator should be satisfied that bleeding on the first side has completely stopped; once a sizeable haematoma has developed, effective arterial compression is difficult and widespread pressure on the side of the neck is necessary, which displaces the trachea and the opposite carotid sheath and which may dislodge a needle in the other carotid artery, causing a bilateral haematoma. Tracheal and carotid body compression and breathing difficulty can arise in this situation necessitating prolonged compression or emergency tracheal intubation, and possibly surgical evacuation of the haematoma.

The blind introduction of a catheter into the common carotid artery is a procedure whose advisability is the subject of debate, owing to the possible dislodgement of a thrombus or atheromatous plaque lying at the internal carotid origin (Fig. 16.06). The author considers this to be a dangerous practice in patients suspected of having cerebrovascular disease, or in any patient over 40.

Translumbar Arteriography. This is largely used in cases of severe disease or blockages of the aortic bifurcation or iliac vessels, where the femoral pulses are poor or absent. This technique has in the past also been used for renal angiography, the 'high lumbar' technique, but has been largely superseded by catheter examinations. This examination dates back to the work of Dos Santos and his colleagues who described their technique in 1929. It can be carried out under local anaesthesia, using modern pain-relieving and tranquillising drugs, without the problems of maintaining general anaesthesia in a prone patient. The level of puncture, approximately at the body of the 3rd lumbar vertebra, is best determined by placing three lead dots on the patient's back when the control film is taken. The angle of entry recommended is 45° to the sagittal plane on the patient's left side, the point of entry being 'a hand's breadth' from the midline. It is left to the experience of the operator to decide if this shall be the width of the

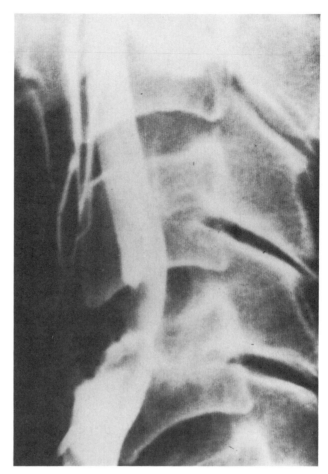

FIG. 16.06. Large thrombus at carotid bifurcation lying at needle tip. Blind introduction of catheter might have dislodged this.

patient's or the operator's hand. Good local anaesthesia is humane; the remote possibility of entering the spinal canal should be borne in mind, and infiltration with local anaesthesia should not be excessive. An 18 gauge Teflon-covered needle of approximately 20 cm should be used. Bony obstruction about 5 cm from the skin suggests that a transverse process has been encountered, whereupon the needle should be aimed slightly higher or lower. The chief point at this time should be to contact the side of the vertebral body, when the needle can be withdrawn slightly and reinserted at a slightly steeper angle. The experienced operator can usually sense the pulsation of the aorta, and its penetration by the needle; frequently, however, the aortic lumen is transfixed, and discovered when the needle or catheter is gently withdrawn after having its stylet removed. Once the aortic lumen is entered, it is sometimes possible to advance the Teflon catheter up or down the aortic lumen by inserting a guide wire with a curved tip. The desirability of this is debatable, depending on how cleanly the aorta has been entered, because the amount of recoil of the catheter during injection is very small because of the large mass of tissue which has been transfixed. Some operators prefer to screen the patient at this point, to determine whether they have entered the aortic lumen or one of its branches, by injection of a small quantity of contrast. In the event of a complete distal aortic blockage, this may shorten the procedure by enabling better timing of subsequent serial film taking.

Once the operator is satisfied that the aortic lumen has been successfully cannulated, he must decide whether to do a hand or pump injection. If he has doubt about the cleanliness of his entry, it is preferable to take a series of films using a hand injection of 20–30 ml of contrast medium. Pump injections can safely be carried out if the catheter has been passed along the aortic lumen.

When a satisfactory series of films has been obtained, the catheter should be withdrawn as soon as possible. Withdrawing a comparatively large catheter from a vessel as large and as remote as the aorta is disconcerting to many radiologists; however, in practice, there appears to be no problem, even though surgeons have sometimes found a 1–2 pint haematoma when carrying out a sympathectomy shortly after. It is advisable to instruct the nursing staff to watch pulse rate and blood pressure for 3 hours after the procedure.

Complications of this procedure include renal or mesenteric artery occlusion, intimal stripping and paraplegia, the latter presumably due to direct injection into one of the lumbar vessels supplying the lower spinal cord. Severe pain in the back directly after the injection suggests that some or all of the contrast medium has extravasated. The pain will subside after a little while and it is unlikely that any damage will ensue. Entry into the spinal canal has been recorded also. Considering the other possible hazards, such as damage to intestine, the technique has enjoyed very wide use by many operators of widely varying experience, and can be regarded as an acceptably safe clinical procedure.

Brachial or Axillary Puncture. These have limited application; they can be used for retrograde or distal examination, but have largely been superseded by catheter examinations via femoral puncture. The brachial artery has a considerable potential for spasm and, if injured above the origins of its lower branch vessels, can have ischaemic effects in the hand. The axillary artery appears to be a safer artery but, lying in close proximity to the axillary plexus nerves, it offers considerable scope for a painful procedure in the non-anaesthetised patient, particularly as extensive anaesthetic infiltration is to be avoided, and the abducted arm has to be held in a fairly critical degree of rotation if the arterial pulsation is to be easily and stably felt. It can be a useful artery to use in patients in whom a

dissecting aortic aneurysm is suspected, in patients whose vertebral arteries are otherwise inaccessible and in those patients whose lower aorta is blocked and a translumbar approach is inadvisable or has failed.

Catheter Arteriography

This is the preferred method of introducing contrast medium into arteries in many cases, as it allows a controlled introduction of contrast into quite small branches of major vessels – 'selective arteriography'. The development of percutaneous introduction of catheters into arteries by Seldinger (1953) can be regarded as one of the milestones of radiology, not just of angiography. The alternative, direct introduction of a catheter into an artery by arteriotomy following surgical dissection, has the merit of allowing the introduction of a blunt ended catheter in which the absence of a terminal hole reduced recoil during forceful injections, but requires surgical skill, an open wound with its possible septic complications, and the facilities for a fairly long procedure. It is largely employed for angiocardiography and some types of coronary angiography.

The Seldinger Technique. This is a brilliantly simple technique, consisting of entry of the vessel with a hollow needle, the introduction of a flexible guide wire through the needle, and the subsequent introduction of a flexible open-ended catheter over the guide wire once the needle itself has been withdrawn. The series of stages are shown in the diagram (Fig. 16.07).

Since the introduction of the technique, each part of it has enjoyed a series of refinements.

The needle. During its introduction the lumen of the needle is occupied by a matching obturator or stylet. The length of the needle is usually about 7 cm, and the gauge of the needle is matched with that of the guide wire and catheter to be employed. A wide variety of needle combinations is now available, disposable or otherwise, whose bevelled sharpness can be guaranteed. Also important is for the needle to have a bevelled entry from its wide mouth into its lumen to facilitate the passage of the guide wire or re-entry of the stylet. The diameter of the needle should be no greater than is necessary, but should allow sufficient rigidity to enable the operator to guide the needle through the soft tissues and to chase a mobile artery.

The guide wire. Many types are available. Most consist of a central core with a spirally wound metal covering. The core may be metal or plastic. Some guides are solid plastic. The terminal portion of the wire has a much less rigid core, so that it is more flexible than the rest of the catheter. This is the tip which is advanced into the vessel and the flexibility is intended to guide the wire around curves in vessels, and also to prevent damage to the arterial intima and any atheromatous plaques thereon. One advance was the introduction of guide wires with preformed curved tips, and currently popular

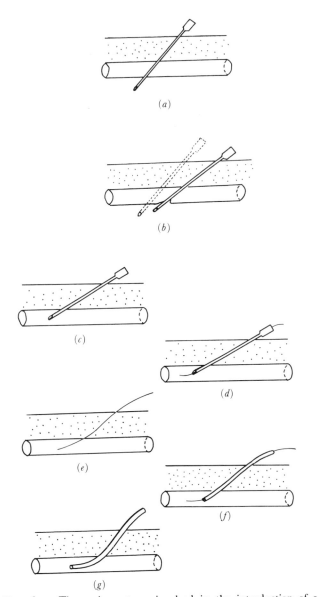

FIG. 16.07. The various stages involved in the introduction of a catheter into a vessel using the Seldinger technique.

has become kinked, because one of the hazards of Seldinger arteriography is detachment of the tip of a guide wire. An important consideration is the smoothness of the surface of the guide wire (and catheter). Even a short exposure to blood results in a deposition of fibrin and platelets on their surfaces, and roughness increases this deposition. It is important, therefore, for guide wires to be as smooth as is reasonably possible, and this is one reason why 'plastic' wires have been considered an advance.

The Catheter. Originally, catheters were not radio-opaque, and their position was determined by opacifying them with contrast injections. A marked advance was the introduction of a radio-opaque material into their wall, allowing much easier selective arterial entry, particularly as this advance came about before the introduction of image intensifiers. Opaque and non-opaque catheters in an infinite variety of sizes and pre-formed shapes are now available, to be chosen depending on their intended use and the preference of the individual operator, and some radiologists still prefer to preform catheters to their own requirements by bending a boiled segment of catheter to a particular shape and allowing it to cool. Many catheters have sideholes near their tips; these tend to reduce recoil due to the jet effect associated with purely end-hole catheters, and increase the flow rates where the catheter tip has a marked taper. However, the operator should remember that a clot can form between the terminal side-hole and the catheter tip, so that the catheter should be flushed vigorously with heparinised saline at fairly frequent intervals.

Contrast Media

These are not specific to arteriography, and manufacturers of media are very ready to point out the wide variety of uses of their newer, more expensive products. Most experienced arteriographers will be directly aware of the improvements which currently available media have produced due to reduced toxicity and better patient-acceptability. Important physical factors in contrast agents are low viscosity, to promote rapid injection rates, and good miscibility to reduce the risk of contrast-layering which can cause artefacts and possibly damage to nervous tissue.

The original contrast medium used for vascular examinations was a solution of thorium dioxide ('thorotrast'). This substance was taken up by the reticulo-endothelial system rather than being excreted (Fig. 16.08) and being slightly radioactive, it gave rise to malignant reactions in spleen, liver and abdominal lymph glands in a number of patients, and its use ceased. This complication was unfortunate; unlike the subsequently used iodine-containing ionic media, thorotrast did not cause cardiovascular reactions.

The original iodine-containing media, mainly sodium iodide, were extremely irritant, giving rise to consider-

guide wires have a flexible tip whose length and curvature can be controlled by moving the core within the guide wire from the outside end of the wire. Using these 'J tipped' guide wires, it is possible to traverse the most tortuous iliac vessels; failure to do so easily suggests complete arterial blockage, and the experienced operator does not persist in trying to force such a guide wire where it clearly cannot readily pass. Occasionally, the tip of a guide wire will enter a branch vessel and the wire will become bent over itself, causing a partial fracture. The wire will not then advance and should be withdrawn and discarded if it is seen that it

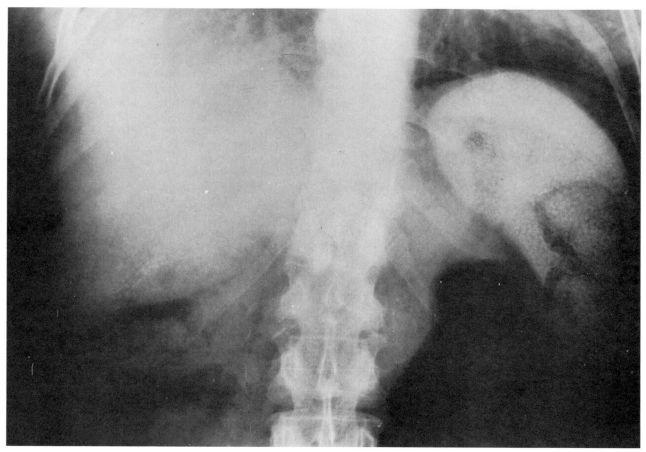

FIG. 16.08. Thorotrast liver and spleen. 25 years after carotid angiography. Malignant changes present in upper abdominal lymph glands.

able pain, nausea and vomiting, as well as on occasion an iodine sensitivity allergic-type reaction, whose severity might vary from mild urticaria to fatal cardiovascular collapse. Subsequently, the iodine was bound to various organic compounds to form salts. The effect of this was to reduce their irritative nature, but to increase their viscosity, thus reducing the rate at which they could be injected. Various mixtures of sodium and organic iodides are available, with different iodine concentrations, and are suitable for all vascular examinations. They are marketed under different trade names in different countries.

'Nonionic' contrast media are the most recent contrast innovation. These low osmolaric agents were introduced originally for intraspinal or nervous system opacification, but they have subsequently been used for other applications such as peripheral arteriography where they produce less pain on injection than hypertonic media. Currently, they are expensive by comparison with conventional media, and could not be recommended in situations where cost is a deciding factor as to whether arteriography should be carried out or not.

The situation is rapidly changing and the new nonionic media may well prove cost effective if they reduce the need for the presence of anaesthetists.

Anaesthesia

As with contrast media, personal preferences may be strong. It is almost axiomatic that the need for general anaesthesia varies inversely with the skill of the arteriologist; a good knowledge of currently available sedatives, tranquillisers and analgesics, plus an awareness that these each need separate consideration, will obviate the need for general anaesthesia in most peripheral examinations, particularly if the nonionic media can be justified on cost grounds. If general anaesthesia is employed, the anaesthetist should be instructed on the objectives of the technique so as to avoid the use of techniques which might introduce artefacts in the radiological appearances (such as hyperventilation).

Complications of Arteriography

Leaving aside complications related to the contrast media, most complications are specific to the technique employed and have been discussed above. One general hazard to be avoided is the inadvertent injection of fluid intended for skin sterilization instead of saline or contrast medium; this can happen when open bowls are used on the nursing trolley, particularly in a darkened room. All sterilizing fluids should be coloured and kept separate from fluids to be injected. Similarly, care should be taken to avoid the injection of air into the arterial system, particularly in the carotid circulation, although there is no factual information as to how much air can be introduced into the circulation without danger.

Complications of arterial puncture. Trauma to the intima may result in it stripping, so occluding the vessel lumen. This can happen without obvious evidence in the common carotid artery, because the tip of the needle lies proximal to the occlusion, and there is good arterial return from the needle. It is less likely with femoral puncture, where poor arterial return gives a rapid indication that the needle is not properly within the lumen. Sometimes, a carotid artery puncture can result in a carotid sheath haematoma. This probably results from bleeding due to a previously unrecognised arterial entry or inadequate compression of a previous puncture. Being comparatively unyielding, the carotid sheath can build up a substantial pressure and this can produce a good return of blood, fairly pulsatile, which can confuse even an experienced operator. Once a haematoma forms in this way, it is wise to try to postpone the procedure (a very large haematoma can cause tracheal compression) and bilateral examination in these circumstances can be disastrous. The injection of hyalase is claimed to speed the resolution of clot; one fortunate sequel of haematoma is that an artery which has been 'fixed' in position by clot for a week becomes a much easier vessel to penetrate subsequently, except that repeated examinations of the same vessel over the years can result in its becoming encased by an almost impenetrable sheath of fibrous tissue.

Clumsy penetration of the arterial wall, especially if a catheter tip has become damaged and blunted at a previous attempt, may result in a small tear in the arterial wall. This can cause continued bleeding at the puncture site throughout the procedure, particularly if the catheter is changed for a smaller one, and either cause a haematoma or give rise to excessive bleeding when the catheter or needle is withdrawn. In a retrograde femoral examination, the puncture in the artery may be 2–3 cm above the obvious skin puncture, and conversely in a carotid injection, which is an antegrade injection, the puncture in the skin may be well below the arterial puncture. As mentioned, assistants should be informed accordingly. Excessive use of local anaesthesia should be avoided. In particular the wall of the artery should not be infiltrated directly because the anaesthetic agent has a spasmolytic effect which tends

to cause excessive and prolonged bleeding. A well recognised, but fortunately rare, complication of arterial puncture is the formation of an arteriovenous fistula. Pseudo-aneurysm is another such complication.

The guide wire. Loss of the tip has been mentioned. Another possibility is knotting of the guide wire, which can happen where excessive force is used by an operator whose hands are not sufficiently experienced to indicate that the whole guide wire is not moving smoothly along the artery, and that its tip has become impacted. Insertion of a short, stiff catheter may facilitate the undoing of the knot but, occasionally, surgical aid has to be sought. Coating of the guide wire with platelets and fibrin has been mentioned. A rare complication of femoral angiography has been a cotton granuloma in the leg, due to cotton shreds from a gauze swab used to clean the guide wire, becoming attached to it and then being introduced into the vessel with the catheter tip.

The catheter. Kinking, fracture and knot formation can occur as with guide wires. It cannot be emphasised too strongly that experience is the best guide, and the inexperienced radiologist should beware of undertaking anything other than simple procedures without the direct supervision of a more experienced person. The use of excessive injection pressure will cause catheters to rupture adjacent to the connection to the pump rather than within the body, and there is no evidence that intra-arterial injection has any direct effect upon blood pressure (although reaction to anaesthetic and contrast agents are well known).

Haemorrhage. Excessive open blood loss is usually an indication of inexpertise in the operator, rather than a risk to the patient's life. A simple femoral retrograde catheterisation can be carried out with no more loss of blood than can be absorbed on a single swab, particularly if the operator has an experienced assistant. Uncontrolled blood loss occurs while trocars are removed and a flexible connector fixed. Careful preparation of flushed connectors and taps will ensure minimal blood loss in other circumstances. The need for assistance from a person who is aware of the demands of the procedure cannot be stressed too highly. This is particularly so when the radiologist has to divide his efforts between operating sterile catheters and syringes, and nonsterile controls of fluoroscopic apparatus.

Complications of contrast media. These are numerous, ranging from local pain, nausea, vomiting and mild urticarial rash to cardiac arrest, complete circulatory failure or respiratory failure, either central or due to laryngeal and tracheal oedema.

All patients should be asked if they are sensitive or allergic to iodine or have any other allergies. If the response is positive, or equivocal, the prudent radiologist will administer both an antihistaminic agent and hydrocortisone intravenously a few minutes before the contrast injection. In any case, these substances, together with full resuscitative procedures, should be available before introducing a large amount of iodine-containing contrast agent into the circulation; a small test dose was once considered mandatory, but is now only given where there is some doubt about the patient's allergic state. It is important that cannulae and connections used for preliminary sedation and analgesia be left in place throughout the procedure, so that they can be used for resuscitative measures should they become necessary.

OTHER MODES OF VASCULAR IMAGING

Computer tomography and digital vascular imaging have been mentioned.

One of the more recent realisations about arterial disease is the importance of the amount of flow possible to a structure under physiologically important conditions; mainly what is the peak flow possible to something like a limb, whose blood supply can vary tremendously depending on whether it is at rest or exercising violently? The work of Brice *et al.* in 1964 highlighted the fact that a simple stenosis in a vessel, until it obliterated about 70% or more of the lumen, did not actually cause a reduction in flow in major arteries, indicating that normally, flow regulation was at small-vessel level, rather than within major arteries. Arteriography can give a precise geographical map of an area, but not a schedule of the local transport timetable, and is almost always carried out under virtually basal functional conditions.

Ultrasonography

The introduction of ultrasound into medical practice (where it is thought to be physiologically inert) has resulted in the availability of techniques giving information about arterial function as well as morphology, and this has reduced the reliance of clinicians upon arteriography, improving their clinical assessment of a patient based upon clinical history, detection of pulses and bruits, etc., aided by a knowledge of flow characteristics derived principally from ultrasonic measurements and recently, nuclear techniques.

The principal technique in the assessment of flow is the pulsed Doppler technique, which can continuously indicate flow velocities within superficial arteries such as the femoral and carotid (Fig. 16.09). A refinement of this technique allows actual imaging of the vessel lumen similar to B mode ultrasonic imaging of intra-abdominal structures and can be used to demonstrate the presence of atheromatous or other narrowings in vessels. This technique relies on reflection of ultrasound from moving blood particles; it remains to be seen whether the moving particles are more important than those which are stationary but not yet incorporated into the vessel wall as thrombus or atheroma.

B-mode ultrasound. This technique rapidly gained acceptance as a safe, noninvasive method of determining whether internal structures are solid or fluid filled. Unlike CT, which gives cross sectional images, ultrasound (US) can scan in transverse, longitudinal or oblique directions. It is particularly useful in the repeated assessment of aortic aneurysms, as it shows not only the patent portion of the lumen but also the amount occupied by thrombus (Fig. 16.10).

Isotope Techniques. Unlike the pulmonary circulation, where isotopes provide an effective means of detecting vessel occlusion, the arterial system does not, as yet, have imaging techniques which appear likely to supplant conventional arteriography. The inherent unsharpness of nuclear techniques makes it unlikely that they will become of value in atheromatous disease, where precise delineation is desirable because of its therapeutic implications, but isotope-labelled particles injected into vessels may have a potential in determining abnormalities of flow, and in determining the extent of ischaemic or neoplastic tissue.

Nuclear Magnetic Resonance. This imaging technique allows the delineation of hollow structures, and may prove to be of value in the assessment of gross disease of large arteries such as the aorta. It is doubtful whether its resolution will be sufficient to give an accurate portrayal of the patency or otherwise of small limb vessels, and its chief value may be in tissue differentiation.

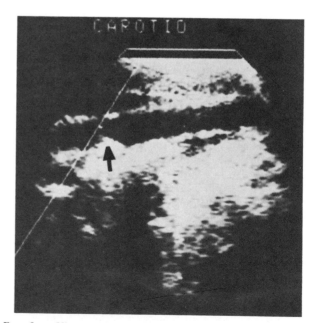

FIG. 16.09. Ultrasound sector scan of a common carotid artery. A large atherosclerotic plaque is present (arrow). The straight line and its mark show the position of a Doppler sample (as described in Chapter 4).

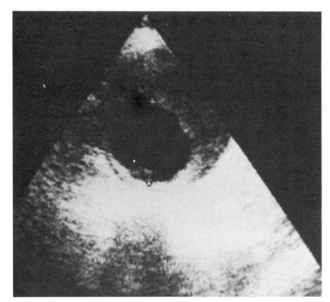

FIG. 16.10. US Transverse section of an abdominal aneurysm. Note wall, clot and lumen. Markers + denote AP diameter of lumen. (See also Fig. 16.43.)

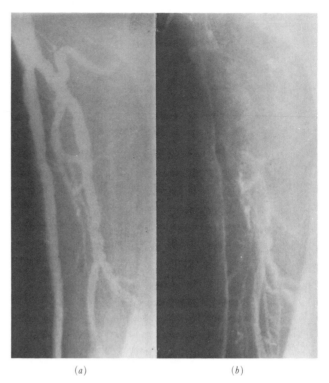

(a)   (b)

FIG. 16.11. (a) Oblique views of the femoral artery and its bifurcation showing atheroma of the profunda origin, and contrast statis on the dependent wall of the superficial femoral artery. The film was taken with a horizontal x-ray beam. (b) Shows contrast layering on the dependent wall, and some stasis at the profunda femoris origin.

A practical result of new techniques, plus a growing awareness of the overall limitations of surgery for atherosclerotic disease has resulted in a reduced demand for arteriographic investigation of ischaemic limbs over the past 10 years.

ARTEFACTS IN ANGIOGRAPHY

Subintimal injection, usually with needle injections, is where the introduction of the needle has lifted a flap of intima which is only realised because of poor opacification of the vessel to be examined. A local film may show a curled line along the vessel, with a greater concentration of contrast below the line and little contrast above. Neuroradiologists who have gained much experience with direct puncture examinations of the common carotid artery will be aware of the phenomenon, and also that it is unlikely to be of consequence to the patient, as the intimal change does not involve the whole of the lumen, the clinical status of the patient is unchanged, and that the lesion will not be apparent at a subsequent examination.

Contrast stasis seen on a horizontal ray examination (usually in the carotid vessels) has in the past been confused with vascular spasm. Extending along the length of the vessel, rather than the localised stasis associated with atheroma, it is an indication that flow in the vessel is so slow that the contrast medium, being heavier than blood, has layered along the dependent wall of the vessel (Fig. 16.11). The flow in the vessel may be slow because of blocked distal vessels or over-

enthusiastic ventilation by an inexperienced anaesthetist (Fig. 16.12) or it may occur in the internal carotid arteries of a moribund patient (Fig. 16.13) whose intracranial pressure is sufficiently high as to approach systemic blood pressure due to tumour or haemorrhage, in which case death is predictably imminent (but not due to the angiogram!).

Stationary waves. Occasionally, a wave-like appearance of the contrast medium is seen extending along the course of an opacified vessel (Fig. 16.14) which is surprisingly regular and which does not indicate the state of the vessel lumen. Waves in fluids generally can be caused by an 'interface' phenomenon, where fluids of different composition and viscocity induce an altered shape or velocity in one another (e.g. air blowing over a lake can induce waves in the water). It is thought that stationary waves in arteries are due to incomplete mixing of contrast medium and blood, not due to contrast layering within the vessel but due to contrast entering the cylindrical boundary of the lumen, with blood passing at a different velocity (faster) down the central part of the vessel lumen. The author has seen this phenomenon in renal, visceral, brachial, iliac and femoral arteries, and repeatedly in the same patient

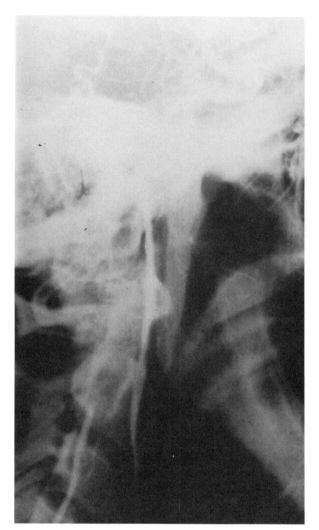

Fig. 16.12. Contrast layering in the internal carotid artery due to hyperventilation. Some reflux has occurred into the vertebral artery.

during one examination, but the phenomenon is so uncommon that its precise cause is conjectural. The differential diagnosis is from fibromuscular hyperplasia, but the latter has an asymmetrical irregularity which is constant rather than the symmetry of stationary waves, and which may not be seen on a subsequent examination.

Incomplete mixing of contrast medium and blood is sometimes seen in the anterior cerebral arteries, due to a dual supply via the anterior communicating artery. A similar 'wash-out' appearance is sometimes seen in femoral arteries because of slow clearance of contrast medium from the vascular boundary-layer. Of no clinical significance, unless localised, the appearance should be noted by arteriographic researchers into vascular diameters.

ARTERIAL DISEASE

By far the most common arterial disease is the occlusive variety, due to partial or complete luminal obliteration of major vessels by the build up of deposits of thrombus or atheroma or both within them. Less commonly, a sudden arterial occlusion can occur due to embolism as when a patient with a cardiac abnormality such as mitral valve disease or coronary artery disease changes rhythm and discharges a thrombus into the aorta or one of its major branches, causing fairly acute localised symptoms depending on the site of embolic arrest (Figs 16.15, 16.16). Much less frequently, arterial insufficiency can result from extrinsic compression as by a cervical rib or band, or from compression by the inguinal ligament or even within the adductor canal. Another disease of arteriographic interest is vascular sclerosis or 'arteriosclerosis' which is a condition different from atherosclerosis; the one affects the structure and function of the wall and the other the state of its inner lining. Although they frequently co-exist, and both may have hypertension and smoking as causative factors, they must be regarded as separate pathological conditions. A further cause of arterial disease is a change in the vessel wall due to fibromuscular hyperplasia, which results in luminal restriction and probably altered pulsatility, producing relative ischaemia. This disease may affect one or several arteries. An occasional congenital abnormality is disproportionate vascular size, usually seen in females, where arterial diameters are far smaller than the body size would seem to demand. Congenital anomalies of branch vessel origins are fairly frequent, and cannot really be considered as arterial disease. Most can be readily explained with embryological knowledge (see Chapter 15).

Inflammatory Disease of Arteries

In the past syphilis, particularly in the ascending aorta, commonly might result in a multiplicity of symptoms of which few would be due to reduced flow, but more probably to pressure on adjoining structures. Arteritis of the temporal arteries (aetiology uncertain) causes localised pain, but obliteration of the lumen of these arteries appears not to be of functional importance, as the diagnosis is established by biopsy of the whole section of the vessel. Vasculitis in small renal vessels is of considerable clinical significance, but this condition in peripheral small vessels is not of arteriographic interest. Rarely, localised arteritis of clinical significance might result from adjacent inflammatory disease (Fig. 16.17) (see also Chapter 10).

Atheromatous Disease

For very many years, there has been vigorous debate as to whether atheroma results from hypercholesterolosis causing localised deposits of cholesterol, which is a

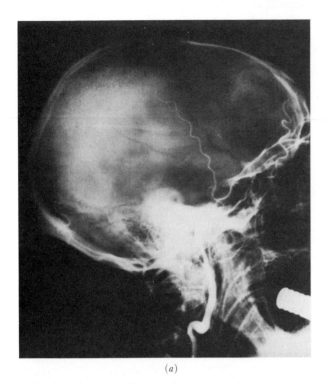

(a)

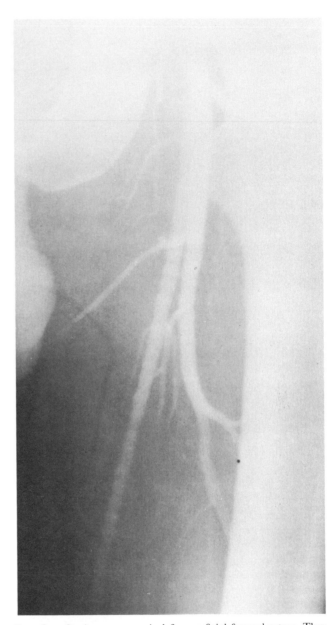

FIG. 16.14. Stationary waves in left superficial femoral artery. They were seen on repeated injections in this patient.

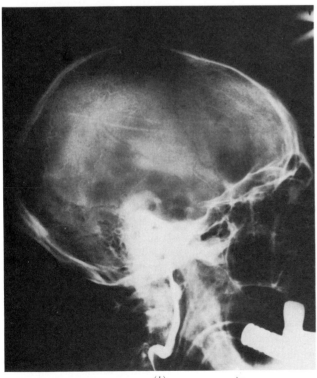

(b)

FIG. 16.13. Serial views during carotid arteriography in a patient with a large cerebral tumour. The contrast failed to pass into the skull, and the contrast layering in the internal carotid artery simulates spasm. It is easily recognised as layering if the films are viewed turned on their side.

major constituent of established atheromatous deposits, or intra-arterial thrombosis of blood constituents such as fibrin and platelets, with the resulting thrombus becoming incorporated into the wall. This second theory has persisted despite a prolonged period of research into abnormalities of cholesterol metabolism because pathologists and vascular surgeons are constantly presented with thrombus on the surface and in the vicinity of established cholesterol-containing atheromatous plaques. The focal nature of atheroma, its association with altered intra-arterial pressure gradient (hyperten-

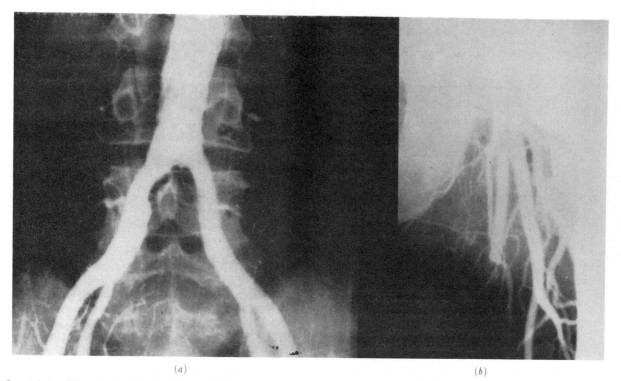

(a)   (b)

FIG. 16.15. (a) A saddle embolus of aortic bifurcation. Note involvement of inner walls of bifurcation branches, not the outer ones as in atheroma. (b) Same patient. Complete occlusion of superficial femoral artery at a non-atheromatous site. Sudden onset of left leg ischaemic symptoms.

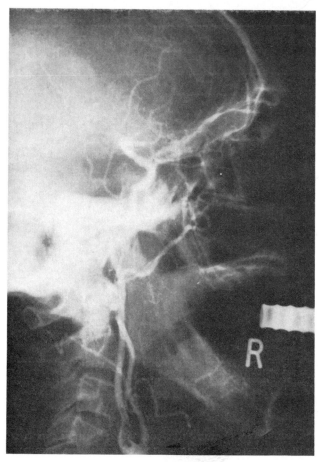

FIG. 16.16. Thrombus arrested within origin of internal carotid artery. Note relative slowness of internal carotid filling compared with the external, and the paucity of intra cerebral contrast.

sion in both pulmonary and systemic circulations is associated with an increased incidence of atheroma), its absence in veins carrying blood with similar cholesterol concentrations, and an improved knowledge of intra-vascular flow patterns suggest that atheroma has a multifactorial aetiology in which cholesterol abnormalities are a minor part. It has been suggested that adverse pressure gradients can occur in arteries due to several reasons (Fox and Hugh, 1966) and that because of the altered pressure gradient the calibre of major vessels ceases to be appropriate, resulting in zones of stasis at the origins of major vessels, and in certain areas within curved vessels. The more recent work of Vane and co-workers (1976) has explained both why these zones of stasis can be not only locally thrombogenetic due to prostaglandin abnormalities, but also self-perpetuating because of the release of a vasoconstrictive agent which will tend further to increase the adverse pressure gradient within that particular vessel. Hypertension is a recognised predisposing condition in the development of atheroma; less understood is the importance of an increased blood viscosity (altered thixotrophy) which could also alter pressure gradients within major vessels, and it is here that cholesterol abnormalities could be of primary importance.

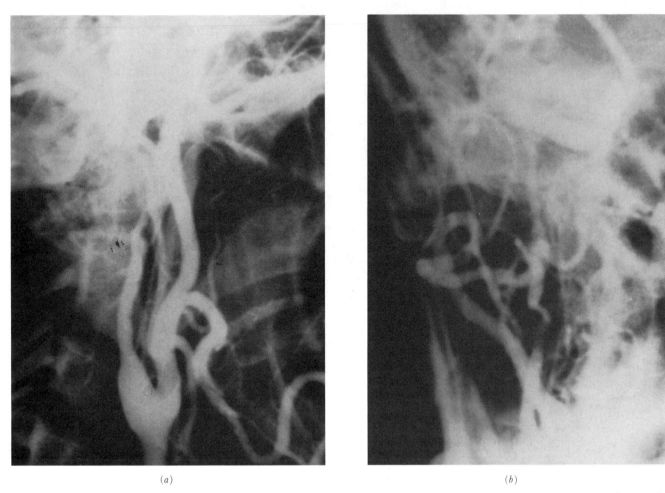

(a)   *(b)*

FIG. 16.17. (*a*) Lateral view, (*b*) AP view. Female patient of 32 years developed an abscess in the neck following dental treatment of a carious tooth. Three weeks later presented with hemiparesis, with irregular narrowing of the internal carotid artery in the neck at the level of the abscess.

Atheroma is clinically of importance in two ways. Firstly, impairment of the lumen may obviously be an impediment to flow and be associated with ischaemia. Secondly, atheromatous irregularities within arteries offer a nidus for the development of thrombi owing to the development of zones of stasis downstream and sometimes upstream of a plaque (Fig. 16.18) resulting in embolisation.

Atheromatous disease, although almost always a multivessel disease, has similar patterns of development in the carotid arteries and in the femoral artery. It has a peculiar predilection for the outer aspect (Fig. 16.19) of the internal carotid vessel origin (outer implying that part of the intimal surface opposite the external carotid origin), sparing the comparatively long part of the internal carotid artery in the neck, with a second site of predilection within the syphon (Fig. 16.20), and the external carotid artery and its branches tend to be spared. Similarly, the origin of the superficial femoral

artery is involved more frequently than the profunda femoris (although oblique views show more involvement of the latter than was once supposed (Fig. 16.11 (a)). Unlike the internal carotid artery, the superficial femoral artery tends to develop plaques along its length, but this is possibly an indication of the differing time scale involved; internal carotid disease produces rather dramatic symptoms earlier because of transient ischaemic attacks (e.g. amaurosis fugax) due to the release of emboli, whereas the sedentary patient might be unaware of a developing ischaemic state in his legs for a long period.

Atheroma of aortic arch vessels. Atheromatous changes in the major vessels arising from the arch of the aorta are not uncommon, with predictable effects, but occasionally, they can produce dramatic effects, the most interesting being the subclavian steal syndrome. Here, blockage of the proximal part of the left subclavian artery results in the left arm being supplied by retro-

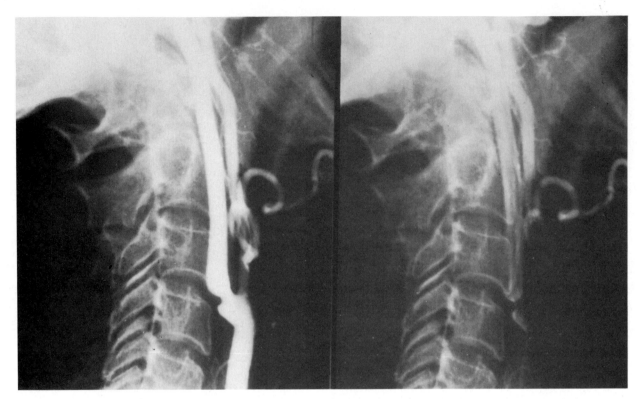

FIG. 16.18. Atheroma at carotid bifurcation. Note contrast stasis both up and downstream of the atheromatous lesion.

grade flow down the left vertebral artery. A similar syndrome is illustrated in Fig. 16.21. If the other major vessels (carotid arteries) supplying the brain are impaired or blocked, sudden exercise of the arms can so reduce flow to the hindbrain as to produce transient blackouts or other neurological symptoms. Awareness of this syndrome highlights the extent to which the brain is protected from ischaemia by its multiple sources of supply. It is not uncommon to find patients presenting with comparatively minor neurological symptoms, who have severe impairment or complete occlusion of both internal carotid origins, but with no history to suggest a sudden calamitous occlusion of a major source of arterial supply.

Radiographically, the arteries leaving the aorta for the head, neck and arms can be demonstrated quite simply by an injection into the arch of the aorta through a slightly curved catheter inserted transfemorally by the Seldinger technique. Detail of the important internal carotid origins is not as well displayed as by selective injection, but adequate information is usually obtained provided that both oblique projections are taken; the disposition of the various major branch orifices is such that if only a single oblique projection is used some of the branch mouths will be obscured by other vessels (Fig. 16.22), particularly if they have become tortuous.

The patient should be turned approximately 30° from the supine position by the use of firm triangular wedge pads under the appropriate shoulder while the injection is made. A pad under the left shoulder facilitates correct positioning of the arch catheter, and subsequent selective entry of its major branches. For the midstream injection, the side-holed catheter should have its tip placed just upstream of the innominate origin, and a pump-assisted injection is virtually obligatory, owing to the rapid and reversible flow in this part of the aorta.

Atheroma of the internal carotid origin. This is an important condition, as it is amenable to surgical correction. It may present with transient cerebral ischaemic attacks (small temporary strokes, loss of consciousness, visual disturbances) probably due to the release of small thrombi formed in the downstream shadow of an atheromatous plaque or as a major stroke. Careful localised views of the carotid bifurcation in the neck can demonstrate the precise localisation of the plaque; oblique views may be necessary to assess the condition fully, and to demonstrate the presence of superadded thrombi. Stasis localised to the mouth of the internal carotid origin, indicating impaired flow adjacent to the endothelium, may have thrombi and atheroma associated with it. A horizontal beam and a series of films taken over 6–8 seconds are necessary to

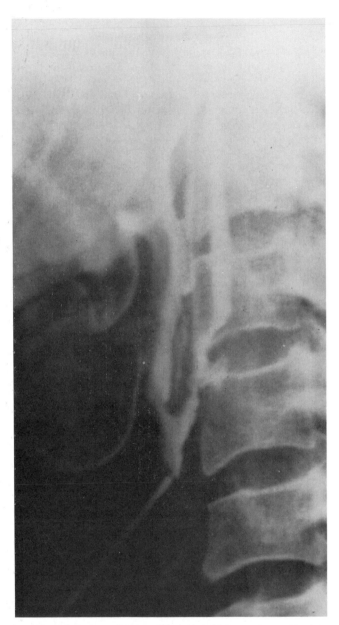

FIG. 16.19. Severe ulcerative atheroma at the internal carotid origin with some involvement of the external carotid artery origin. Note involvement chiefly of the outer walls of the bifurcation vessels.

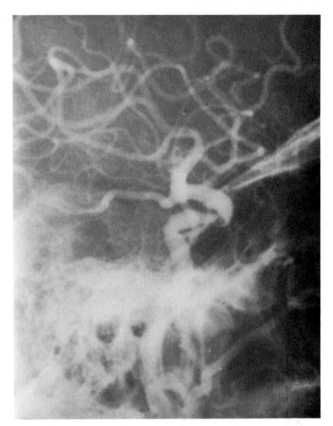

FIG. 16.20. Atheroma and thrombus in the carotid artery siphon. Direct origin of the posterior cerebral artery from the carotid artery.

assess fully the severity of stasis, and to distinguish localised stasis at the mouth of the vessel from generalised stasis along the length of the internal carotid artery due to severely raised intracranial pressure or hyperventilation anaesthesia (Fig. 16.12). It is unfortunate that some highly specialised apparatus developed for rapid film studies of the cerebral vessels does not allow simultaneous visualisation of the neck vessels. Localised stasis of contrast medium at the mouth of the internal carotid origin indicates that 'mixing forces' in this region are disturbed, probably due to boundary-layer separation. The late films, up to 8 seconds after injection, will indicate the degree of this abnormality (Fig. 16.23), and will alert the radiologist to the fact that the ratio of vessel diameter to vessel flow has become physiologically abnormal. Stasis downstream of a stenosis is seen quite frequently. Upstream stenosis, with the attendant possibility of formation of a thrombus which can block the stenosis, is less commonly seen (Fig. 16.18). The mechanisms whereby arteries withstanding high pressures can block completely have not been fully investigated; slowed flows, due to altered pressure gradients, clearly are of importance but the actual occlusion is presumably embolic. Occasionally, atheroma may be seen in the mouth of the external carotid artery but it is always less marked than in the internal carotid origin.

Thrombus formation at the mouth of the internal carotid artery may be observed with or without the concurrent presence of an atheromatous plaque or ulcerated plaque. Fig. 16.24 demonstrates a large thrombus at the internal carotid origin, shown on multiple injections taken with differing projections, none of which showed evidence of atheromatous change, and Fig. 16.25 shows a pedun-

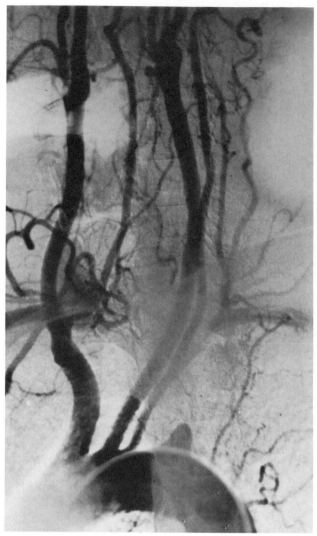

FIG. 16.21. Aortic arch injection; subtraction film. Complete occlusion of left subclavian artery; left vertebral artery arises directly from aortic arch and feeds cervical vessels which then supply the left arm.

and stems compared with the other kidney on IVU (Fig. 16.26). Sometimes the stenosis is bilateral (Fig. 16.27), and a midstream injection is always desirable both to exclude this as well as the possibility of the presence of multiple arteries. Selective injection is necessary to give optimum detail of the small intrarenal arteries, which in hypertension can become tortuous and lengthened, giving a beaded appearance. Poststenotic dilatation is usually seen associated with severe stenosis (Fig. 16.28) and is referred to later. Discovery of an occlusion should lead to close scrutiny of the later films of a series, because the distal artery may refill through branch and capsular vessels, as well as anastomotic vessels running up the ureter (Fig. 16.29) which can give it a beaded appearance on IVU.

Atheromatous disease of the lower aorta and its branches. Ischaemic signs and symptoms are the usual indications for arteriography. Leg pain on exercise, at rest and overt gangrene usually give a reasonable indication of the likely arteriographic findings. One purpose of arteriography is to indicate the level of blockage (which can usually be predicted from a clinical examination of the pulses in groin, popliteal fossa and dorsum of foot) and more important to show whether the 'run-off' vessels are in reasonably good condition, particularly those in the calf. Major arterial by-pass surgery is a time-wasting, frustrating exercise if there are no reasonable small vessels to receive a potentially good flow of blood from a by-pass or opened out blockage in a major proximal vessel.

As in the carotid system branch vessel origins are the prime site for the formation of atheroma (Fig. 16.30), but quite frequently, long straight vessels may show marked atheromatous change. At the aortic bifurcation both common iliac vessels usually show signs of disease but one may be more heavily involved than the other. Sometimes one vessel may be completely blocked, the flow to the limbs being supplied by collateral vessels crossing the floor of the pelvis and the perineal and buttock regions, either into the internal iliac artery or into the profunda femoris artery on the blocked side. Complete occlusion of the lower aorta and the proximal iliac arteries may produce the 'Leriche' syndrome, consisting of symptoms of ischaemia in the legs extending up to the buttocks, together with impotence in males. Examination by a fairly high translumbar approach, or by catheter from the axilla, is necessary for the full assessment of this condition (Fig. 16.31). One of the most frequent casualties is the origin of the superficial femoral artery; collateral vessels arising from profunda femoris branches may feed into the lower part of the superficial vessel, or into the popliteal artery at its origin, or halfway along its length. Obliteration of the lower part of the popliteal artery and its tibial branch origins is usually a contra-indication to major arterial surgery and an attempt should always be made

culated thrombus at one internal carotid origin in a patient with a completely blocked vessel on the other side, occluded at the same level as the thrombus.

The association of stasis, thrombus formation and atheroma at the same situation in the origin of a vessel which is otherwise free of disease suggests that there is a strong haemodynamic factor concerned in the aetiology of atheroma.

Renal artery stenosis. This is an important condition as the hypertension which it can cause may be amenable to surgery or balloon dilatation. Clinically significant stenosis may produce reduced urine flow in the affected kidney, which may be of reduced volume and show hyperconcentration and underfilled calyces

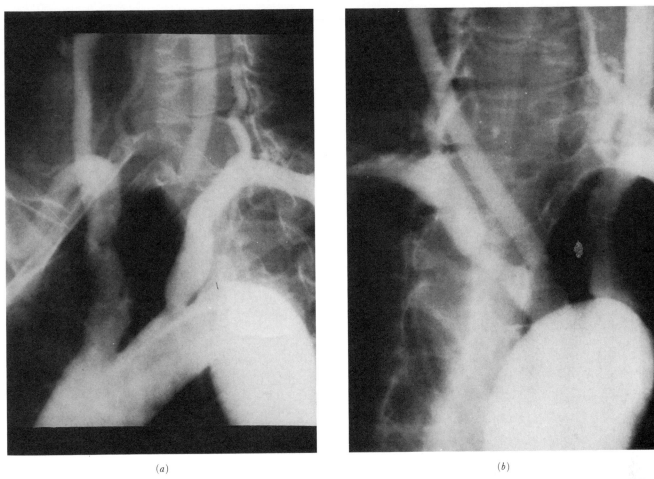

(a)   (b)

FIG. 16.22. (a) Lying behind the right common carotid artery, the stenosis of the right subclavian artery is concealed in the left anterior oblique projection. (b) Right anterior oblique projection: the stenosis and post-stenotic dilatation are well displayed.

to demonstrate these vessels as part of a full pre-surgical assessment (Fig. 16.32).

Blockage of smaller vessels beyond the mid-calf region without major changes in the larger proximal vessels is usually embolic or a sign of a metabolic abnormality, frequently diabetes or Buerger's disease, rather than being primarily an atheromatous disorder; arteriography may be useful in indicating the optimum site for amputation.

Occasionally, it is clinically difficult to decide whether leg pain on exercise is due to arterial disease or to spinal stenosis or some other abnormality of the nervous system. This possibility should be borne in mind when a surgical patient is being investigated, and a healthy arterial system is demonstrated.

Non-atheromatous Occlusive Conditions

Occasionally, arterial occlusion can result from extrinsic compression of a vessel, e.g. of a subclavian

vessel, due to a cervical rib or band (Fig. 16.33). To demonstrate this it is important to place the arm in the position causing the maximum arterial compression during arteriography, the patient's history and close attention to the radial pulse being important during investigation of this condition. Arterial compression by other extrinsic masses can occur but clinically is of less importance than the accompanying venous or nervous involvement, e.g. in the superior mediastinum.

Arterial blockage due to embolus. This is usually a sudden, clinically diagnosable event, largely because of an underlying predisposing condition such as mitral valve disease or arrhythmia (Fig.16.15). Occasionally, investigation of a patient with intermittent ischaemic symptoms may disclose a localised vascular blockage with otherwise healthy vessels and should raise the suspicion of an embolus rather than a primarily atheromatous lesion, so that search will be made for a source of emboli and appropriate therapy undertaken.

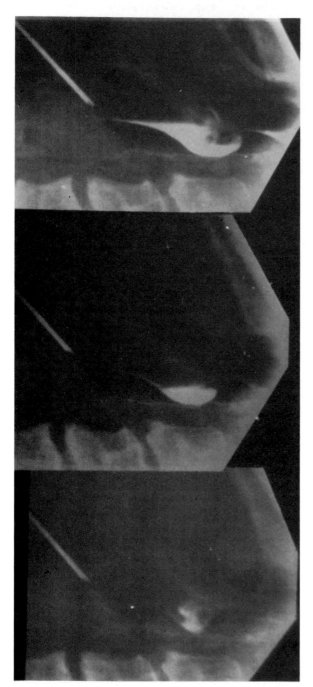

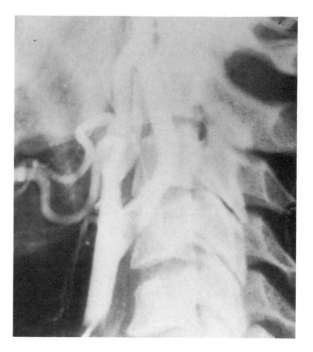

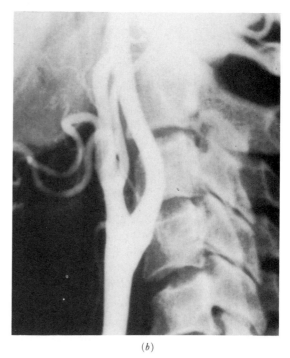

FIG. 16.23. A trickle injection of dense contrast medium into the common carotid artery demonstrates a thrombus and 8-second stasis at the origin of the internal carotid artery in a patient with T.I.A.'s.

(b)

FIG. 16.24. (a) Large thrombus in origin of internal carotid artery in a patient with history of T.I.A.'s. (b) Three weeks later thrombus has disappeared but patient had had no further symptoms.

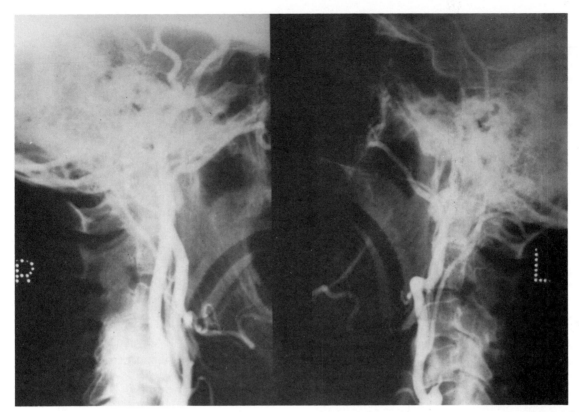

FIG. 16.25. Bilateral carotid artery examination. On the right side there is a pedunculated thrombus protruding into the lumen of the internal carotid origin. On the left side the vessel has occluded completely.

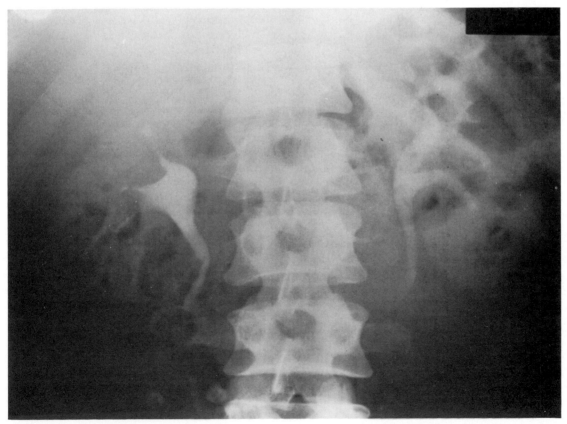

FIG. 16.26. Right renal artery stenosis. Renal volume looks normal, but there is increased contrast density on the right, with 'spastic' calyceal stems, due to the reduced blood and urine flow through the right kidney. Hypertensive patient.

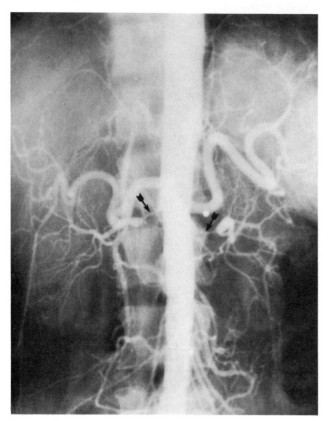

FIG. 16.27. Severe bilateral renal artery stenosis in a hypertensive patient.

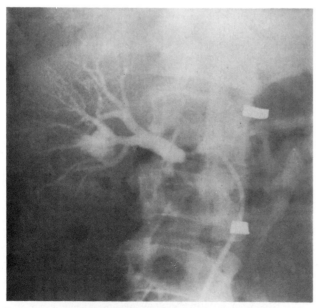

FIG. 16.28. Severe renal artery stenosis with some poststenotic dilatation. A small lower polar vessel was also present.

Congenital Abnormalities

Major arch abnormalities are considered in Chapter 15. Congenital anomalies of the origins of the great vessels are not uncommon; simultaneous origin of the left common carotid and the innominate artery is sufficiently common for it to pass unreported (Fig. 16.34), but can cause a slight problem when attempting selective catheterisation.

Other congenital abnormalities of radiological importance in the head and neck are an abnormally low bifurcation of the common carotid artery in the neck, which can cause a problem if the origin of the internal carotid artery is to be shown by a direct puncture examination, and persistence of some of the branchial arch vessels. A persistent trigeminal artery is the most frequent of these (Fig. 16.35) and, occasionally, persistent hypoglossal and acoustic arteries are found; the practical result is simultaneous filling of the basilar artery and the carotid vessels, from a carotid injection.

The vertebral artery, usually the left, frequently has an anomalous origin, the most common being direct from the aortic arch between the left common carotid and the left subclavian arteries (Fig. 16.21). The relative sizes of the two vertebral arteries can vary considerably; once of importance, when vertebral examinations were usually carried out by direct puncture in the neck, this variation is probably of little clinical significance.

In the limbs, congenital abnormalities are not uncommonly seen, and are of little clinical interest. A high brachial artery bifurcation is of some concern to those who catheterise this vessel, and a high origin of the posterior tibial artery, usually at the level of the mid-popliteal artery, is worth reporting in case surgical grafting is considered.

In the abdomen, the most common variation is multiple renal arteries. A lower polar artery is sufficiently common for it always to be looked for when selective renal angiography is carried out without a preliminary midstream injection (Fig. 16.36), and the latter occasionally shows the presence of three or even four renal arteries on one side.

A chance finding on abdominal aortography is a large vessel leading upwards through the diaphragm to supply a *sequestrated portion* of lung, usually dissociated from an air supply as well as a pulmonary artery supply, thus showing as an opacity at the lung base behind the heart, usually on the left side. Clinically, these are frequently associated with recurring chest infections.

Variations in the origins of the *splanchnic vessels* occur occasionally and are mentioned elsewhere. Because a lateral view is required to demonstrate them they are not usually seen on routine lumbar-femoral angiograms.

The aortic bifurcation and the iliac bifurcations can vary considerably in position; a fact to remember when trouble is experienced with both translumbar and

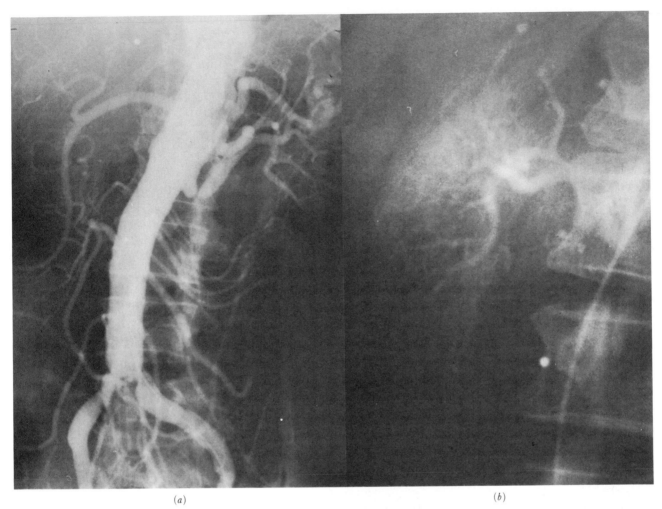

(a)   (b)

FIG. 16.29. (a) Renal angiogram in a hypertensive patient. Mid-stream injection. Severe stenosis on left. Complete occlusion of origin of right renal artery. Severe iliac stenosis also. (b) The distal part of the right renal artery and its branches have filled through collaterals on this later film. Multiple small arteries are seen running up the ureter.

FIG. 16.30. Complete occlusion of left external iliac artery origin. Re-filling via internal iliac branches into profunda vessels.

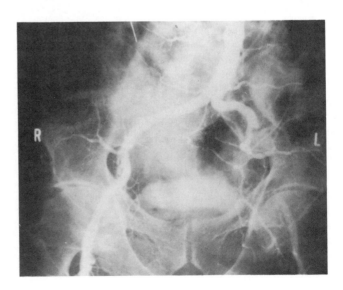

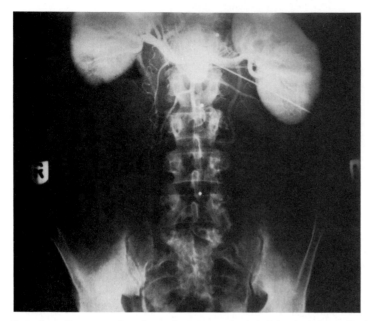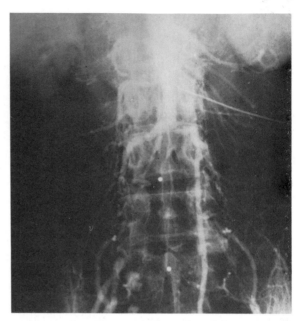

FIG. 16.31. Two examples of complete obstruction of abdominal aorta (Leriche syndrome). One shows gradual tapering of the aorta to the occlusion, whereas the other was abrupt.

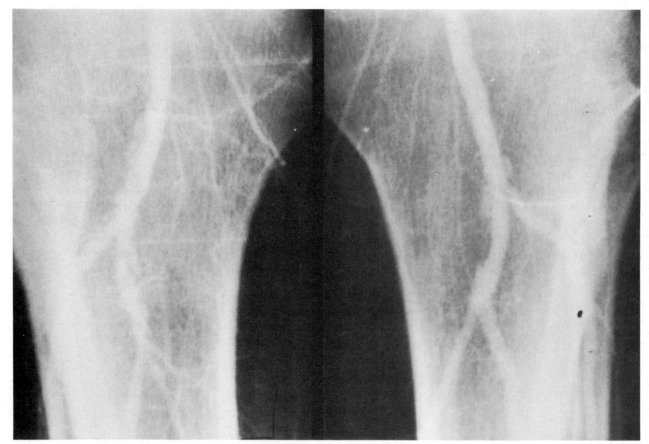

FIG. 16.32. Bilateral ulcerative atheroma at the popliteal bifurcations.

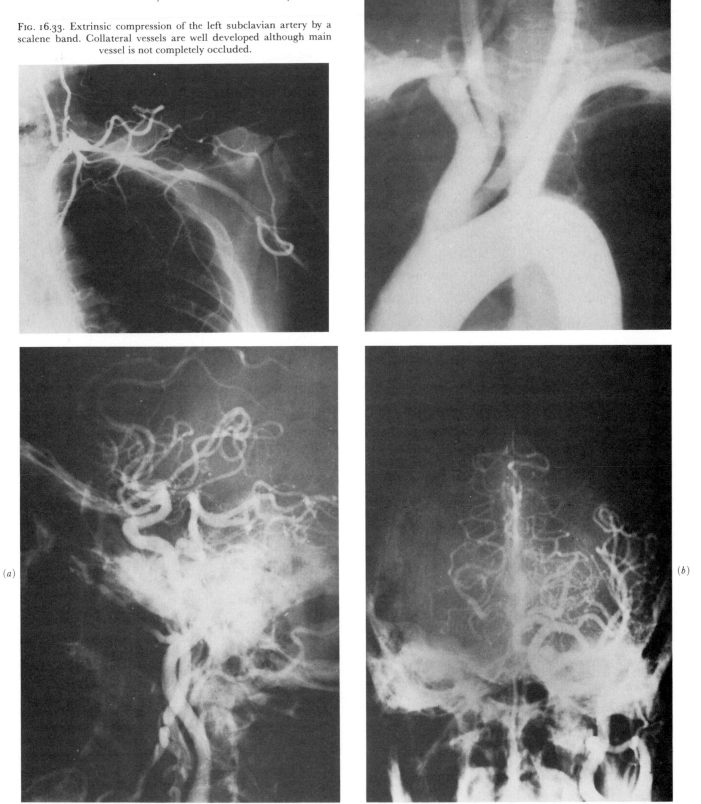

FIG. 16.34. Arch aortogram. Common origin of innominate and left common carotid artery. Absent left vertebral artery.

FIG. 16.33. Extrinsic compression of the left subclavian artery by a scalene band. Collateral vessels are well developed although main vessel is not completely occluded.

(a)

(b)

FIG. 16.35. (a) Persistent trigeminal artery. Common carotid injection produces filling of basilar and both posterior cerebral arteries. (b) AP view shows filling of left anterior and middle cerebral arteries and of both posterior cerebral arteries.

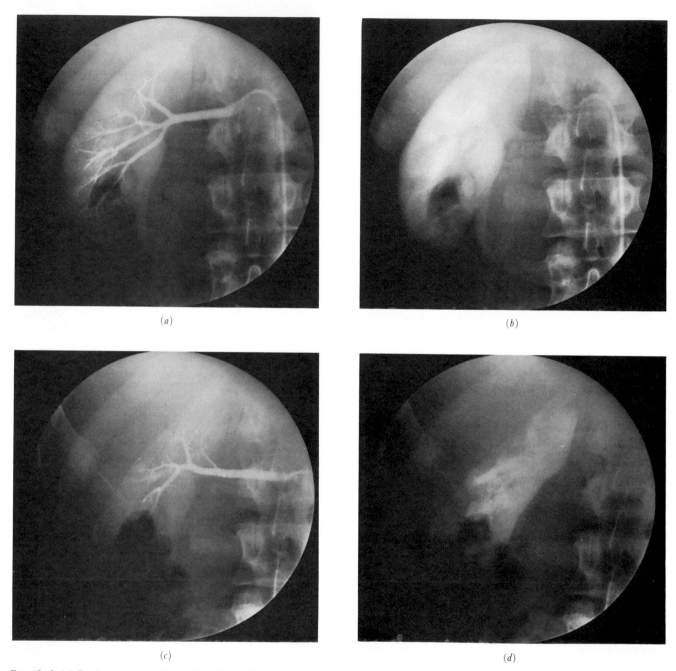

FIG. 16.36. (a) Dual arterial supply to right kidney. Upper pole vessel appears to supply all the kidney, because of the oblique diversion of the vascular supply within the kidney. (b) Nephrographic phase following selective injection of the upper renal artery. (c) Selective injection of the lower polar renal artery. This supplies the dorsal part of the lower part of the kidney. (d) Nephrogram following lower polar artery injection. (*Courtesy Dr. W. N. Boyd.*)

catheter approaches. Failure to visualise the opposite iliac artery could be due to the bifurcation being appreciably higher than the catheter tip, rather than a blocked vessel.

The small vessel syndrome (disproportionate arterial size). This infrequent condition causes ischaemic changes in patients who are appreciably younger than those usually involved in ischaemic disease due to atheroma, i.e. 20–40 years. The condition consists of arteries whose diameter is appreciably less than normal (involving the aorta and its major branches) in which either minor atheromatous change or even simple arterial insufficiency causes ischaemic symptoms or signs. The upper or lower halves of the body may be affected, or both, and when atheroma is not present, the large vessels have a smooth narrow outline unlike fibro-muscular hyperplasia, which produces a beaded appearance.

Takayasu's Disease, which tends to involve large vessels in the upper part of the body, also produces localised stenoses but may have generally narrow vessels as well, possibly a result of low arterial pressure. Experimentally, in animals it can be readily shown that arterial size is a function of intra-arterial pressure. Smoking cannot be incriminated as a cause of the small vessel syndrome, although it is important in the common atheroma/ischaemia syndrome.

Marfans Syndrome is discussed in Chapter 10. Involvement of the peripheral arteries is rare. Occasionally, a 'mega-artery' syndrome is seen, where some or all large arteries are both lengthened and dilated but where there is no involvement of other connective tissues, and no other stigmata of Marfan's syndrome (Fig. 16.37). The vascular tortuosity can give rise to pressure symptoms within the skull, and subarachnoid haemorrhage is an occasional complication of this rare abnormality.

Arterial trauma. Various body traumas may be associated with major vascular injury; common examples are motor cycle injuries, producing brachial plexus

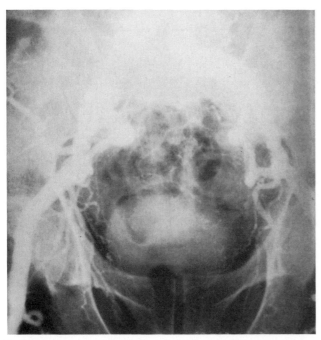

FIG. 16.37. Arteriosclerotic tortuosity of iliac vessels with some generalised dilatation and aneurysmal dilatation in mid part of the right internal iliac artery. Configuration of common iliac arteries sometimes called 'dancing-man' appearance.

avulsion and subclavian damage, flexion injuries of the spine complicated by partial or complete aortic rupture, and limb fractures with possible vascular rupture, dissection or blockage due to haematoma. Each injury has to be assessed clinically and arteriography, if necessary, has to be carried out in an appropriate fashion. Occasionally, single film angiography may be carried out within an operating theatre so that an on-the-spot decision can be made whether amputation or restoration should be carried out.

Stab wounds not infrequently cause arterial trauma, and this may be associated with trauma to an adjacent vein leading to either an immediate or a delayed arteriovenous fistula. The history usually indicates the aetiology, and appropriate arteriography is helpful in the surgical management. Iatrogenic stab wounds can cause arterial trauma, resulting in aneurysmal change, e.g. in liver or kidney biopsy.

Small vessel disease in the kidneys. In recent years, attention has been directed to a number of clinical syndromes in which abnormalities have been described in the smaller radiologically visible arteries in the kidneys. The syndromes include loin pain and haematuria, and hypertension in younger patients, particularly female ones and various aetiologies have been described, including the use of analgesics and oral contraceptives. The radiographic abnormalities consist of tortuosity and beading of the subcortical arteries with contrast stasis, and are associated with inflammatory changes in small vessels on renal biopsy.

Arterial Aneurysms

Aneurysms are of two clinical types:
  (i) where they are of clinical importance;
  (ii) where they are very small, and are discovered in the course of 'routine angiography'.

Aneurysms causing pressure. These produce signs or symptoms because the vascular enlargement impinges upon other significant body structures so as to affect their function or well-being, e.g. intracranial aneurysms can cause cranial nerve abnormalities. Intrathoracic aneurysms can cause abnormal physical signs (the pulsating sternum of ascending aortic aneurysms) or the 'aneurysm of symptoms', where the aneurysm of the horizontal/upper descending thoracic aorta impinges upon nearby nerves, particularly the left recurrent laryngeal nerve, causing hoarseness. Lumbar aneurysms can cause abdominal and back pain due to pressure on vertebrae (and probably leakage also). Aneurysms of the lower dorsal and upper lumbar aorta can cause pressure indentation on the anterior margins of the vertebral bodies; the resilient intervertebral discs support the upper and lower margins of the vertebral body resulting in a striking vertebral body concavity when viewed laterally. Associated soft tissue calcification usually provides the diagnostic clue in these cases, where pain is usually the dominant clinical feature. Both aortic and iliac artery aneurysms can involve the ureters, causing pressure and obstruction leading to renal failure as seen in Figs 16.38 and 16.39.

Rupture and Dissection. *Intracranially*, they may cause dramatic head pain and nervous system signs. Investigation has to be directed to confirm that the bleeding is actually from an aneurysm, rather than an arteriovenous malformation and, if so, the precise location and position of the neck of the aneurysm or aneurysms, with a view to appropriate clipping.

Intrathoracic. In Western countries, the clinically significant aneurysm of 'signs' and 'symptoms', i.e. the syphilitic and arteriosclerotic ones, respectively, have largely disappeared (other than from radiological libraries) owing to modern therapy for infection and hypertension (Fig. 16.40). More important are those patients who develop sudden severe chest pain, quite possibly due to a coronary artery blockage, where a chest X-ray shows a wide upper mediastinum.

A dissecting aneurysm of the aorta can start in the mid-aorta, and extend back or down to involve the origins of the coronary or renal vessels. If backward extension has involved the origin of the coronary arteries, there may be ECG changes, resulting in confusion with a straight-forward coronary artery impairment due to thrombo-embolus and atheroma. Chest radiographs taken with portable apparatus on semi-recumbent patients (AP not PA) can give confusing views of the superior mediastinum, the AP projection of the superior mediastinum simulating enlargement, and the radiologist may be called upon to carry out aortography. In this situation, if the femoral pulses are difficult to feel because of either cardiac embarrassment or aortic occlusion, the axillary approach to aortic visualisation may be necessary. The resulting angiograms may well show if there is coronary involvement and also in a true downward dissection, whether one or both renal artery origins are involved; obviously a major consideration if massive corrective surgery is involved. In this case, it is important to define the distal extent of the dissection if a 'fenestration' type of operation is contemplated. This topic is also discussed in Chapter 10.

In the other large aneurysms of the aortic arch angiography may be necessary to confirm that a mediastinal mass is, in fact, an aneurysm, and then to define its extent and relation to the major branch orifices. Dynamic CT scanning is a valuable diagnostic tool if available (Fig. 16.41).

Rupture of a lumbar aneurysm other than dissection is usually a striking clinical event; it may be preceded by some days of pain due to mild leakage, and lumbar aneurysms can usually be palpated. Lateral radiographs are usually recommended to detect calcification; aortography was of diagnostic importance but has been superseded by ultrasound and CT in the assessment of

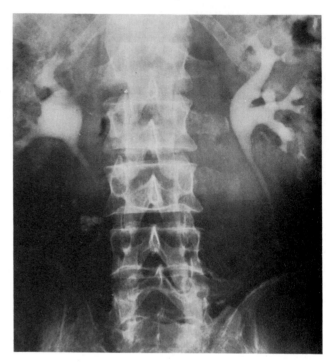

FIG. 16.38. Aortic aneurysm. Wall calcification and lateral displacement of left ureter.

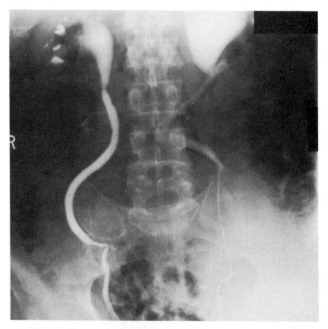

FIG. 16.39. Displacement and obstruction of ureters by bilateral common iliac artery aneurysms. Retrograde examination.

the size and clot-lumen ratio of the affected vessels (Figs 16.42, 16.43, 16.44). Aortography remains of value in discriminating between aneurysm, vascular tortuosity

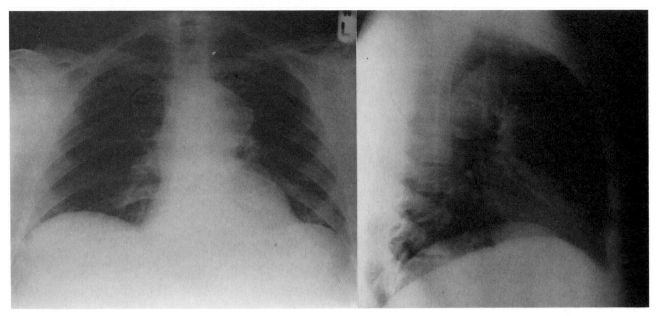

FIG. 16.40. PA and lateral view of chest showing calcification in aneurysm of horizontal and upper descending parts of aortic arch. W. R. negative therefore presumed arteriosclerotic.

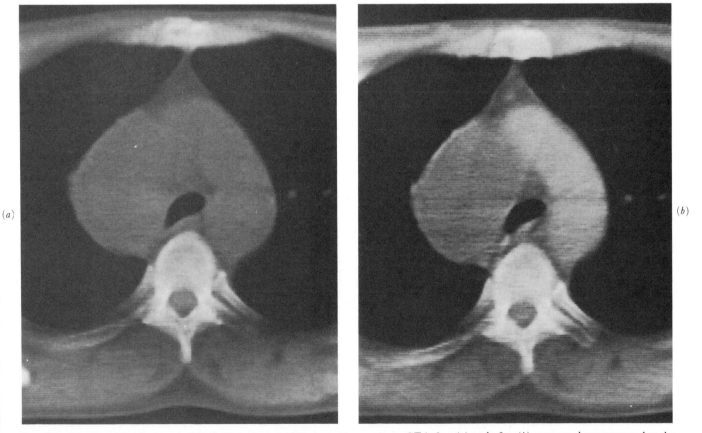

(a)

(b)

FIG. 16.41. Upper mediastinal mass. Clinically suspected to be an aortic aneurysm. CT before (a) and after (b) contrast demonstrates that the mass is quite separate from the aortic arch. See also Fig. 10.05.

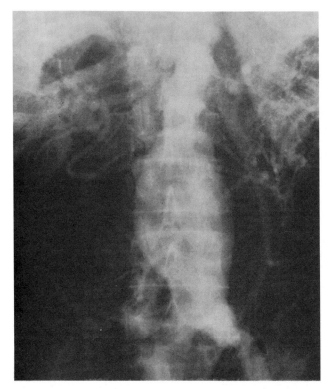

FIG. 16.42. Angiographic demonstration of aortic aneurysm. The displacement of the superior mesenteric artery is greater than would be expected from the size of the opacified lumen due to the presence of clot.

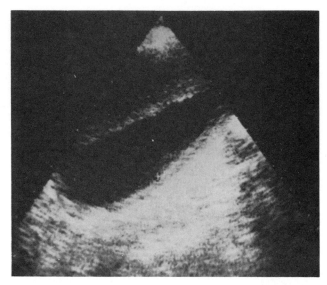

FIG. 16.43. Real time ultrasound demonstration of abdominal aortic aneurysm. Longitudinal section. (Transverse section shown in Fig. 16.10.)

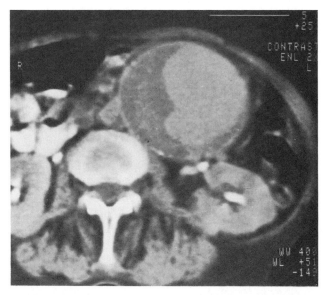

FIG. 16.44. CT demonstration of abdominal aortic aneurysm following IV contrast injection. Note the extensive clot within the aneurysm, calcification in its wall, and displacement of the left ureter.

and an intervening solid tumour, but CT and ultrasound may well be more specific in diagnosing the latter condition.

Peripheral aneurysms. Of several aetiologies, the once common (and presumed) mycotic aneurysm has probably been replaced in frequency by post-surgical ones. The latter usually occur where grafts have been attached, and may be more strictly regarded as pseudo-aneurysms due to leakage and the formation of a false vascular wall. Vein grafts are strikingly able to withstand arterial pressure without undue distension. (See Arteriography following surgery.)

Mycotic aneurysms are much less common than in the past, usually being associated with, or a complication of, sub-acute bacterial endocarditis. They were usually found at vascular branchings, presumably developing in relation to zones of stasis, might involve any large vessel, and could increase in size very rapidly, with rupture being a not uncommon complication.

Renal and splenic artery aneurysms are a chance finding in most cases; both usually calcify, which is why they are found (Fig. 16.45). Renal artery aneurysms are probably not of clinical significance but it has been

stated that splenic artery aneurysms constitute a surgical emergency because of the risk of rupture.

Syphilitic aneurysms are much less frequently seen in Western countries than in the past. They are due to bacterial involvement of the arterial media, producing weakening and consequent dilatation. Although the ascending and horizontal parts of the aortic arch were

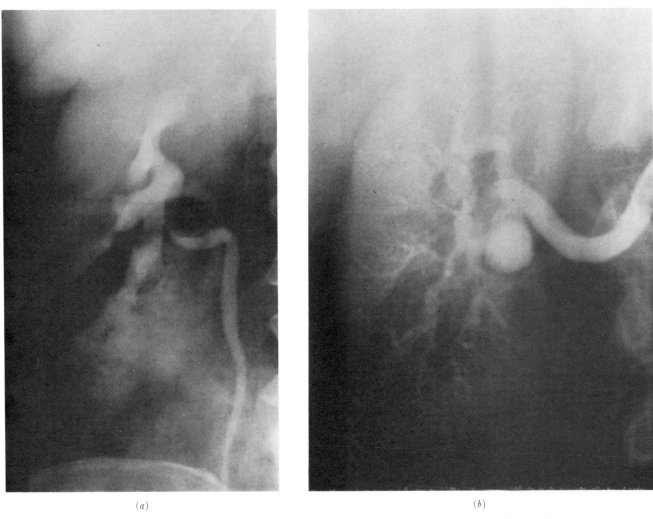

(a)   (b)

FIG. 16.45. (a) Renal artery aneurysm in renal hilum with ring calcification on IVU. (b) Angiogram of same.

favoured sites, any artery might be involved. Calcification might be present in the larger aneurysms but is not specific to syphilitic aneurysms. The mode of presentation obviously depends on the size and site of the aneurysm.

Traumatic aneurysms (see also angiomas and arteriovenous abnormalities). These are usually related to stab-wounds, due to partial severance of the vessel wall. Their aetiology is usually obvious and their precise anatomy is usually demonstrable by angiography. One variety which is likely to increase in incidence is the iatrogenic one, due to the increasing use of blind biopsy procedures.

Post-stenotic dilatation. Most dilatations of this sort can barely be called aneurysms, consisting merely of a mild expansion of the vessel downstream of a constriction, usually atheromatous. They are quite frequently seen in the renal arteries associated with atheroma

(Fig. 16.28), and in the subclavian arteries where the arterial narrowing may be extrinsic due to a band or developmental anomaly of the scalene muscles (Fig. 16.33). They are rarely seen in the lower aorta and legs, if at all, presumably because flow rates are not high. Poststenotic dilatation is usually an indication that the occlusive lesion is 'significant', i.e. that it is a serious impediment to flow (it has been shown that some arteries, e.g. carotid, can sustain an 80% reduction of their lumen without reducing flow, but this does not apply to all arteries) and, in this case, it is accompanied by a thrill and bruit. Stenoses may also have clinical significance without flow-reduction because they can, nevertheless, be a source of micro-emboli.

Incidental aneurysms differ from 'clinical' aneurysms in that they are chance findings and do not, in themselves, cause signs or symptoms. An example already mentioned is the small intrarenal aneurysm following renal biopsy. Multiple small intrahepatic aneurysms have been described in polyarteritis nodosa and other collagen diseases, and occur in the kidney also. They are presumably due to localised arteritis affecting small vessels rather than being embolic or mycotic from lesions elsewhere, and may resolve with effective therapy. Small aneurysms have also been described in the brain, usually in hypertensive patients, and their rupture has been suggested to be the cause of subarachnoid haemorrhages or other vascular incidents in these patients.

Pulmonary artery aneurysm (other than postvalve dilatations) is a rare condition of multiple stenoses affecting the branches of the pulmonary arteries within the lungs. These may be accompanied by poststenotic dilatations which can resemble small 'coin' lesions in a chest radiograph. The combinations of these plus stigmata of pulmonary hypertension should bring this rare condition to mind. A CT examination with appropriately timed contrast injection should be dramatic.

Fibro-muscular Hyperplasia

In this condition, one or several arteries may be involved. The renal arteries appear to be quite frequent victims, although it is possible that the resulting hypertension results in a disproportionate investigation of these particular vessels. Hypertrophy of the muscular and fibrous tissue in the walls of the affected vessel reduces the size of the lumen, and can reduce flow volumes thereby. In a flow-sensitive vessel, this may produce signs or symptoms (which is perhaps why the renal vessels appear to be particularly prone to this condition), but to date no particular predisposing agent or cause has been suggested. In the renal arteries the condition is four times as common in females than in males. Arteriographic appearances may simulate atheromatous disease, but the latter is usually localised, whereas fibromuscular hyperplasia tends to involve an appreciable segment of the vessel (Fig. 16.46). The carotid arteries seem to have an appreciable incidence of this condition, but it is possible that this incidence is exaggerated by the ease with which the condition can produce clinical effects which result in arteriographic investigation because of the obviously vascular nature of the underlying condition.

Arteritis of the temporal and digital vessels can have similar

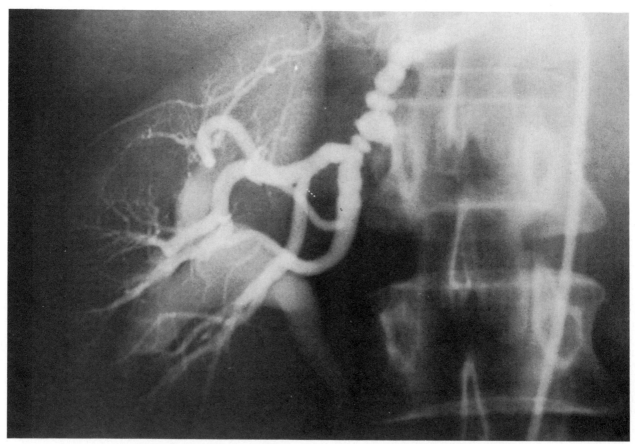

FIG. 16.46. Fibromuscular hyperplasia in right renal artery in hypertensive female patient.

arteriographic appearances as fibromuscular hyperplasia, but the causative condition is more readily explainable than it is in the latter. Angiography has been employed in patients with *Raynaud's disease*; beading and obliteration of digital arteries may be seen, but the procedure does not appear to have much clinical value. Similar angiographic changes have been described in patients with severe rheumatoid arthritis and in other collagen diseases, and the underlying pathological lesion is probably similar to that seen in so-called 'Buerger's disease', probably an immune condition of some variety.

Tumour Angiography

Arteriography is occasionally requested in the preoperative assessment of *bone tumours*, prior to amputation or radiotherapy, because some tumours extend proximally further than is suggested by plain film appearances. Some bone tumours are very vascular (Fig. 16.47), but vascularity per se is of little value in establishing a histological diagnosis. The degree of extension into soft tissues may be demonstrated if this is of clinical value where conservative therapy is indicated because of the presence of metastases (Fig. 16.48). CT offers a better radiological means of assessing tumour extent in bone.

Angiomas and arterio-venous abnormalities do not necessarily have a very active blood supply and angiography may be disappointing in their assessment if peripheral, or discovery if visceral. Nevertheless, angiography is occasionally requested to ascertain the supply vessels of peripheral angiomatous malformations (Fig. 16.49).

Visceral angiography may reveal an otherwise untraceable cause for gastro-intestinal haemorrhage and isotopes have a place in detecting ectopic gastric mucosa

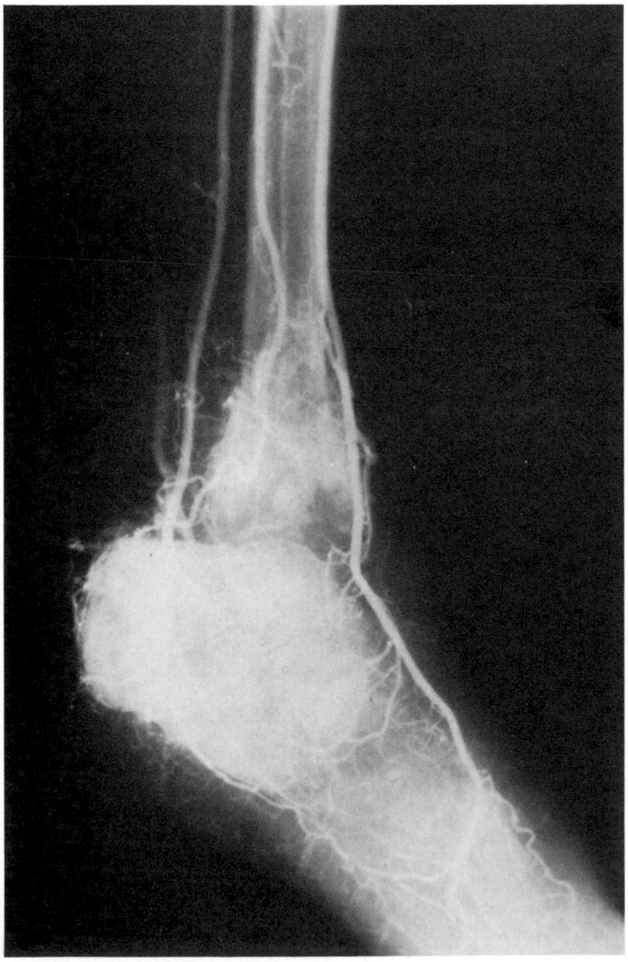

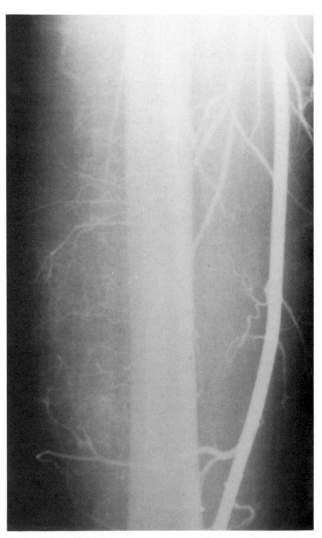

FIG. 16.47. Very vascular tumour in calcaneum. Secondary deposit from cancer of cervix. All feeding vessels dilated and there was extremely rapid venous return.

FIG. 16.48. Fibrosarcoma of thigh. Angiography shows extent of tumour and its vascular nature.

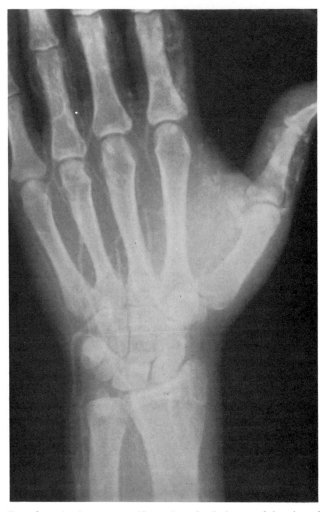

FIG. 16.49. Angiomatous malformation of soft tissues of thumb and index finger.

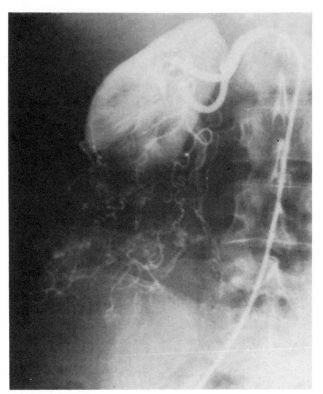

FIG. 16.50. Selective injection of right renal artery demonstrates a large vascular tumour in the lower pole of the kidney.

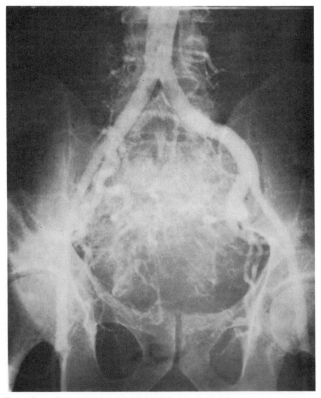

FIG. 16.51. Retroperitoneal tumour: lower abdominal mass confirmed to be retroperitoneal by arteriography. Note enlargement and tortuosity of the internal iliac arteries.

in Meckel's diverticula. Renal tumours were once routinely assessed or diagnosed by arteriography (Fig. 50) but ultrasound and CT offers less invasive alternatives. Angiography occasionally may help in the surgical assessment of retroperitoneal tumours (Fig. 16.51).

Arteriography for Mass Lesions

Mass lesions occasionally present in various parts of the body whose nature is not obvious but whose vascularity is suspect because of their pulsatility; pulsatility may be transmitted from a nearby vessel, from an aneurysm, or from a very vascular tumour. Where conventional arteriography would once have been the first radiological investigation after plain films, the modern sequence would be an ultrasound examination, if the mass were not surrounded by gas-filled organs, probably followed by a CT examination without and then with contrast, particularly if dynamic scanning was available. An example of a vascular carotid body tumour is given in Fig. 16.52, and Fig. 16.5 shows the value of CT in defining the relation of a recurrent tumour in the tonsillar bed to the internal carotid artery, clearly of vital importance to the surgeon in preparing for his operation. CT not only defines the extent of the tumour, but also its relationship to vascular structures nearby (Fig. 16.53). If conventional angiography is performed, lesions low in the neck are best

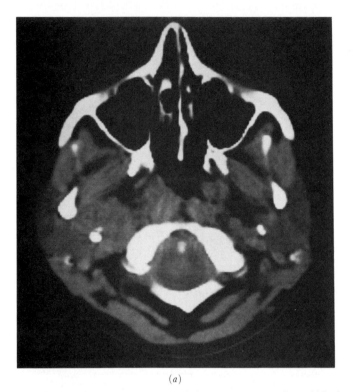
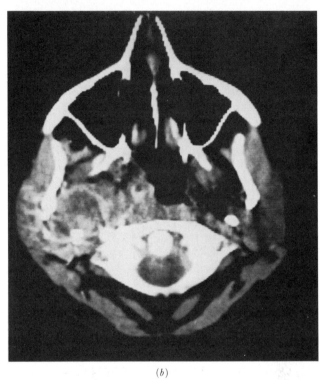

(a) (b)

FIG. 16.52. (a) Very large mass in neck due to recurrence of carotid body tumour. (b) Repeat CT scan of neck with contrast injection into the right common carotid artery. The mass is only moderately and irregularly vascular and the posterior displacement of the carotid artery against the vertebral body is shown.

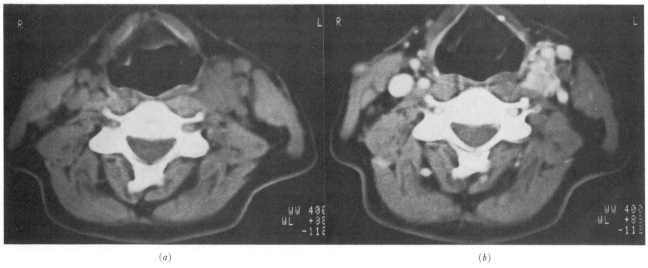

(a) (b)

FIG. 16.53. (a) Transverse CT of neck. Patient with mass on left side. (b) CT during contrast injection into the aortic arch. The mass has enhanced and the displaced internal carotid artery and branches of the external carotid artery are clearly shown. Carotid body tumour.

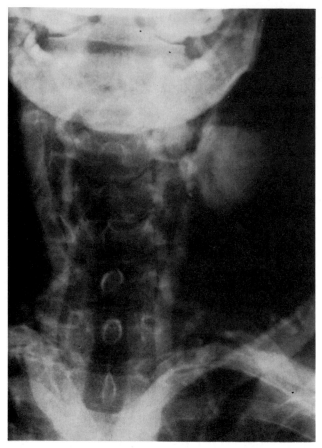

Fig. 16.54. Aortic arch injection to demonstrate carotid artery aneurysm.

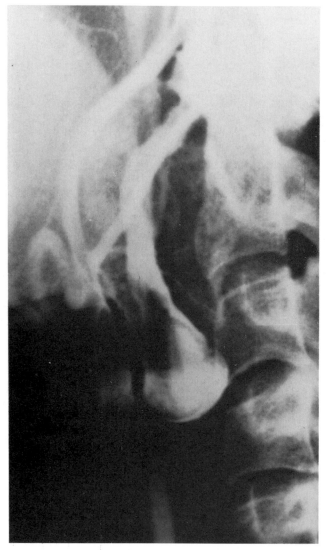

Fig. 16.55. Extensive aneurysm of the internal carotid artery in the neck. The aneurysm extended up to the skull base, although the opacified lumen appeared to be of normal size just beyond the carotid bulb. Neck injection.

approached by catheter (Fig. 16.54), but it is possible to examine lesions high in the neck by a low carotid needle puncture.

Carotid body tumours may have a demonstrable intrinsic vascular 'blush' and their intimate relation to the carotid bifurcation can be well defined with several oblique views and CT (Fig. 16.55). Mass lesions on the face and side of the head can be investigated by selective injection of the external carotid artery, using a curved catheter inserted via the common carotid or femoral artery. Flow in the external carotid artery is normally appreciably slower than in the internal carotid system, and the timing of films is altered appropriately.

An extremely kinked internal carotid artery may present as a pulsatile mass in the neck. In arteriosclerosis (a disease of the whole vessel wall rather than atheroma, which affects the intima) vessels can lengthen appreciably (but do not necessarily dilate much) and where the distal end of a long vessel is constrained, as is the internal carotid artery where it enters the skull, the lengthening can only be accommodated by tortuosity. The internal carotid artery is such a vessel, and on occasion it may perform a complete loop in the neck, resulting in the presence of a pulsatile mass, usually bilateral. This is sometimes termed a 'Corrigan's Kink'. Angiography is diagnostic (Fig. 16.56) and sometimes provides a remarkable demonstration of the difference between 'arteriosclerosis' and 'atheroma', although both appear to be hypertension-related. The dorsal aorta can kink similarly, in the region where it becomes related and presumably fixed to the dorsal spine; this results in an opacity in the left hilar region on a PA film. The change can usually be diagnosed with a lateral film and careful fluoroscopy.

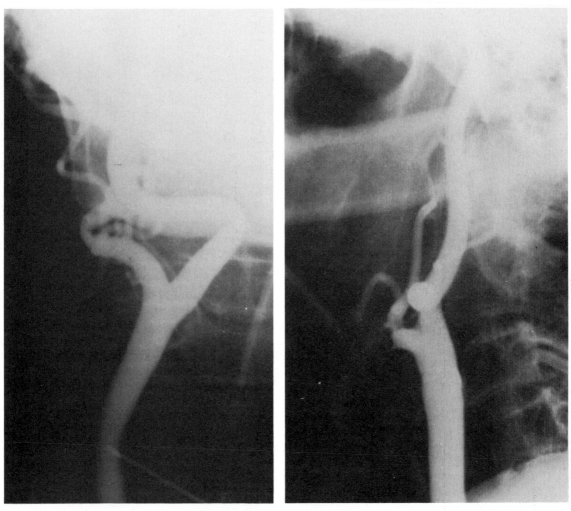

FIG. 16.56. Arteriosclerosis of the carotid arteries has resulted in vascular kinking, causing a pulsatile 'mass' in the neck.

A popliteal swelling which can cause some diagnostic difficulty is a popliteal aneurysm. Pulsatility may be discernible but transmitted, making the diagnosis between cyst and aneurysm difficult. CT and ultrasound are the examinations of choice as they may demonstrate the amount of clot present, but femoral angiography may be necessary for absolute confirmation (Fig. 16.57). Most popliteal cysts communicate with the knee joint, and will be demonstrated by arthrography.

Abdominal aneurysms, presenting on routine clinical examination or because of abdominal pain due to partial leakage, are mass lesions in which conventional arteriography and the newer imaging techniques all have a place in diagnosis and management. The clinical finding of a pulsatile abdominal mass is an indication for CT or ultrasound examination (Figs. 16.10, 16.43, 16.44), which will confirm the diagnosis and both will indicate the amount of clot within. Pancreatic tumours can also

be excluded. Excess bowel gas may be a problem in an ultrasound examination and here a CT examination will give an accurate diagnosis without delay, if apparatus is available. Arteriography by catheter from below or from above will give an indication of whether the renal arteries are involved, an important surgical consideration, and will show whether the aneurysm extends into the iliac vessels, but will not show the amount of clot within the aneurysm (Fig. 16.42). It also provides a small chance of clot dislodgement, but gives an indication of the extent of atheroma and the tortuosity of the vascular system generally. It is likely then that if surgical intervention is considered, ultrasound or CT together with arteriography will be carried out. Both ultrasound and CT provide an excellent means of assessing the progress of an aneurysm if it is treated conservatively.

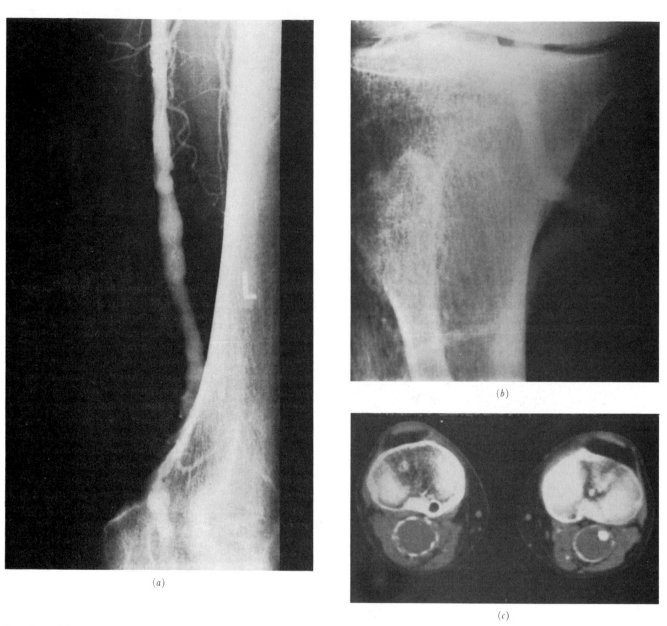

Fig. 16.57. (a) Ragged dilated femoropopliteal artery on left side. Complete occlusion of the vessels at the same level on the right. Some calcification visible on the plain films. (b) Very tortuous 'popliteal' artery. This was the remains of the lumen in a popliteal aneurysm. (c) Same patient as in (a) and (b). Bilateral popliteal aneurysms. Aortic bifurcation contrast injection. Wall calcification, clot, and collateral vessels are seen, together with an irregular lumen on the left side. Complete occlusion on the right side.

THERAPEUTIC ANGIOGRAPHY

There are a number of ways in which techniques originally designed to delineate the vascular system are now being exploited for therapeutic purposes. These include deliberate embolisation of selected vessels; transluminal dilatation of atheromatous narrowings and selective delivery of various therapeutic agents, e.g. cytotoxic and vasospastic agents.

Embolisation techniques have been used particularly in the kidney to infarct large tumours, either to reduce haemorrhage in inoperable cases or to facilitate surgical removal of large vascular tumours. In the periphery they have been employed in arteriovenous malformations to reduce size and tendency to haemorrhage. Various embolic agents have been employed for this; the patient's own blood, clotted with the aid of E.A.C.A., or dura or gel-foam cut into small pieces or small

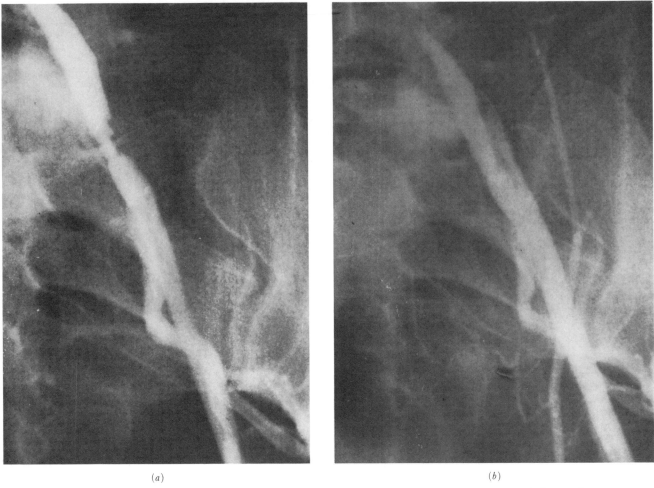

(a)   (b)

FIG. 16.58. (a) Common iliac stenosis, before dilatation. (b) Common iliac stenosis following dilatation by balloon catheter.

metallic coil springs, and also adhesives of the rapid setting variety. Neat ethanol is currently popular.

Transluminal dilatation or angioplasty has recently been used with considerable effect in coronary, renal, iliac and femoral vessels. The technique consists of passing balloon-tipped catheters up or downstream usually via a femoral approach, using the Seldinger wire as a guide after various dilating catheters have dilated the entry into the artery. The guide wire may be straight or have a curved end, and it is surprising how a completely blocked vessel may be penetrated by a guide wire with a flexible tip, and dilated for several centimetres by the progressive introduction of a balloon catheter which is repeatedly dilated after being thrust into the narrowed segment of artery. Demonstration of the arterial lesion by arteriography, preferably with appropriate opaque markers on the skin, must precede this procedure. Balloons of various diameter and length have to be

available to suit the precise size and length of the narrowing to be dilated; balloon catheters tend to be costly but against this must be offset the cost of the alternative surgical procedure. For single short significant arterial strictures of atheromatous nature they are an excellent means of improving blood flow (Fig. 16.58). Multiple stenoses are a relative contra-indication, but a completely blocked segment of vessel is not a complete contra-indication if a guide wire can be passed through the obstructed segment.

Selective introduction of pharmacologically active agents is not commonly practised in the peripheral arterial system, being of principal use in the liver and alimentary tract. It is possible, however, that the improving awareness of the factors underlying atherogenesis may produce pharmacological substances which will need selective arterial introduction. At present, haemostasis in oesophageal varices, bleeding peptic ulcer and colonic

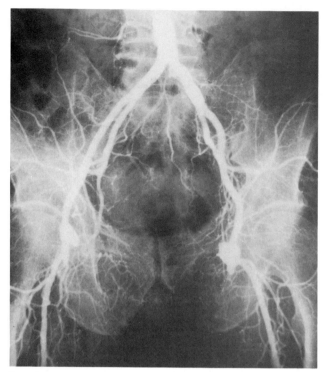

FIG. 16.59. Small aneurysms have formed at insertions of failed cross over femoro-femoral venous graft.

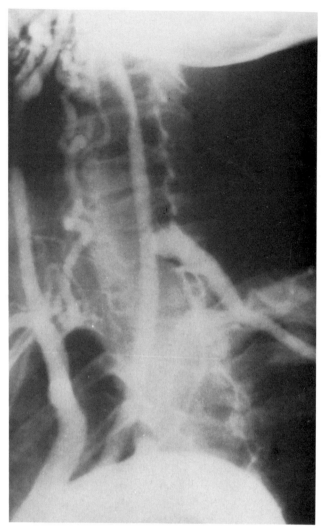

FIG. 16.61. Post surgical angiogram. Complete occlusion of the left subclavian artery near its origin. A venous graft has been inserted between the left common carotid artery and the distal part of the subclavian artery. Graft still patent 6 years later.

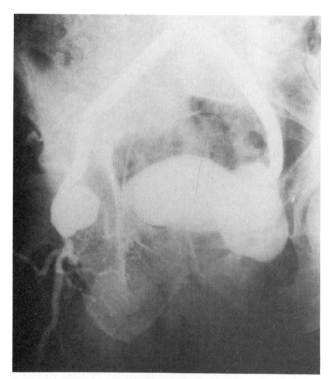

FIG. 16.60. Bilateral aneurysms have formed where a venous crossover graft was placed from one femoral artery to the other. Graft failed after some years. Severe atheromatous disease in each leg below the inguinal ligament level.

lesions provide most patients for this type of therapeutic treatment. Sub selective angiography is of considerable value in this.

ARTERIOGRAPHY FOLLOWING VASCULAR SURGERY

Radiologists are sometimes requested to carry out angiography on patients who have already had vascular surgery. The circumstances vary; a previous operation may have failed, or the patient may have developed evidence of disease elsewhere. In this circumstance, to deal most appropriately with the patient, it is important to ascertain exactly what operative procedure was

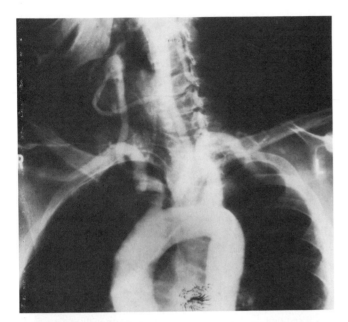

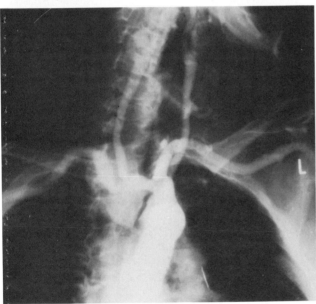

FIG. 16.62. Cross over graft from left common carotid to right bifurcation.

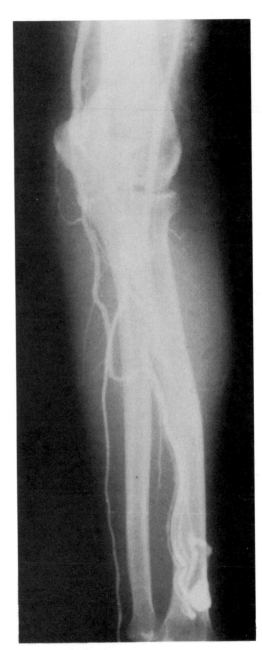

FIG. 16.63. Arteriovenous shunt created in forearm for dialysis. Intermittent shunt function, therefore angiogram. Note aneurysms at junction of artery and vein, and rapid venous return.

carried out, what is the current clinical state of the patient, and what exactly the surgeons now require to know. All this information must be obtained before carrying out any procedure.

One of the most common requests concerns a failed vein-graft by-pass operation in the leg where the patient again has ischaemic signs and symptoms in the foot and leg. Careful palpation for pulsation in each groin will enable the radiologist to decide whether a direct puncture or Seldinger procedure is possible. Entry on the currently diseased side is to be avoided if possible, but may be carried out if this offers the better pulse. In this case a simple stab of the femoral artery may be sufficient to provide the necessary information namely that the graft has occluded, and that there are or are not patent vessels in the popliteal region to which a fresh graft could be attached. Delayed films, even up to 20 or 30 seconds, may be necessary to establish this. One of the features of veins being attached to the femoral artery near the groin is the development of aneurysms or pseudo aneurysms at the site of attachment (Figs. 16.59 and 16.60).

Occasionally, surgery is performed for ischaemia in the arm (Fig. 16.61); clearly, knowledge of the surgical procedure is essential for the correct arteriographic approach to be planned.

Surgery is sometimes performed for cerebral ischaemia due to atheroma at the internal carotid origin; the operation may consist of endarterectomy with or without a vein-patch graft and angiography will show a dilated roughened segment of vessel if it is still patent. Rarely, a cross-over graft is performed for this condition (Fig. 16.62).

Other vascular surgery may result in a request for subsequent angiography. Fig. 16.63 shows an angiogram performed because of intermittent function of an arteriovenous fistula carried out in a dialysis patient. It was thought that the obstruction was due to the aneurysm which developed following surgery.

REFERENCES

BRICE, J. G., DOWSETT, D. J. & LOWE, R. D. (1964) Haemodynamic effects of carotid artery stenosis. *Brit. Med. J.*, ii, 1363.

FOX, J. A. & HUGH, A. E. (1966) Localization of Atheroma: A Theory Based on Boundary Layer Separation. *Brit. Heart J.*, **28**, 388–399.

MONCADA, S., GRYGLEWSKI, R., BUNTING, S. & VANE, J. R. (1976) An Enzyme Isolated from Arteries Transforms Prostaglandin Endoperoxides to an Unstable Substance that Inhibits Platelet Aggregation. *Nature*, **263**, 663–665.

SELDINGER, S. I. (1953) Catheter Replacement of the Needle in Percutaneous Arteriography. *Acta Radiol.*, **39**, 368–376.

CHAPTER 17

PHLEBOGRAPHY OF THE LIMB VEINS

M. Lea Thomas

INTRODUCTION

The term phlebography alone generally refers to contrast phlebography which until recently was the only method available and is used in this way throughout the chapter. The derivation of the word does not, however, preclude its use for any imaging technique but to avoid confusion it is usual to preface other types of investigation to indicate the method being employed, i.e. isotope phlebography, impedance phlebography, etc.

Whilst this chapter is largely concerned with contrast phlebography, for completeness some of the more recently evolved imaging techniques will be briefly discussed.

The earliest description of phlebography appeared in 1923 using strontium bromide but it was not until less toxic contrast media became available, diodone in the 1930's and the triple iodine containing organic compounds such as sodium or meglumine diatrizoate iothalamate or metrizoate in the 1950's, that phlebography became widely employed.

PHLEBOGRAPHY OF THE LEGS

(A) Ascending Phlebography

This is a basic standard technique and is suitable for 95% of clinical situations in which phlebography is indicated.

(i) **The contrast medium.** All the currently available high osmolality contrast media cause mild pain on injection, the severity depending largely on the hyperosmolality and the sodium content of the contrast media. Routinely, meglumine iothalamate 60% is used for phlebography of the peripheral parts of the limbs, but for the pelvis, abdomen and chest a more concentrated medium such as sodium iothalamate 70% may be required. Dilution of the contrast medium say to 40%, will reduce its osmolality and produces diagnostic phlebograms in the thinner parts of the limbs but the proximal large veins are rarely adequately opacified and for this reason routine dilution of the contrast medium is not recommended.

It is already clear that as soon as they become available the new low osmolality contrast media, either non-ionic or dimeric, for example metrizamide, iopamidol or ioxaglate will supercede the currently used media because they are virtually painless on injection and give rise to far less post phlebographic thrombosis. In fact, at the time of writing the author has already abandoned the use of the hyperosmolar media in favour of a low osmolality one of similar iodine content.

The amount of contrast medium needed for a particular examination varies considerably depending on the part of the body being examined, the size of the patient and the type of information required. As a rough guide about 50 ml of contrast is usually sufficient for each leg in ascending phlebography but a total of four times this amount may be required to show the more proximal veins or if doubtful areas have to be re-examined. No complications from these larger quantities have been encountered. The poor quality examinations of the early phlebographers were due to their inability to inject sufficient contrast because of side effects. This restraint no longer applies today and the commonest cause of undiagnostic phlebograms is due to the use of too little contrast medium.

(ii) **Radiographic apparatus.** Special radiographic apparatus for phlebography is not required, but there are certain important features. A tilting table is essential, image intensification and an automatic exposure device are desirable. The use of image intensification combined with television monitoring has considerably improved the diagnostic accuracy of phlebography. It enables the phlebographer to see the direction of flow of the contrast medium, and enables him to take radiographs when the veins are well filled, thus avoiding artefacts. The newer small focal spot X-ray tubes produce almost as good radiographic detail as was previously obtained by the larger focus-film distance possible with an over-couch tube. There is now no justification for the use of 'blind' non-fluoroscopic techniques. The quality of the fluoroscopic method can be further improved by the use of equipment with a fixed focus-film distance of 1 metre such as that on remote control fluoroscopy tables.

In addition to a fluoroscopy table a rapid serial film changer allows sequential exposures which in some situations are necessary to obtain maximum information. Cine radiography has a limited place in dynamic studies of the venous system.

(iii) **The position of the patient.** Ideally, ascending phlebography of the lower limbs should be carried out with the patient in the vertical position as in this position the deep venous system always fills provided it is patent, and there is maximum mixing of the contrast medium with the blood, preventing artefacts. However, such a position is frequently not tolerated by ill patients and even in healthy ones, vaso-vagal attacks are relatively common. For this reason the maximum tilt used is 60° foot downwards but very slight tilt, 20°–30° are often sufficient when combined with tourniquets.

When examining the calf for thrombosis it is important to instruct the patient not to bear weight on the leg being examined, otherwise calf muscle contraction prevents adequate filling of the soleal muscle veins.

(iv) **Venepuncture.** Any vein over the dorsum or distal part of the forefoot is suitable for puncture. The most constant vein is the medial digital vein of the great toe. Another advantage of this site is that any extravasation can easily be detected. Oedema may make intravenous injection difficult. Prolonged pressure will often disperse oedema from over a vein. Vasodilatation can be encouraged by use of warm packs or more effectively by sitting the patient with the legs dependent with the feet in a bowl of warm water. If the examination is not urgent elevation of the legs for about 24 hours beforehand will usually make a percutaneous examination feasible.

Routinely, a 21 gauge 'butterfly' needle is used, but for very small veins a 23 gauge may be required in which case some form of mechanical injector is helpful. Plastic cannulae instead of needles have been recommended by some phlebographers as these can be threaded into the vein minimising extravasation. Such cannula systems are never as sharp as a needle and in the author's view the discomfort to the patient outweighs the marginal advantage of minimal contrast extravasation.

(v) **Tourniquets.** Strictly speaking, as already mentioned, an ankle tourniquet is not necessary to fill the deep venous system provided a sufficiently steep foot-down table tilt is used. However, if the superficial veins are not occluded by a tourniquet, a confusing phlebogram with overlapping of the deep and superficial systems is produced. In certain situations, particularly in the identification of incompetent communicating veins it is essential to occlude the superficial venous system, otherwise the direction of flow in the incompetent communicating veins cannot be appreciated. There are anatomical reasons why an ankle tourniquet is desirable to fill the deep venous system. In the foot both the superficial and the deep veins drain by a common plexus, the superficial dorsal arch, which fills the long and short saphenous veins preferentially. This is why demonstration of the veins in the venous phase of a leg arteriogram is not adequate unless an ankle tourniquet is employed.

The tourniquet is usually placed just above the ankle and its tightness adjusted during injection and television observation to ensure deep venous filling occurs. When looking for incompetent communicating veins at the level of or below the ankle, or when venous ulceration prevents the application of a tourniquet there it may be applied around the forefoot. Although, the lower the tourniquet is applied the more deep veins are shown, as long as the tourniquet is applied proximal to the needle it will assist deep venous filling below the site of injection. Such a high position of the tourniquet may be required when examining patients with leg trauma, ulceration, or if no veins are visible lower down. A steep, foot-down table tilt is useful to utilise the hyperbaric properties of contrast media which fills the more dependent veins by gravity.

A tourniquet above the knee, while not essential, delays emptying of the calf veins, thus improving venous filling.

(vi) **Technique.** With the tourniquets in position films are taken during the injection of contrast medium under fluoroscopic control from the foot to the lower inferior vena cava. Straight projections alone are sufficient when examining for incompetent perforating veins and thrombotic changes but lateral views obtained by turning the patient so that the calf lies flat on the table are desirable to display the muscle veins of the calf in the search for thrombus. When adequate films of the calf have been obtained the tourniquets are released and films from the knee upward exposed. The Valsalva manoeuvre can be useful in phlebography. If the manoeuvre is carried out by the patient when the common femoral vein is seen to be filled with contrast medium the profunda femoris vein will be demonstrated as far as competent valves permit. There is a theoretical objection to the use of the Valsalva manoeuvre is that it may dislodge thrombus and produce pulmonary embolism. The author has not experienced this complication and the advantage of adequately demonstrating as much of the venous system as possible in patients with suspected pulmonary embolus outweighs this theoretical hazard.

(B) Variations of Ascending Phlebography

(i) **The bolus technique.** Calf compression to produce a bolus of contrast is useful to obtain better filling of any part of the venous system but it is particularly valuable to demonstrate the iliac veins and lower inferior vena cava.

A tourniquet is applied tightly around each knee and 50 ml of contrast medium injected simultaneously into each foot vein. The table is then tilted slightly head downwards, the tourniquets are released, and firm pressure applied immediately to both calves while an exposure of the pelvis is made. This bolus method gives adequate opacification of the iliac veins and lower

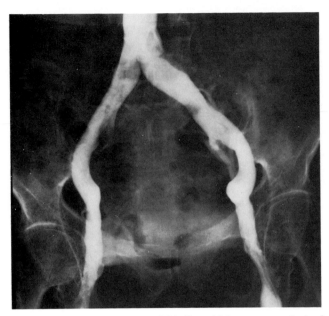

FIG. 17.01. The bolus technique. This iliac phlebogram was obtained by calf compression after foot injections of contrast medium. The iliac veins and lower inferior vena cava are well shown and a significant lesion is excluded.

inferior vena cava in about 95% of patients (Fig. 17.01). In the remaining 5% separate iliocaval phlebography is required. Calf compression can be criticised as liable to dislodge thrombus from the calf veins. The author has not encountered this complication probably because the pressure rise in the veins produced by calf compression is not greater than that caused by normal muscular contraction.

(ii) **Tilt phlebography.** This variant of ascending phlebography involves tilting the patient foot down immediately after injection in order to temporarily arrest upward blood flow and to reverse the hydrostatic gradient so as to sharply identify venous valves and their competence. Similar information can be obtained by the use of ascending phlebography with a Valsalva manoeuvre or by descending phlebography.

(iii) **Exercise phlebography.** This technique involves combining the foot down posture with leg muscle exercise. In this way the deep veins are positively filled by the pumping action and the competence of incompetent communicating vein valves are directly tested. Incompetent communicating veins can be more simply demonstrated by the use of a tourniquet to occlude the superficial venous system, so that the reverse flow of blood from deep to superficial veins indicates incompetence.

(iv) **Intraosseous phlebography.** This route produces excellent demonstration of the deep leg veins. It involves the injection of contrast medium into the bone marrow. Its main disadvantage is that, being painful, a general anaesthetic is usually required and there is a risk of osteomyelitis unless a scrupulous aseptic technique is employed. Its main use is for the demonstration of the pelvic veins and is described in detail later. Its value in ascending phlebography of the legs is when accessible subcutaneous veins are not available, either because of occlusion by thrombus or oedema. Injections into the malleoli or os calcis show the deep veins of the legs and is particularly useful in the demonstration of incompetent communicating veins as the deep veins fill preferentially from the bone marrow. It is also useful in demonstrating angiomas by injecting into the bone marrow of a nearby bone.

(v) **Descending phlebography.** The femoral vein is punctured in the groin using a cannula which can be threaded a short distance into the vein and strapped in position. Femoral vein puncture is easier if the patient carries out a Valsalva manoeuvre to distend the vein. Ideally the femoral puncture should be made below the inguinal ligament as it is easier to promote haemostasis by pressure at this point, but in practice the vein is punctured medial to the maximum pulsation of the femoral or external iliac artery.

The examination is carried out with a 60° foot down table tilt. Fifteen ml of contrast medium is injected as a bolus under fluoroscopic control and a control film taken. Immediately after the injection the patient is asked to perform a Valsalva manoeuvre. This is standardised at 40 mm Hg and maintained for 12 seconds. At the end of the Valsalva manoeuvre films are taken from the needle downwards, to see the level to which the contrast has descended.

This method is used for assessing the competence of the femoral venous valves. In the normal patient contrast medium is stopped by the first or second valve. An arbitrary grading of the degree of incompetence is used, i.e. grade 1 when the contrast medium is held up in the upper thigh; grade 2 when the contrast is held up above the knee; grade 3 when the contrast passes into the upper calf, and grade 4 when the contrast medium reaches the ankle. The significance of these gradings is difficult to interpret in practice. Venous valves, unlike arterial ones, are normally partially incompetent in the resting position and when contrast is injected into veins because it is heavier than blood it tends to gravitate downwards. The author believes that a standardised Valsalva manoeuvre is an essential aspect of the test as this closes normal valve cusps tightly rendering them competent.

(vi) **Retrograde phlebography.** This is a modification of descending phlebography and is often carried out after pulmonary angiography to exclude thrombus in the large proximal veins.

A catheter is passed from the arm through the right atrium down the inferior vena cava and into the femoral vein. The catheter can also be positioned in either internal iliac vein. As the catheter is directed under fluoroscopic control small injections of contrast medium are made by hand at various levels and the state of the veins recorded on spot films. In this way the whole of the inferior vena cava, the common iliac and external iliac veins and the internal iliac veins can be clearly demonstrated.

(C) Iliocaval Phlebography

(i) **Femoral vein injections.** The injection of contrast medium by hand into the femoral veins with the patient in the horizontal position produces excellent opacification of the femoral and iliac veins. This technique is the method of choice if the femoral vein is known to be patent. Bilateral simultaneous injections of 50 ml of contrast medium gives better opacification of the lower inferior vena cava.

The femoral veins are punctured with a needle or cannula as described above (see descending phlebography). The examination is carried out using a serial film changer. Films of the pelvis are taken to show the iliac veins and of the abdomen to show the inferior vena cava. The inferior vena cava is better shown in a slightly oblique projection so that the cava is projected to the right of the vertebral column and thus not obscured by bone. To show the internal iliac veins a Valsalva manoeuvre is carried out about half-way through the injection of contrast medium.

(ii) **Intraosseous injections.** Intraosseous injections are indicated, when it is thought or known that the femoral vein is occluded to demonstrate the upper limit of such an occlusion. To facilitate the examination the author has devised a cannula with a three faceted drill tip for easier penetration of the cortex of the bone (Fig. 17.02). To demonstrate the iliac veins or the inferior vena cava the greater trochanters are the site of injection. Simultaneous injections of 50 ml of contrast medium are made using a pressure pump at 50 p.s.i. A serial film changer is used and about 10 films taken at the rate of 1 per second, starting at the beginning of the injection. Two pressure injectors are employed because a single pressure injector with a 'Y' connection is not satisfactory because the contrast medium tends to enter the side giving the least resistance. If the inferior vena cava is being examined the films are centred over the abdomen the same way as for the femoral vein injection technique.

A combination of percutaneous femoral injection on the patent side and an intraosseous injection on the obstructed side is often used. As contrast medium is hyperbaric and tends to fill the more dependent veins, better filling of the external and common iliac veins is

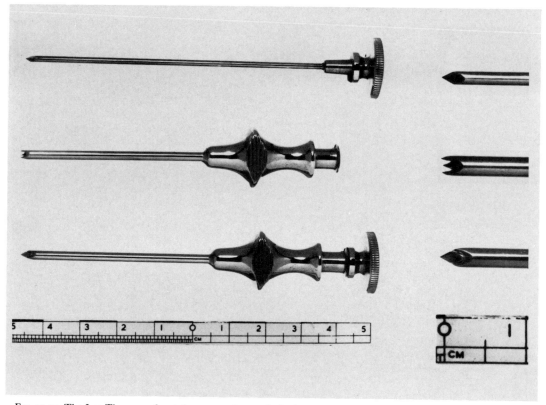

FIG. 17.02. The Lea Thomas 3 faceted trocar and cannula for intraosseous injections. The tip is shown in close up.

obtained with the patient in the *prone* position and of the internal iliac veins with the patient in the *supine* position.

After all phlebographic examinations the veins should be cleared of contrast by injecting 100 ml or more of physiological saline to minimise the irritating effect on the intima.

(D) Variations of Technique According to Clinical Need.

(i) **Deep vein thrombosis.** When phlebography is undertaken to confirm the presence of deep vein thrombosis the standard technique of ascending phlebography should be followed with a special emphasis on the following objectives:

(a) If the suspect limb is found to contain thrombus, the other clinically normal limb must be examined because there is a 50% chance that it will also contain thrombus.

(b) The upper limit of any thrombus or occluded vein must be displayed, if necessary with supplementary perfemoral or pertrochanteric injections.

(c) More than one film must be taken of each segment of the venous tree to confirm that any filling defects are persistent and of constant shape indicating that they are not artefactual.

(d) As many deep calf and thigh veins as possible should be filled, especially any collateral channels which may by-pass occluded veins.

(e) The ankle tourniquet must not be so tight that the superficial veins are completely obstructed, otherwise superficial vein thrombosis can be missed.

(ii) **The investigation of pulmonary thromboembolism.** The search for the source of pulmonary emboli should include a full ascending phlebogram of *both* limbs. Views should be taken of the feet and every attempt made to fill the profunda femoris and internal iliac veins. If it is thought essential to show the whole internal iliac system a bilateral pertrochanteric phlebogram in the supine position should be performed. For absolute completeness, especially if no thrombus has been found in the limbs, an angio-cardiogram of the right atrium, ventricle and pulmonary arteries is necessary.

(iii) **Incompetent communicating veins.** Before surgery or sclerotherapy the clinician may wish to know about the presence and the precise location of incompetent communicating veins in order to plan treatment. The technique for ascending phlebography is modified by applying the ankle and above knee tourniquets tightly so that they completely occlude the superficial veins and allow the radiologist to see with fluoroscopy any reverse flow from the deep to the superficial veins through incompetent communicating veins.

Self fastening rubber tourniquets are usually adequate if applied tightly enough, but pneumatic cuffs which are attached to a manometer so that the cuff pressures can be measured are particularly useful. Usually the lower cuff is placed just above the ankle but can be applied around the forefoot if a submalleolar incompetent perforating vein is suspected. The upper cuff should be above the adductor hiatus otherwise an incompetent communicating vein in Hunter's canal may be occluded. The ankle cuff is inflated to 120 mm Hg and the mid thigh cuff to 200 mm Hg. These pressures do not occlude the arterial flow because the cuffs are narrow. When the superficial veins are opacified inadvertently because of too loose an ankle tourniquet, or through an incompetent communicating vein, the deep veins are cleared of contrast medium with physiological saline and a second more proximal tourniquet applied before continuing the examination. As a rule only straight films are required as lateral films are difficult to interpret if there is superficial vein filling. Nearly all the clinically important communicating veins connecting the posterior tibial and peroneal veins to the superficial veins are shown on the straight projections. Early films, judged by fluoroscopy, are taken to show the *origins* of the incompetent communicating veins; late films with too much superficial venous filling are unhelpful. Oblique views are occasionally necessary to distinguish a superficial from a deep vein. The former move in a wider arc during rotation of the leg than the latter which are closely applied to the tibia and fibula (Fig. 17.03).

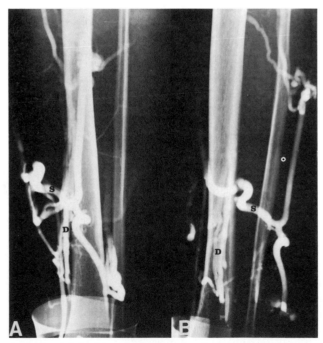

FIG. 17.03. (A) In this straight projection the superficial (S) and the deep veins (D) are superimposed. (B) Rotation of the limb separates the two sets of veins, the deep veins remaining close to the bones.

An incompetent communicating vein in the thigh can sometimes only be shown by a Valsalva manoeuvre carried out when the femoral vein in the adductor canal region is filled with contrast medium.

As mentioned previously an intraosseous injection is an accurate method of demonstrating incompetent communicating veins, and can be conveniently carried out in the operating theatre immediately before surgery.

(iv) **Congenital malformations.** These malformations display such a wide clinical spectrum that each case has to be considered separately. If the venous abnormality is localised, direct injection of contrast medium into the dysplastic veins to show their size and tributaries may be all that is required. In the relatively common Klippel Trenaunay syndrome the main problem is to confirm that the deep venous system is patent before surgical removal of any superficial veins. In this condition direct injection of the superficial venous channels to demonstrate their site of connection with the deep venous system is often also required.

In some instances introsseous phlebography at a site close to the malformation may give the maximum information and in the more complex angiomas arteriophlebography, that is arterial injection with follow through to the venous phase, may be the only way to demonstrate the full extent of the lesion. Because of the size of some of these lesions a large volume of contrast medium may have to be used. Even so visualisation of the veins is often poor and the subtraction technique may be useful to enhance the quality. It is possible that the recently developed digital subtraction angiography will overcome this difficulty.

Complications of Phlebography

Only those complications which may occur as a direct result of phlebography are discussed here. Systemic and idiosyncratic reactions due to the contrast medium obviously have the same incidence as they have when used for other radiological examinations.

(i) **Local extravasation.** Contrast medium which extravasates into the tissues causes a chemical cellulitis (Fig. 17.04). Very rarely (0·4%) this may progress to ulceration, soft tissue necrosis and even gangrene (Fig. 17.05). Although rare, these complications may need to be treated by skin grafting and even amputation. For this reason extreme care should be taken over the venepuncture, and the position of the needle checked by a small test injection before the full examination is carried out. Throughout the examination the injection site should be inspected for swelling and examined with a fluoroscope for evidence of extravasation. Should the patient complain of pain the site should immediately be examined. If extravasation is present another venepuncture should be made leaving the first needle in position to minimise leakage from the first puncture site. If severe, the examination should be terminated.

Ankle tourniquets applied too tightly cause fragile distal veins to rupture with considerable extravasation of contrast medium. When examining for incompetent communicating veins the tourniquet needs to be tight enough to occlude the superficial venous system but if excessive tightness is required and particularly if the

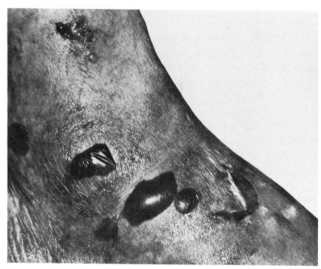

FIG. 17.04. Superficial skin necrosis and blistering following extravasation of contrast medium.

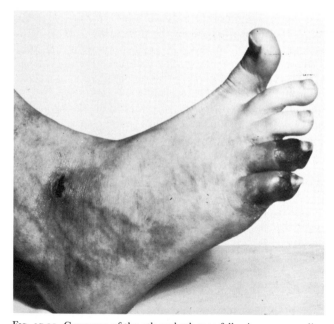

FIG. 17.05. Gangrene of the 4th and 5th toes following an ascending phlebogram. The patient has Klippel-Trenaunay syndrome with absent deep veins of the calf preventing clearing of the contrast from the foot. The site of the cut down for the phlebogram can be seen in front of the lateral malleolus.

patient complains of a severe bursting sensation below the tourniquet this should be released and the examination abandoned. An intraosseous examination can be carried out instead.

Tissue necrosis from extravasated contrast medium is particularly likely to occur in patients with chronic arterial or venous insufficiency and great care is required when examining such patients.

If extravasation occurs an attempt should be made to disperse the contrast medium to prevent localised concentration beneath the skin or in the soft tissues. This is best done by gentle local massage and diluting the contrast medium in the tissues by injecting physiological saline. Hyaluronidase is probably contraindicated as the combination of this drug with contrast medium will increase the risk of tissue damage.

(ii) **Thrombosis.** Contrast media are known to damage the venous intima, and thrombosis at the site of injection in the superficial vein is quite common, occurring in about 20% of patients. Post phlebographic deep vein thrombosis which is clinically manifest is rare occurring in only about 1% in the author's experience. Recent studies using the I[125] fibrinogen test following phlebography has disputed this view and it is now suggested that as many as a third of patients develop deep vein thrombosis following phlebography using the currently available hyperosmolar contrast media.

Every effort must be made to prevent thrombosis by clearing the contrast media from the veins by injecting physiological saline and encouraging active movement. The clearance of contrast media from the veins should be confirmed by fluoroscopy. Routine use of heparinised saline is not necessary except in patients with a high thrombogenic tendency such as those with carcinomatosis.

(iii) **Complications of intraosseous phlebography.** These include pain at the site of injection, caused by extravasation, osteomyelitis, ischaemic bone necrosis and fat embolism. The latter should be suspected in patients who develop neurological signs after the examination.

Anatomy

(i) **The foot.** There are two venous systems in the foot, the superficial dorsal system, i.e. the long saphenous veins joined together by the dorsal venous arch, and the deep venous system of the sole. The deep and superficial networks are connected by a series of communicating veins.

(ii) **The deep veins of the leg.** The deep veins of the lower leg consist of three sets of paired veins accompanying the arteries, the anterior and posterior tibial veins and the peroneal veins (Fig. 17.06).

In a film taken in a straight projection with the foot internally rotated the peroneal veins lie between the images of the tibia and fibula; the anterior tibial veins

more laterally, often over the fibula, the posterior tibial veins medially, running obliquely upwards to cross the lower third of the shaft of the tibia. The individual veins are often easier to identify in the lateral view (Fig. 17.07 A & B).

The veins of the calf muscles are either large, baggy and valveless, the so called sinusoidal veins, or thin and straight with valves. The former predominate in the soleus muscle, the latter in the gastrocnemius muscle. The veins from the gastrocnemius muscle drain into the upper part of the popliteal vein.

In the upper calf these paired veins merge into single trunks and then unite at different levels to form the popliteal vein, usually below, but sometimes above, the

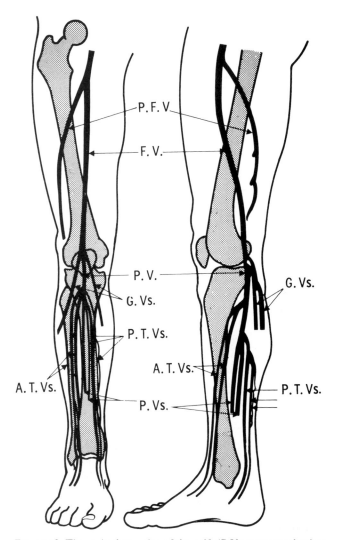

FIG. 17.06. The main deep veins of the calf, (P.Vs. = peroneal veins; A.T.Vs. = anterior tibial veins; P.T.Vs. = posterior tibial veins; G.Vs. = gastrocnemius veins; P.V. = popliteal vein; F.V. = superficial femoral vein; P.F.V. = profunda femoris vein) (*After May & Nissl, 1959*).

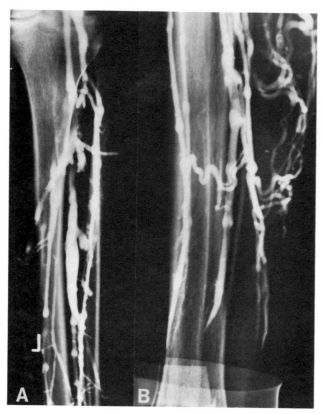

FIG. 17.07. (A) Straight projection of calf. The three sets of stem veins can be identified. (B) In the lateral projection the three sets are more clearly identified. The posterior tibial veins are the ones a short distance behind the tibia and fibula, above the ankle.

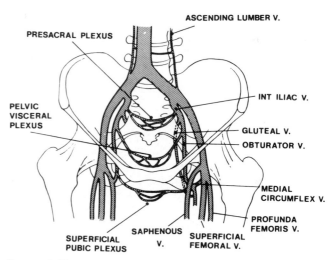

FIG. 17.08. Diagram of potential collateral pathways in parietal pelvic vein obstruction (*After Mavor & Galloway, 1967*).

knee joint. Double popliteal and superficial femoral veins are common.

(iii) **Deep veins of the thigh.** The superficial femoral vein is a continuation of the popliteal vein and passes obliquely upwards and medially across the lower third of the femur. Below the inguinal ligament it receives the profunda femoris vein which is only demonstrated fully in about a third of patients where there is a direct loop connection between the superficial and the deep veins.

The common femoral vein is formed by confluence of the superficial femoral and profunda femoris veins. This vein has a number of small tributaries which become important collaterals when the iliac vein is obstructed.

(iv) **The pelvic veins and inferior vena cava.** The external iliac veins are the continuation of a common femoral vein. They run from the inguinal ligament to the sacroiliac joints where they are joined inferomedially by the internal iliac veins emerging from the true pelvis.

The main tributaries of the external iliac vein anastamose with their fellows of the opposite side and form important collaterals in iliac vein obstruction (Fig. 17.08). The internal iliac vein is formed in the

floor of the true pelvis by the union of the pelvic veins and the parietal and pelvic visceral plexuses. The common iliac veins are short wide trunks which pass upwards from the sacro-iliac joints to unite on the right side of the 5th lumbar vertebra to form the inferior vena cava. The right common iliac vein and the inferior vena cava run upwards in a straight line, whereas the left common iliac vein joins the right common iliac vein at a right angle. At this point the common iliac vein is pushed forwards by the convexity of the lumbosacral junction and crossed by the right common iliac artery. This causes a variable degree of anteroposterior compression of the termination of the left common iliac vein (Fig. 17.09) which appears as a radiological filling defect in about 50% of phlebograms. Excessive compression at this site may predispose to venous thrombosis producing the so called Cockett–Lea Thomas Syndrome.

The only tributary of the common iliac vein is the iliolumbar vein which is larger on the left than the right. Its iliac tributary provides an important collateral pathway around an external iliac vein obstruction and the ascending lumbar vein in inferior vena caval obstruction through its numerous communications with the vertebral venous plexuses and the azygos and hemiazygos venous systems. The inferior vena cava ascends from the 5th lumbar vertebra to the right atrium to the right of the vertebral bodies. It receives a variable number of pairs of short wide lumbar veins which connect with the vertebral venous plexuses.

(v) **Venous valves.** The common iliac veins and the inferior vena cava are valveless. Valves are occasionally found in the external iliac vein and usually in the main trunk of the internal iliac vein and its tributaries.

There are many valves in the distal deep veins of the

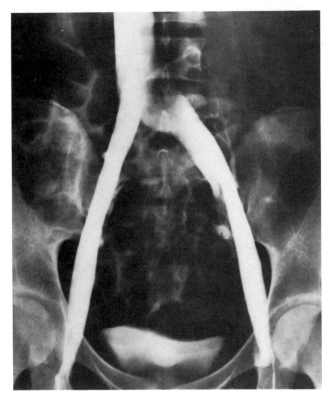

FIG. 17.09. Iliac phlebogram. There is a translucency at the junction of the left common iliac vein with the inferior vena cava caused by compression between the right common iliac artery in front and the sacro-iliac spine behind. This is present in about 50% of phlebograms and is of no significance. More severe compression may lead to thrombosis and the iliac vein compression syndrome.

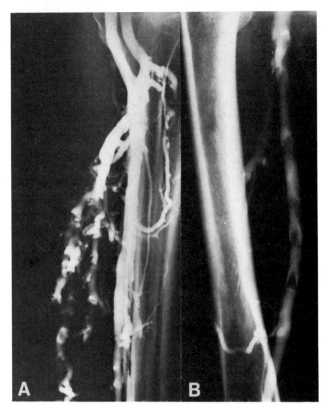

FIG. 17.10. (A) There are numerous valves in the stem and muscle veins of the calf, but the valves become progressively fewer in the more proximal veins. The external and common iliac veins and the inferior vena cava are almost always valveless. Valves are present in the internal iliac veins preventing retrograde filling. (B) Normal bicuspid valves in the femoral vein shown during a Valsalva manoeuvre.

limb but they become progressively fewer in the proximal veins such as the superficial femoral and profunda femoris veins. There are no valves in the baggy sinusoidal veins in the soleal muscles, but the venous arcades which also drain the soleus and gastrocnemius muscles have many valves (Fig. 17.10A & B).

All the communicating veins in the lower part of the calf and all the veins connecting the deep and superficial veins in all parts of the lower limb have valves and ensure that blood can pass only from the superficial to the deep system.

(vi) **The superficial veins.** The *long saphenous vein* is formed by the union of veins from the medial side of the sole of the foot and the medial plantar vein. It runs upwards in front of the medial malleolus, along the length of the antero-medial aspect of the limb to join the common femoral vein at the groin (Fig. 17.11).

The *short saphenous vein* begins at the outer border of the foot behind the lateral malleolus. It is formed by the union of the lateral plantar vein with small veins draining the outer part of the heel, and enters the popliteal space between the two heads of the gastroc-

nemius muscle. Phlebographically the vein is best seen in the lateral projection of the calf where it can be seen superficially following the curve of the calf muscles. Its precise terminations can be extremely variable. Usually it unites with the popliteal vein in the popliteal fossa a few centimetres above the level of the knee joint but it may join at any site, sometimes as high as the upper part of the femoral vein. It is for this reason that phlebography of the short saphenous vein is often required to show its exact termination if ligation for varicose veins is being considered (Fig. 17.12A & B).

(vii) **Anatomical variations.** Because of the complicated embryology congenital abnormalities of the superficial and deep venous systems are extremely common. These consist, for the most part, of reduplications of the veins, accessory veins and abnormalities of the position and site of termination of the veins. These variations are not usually, in themselves, of any significance but need to be appreciated if surgical treatment is being carried out and may need to be demonstrated by superficial or deep phlebography.

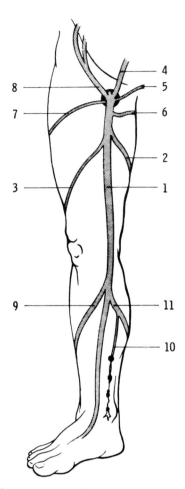

FIG. 17.11. The long saphenous vein and its connections. 1. Main long saphenous vein. 2. Medial accessory saphenous vein. 3. Lateral accessory saphenous vein. 4. Superficial epigastric vein. 5. External pudendal vein. 6. Medial circumflex femoral vein. 7. Lateral circumflex femoral vein. 8. Superficial circumflex iliac vein. 9. Anterior vein of the leg. 10. Posterior arch vein. 11. Anastomosis with the short saphenous vein (*After May, 1979*).

It has been estimated that about 1% of otherwise normal subjects have congenital abnormalities of the inferior vena cava.

(viii) **The communicating veins.** The largest communicating veins are the terminations of the long and short saphenous veins where they join the deep venous system. They are however, only a part of a series of communicating veins. There are numerous communicating veins which are not of great clinical significance as bi-directional flow between the superficial and deep veins normally occurs.

In the lower leg the medial and lateral communicating veins are of considerable clinical importance. The medial communicating veins penetrate the deep fascia and empty directly into the lower tributaries of the posterior tibial veins. There are three constant medial

communicating veins, one just above the tip of the medial malleolus and two others approximately 6 cm apart just behind the posteromedial border of the lower half of the tibia. These veins are linked to each other making an arcade known as the posterior arch vein and do not drain directly into the long saphenous vein (Fig. 17.13).

In the thigh there is a constant long communicating vein which joins the long saphenous vein, or one of its tributaries, to the superficial femoral vein in the lower part of the subsartorial canal. Incompetence of this vein can be shown phlebographically by ascending phlebography combined with a Valsalva manoeuvre.

While some communicating veins are relatively constant in position (Fig. 17.14) there are many others which may become incompetent and it is for this reason that accurate localisation by phlebography is often required.

Artefacts

These usually result from streaming of contrast along the vein wall, uneven mixing of the hyperbaric media with blood, and entry of non-opacified blood from tributaries. These may resemble thrombus (Fig. 17.15A & B) or post thrombotic changes (Fig. 17.16A & B).

They can be minimised by using ample contrast medium and by the use of fluoroscopy to ensure that films are taken when the veins are optimally filled.

They can be distinguished from pathology because they are inconstant in appearance.

Appearances of Thrombus

Thrombus shows as a constant filling defect in an opacified vein which is the same size and shape in at least two films with an interval between them. It is important for accurate diagnosis to try and outline the thrombus itself and not rely solely on non-filling of veins. The ends of an unfilled vein should be carefully examined for a little thrombus projecting from one or other end (Fig. 17.17). However, a constantly unfilled segment using a correct phlebographic technique is very suggestive of thrombus. Clearly, the exact site of thrombus is also important (Fig. 17.18A, B & C).

If the thrombus is very fresh it will not be adherent to the wall and will appear as a translucent defect separated from the wall by a thin line of contrast medium (Fig. 17.19). Obliteration of this line indicates the adherence of the thrombus to the wall (Fig. 17.20). When a thrombus completely occludes a vein there is no contrast around it but there is contrast medium in the vein above, below it and in the collateral vessels beside it (Fig. 17.21). Thrombus, as it ages, becomes smaller and there is a thicker layer of contrast surrounding it making its surface more clearly defined (Fig. 17.22). The process of adherence and retraction occurs simultaneously. When a vein re-opens as a result

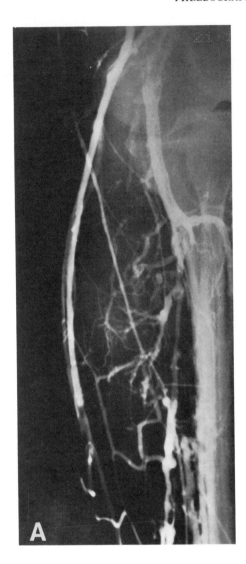

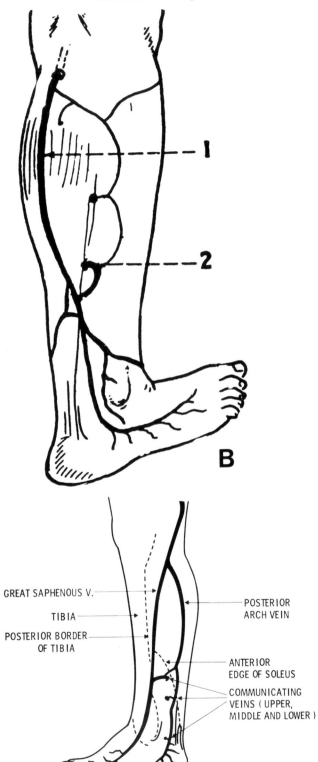

FIG. 17.12. The short saphenous vein. (A) Ascending phlebogram. (B) Diagram. 1. The short saphenous vein. 2. The large constant ankle communicating vein.

FIG. 17.13. The sites and superficial connections of the medial communicating veins. Note that the three main communicating veins are not directly connected to the long (great) saphenous vein and are not affected by stripping operations.

GREAT SAPHENOUS V.

TIBIA

POSTERIOR BORDER OF TIBIA

POSTERIOR ARCH VEIN

ANTERIOR EDGE OF SOLEUS

COMMUNICATING VEINS (UPPER, MIDDLE AND LOWER)

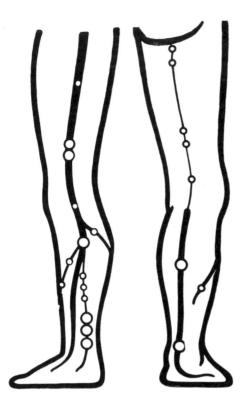

FIG. 17.14. The common sites of the communicating veins. The sites of those marked on this figure are relatively constant but there are many communicating veins at other sites (*After May, 1979*).

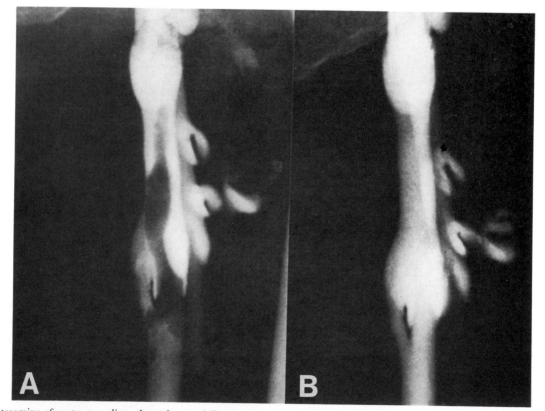

FIG. 17.15. (A) Streaming of contrast medium through a partially opened valve resembling a thrombus with a 'loose tail'. (B) A subsequent film shows the vein is normal.

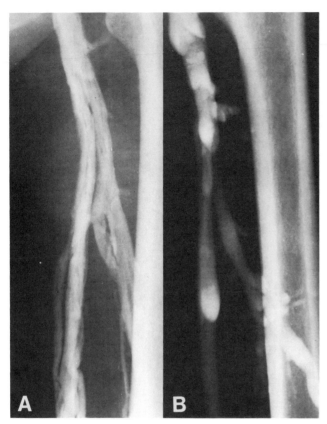

FIG. 17.16. (A) Gross failure of mixing resembles recanalisation changes in the superficial and deep femoral veins. (B) A later film during a Valsalva manoeuvre indicates the veins are normal.

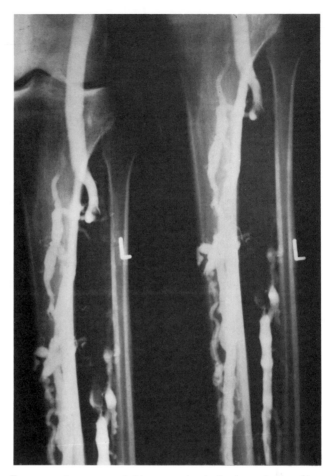

FIG. 17.17. A segment of this peroneal vein is absent in two films taken with an interval between them. Careful examination of the segment shows that there is a little thrombus at each end of the unfilled segment indicating that it is occluded by thrombus.

of retraction of the thrombus, so called recanalisation, the lumen is irregular and often reduplicated and the valves are damaged or destroyed (Fig. 17.23). Such recanalisation changes do not always follow thrombosis.

An important feature of a thrombus is its proximal extremity. It may have a 'floating tail' which may become detached and embolise (Fig. 17.24) or it may have a horizontal 'square cut' shape indicating that a portion has already broken off and embolised (See Fig. 17.18B). It is possible to make a crude estimate of the age of a thrombus. In the first week a thrombus is smooth and loose and almost fills the whole vein allowing only a thin line of contrast medium to surround it. Over the next fourteen days it becomes adherent to the vein wall and retracts with a thicker layer of contrast around it and its edge more clearly defined. Further retraction and resorption make the surface of the thrombus irregular and produces slowly progressing recanalisation changes over several months. An estimate of looseness or adherence of the thrombus is important in the management of deep vein thrombosis as the former is likely to embolise.

A vein may remain totally occluded following throm-

bosis or recanalise with no, or variable, damage to valves. It is not possible to predict the final outcome from the original phlebogram. When permanent venous obstruction occurs the collateral veins which may develop may be enlarged venae commitantes which may be recognised because they are always slightly smaller but in the same line as the veins they replace, or nearby non-obstructed veins.

The Post Thrombotic Syndrome

Following thrombosis of the deep veins of the calf recanalisation almost invariably occurs but in the process the valves are frequently damaged and become incompetent.

This distorts the normal function of the calf muscle pump and high pressure during exercise is transmitted to the superficial veins through incompetent communicating veins. This high pressure, probably combined with additional factors such as tissue response, even-

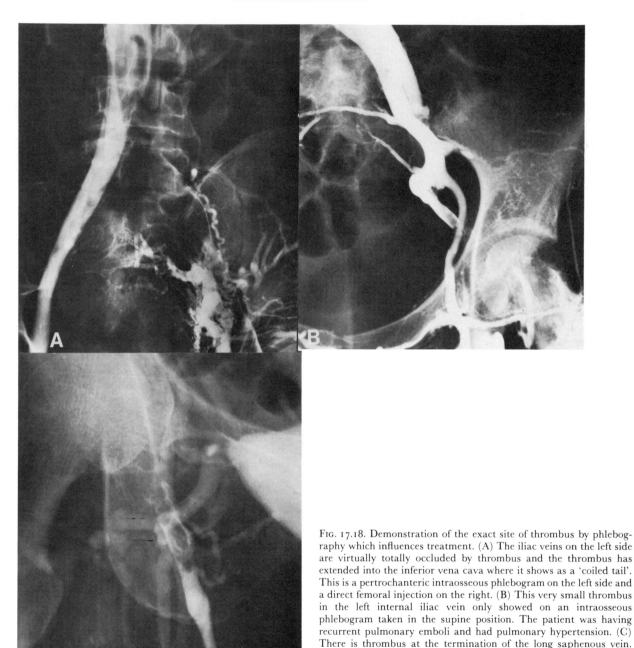

FIG. 17.18. Demonstration of the exact site of thrombus by phlebography which influences treatment. (A) The iliac veins on the left side are virtually totally occluded by thrombus and the thrombus has extended into the inferior vena cava where it shows as a 'coiled tail'. This is a pertrochanteric intraosseous phlebogram on the left side and a direct femoral injection on the right. (B) This very small thrombus in the left internal iliac vein only showed on an intraosseous phlebogram taken in the supine position. The patient was having recurrent pulmonary emboli and had pulmonary hypertension. (C) There is thrombus at the termination of the long saphenous vein. Embolism probably does not occur from the long saphenous vein but propagation into the common femoral vein and beyond does occur and treatment is therefore necessary.

tually leads to skin necrosis and ulceration around the ankle.

It is generally thought that thrombosis destroys the valves of the deep veins and the communicating veins. However, phlebographically incompetent communicating veins are often demonstrated when the deep veins appear normal. When the deep veins are damaged they show typical changes of recanalisation with irregular, reduplicated lumens and destroyed valves (Fig. 17.25A & B). Valve function is best shown phlebographically by descending phlebography (Fig. 17.26A & B). While any vein in the deep venous system may remain obstructed after thrombosis the common sites are the left common iliac vein, the proximal part of the superficial femoral vein in the adductor canal region and the inferior vena cava. These occlusions are frequently

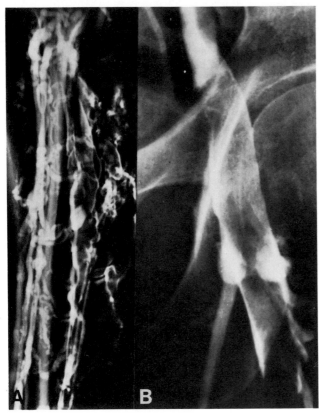

FIG. 17.19. Examples of recent thrombus, probably less than three days old. (A) In the calf. (B) In the superficial and common femoral veins. In both cases the thrombus is surrounded by a thin white line of contrast medium indicating that it is not adherent to the wall. The 'square cut' end of the thrombus in B indicates that an embolus has already occurred.

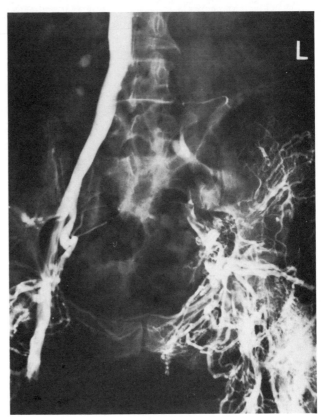

FIG. 17.20. A left intraosseous phlebogram showing total occlusion of the external and common iliac veins with a little thrombus extending into the inferior vena cava showing as an irregular margin. Thrombus is also shown in the left internal iliac vein. The right intraosseous phlebogram shows that there is no thrombus on this side. Intraosseous phlebography in the only satisfactory method of showing the ilio-caval segment when the femoral vein is occluded.

accompanied by extensive deep vein damage in the calf and elsewhere (Fig. 17.27A & B).

The collateral pathways which may open following venous obstruction are an important confirmation of the site and significance of the obstruction.

Varicose Veins

It is convenient to classify varicose veins into primary, where the cause is unknown, and secondary, when they are due to known venous pathology usually past deep vein thrombosis.

Phlebography plays little part in the diagnosis and management of primary varicose veins as the diagnosis is readily made clinically. These veins can be demonstrated phlebographically if required either by ascending or descending phlebography, or by direct injection into the varicose veins, so called varicography (Fig. 17.28).

If there is doubt as to whether varicose veins are primary or secondary or have a mixed aetiology, phle-

bography is useful in identifying the presence of incompetent or obstructed deep veins and incompetent communicating veins. Phlebography is particularly valuable when assessing recurrent varicose veins following surgery or sclerotherapy to show any large incompetent communicating veins which have been missed by the treatment.

Incompetent communicating veins are readily recognised by ascending phlebography. In addition to retrograde flow, from deep to superficial veins they do not have normal valves, are abnormally wide and tortuous and frequently dilated at their distal end where they join a varicose vein. Communicating veins without these features should be considered normal as sometimes a normal vein allows contrast to pass from a deep to a superficial vein.

Accurate localisation of a site of incompetent communicating veins is helped by placing a plastic ruler containing radiopaque ball bearings at 1 cm intervals beneath the leg during phlebography. The sites of the

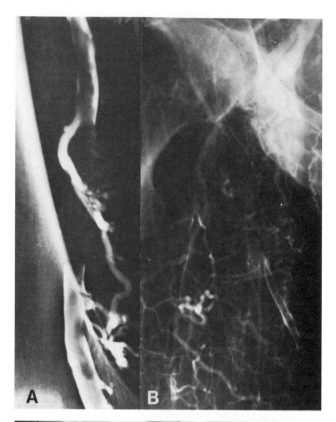

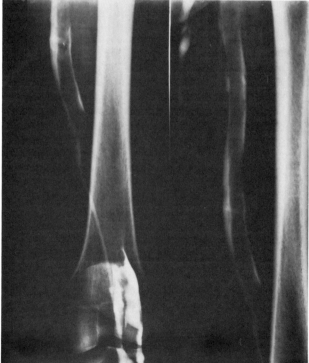

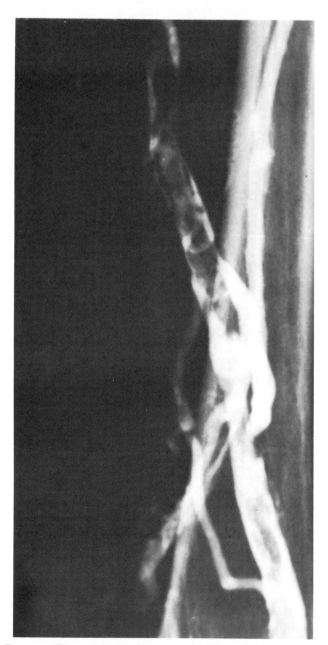

FIG. 17.21. Examples of collateral formation in venous occlusion. Collaterals arise very rapidly when veins are obstructed and they do not indicate chronicity as they do in arteries. (A) This segment of the superficial femoral vein is occluded by thrombus and by-passed by a very large collateral vein. (B) In this examination the femoral vein can just be made out with a little contrast lying along its outer side and thrombus can be seen in a segment of the long saphenous vein. There is virtually total occlusion of the deep venous system however and there are a vast number of collateral veins which include superficial veins, deep veins and communicating veins.

FIG. 17.22. Ageing of thrombus. The changes are most marked in the popliteal vein where the thrombus has contracted considerably and is surrounded by a thick margin of contrast medium. More proximally on the medial aspect of the femoral vein the retraction is shown by the thicker line of contrast medium and on the lateral aspect of the femoral vein in two places the contrast line is completely obliterated indicating adherence at these sites.

FIG. 17.23. The thrombus in this popliteal and femoral veins is several weeks old. The lumen is irregular and narrowed and no valves are visible. The vein is occluded in the adductor canal. The damage created by this thrombus is almost certainly irreversible.

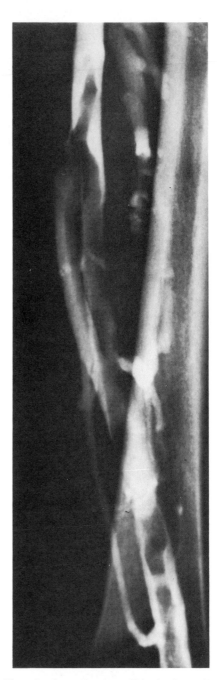

FIG. 17.24. There is a loose 'floating tail' in the femoral vein above a recent thrombus. Such a loose thrombus is likely to embolise but the amount of damage it would do in the lung depends on the size. Most of the thrombus demonstrated here is adherent and unlikely to embolise.

veins can then be defined in centimetres above the tip of the medial or lateral malleolus and thus more easily identified at surgery. When carrying out ascending phlebography early films are particularly important to demonstrate the origins of the veins (Fig. 17.29A, B & C).

Extrinsic Compression

Veins, being thin walled, are readily deformed by adjacent structures. Mention has already been made of compression of the left common iliac vein by the right common iliac artery.

Tumours occurring near a vein may deform, displace or obstruct it. The commonest examples of compression by tumour are seen in the iliac veins and lower inferior vena cava. Enlarged lymph nodes whether secondary to distant malignant disease or primary reticuloses may cause a lobulated indentation which may be a clue as to their nature (Fig. 17.30A, B & C). Benign masses tend to smoothly deform or displace the vein (Fig. 17.31) whereas malignant tumours invade the wall and appear as irregular filling defects within the opacified lumen (Fig. 17.32). As obstruction leads to stasis, thrombosis may be the only demonstrable abnormality (Fig. 17.33). Nevertheless venous deformity may be a useful indication of the site, if not the nature of the lesion.

Phlebography does not indicate the nature of the lesion because it does not reveal a pathological circulation as does arteriography. Consequently it has a limited place in the diagnosis of mass lesions but it may be the first indication of the presence of a tumour.

Congenital Malformations

The congenital angiodysplasias present a wide range of malformations from small and insignificant capillary naevae to large and haemodynamically important arteriovenous fistulae. Within this extensive group there is a small subgroup, the venous dysplasias in which the vascular abnormality is solely in the venous system and the arterial and lymphatic systems are normal.

Within this group of venous dysplasias are included venous aplasia, hypoplasia, reduplications, venous aneurysms, localised venous angiomas and extensive ramifying angiomas extending throughout the tissues of the limb and producing secondary effects in soft tissues and bones.

The commonest complex venous angiodysplasia is the Klippel-Trenaunay syndrome in which there is a cutaneous naevus, varicose veins on the same side and mild hypertrophy of bones and soft tissues but no evidence of arteriovenous fistulae. A fairly constant feature of this syndrome is the persistence of the primitive lateral vein of the leg as a valveless, dilated, tortuous channel which may join the profunda femoris vein, the superficial femoral vein, the iliac veins or the inferior vena cava, frequently by multiple connections (Fig. 17.34). The most important aspect of the investigation of these patients is to demonstrate the state of the deep veins. If the deep veins are absent or hypoplastic, ligation of the superficial veins will aggravate

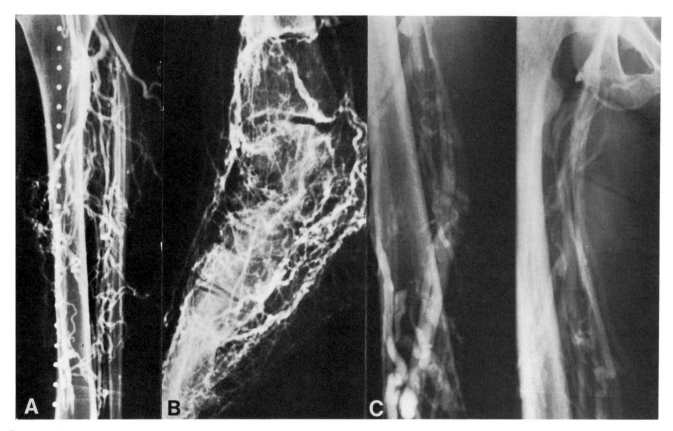

FIG. 17.25. Post thrombotic changes. The veins are irregular, reduplicated, collaterals are present and no normal valves can be seen. Incompetent communicating veins are present in the calf (note the ruler with 1 cm metal markers to relate the sites of the incompetent communicating veins to the patient's leg in A). (A) Foot. (B) Calf. (C) Thigh.

the situation and increase the size and number of varicose veins and oedema.

The phlebographic techniques which may be needed to investigate patients with venous angiodysplasia include ascending phlebography, intraosseous phlebography, varicography or direct injection of the lesion (Fig. 17.35A, B & C). In the extensive venous dysplasias arteriography with follow through to the venous phase may be necessary to show the nature and extent of the lesion (Fig. 17.36A & B). The venous phase can be enhanced by subtraction. Computed tomography is an excellent way of showing the extent of a venous malformation once its nature has been established and it seems likely that digital subtraction angiography (D.S.A.) will have a place in the diagnosis and management of these lesions if only to separate those with arteriovenous fistulae from those without.

OTHER USES FOR PHLEBOGRAPHY

Operative Phlebography
(i) **During thrombectomy.** It is generally recog-

nised that iliofemoral thrombosis is a common and serious event both as regards the possibility of fatal pulmonary embolism and the development of the post thrombotic state. The aims of venous thrombectomy in this situation are to restore patency of the iliofemoral segment so that symptoms of acute and chronic venous insufficiency may be minimised, and to reduce the risk of embolism.

In its simplest form perioperative phlebography involves the injection of contrast distal to the site of thrombectomy and either watching the flow of the medium through the thrombectomised segment with a portable image intensifier, or taking a film as the contrast is injected. The superficial circumflex iliac vein can be divided, preserving the portion leading to the long saphenous vein so that a catheter may be passed through it to the external iliac vein to facilitate postoperative phlebography.

(ii) **Other perioperative situations.** One of the most useful situations for the use of perioperative phlebography occurs in bypass surgery. Not only is it necessary to demonstrate the venous anatomy beforehand but it is also desirable to confirm the functional

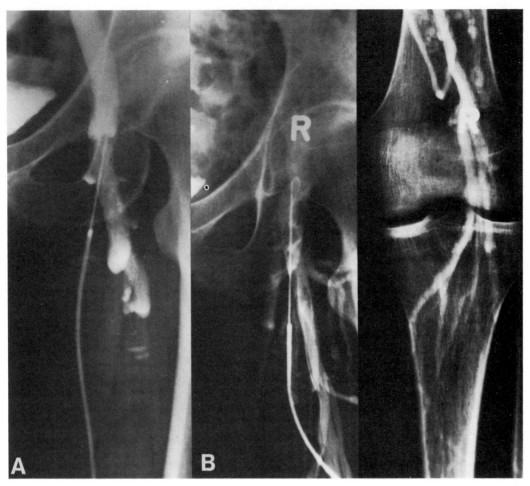

FIG. 17.26. Descending phlebograms. (A) A normal descending phlebogram showing that the contrast medium is held up in the upper part of the femoral vein by competent valves. (B) Venous incompetence. The contrast medium passes downwards below the knee indicating at least Grade 3 deep vein incompetence.

success of the reconstructive procedure. Phlebography may also be required following various surgical procedures performed for varicose veins, particularly if surgical damage to the deep veins is suspected or if there is rapid and unexpected recurrence of varicosities. Venous angiodysplasias often require preoperative and perioperative phlebography to demonstrate their extent and connections, as well as post excision phlebography to confirm complete removal.

Since elaborate serial changes and sophisticated television monitoring systems are not often available in operating theatres, single film radiography is usually all that can be carried out. For this reason the timing of the film is critical. A relatively large volume of contrast medium, i.e. 50 ml of 60% meglumine iothalamate, should be injected continuously by hand and a film taken towards the end of the injection. In this way diagnostic results can be obtained with a minimum of delay, avoiding repeated injections if the critical phase is missed.

(iii) **Anticoagulant and thrombolytic therapy.** Heparin is usually given in the initial therapy of venous thrombosis while oral anticoagulation is being established. Heparin is not a thrombolytic agent but in the correct dosage prevents propagation of thrombus. This may stop established thrombus reaching lethal proportions. It will also minimise the extent of post thrombotic damage to the valves and the veins themselves, which is particularly important in the large veins above the calf.

Thrombolytic agents such as streptokinase and urokinase will lyse thrombus provided it is in a free flowing bloodstream. The phlebogram is repeated on about the 5th day of a standard course of therapy. Further thrombolytic therapy is determined by comparison of the two examinations to assess progress.

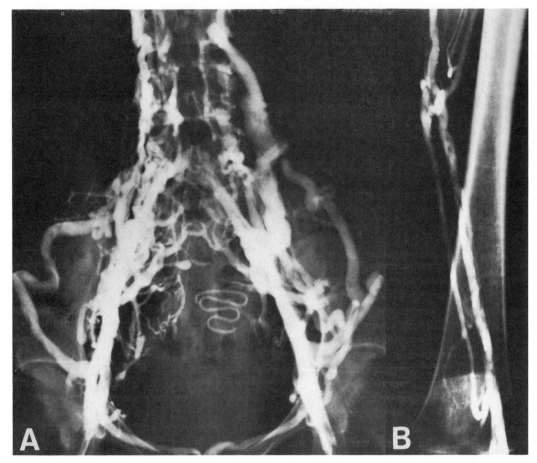

FIG. 17.27. A combination of obstruction and valve incompetence. (A) The inferior vena cava is occluded with collateral formation. (B) The superficial femoral vein is narrowed, irregular, by-passed by collaterals and the valves are destroyed.

(iv) **Clinical trials.** Phlebography has a very small morbidity and it is therefore justifiable to use it for clinical trials with the patients' understanding and permission. Thus, it has been employed in assessing the radiological progression of deep vein thrombosis and in comparing the results of surgical and medical treatment of venous thrombosis. Phlebography has been used to assess the generalised and local side effects of the new low osmolality contrast media by comparing them with the conventional hyperosmolar media in current use.

About half the patients asked to undergo repeat phlebography for clinical trials do so.

(v) **Superficial phlebography.** The essence of the technique is to inject directly the long or short saphenous vein or one of their tributaries at or around the ankle with the patient in the supine position and without tourniquets which direct the contrast into the deep venous system. As the contrast medium passes centrally its progress is followed on a television monitor and spot films taken of the superficial veins. Apart from the use of superficial phlebography to demonstrate varicose veins and to demonstrate venous angiomas and their tributaries together with any deep connections, there are other situations in which superficial phlebography may be useful. Superficial phlebography may be required to demonstrate a suitable vein for an arteriovenous shunt in patients with chronic renal failure. Another use is to identify suitable segments of veins for use in arterial bypass surgery both in peripheral arterial disease and in coronary artery disease (Fig. 17.37).

(vi) **Venous trauma.** Trauma to the venous system is common but produces less dramatic and immediate effects than arterial trauma. For this reason it has received less consideration, management usually being confined to tying off bleeding veins. Improved phlebographic techniques have drawn attention to the late sequelae of the ligation of main veins especially in the form of the post thrombotic syndrome, and more recently interest has been focussed on reconstructive procedures.

Phlebography may be used to assess the site and the extent of an acutely injured vein. It can also be used at

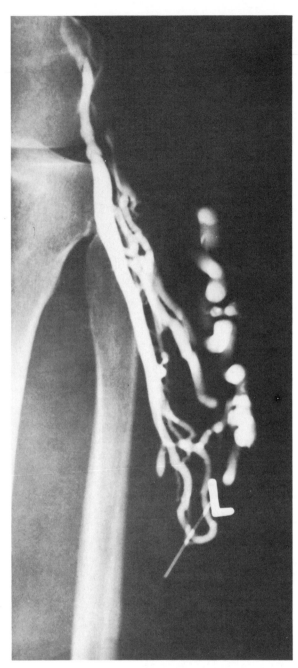

FIG. 17.28. A varicogram. Direct injection of these varicose veins show that they connect with the short saphenous vein which is, itself, normal. This indicates that simple excision of the varicose veins is likely to produce a good result. Varicography is particularly useful in recurrent varicose veins and may indicate a communicating vein which has been missed at surgery.

a later stage following venous injury to assess the long term effects of emergency therapy such as major vein ligation. Venous injuries may result from penetrating trauma including surgery, blunt trauma, compression by haematomas or fractures and direct injury due to stretching associated with dislocations. The long term effects which concern the vascular surgeon are the post thrombotic syndrome, arteriovenous fistulae and aneurysms. In these acute and chronic situations phlebography plays an important part in management.

The technique of phlebography has to be tailored to the particular circumstance. Injured patients may be unable to stand so that steep table tilts cannot be employed, and tourniquets may have to be placed on unusual sites. As long as they are proximal to the site of injection they assist deep venous filling. A single film after the injection of 50 to 100 ml of contrast medium is often all that can be obtained in the casualty department or operating theatre (Fig. 17.38).

Iliofemoral thrombosis is common after hip replacement surgery, but in addition postoperative immobility results in venous stasis with a possibility of calf vein thrombosis. For this reason an ascending phlebogram in suspected venous thrombosis in these patients should be carried out to show the whole of the deep venous system of the legs and pelvis.

(vii) **Reconstructive surgery in iliac vein obstruction.** The principle of these bypass operations, which have now become a practical possibility as a result of the work of Palma, is to divide a saphenous vein on the healthy side at the level of the knee, free it from all collateral vessels to its junction with the femoral vein, and transpose it in a subcutaneous tunnel across the pubis to the diseased side where it is anastamosed with the femoral vein (Fig. 17.39). The shunt may be kept open by a temporary arteriovenous fistula.

The long term benefits of this therapy have yet to be evaluated, but if patient selection is limited to those with diseased pelvic veins and where the distal leg veins are well preserved, reasonably good symptomatic results may be expected.

To demonstrate the patency of the bypass graft an ascending phlebogram of the affected leg is carried out when contrast is shown to drain from the affected leg into the opposite common femoral vein. Alternatively the vein below the bypass may be injected directly.

PHLEBOGRAPHY OF THE UPPER LIMBS

Anatomy

(i) **The superficial venous network.** The superficial veins drain the dorsal aspect of the hand laterally through the cephalic vein and medially through the basilic vein. At the elbow the veins join through the median cubital vein and the blood is carried proximally by the cephalic and basilic veins which join the deep veins at different levels near the shoulder.

(ii) **The deep veins.** This system drains the palmar surface of the hand, the arch formed continued as paired

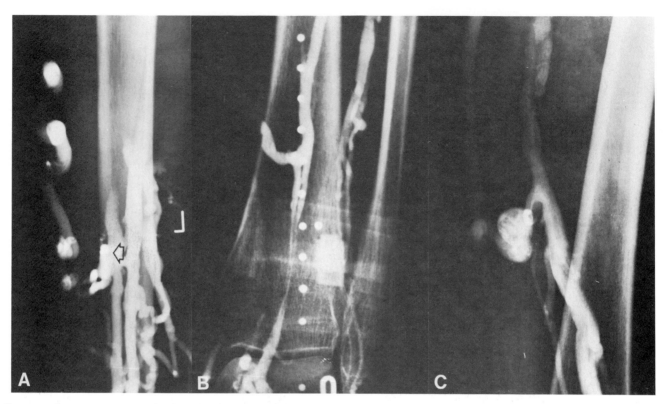

FIG. 17.29. Incompetent communicating veins. (A) A typical large, medial, incompetent perforating vein joining a varicose vein. The deep venous system appears normal. (B) An early film showing the origin of a medial incompetent communicating vein. Early films are essential as the origin is what interests the surgeon. A ruler with ball bearings at 1 cm intervals allows more accurate localisation. (C) An incompetent communicating vein in Hunter's·canal. There are recanalisation changes in the deep veins. The communicating vein is extremely dilated and connects with the long saphenous vein. The direction of flow can be appreciated because the contrast medium in the long saphenous vein above the communicating vein is more dense than that below. A grossly incompetent adductor canal communicating vein like this is easy to demonstrated by ascending phlebography but smaller ones may require a tourniquet above Hunter's canal or varicography at the suspected site. The phlebographic appearances of a communicating shown by varicography may suggest incompetence. If there is doubt this can be confirmed by the Doppler ultrasound technique.

venae commitantes of the radial and ulna arteries. A third group of deep veins, the intraosseous veins join with the radial and ulnar veins to form a pair of brachial veins which become in turn the axillary, subclavian and innominate veins. The right and left innominate veins unite to form the superior vena cava (Fig. 40, 41 A & B). The superficial and deep systems are linked by a few anastamoses. One of the most important of these is a valveless communicating vein in the region of the elbow. The cephalic vein frequently anastomoses with the brachial or axillary vein, either directly or to a collateral such as the circumflex humeral vein. There are communicating veins in the forearm and both the superficial and deep networks have valves. In contrast to the lower limbs the superficial circulation is the more important of the two. The valves do not play an important part of the circulation of the upper limbs and there is no equivalent of the calf and thigh muscle pumps. Venous drainage is largely due to cardiac

function. These differences explain why pathological conditions of the upper limb are uncommon. Only a few patent veins are required for an adequate venous return and most venous occlusions are rapidly compensated by collaterals and few, if any, symptoms occur.

Thromboses in upper limb veins damage the valves as they do in the lower limbs but in generaly leave few sequelae. Valvular incompetence does not produce symptoms in the upper limb.

Phlebographic Techniques

There is rarely any clinical indication for demonstration of the veins of the hand and forearm except in the presence of suspected or known venous malformation. The only practical way of demonstrating those veins is by arterial injection and follow through, the venous phase sometimes requiring enhancement by the subtraction technique.

Most pathology occurs in the axillary, subclavian and

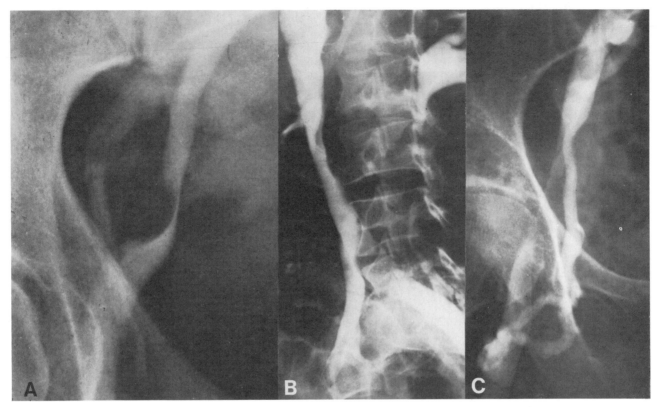

Fig. 17.30. Examples of lymph node enlargement. (A) Lymph nodes compressing the external iliac vein. (B) Lobulated filling defects on the posterior aspect of the inferior vena cava are due to enlarged, para-aortic lymph nodes. (C) The common femoral vein and the external iliac vein are compressed by enlarged inguinal lymph nodes. The obturator vein is functioning as a collateral.

innominate veins and in the superior vena cava. The simplest way of demonstrating these large proximal veins is by an injection of about 50 ml of contrast medium through a large bore needle (16 gauge) introduced into a vein in the antecubital fossa. A hand injection is satisfactory, the contrast being introduced at about 10–15 ml per second. Tourniquets are not generally required, both the superficial and the deep veins filling together. In order to show the superior vena cava bilateral injection should be made.

Patients in whom a suitable vein cannot be identified in the antecubital fossa, either because of oedema or because of subcutaneous tissue, a smaller needle may be introduced into a vein of the hand or wrist and a bolus technique similar to that used in the leg employed. A fairly tight tourniquet is applied at the elbow and after completion of this injection this is quickly removed and pressure applied to the forearm muscles (Fig. 17.42). Another useful method in some patients is the intraosseous technique. A smaller version of the intraosseous cannula measuring about 3 cm in length is introduced into a suitable bone such as the olecranon process or the greater tuberosity of the humerus (Fig. 17.43 & 44).

Whatever method of phlebography is used a short series of films at a rate of 1–2 per second is always desirable because in the absence of obstruction the venous flow may be very rapid and obtaining films when the veins are properly filled can be difficult and artefacts due to streaming are common on a single film.

Catheterisation techniques are advocated by some, but in general the author considers these should be avoided. Pressure injections into small capacity veins can cause bursting, particularly in the presence of obstruction and it is safer as in the lower limb to avoid these selective methods if possible.

Should catheters be used they should be introduced into the basilic vein and positioned by fluoroscopy and test injections of contrast medium made. If an obstruction is encountered the catheter is withdrawn a few centimetres before the main injection is made to minimise the risk of rupture. The cephalic vein joins the axillary vein almost at a right angle and it is often impossible to negotiate this angle with a catheter.

The demonstration of the azygos system is possible in several ways, the easiest one being to perform an intraosseous phlebogram of one of the lower dorsal vertebral spinous processes or one of the lower ribs.

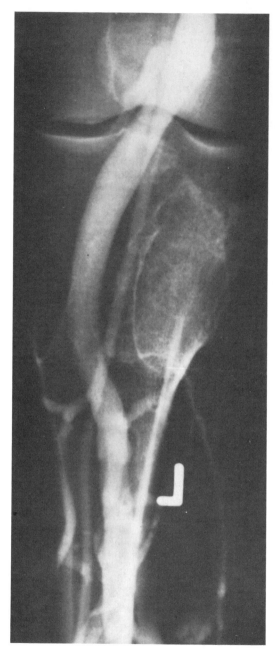

FIG. 17.31. The popliteal vein is smoothly displaced by an osteochondroma.

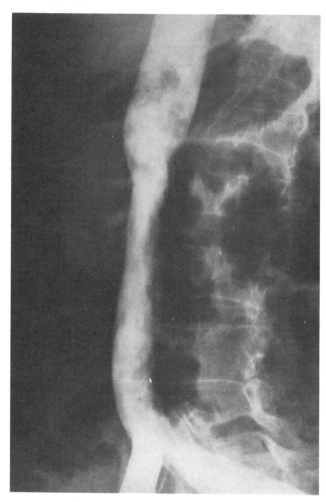

FIG. 17.32. The irregularity of the posterolateral aspect of the inferior vena cava is due to malignant invasion by a renal carcinoma.

Direct catheterisation using a suitably shaped catheter introduced from the femoral vein into the superior vena cava and advanced on down the azygos vein for a few centimetres can also be used. Injection of contrast medium shows the azygos and hemi-azygos systems clearly by retrograde flow of the contrast medium. The indications for azygosography are very limited and it is rarely requested.

Pathological Conditions

(i) **Thrombosis.** Acute thrombosis presents exactly the same appearances in the upper limbs as in the lower limb (Fig. 17.45). Such thromboses generally subside without specific treatment leaving no symptoms. Rarely, pulmonary emboli arise from the proximal arm veins and these may need to be examined as part of the general examination of the venous system in the search for the source of pulmonary emboli.

Compression of the subclavian vein at the thoracic outlet in extreme positions of the arm can be demonstrated phlebographically in a significant number of healthy individuals. Sometimes acute subclavian vein thrombosis, a consequence of thoracic outlet syndrome is encountered. The narrowing occurs in the costoclavicular space and is often associated with fibromuscular bands. In order to assess the degree of obstruction at phlebography the patient should be examined with the

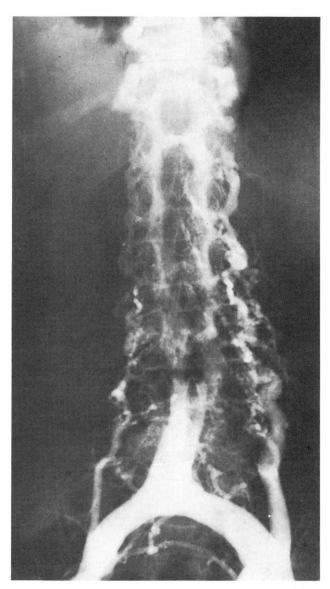

FIG. 17.33. The inferior vena cava is totally occluded with collateral flow through both ascending lumbar veins and the vertebral plexuses. While the appearances could be due to iliopathic caval thrombosis the square, irregular end raises the possibility of extrinsic invasion. The patient had metastases from a leiomyoblastoma of the stomach.

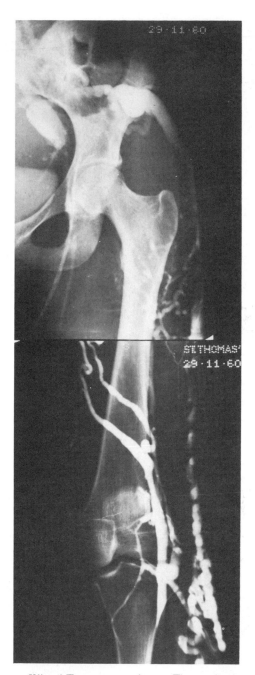

FIG. 17.34. Klippel-Trenaunay syndrome. The persistent primitive valveless lateral channel has been injected in the calf (varicography). The abnormal channel joins the internal iliac vein in this patient.

arms neutrally by the side and in hyperabduction (Fig. 17.46). While most of these patients respond to conservative treatment alone (bedrest, elevation of the arm, anti-coagulants, etc.), a small minority of patients complain of pain and swelling of the arm and new episodes of thrombosis occur (Fig. 17.47A & B).

Surgical intervention consists of thrombectomy in the acute phase if loose thrombus is present, and decompression by resection of the first rib with scalenectomy and excision of all anomalous fibrous bands. It should be noted however that thrombosis of the upper limb

accounts for only 1–2% of all venous thromboses. Iatrogenic thromboses are fairly common following catheterisation techniques and intravenous infusions.

(ii) **Venous malformations.** The superficial and deep veins of the arms are fairly constant in position compared with the lower limb but nevertheless variations in number, position and site of termination do

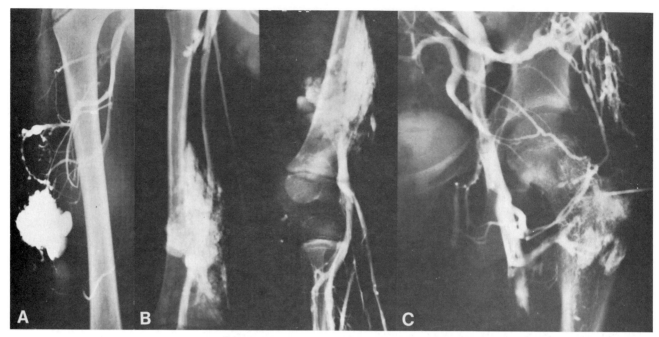

Fig. 17.35. Methods of investigating venous angiodysplasias. (A) Direct injection. (B) Ascending phlebography. (C) Intraosseous phlebography. The malformation in the patient is in the buttock, and can be seen in the upper right hand corner.

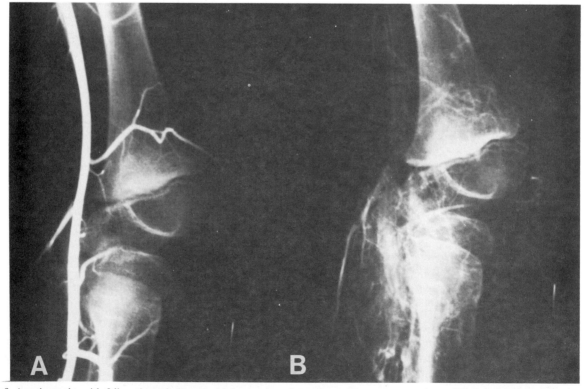

Fig. 17.36. Arteriography with follow through (arteriophlebogram) to show an extensive venous angioma. (A) Arterial phase. The femoral and popliteal arteries are of normal size. A few small branches supply the angioma. (B) Venous phase. This shows that the angioma is mainly situated in the popliteal fossa but it also extended into the knee joint, the patient presenting with a haemarthrosis. This is *not* an arteriovenous fistula.

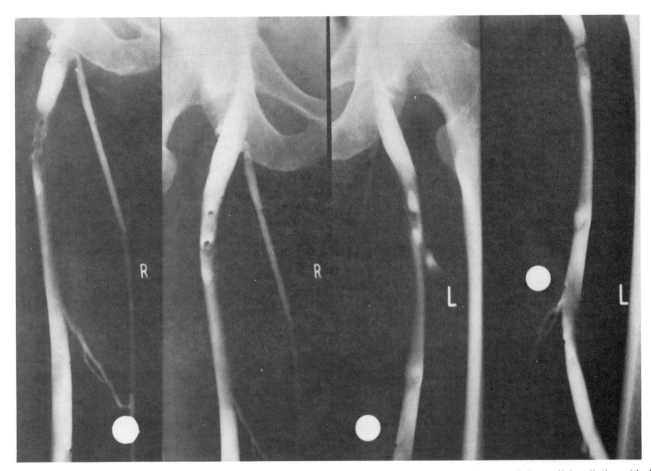

FIG. 17.37. Saphenogram. This examination was carried out by injecting the long saphenous vein just in front of the medial malleolus with the patient supine and using no tourniquets. The long saphenous vein on both sides is shown. The one on the right side has a good lumen and is suitable for surgical by-pass but the one on the left is too small. The round metal markers placed on the patients leg enable an exact measurement of the calibre of the saphenous veins to be made.

occur and although not of clinical significance may affect the approach for phlebography and surgery.

The only congenital variation of importance occurs in the superior vena cava which may be left sided, double, or absent with azygos continuation. When the cava is left sided it drains into the coronary sinus and when it is double the right cava drains normally while the left drains into the coronary sinus.

Simple venous dysplasias occur in the upper limb as they do in the lower and are best demonstrated by direct injection (Fig. 17.48). Before surgical removal is contemplated views of the deep venous system are required to make certain that the venous drainage would be adequate after removal of the malformation. Complex venous anomalies also occur and these can be shown, either by direct injection at a number of sites into the malformation itself, or draining veins, or by injecting into a vein below the malformation with a tourniquet above to direct the contrast into the malformation.

Finally, as mentioned previously arterial injections with follow through to the venous phase may be the only way to show the full extent of these malformations (Fig. 17.49).

The Klippel-Trenaunay syndrome, which is the commonest complex venous dysplasia of the lower limb, rarely occurs in the upper limb although it may occur in one or both upper limbs in conjunction with a similar lesion in one or both lower limbs. The investigation and management is the same, irrespective of the site.

(iii) **Traumatic lesions.** Veins can be damaged as a result of fracture, dislocations and by surgical intervention and these may need to be demonstrated using the techniques of ascending phlebography of the arm as described earlier.

Tumours and Inflammatory Lesions

(i) **Benign lesions.** The veins of the upper limb, usually in the brachiocephalic segment are readily

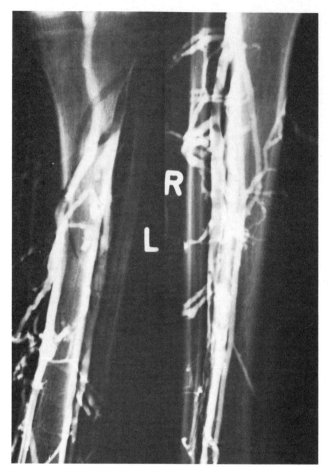

FIG. 17.38. Modification of ascending phlebography in trauma. Despite the fracture on the left an ankle tourniquet to direct contrast into the deep venous system was possible. No thrombus has been demonstrated on this side. On the right side there is extensive recent thrombus. The patient had had a small pulmonary embolus. It is important to examine both sides in such patients.

deformed by adjacent masses arising from nearby soft tissues or bones. Such compression as in the thoracic outlet syndrome may give rise to arm oedema and is investigated by ascending phlebography (Fig. 17.50).

(ii) **Malignant lesions.** The superior vena cava may be displaced by mediastinal masses, narrowed by involvement in fibrotic conditions such as reticuloses, invaded by malignant neoplasm or thrombosed following malignant invasion (Fig. 17.51 & 52). When the superior vena cava is completely obstructed drainage from the arm occurs by means of the posterior intercostal veins to the azygos system and thence to the superior vena cava and right atrium. If the superior vena cava thrombosis involves the azygos vein, drainage is by the thoraco-abdominal veins to the iliac veins and the inferior vena cava.

Azygosography, briefly referred to earlier may help to distinguish between simple and malignant mediastinal tumours, and possibly determine the operability of lung cancer. This indication for phlebography of the upper limb is now rarely used being superceeded by such investigations as computed tomography, possibly combined with simple ascending phlebography of the arm. One of the commonest causes of oedema of the arm follows the treatment by excision and radiotherapy for breast carcinoma. Lymphatic and venous factors often co-exist the former being the most important in most patients. The venous component of such a cause of limb swelling can be readily demonstrated by conventional arm phlebography (Fig. 17.53).

As in the lower limb, phlebography plays only a minor part in the diagnosis of masses in the upper limb because the nature of the lesion, other than primary venous abnormalities such as angiomas, cannot be ascertained by this method. However, thrombosis alone or compression or indentation of the veins may be the first indication of the site of an abnormality allowing appropriate further investigation to be carried out (Fig. 17.54).

NON-CONTRAST PHLEBOGRAPHY

(i) **Radionuclide Phlebography**

This it can be useful in acute venous thrombosis where the isotope adheres to its surface or venous obstruction traps the isotope below the blocked vein (Fig. 17.55).

A needle is inserted into a dorsal vein of each foot. Tourniquets are applied above the ankles and knees to occlude the superficial veins. The patient is positioned under a gamma camera. A bolus of 0·5 mCi 99 mTc human albumin microspheres is injected simultaneously into each foot before each polaroid photograph. The patient is positioned so that the veins from the abdomen to the ankle are visualised. The tourniquets are then released and the patient is asked to exercise by flexion of the foot, and the photographs repeated to see that an accumulation of activity is due to thrombus and not to stasis (Fig. 17.56). The procedure is relatively safe but care should be taken in patients with reduced lung function in the same way as for perfusion pulmonary scans.

An advantage of using albumin macroaggregates is that a lung scan can be obtained at the time of the phlebogram. The radiation hazard of this investigation is negligible. In most studies where isotope phlebography has been compared with contrast phlebography it has been suggested that there is an 80% accuracy rate but the method does not give an accurate indication of the site and age of the thrombus and false negatives are common with small thrombi which do not obstruct the venous flow. False positives results when there are areas

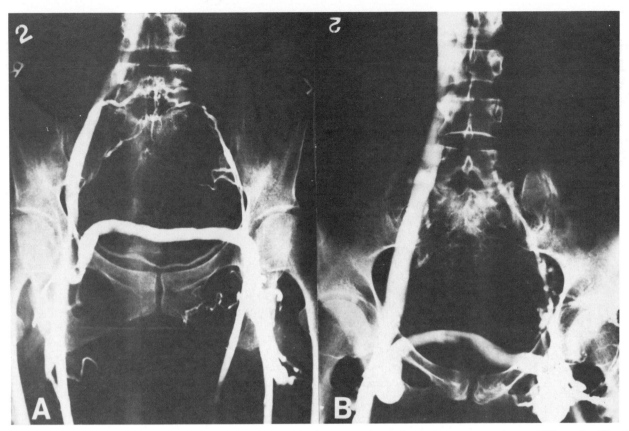

FIG. 17.39. Two examples of Palma's operation. In both instances there is a severe obstruction to the common and external iliac veins. The right long saphenous vein has been transposed and joined to the left femoral vein in order to provide venous drainage of the left lower limb. (A) An example five years after the operation with the patient's by-pass demonstrated by an ascending phlebogram. (B) An example twelve years after surgery in which the patient by-pass has been shown by direct left femoral vein injection (*Radiographs by courtesy of Dr Robert May*).

FIG. 17.40. Diagram of the main veins of the upper limb (*by courtesy of Dr John Dow*).

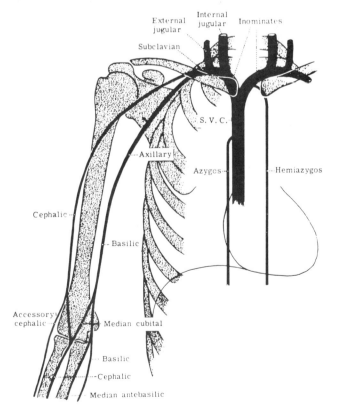

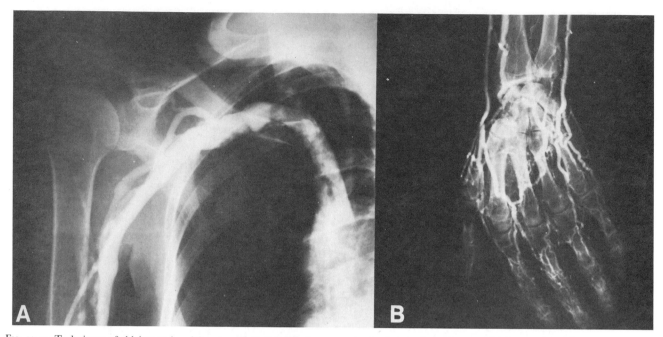

FIG. 17.41. Techniques of phlebography of the upper limb. (A) The large proximal veins are shown by a rapid injection through a large bore needle in the median cubital vein. (B) These hand veins were shown by arterial injection and follow through to the venous phase.

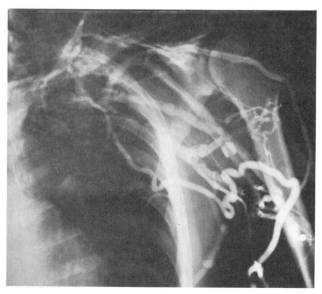

FIG. 17.42. This patient had a very swollen arm and no vein could be found in the antecubital fossa. A needle was introduced into a vein on the back of the hand and the bolus technique used. The examination shows a total occlusion of the left sub-clavian vein with collaterals.

of inflammation or oedema. The ability to screen the limbs and get a lung scan from a single intravenous injection has obvious advantages.

(ii) Fibrinogen Uptake Test

This test is used to detect venous thrombosis. The method depends on the incorporation of circulating radioactive fibrinogen into a forming or recently formed thrombus so concentrating the radioactivity to a degree that makes it detectable by external scintillation counting. The important points of the technique are as follows: The thyroid gland must be saturated with iodine before giving the labelled fibrinogen, by giving oral potassium iodide to stop it taking up any radioactive iodine. Higher count rates are obtained over the thrombus if the labelled fibrinogen is given before the thrombus forms. This means that the method is most useful for surgical patients when the labelled fibrinogen may be given before or immediately after the operation. The legs can be examined with a scintillation counter technique. The results are expressed as a percentage of the pre-cordial count. The diagnostic criteria vary slightly according to the method used. A difference of 15–20% between adjacent count rates indicates a thrombus.

The method can be used to examine the legs only below the middle of the thigh because above this level the background count for the soft tissues, large blood vessels and the bladder masks the relatively small increases in activity that occur in thrombi. Below the middle of the thigh the method is 95% accurate when compared with phlebography and autopsy. False positive readings occur when there is inflammation, hae-

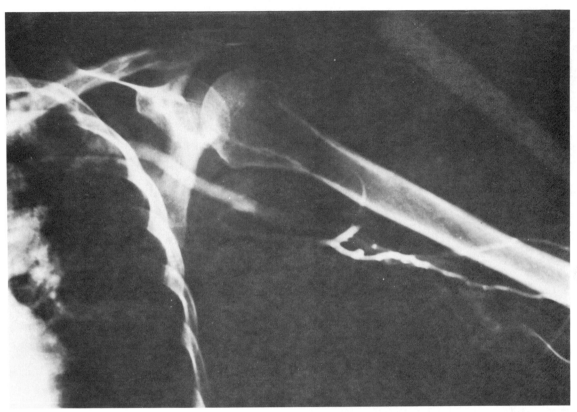

FIG. 17.43. Intraosseous olecranon injection. The venous system is normal. This method was employed because there was gross oedema following a mastectomy. A lymphangiogram confirmed that this was lymphoedema.

matoma or marked oedema. The test is probably more accurate in the calf than phlebography and small accumulations of radioactivity associated with negative phlebograms are thrombi that are too small to be detected by phlebography. The main cause of false negative readings is a thrombus that is more than 5 days old which cannot take up the labelled fibrinogen.

The radiation dose is small and safe in most patients but women of child bearing age are generally excluded from the examination except when the clinical indication is strong.

There is a risk of transmission of viral hepatitis because fibrinogen cannot be sterilised by autoclaving, but careful screening has made the test remarkably safe and many thousands of examinations have been carried out in the United Kingdom without an outbreak of hepatitis.

The method is relatively costly in equipment and materials and in the technicians time. Each examination takes 15–20 minutes and cannot be performed until 24 hours after the injection of isotope making the test useless in urgent clinical situations. The advantage of the technique is that it can be repeated as often as necessary without discomfort to the patient and the author and others have used the method to assess the incidence of post phlebographic thrombosis using the new low osmolality contrast media.

(iii) **Thermography**

It is a clinically observed fact that thrombosed limbs are warmer than normal and this can be detected with an infrared camera. The leg of the patient is exposed, to allow equilibrium between the skin and room temperature, and elevated to empty superficial veins. The heat radiating from the legs is reflected onto the camera by means of a heat reflecting mirror and the results recorded as a polaroid photograph. The test is totally noninvasive and can be repeated as often as the investigator wishes.

The accuracy for calf vein and femoral vein thrombosis is said to be about 90% but the technique cannot detect thrombi in the iliac veins or the inferior vena cava which are not obstructing venous flow and other causes of inflammation give false positive readings.

The method has not been widely adopted for clinical use because the apparatus is expensive and has a limited use in other fields of diagnostic imaging.

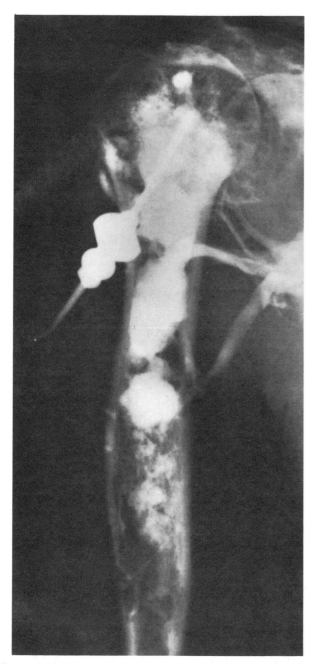

FIG. 17.44. Intraosseous injection into the greater tuberosity of the humerus, to show the extent of bone involvement in a patient with lymphohaemangiomatosis.

(iv) **Computed tomography**

This examination has a very limited place in the diagnosis of venous disease because of the very large number of transverse sections which would need to be taken to visualise the longitudinal venous system and the consequent very heavy radiation dosage. For these reasons computed tomography should never be the primary investigation in suspected abnormality of the venous system. Should thoracic or abdominal scans be indicated for other reasons the superior and inferior venae cavae should be assessed for size, shape and position. Like all veins, the walls being thin, and are easily deformed by external pressure by tumours, gland masses and by thrombus whether primary or secondary to adjacent malignant or inflammatory processes (Fig.17.57A & B). Nearby tumours frequently deform or invade the walls of the cavae giving an indistinct outline and an irregular lumen.

In order to distinguish the cavae from surrounding structures cuts should be taken before and after contrast medium to show if there is any enhancement. To show the superior vena cava an infusion of about 100–150 ml of 60% meglumine iothalamate is infused through an arm vein and a similar amount into a foot vein to show the inferior vena cava. Additional bolus injections of 50–100 ml of contrast medium may be required in some examinations.

The anatomical position of the superior vena cava is just to the right of the aorta and in front of the right main bronchus. It can thus be involved in diseases of the mediastinum whether neoplastic or inflammatory and particularly in carcinoma of the bronchus, with or without enlarged lymph glands.

The inferior vena cava being a longer structure has a variety of anatomical relations throughout its length. In its more proximal part it lies just behind the caudate lobe of the liver and the right lobe itself. Lower down it lies just in front of the right kidney in the region of a vascular pedicle. At both these sites the aorta lies virtually in the mid line just in front of the vertebral bodies.

Identification of the inferior vena cava at these sites is important because lesions in the porta hepatis affect the former and tumour thrombus extending from a renal carcinoma into a renal vein often grows along the wall of the inferior vena cava, a fact which alters the operative approach and the prognosis of the condition.

Enlargement of the inferior vena cava together with dilatation of the contiguous renal vein suggest tumour thrombus from a renal carcinoma. Often the carcinoma of the kidney is shown on the scan. Collaterals in iliac vein or in inferior vena caval obstruction can also be seen on the computed tomogram most easily with contrast enhancement (Fig. 17.58A & B).

Clearly C.T. scan could be used to evaluate anomalies of both the superior and inferior vena cavae although these are better investigated by angiographic techniques.

Ultrasound

For technical reasons this examination plays no place in the investigation of the peripheral veins of the limbs

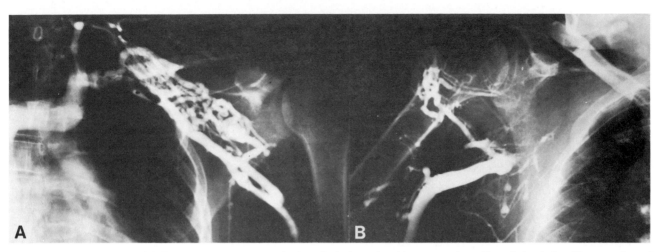

FIG. 17.45. Acute thrombosis. (A) There is recent thrombus in the sub-clavian vein with an extensive collateral circulation. Venous collaterals, unlike arterial ones, only give a very rough idea of how long an obstruction has been present because they open up very quickly. (B) Total occlusion of the axillary vein, so called 'effort thrombosis'.

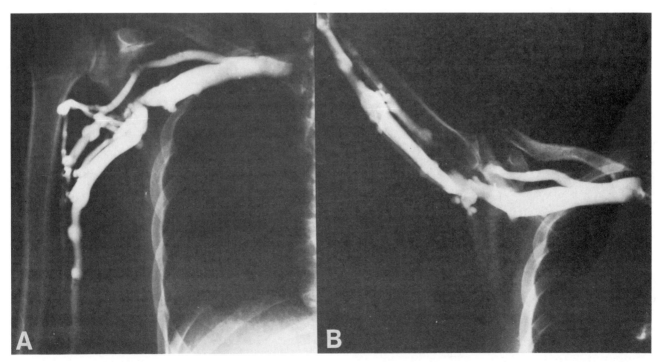

FIG. 17.46. Phlebography in the thoracic outlet syndrome. (A) There is a narrowing in the axillary vein with the arm at the side which is not present when the patient's arm is hyperabducted. (B) The arm should always be examined in these two positions because in other instances the obstruction is only obvious when the arm is abducted. In this patient there is a further permanent narrowing of the sub-clavian vein which remains unchanged in both positions of the arm. This was a congenital abnormality of the vein itself.

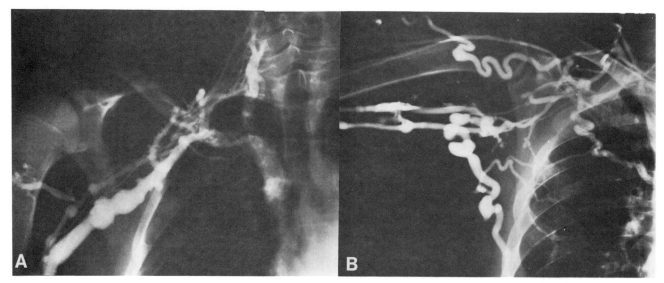

Fig. 17.47. Examples of post thrombotic obstruction. (A) A segment at the junction of the axillary vein with the sub-clavian vein is narrowed with an irregular lumen and the presence of periscapular collateral indicate that the narrowing is causing obstruction. A diagnosis of venous obstruction should never be made in the absence of collateral veins. (B) In this long-standing example the axillary and sub-clavian veins are totally occluded and there is extensive collateral circulation, not only in the periscapular region but also through veins of the chest wall.

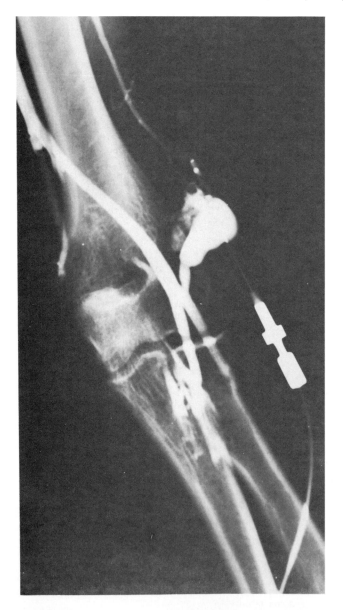

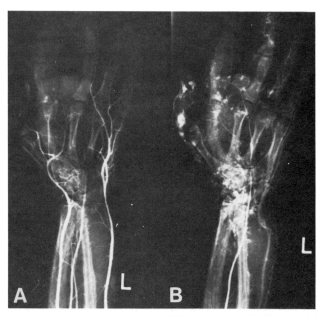

Fig. 17.49. Arterial injection with follow through. (A) The arterial phase. The arteries are of normal size and there is no evidence of arterio-venous fistulae. Phleboliths can be seen in the soft tissues. A surgical amputation of the second finger has been carried out. (B) Venous phase. The extensive venous angioma is noted around the wrist and extending into the palm, the thumb and the middle finger.

Fig. 17.48. A phlebogram by direct injection showing a localised cavernous malformation draining mainly into the median cubital vein.

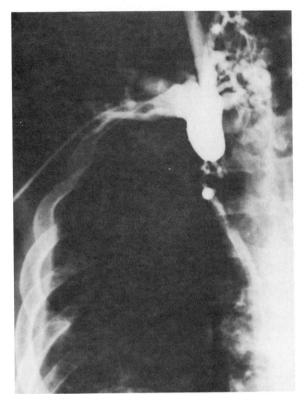

Fig. 17.50. Idiopathic mediastinal fibrosis. There is a tight stricture just at the origin of the superior vena cava and the left innominate vein is totally obstructed with extensive collateral formation. There is no evidence of a mass.

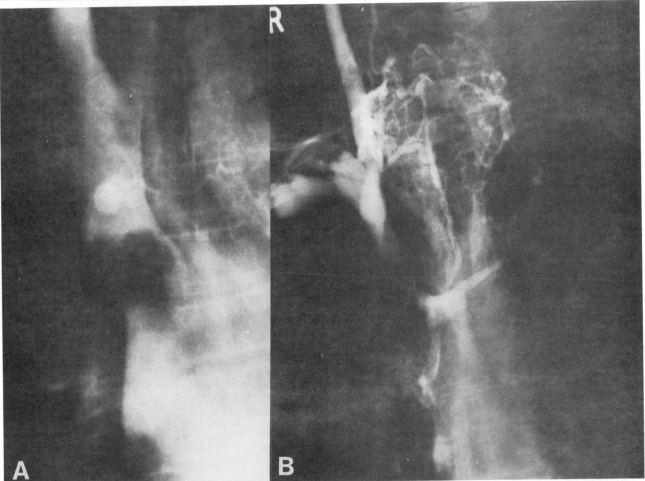

Fig. 17.51. Superior vena cavography in bronchial carcinoma. (A) A lobulated mass is seen within the lower part of the superior vena cava. (B) The superior vena cava contains an irregular filling defect representing invasion by the bronchial neoplasm and secondary thrombosis. The left innominate vein is narrowed and occluded near its junction with the sub-clavian vein. The veins from the left side of the neck are occluded by thrombus. It is not possible to make a firm diagnosis of the nature of the lesions causing these phlebographic appearances but they suggest that they are due to mediastinal invasion by malignant disease.

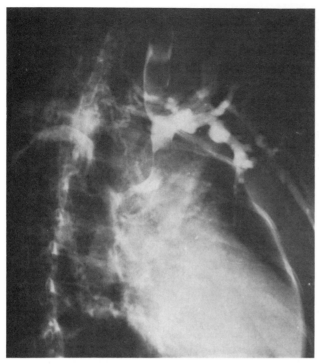

FIG. 17.52. Hodgkin's disease invading the superior vena cava and its tributaries, particularly the left innominate vein. There is thrombus in the left innominate vein and also in the left internal jugular vein.

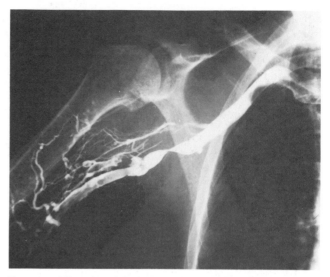

FIG. 17.54. There is a tight stricture at the junction of the brachial vein with the axillary vein with distal thrombus. There is also a little mural thrombus in the axillary vein more proximally. This patient presented with swelling of the arm, the cause of which was not apparent and was assumed to be a primary venous thrombosis. This phlebogram led to biopsy which showed that the causative lesion was a sarcoma arising in the soft tissues.

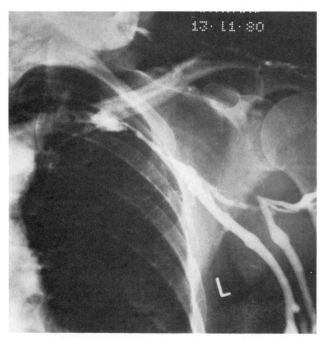

FIG. 17.53. Following a mastectomy and radiation this patient developed a very swollen arm. The phlebogram shows severe narrowing of the left sub-clavian vein with a venous pressure of 34 cm H2O on the left side compared with a normal pressure on the right. In this patient the venous component was the main cause of the patient's post-mastectomy arm oedema.

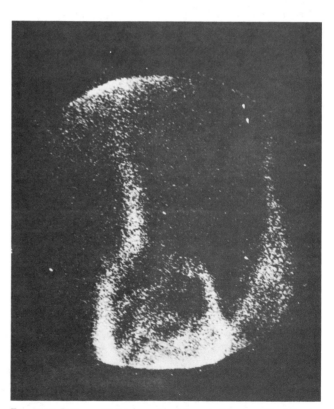

FIG. 17.55. Isotope phlebogram of pelvis and abdomen. The injection was made into the left foot only. There is an obstruction at the junction of the left common iliac vein with the inferior vena cava with extensive pelvic collaterals filling the right iliac veins.

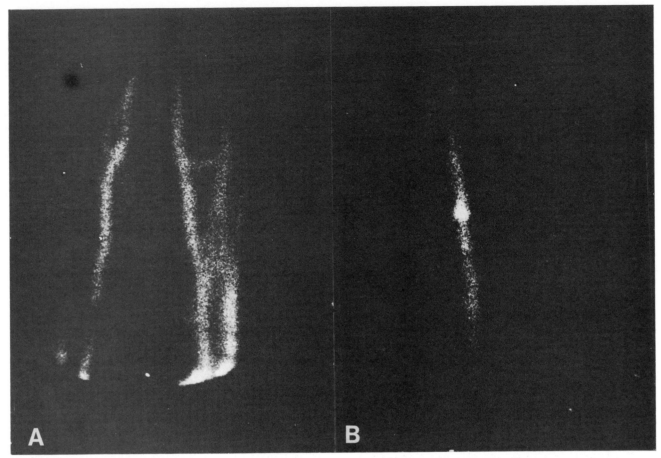

FIG. 17.56. Isotope phlebogram. (A) Static picture. (B) After exercise. There is accumulation of activity in the calf which remains after exercise indicating that this is a thrombus.

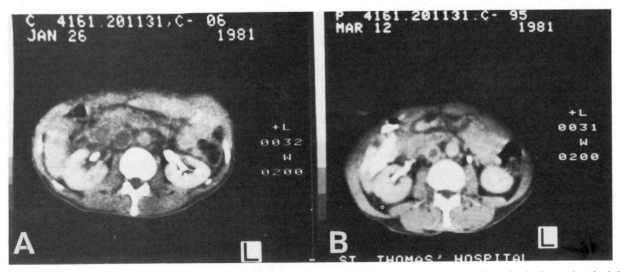

FIG. 17.57. (A) C.T. scan of abdomen (with contrast infusion) at 20 mm intervals showing extensive recent thrombosis obstructing the inferior vena cava. (B) Repeat examination 10 weeks later showing contraction of the thrombus with a smaller diameter of the inferior vena cava. This was an example of idiopathic inferior vena caval obstruction.

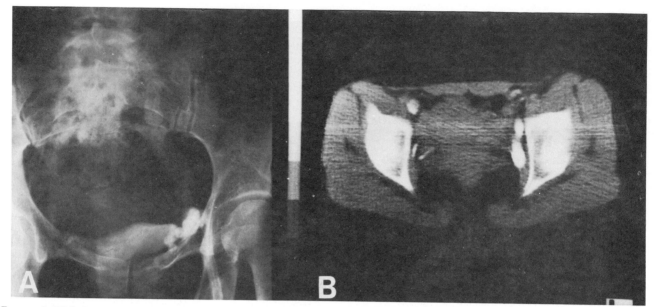

FIG. 17.58. (A) Left iliac phlebogram showing common iliac obstruction with pubic and pre-sacral collaterals. (B) C.T. scan with contrast infusion into the left foot showing some of these dilated collaterals and filling by them of the right external iliac vein (*Radiographs by courtesy of Dr G. Davis*).

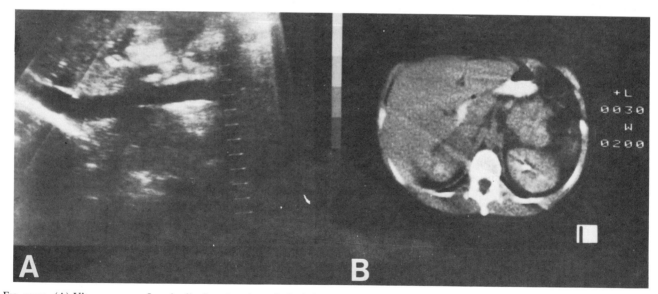

FIG. 17.59. (A) Ultrasonogram. Longitudinal section through the inferior vena cava. This shows the proximal portion of the inferior vena cava is distorted by a mass posterolateral to it. (B) Computed tomogram of the same patient. This examination confirms the position of the mass in relation to the I.V.C. and is shown to lie anterior to the upper pole of the right kidney. This is a phaechromocytoma.

and is of little value in investigating the superior vena cava due to the surrounding structures and the difficulty of access with the ultrasonic probe. It is, however, of some value in the investigation of the inferior vena cava and has the considerable advantage of being totally non-invasive and harmless. The limitations of the technique are largely due to overlying bowel gas.

The longitudinal ultrasonogram about 2 cm to the right of the mid line shows the inferior vena cava in its longitudinal extent. The variations of the calibre of the inferior vena cava can be displayed using the M-mode and if there is no evidence of respiratory variations in the calibre of the cava this may suggest that the inferior vena cava is obstructed. Ultrasound of the inferior vena cava may show extrinsic compression from related structures and masses arising from the liver, pancreas, kidney or adrenal (Fig. 17.59A & B).

Conclusions

Despite the introduction of many new and non-invasive techniques for the investigation of the venous system, some of which have been mentioned here and others including the ultrasonic Dopplergram, impedance phlebography and volumetry, the demand for contrast phlebography continues to increase.

In a recent study it was noted that before a clinical laboratory was established 31% of patients underwent contrast phlebography and that afterwards this had increased to 59%.

It thus appears that contrast phlebography will remain the final arbiter on the anatomical and pathological state of the venous system for the foreseeable future.

Contrast phlebography does have some disadvantages and complications as has been pointed out in this chapter but it is generally simple to perform, well tolerated by patients and gives information not obtainable by any other method.

FURTHER READING

ANSELL G. (Ed.) (1976) *Complications in Diagnostic Radiology.* Oxford: Blackwell Scientific Publications.

BRITISH MEDICAL BULLETIN (1978) Volume 34, Number 2. London: British Council.

DODD, H. & COCKETT, B. (1978) *The Pathology and Surgery of the Veins of the Lower Limb.* Second Edition. Edinburgh: Churchill Livingstone.

KAPPERT, A. (Ed.) (1977) *New Trends in Venous Diseases.* Vienna: Hans Huber Publishers.

LEA THOMAS, M. (1982) *Phlebography of the Lower Limb.* Edinburgh: Churchill Livingstone.

LUDBROOK, J. (1972) *The Analysis of the Venous System.* Vienna: Hans Huber Publishers.

PICARD, J. D. (1975) *La Phlebographie des Membres Inferieurs et Superieurs.* Paris VI: Expansion scientifique française.

SCHOBINGER, R. A. (1977) *Periphere Angiodysplasien.* Bern: Verlag Hans Huber.

SCHMITT, H. E. (1977) *Aszendierende Phlebographie bei tiefer Venenthrombose.* Bern: Verlag Hans Huber.

CHAPTER 18

DIAGNOSTIC IMAGING OF THE LYMPHATIC SYSTEM

E. Rhys Davies

INTRODUCTION

Anatomy

The lymphatic system consists of:

(*a*) Lymph capillaries, which are minute vessels that are formed in the tissue spaces of the body, anastomose freely and ultimately drain into the brachiocephalic veins.

(*b*) Lymph nodes or aggregates of lymphoid tissue into which the lymph vessels enter at some part of their course.

(*c*) Lymphoid tissue in the walls of the gut.

(*d*) Lymphocytes in the circulation.

Lymph capillaries are present in most tissues of the body except the brain, spinal cord, splenic pulp, bone marrow and avascular structures such as hair, nails, etc. These capillaries form tributaries to afferent lymph vessels that drain into regional or sometimes distant lymph nodes, with a few exceptions that bypass these nodes. Efferent lymph vessels lead from the nodes, tending to accompany arteries or veins, eventually draining either into the thoracic duct via the cisterna chyli, and thence into the left brachio-cephalic veins; or into the right lymphatic duct which drains into the right brachiocephalic veins. The lymph channels are punctuated by many semilunar valves arranged in pairs, and the lumen is usually expanded into a small pouch immediately proximal to each valve.

Each lymph node is enclosed by a fibrous capsule which is continuous on its deep surface with a system of trabeculae and reticular tissue. Within this reticulum are macrophages, lymphocytes, and lymphocyte stem cells. Dense aggregates of cells in the cortex are known as lymphatic follicles which contain the germinal centres for small lymphocytes. Usually each node has a small depression on one aspect, called the hilum, through which blood vessels enter and leave. The afferent lymph vessels enter at numerous points on the periphery of the node draining into a marginal sinus from which the lymph usually permeates slowly through the cortex into the medulla before leaving the node in one or more efferent lymph vessels via the hilum.

Physiology

The endothelial wall of the lymph capillaries is permeable to substances of relatively large molecular size and the capillaries are the pathway of absorption of colloid material, cell debris and micro-organisms from the tissue spaces. The lymph draining from most tissues is clear and colourless but that draining from the small gut is white, due to the absorption of chylomicra. This fluid is called chyle and the vessels are called lacteals.

Lymph is propelled as a result of many influences, including the filtration pressure in the tissue spaces, contraction of skeletal muscle, contraction of smooth muscle in the walls of lymph trunks and the thoracic duct, respiratory movement, and possibly arterial pulsations. The lymph nodes generate lymphocytes, macrophages and plasma cells, and also trap foreign material and antigen by phagocytosis.

Pathology

Under intense antigen stimulation the whole node may increase in size and vascularity, demonstrating proliferation of germinal centres, increased production of lymphocytes, macrophages and plasma cells. These are characteristic features of reactive hyperplasia, mediated by antigen, tumour or foreign material such as contrast medium.

In addition to this antigenic stimulus, tumour cells and infected material spread by the lymphatic system and are trapped by the lymph nodes. In the case of tumour, the node is gradually destroyed as it enlarges, and becomes a site of secondary tumour growth. Other tumours arise in lymph node elements.

In many clinical circumstances, it is vital to locate these lesions. Subcutaneous lymph nodes in the limbs and neck can be palpated and moderate enlargement of mediastinal nodes can be detected by chest radiography. Abdominal and pelvic nodes are often more important but can rarely be assessed by palpation or radiography. The technique of lymphangiography by contrast injection was designed to achieve this. It has been supplemented by isotope lymphangiography, computed tomography and ultrasound (Table 18.I). Nuclear magnetic resonance has great potential in this field. Primary or developmental abnormalities of the lymph capillaries and trunks also are amenable to investigation by contrast lymphography, and in these cases it usually provides more detailed information than the supplementary techniques.

TABLE 18.I. Methods of lymph node imaging.
(1) Radiography
    (a) Plain films
    (a) Opacification of adjacent organs
    (c) Lymphography
(2) Computed Tomography
(3) Radio-isotope lymphography
(4) Ultrasound

LYMPHANGIOGRAPHY

Technique

With few variations the early descriptions of lymph-angiography (Kinmonth *et al.*, 1955; Chapman & Nakielny, 1981) established the principles of successful lymphangiography. A diffusible coloured dye is injected subcutaneously so that it can be taken up by lymphatic vessels, in order to colour them and make them suitable for cannulation and injection with radio-opaque contrast agents. This method can be used wherever there is a lymphatic drainage system but in the vast majority of instances it is applied to the feet and to a lesser extent the hands. From the feet the deep abdominal lymph nodes and the thoracic duct can be demonstrated, and from the hands the axillary nodes and brachiocephalic trunks can be shown.

Pedal lymphography is described in detail. It is carried out under local anaesthesia from the age of 12 or 13 years upwards. Sedation is often helpful in younger children but general anaesthesia is rarely necessary over the age of 5 years. Ideally the investigation is done on a table in an X-ray room and is liable to take between 2 and 3 hours from the start to the completion of contrast injection. The investigation is carried out in the following stages:

Outlining Lymphatics. The patient should be fasting and the skin of both feet is prepared with Hibitane spirit, paying particular attention to the inter-digital clefts. A suitable macromolecular dye such as patent blue violet is then injected subcutaneously. It is supplied in a 5 ml ampoule which can be diluted with an equal quantity of 1% procaine before injection in order to obviate the pain. 0·5 ml of diluted dye is injected into each of the web spaces through a 19 gauge hypodermic needle. It is important not to stain the surface of the skin and it helps to draw back the plunger of the syringe as it is being withdrawn from the tissues. The injection sites should be massaged gently and the joints of the limb put through a range of movements passively for 3 minutes or so. Within 10 minutes it should be possible to identify green lines through the skin corresponding to the dye-laden lymph vessels. Obesity and oedema will make the lymphatics less visible.

Cannulation of a Lymphatic. Full aseptic technique is essential. A small incision is made alongside a readily visible lymphatic. Alternatively a transverse incision

may be made on the dorsum of the foot or just below the ankle if the lymphatics are not seen clearly. The stained lymphatic can be distended by proximal pressure on the skin with a finger, and at least 1 cm of the lymphatic is then very carefully cleared of surrounding fat and tissue. Three pieces of black thread of suitable length are placed under the lymphatic, and the proximal one is advanced to the edge of the wound in order to fix and distend the lymphatic. The distal thread can be used to steady the lymphatic. The needle assembly consists of a 26 SWG gauge needle bonded to a polythene cannula which is connected to a syringe and filled with saline. The lymphatic is distended and the needle is gently advanced into the distended lymphatic for about half the length of the needle. Its position can be checked by making a small injection of saline and noting that the lymphatic is distended and the needle can then be tied in position using the final piece of thread. The tubing is taped to the skin and further fixed by passing it between the toes.

Injection of Contrast Agent

(a) *Water soluble compounds.* These can be injected rapidly but diffuse quickly through the lymphatic walls and enter the blood stream at the first group of nodes. Their use is limited to demonstration of afferent lymphatics only. In these circumstances 2–4 ml of contrast containing 280 mg iodine per ml is usually satisfactory.

(b) *Iodised oils.* The usual compounds are Neohydriol fluid (40% iodine) or Lipiodol ultra fluid (37% iodine). These are viscous and can only be injected slowly under pressure. They outline the lymphatic channels, the lymph nodes and thoracic duct. Although most of the agent enters the circulation within 24 hours, enough remains trapped in the lymph nodes to display them radiologically for up to several months. Ideally the contrast is drawn up into a glass syringe and injected by an electrically operated pump calibrated to inject about 5 ml per hour.

As soon as contrast has begun to traverse the needle into the lymphatic, it is essential to take a radiograph of this area to check that the needle is properly sited in the lymphatic, when there will be a characteristic, continuous fine column of contrast. The main hazard apart from extravascular injection is that a small vein has been cannulated in error. This is readily recognised by the broken column of contrast in a venule, or an aggregate of globules in a larger vein (Fig. 18.01).

The total volume of contrast injected must be kept below a safe limit and in an adult the maximum volume injected should be 7 ml in each lower limb. This volume is reduced pro rata for children. A further check is made on the volume injected by radiographing the pelvis and lower abdomen after some 5 ml has been injected. When

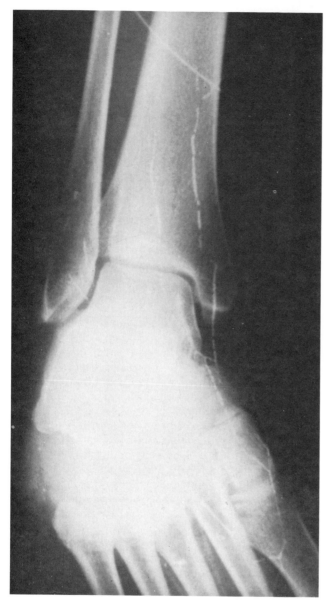

FIG. 18.01. Intravenous cannulation and injection. Note the broken column of contrast.

the column of contrast reaches the ipsilateral lower para-aortic lymph nodes the injection can be stopped. The total volume injected should not exceed 0·2 ml/kg. body weight.

Closing the Incision. The sutures are loosened, the cannula is removed and the distal thread is tied. The wound is swabbed out with normal saline and 2 or 3 silk sutures are used to close it. A dry dressing is applied.

Radiographs to be taken. A *preliminary radiograph* of the chest should be taken as pulmonary lesions may lead to modification of technique. Those radiographs taken during the injection have already been mentioned.

Postinjection radiographs are taken in two stages. The patient should walk gently in the room for 10 minutes or so and a penetrated frontal radiograph of the chest is then taken to demonstrate the thoracic duct. Frontal radiographs of suitable penetration can be taken in an hour or so to show the pattern of abdominal filling.

Radiographs are taken at 24 hrs to show the detailed structure of the abdominal lymph nodes. Frontal and both right and left posterior oblique films of the whole abdomen and pelvis are taken for complete demonstration.

In some circumstances excretion urography is indicated at this stage, adopting the usual technique of injection used in the department. In the first instance a frontal nephrogram and frontal and oblique films at 10 minutes are taken. Other necessary views are determined at that time.

Alternative Sites for Injection

In the leg supplementary injections of dye may be made distal to each malleolus in order to show lymphatics anteriorly or occasionally posteriorly at the level of the ankle.

In the upper limb a technique similar to that used in the leg is applied to the dorsum of the hand. 3–5 ml contrast agent is usually adequate, and the injection should be ended when the radiographs show that contrast has reached the axillary lymph nodes. Direct injection into lymph nodes (e.g. into a superficial inguinal node in order to demonstrate the pelvic lymphatics) has been described but is virtually never used.

Direct exposure of lymphatics in the spermatic cord has the theoretical advantage of being the best way of showing potential metastasis from testicular tumours to pararenal and upper para-aortic lymph nodes. It is rarely, if ever, used.

Sequelae and Complications

Fortunately these are uncommon, provided the described method is used, with particular emphasis on aseptic technique and careful control of the volume of contrast medium injected. Some are an obligatory consequence of the introduction of contrast medium or dye into the lymphatic system, or the use of local anaesthetic. Thus, patent blue violet enters the circulation and is excreted in the urine. The patient and those coming into close contact with him during the 24 hours after lymphography should be warned that his complexion will assume a slaty blue hue and his urine will be discoloured blue-green during this time.

The most important obligatory consequence of lymphography is *multiple pulmonary micro-embolus*. The contrast that is delivered into the brachiocephalic vein is arrested temporarily in the pulmonary capillary network. Its presence is shown well on chest radiographs

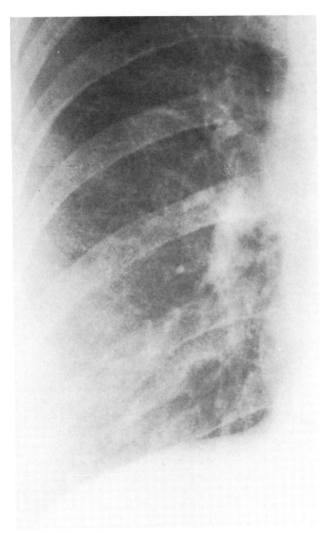

FIG. 18.02. Localised view of right lung 24 hours after lymphogram. Note the numerous punctate oil emboli.

have been noted and occasionally there are subsegmental radiographic densities. True *hypersensitivity* may contribute to the clinical syndrome in the more severe cases, but the most important single contributory factor is pre-existing lung disease. *Death* has been recorded following lymphography, but present contrast agents used in the recommended dosage are unlikely to prove fatal. The breakdown products of fat hydrolysis pass into the systemic circulation and some of the minute emboli may do so also, creating a theoretical possibility of similar reaction in other organs. It is likely that the only recorded clinical example of this was due to massive over-dosage with contrast (Gruweg *et al.*, 1967).

Among the milder reactions to the agents used, the most spectacular is a blue-tinged *urticaria* developing soon after the injection of the patent blue violet. If necessary it can be controlled by antihistamines or steroids. More severe reactions such as *hypotension* and *peripheral circulatory collapse* are rarely due to patent blue violet (Mortazavi & Bussons, 1971) and require immediate resuscitation. Similar reactions are recorded also after the use of local anaesthetic agents, but fortunately are rare following the use of agents such as Lignocaine hydrochloride.

True *allergic* or *anaphylactic reaction* to oily contrast agents is exceptionally rare, but less severe reactions are more common. Occasionally, distention of the lymphatics during injection causes *pain* which is readily controlled by simple analgesics. During the 24 hours following injection superficial lymph nodes in the line of ascent of the contrast medium (e.g. the inguinal nodes during pedal lymphography) often become slightly swollen and tender, the result of inevitable distention of the intercellular spaces and sinuses by deposited contrast. Characteristically there is a foreign body type of reaction with giant cells and histiocytes surrounding the oil deposits. A certain amount of permanent disorganisation of the node structure follows and there may be some fibrosis. This sequence is important to the radiologist because it accounts for small changes in the size of lymph nodes that are frequently observed immediately after the lymphogram. Also it accounts for slightly more marked diffuse increase in size and altered filling of lymph nodes in some instances. These changes are clearly detected histologically and as they are now well recognised they are unlikely to cause any confusion in biopsies from lymph nodes involved in a recent lymphogram. Similar but more marked radiographic changes are observed in the reactive hyperplasia already mentioned.

There is experimental evidence that the lymph nodes are more permeable to particles and cells during this reactive phase but there is no evidence that metastasis is commoner or functional deficit permanent following lymphography. *Lymphangitis*, *cellulitis* and *wound infection* may require rest, elevation and antibiotics, but their

at 24 hours, where minute high density opacities can be shown on careful search (Fig. 18.02). The mechanical effects of this embolisation are unlikely to be significant if the contrast volume is carefully controlled, and it is the chemical effects that have the greater significance. The oil that is the vehicle of the contrast agent is hydrolised to fatty acids which may damage the capillary epithelium and initiate interstitial and intra-alveolar inflammation. Surfactant is reduced and this diminishes resistance to infection. Careful measurement of pulmonary function has shown that there is a measurable fall in CO diffusion (indicating impaired oxygen transfer) which is maximal between 24 and 48 hours and thereafter gradually returns to normal (White *et al.*, 1973). This change usually passes unnoticed, but nonproductive cough, fever, and mild breathlessness instance is reduced to a minimum if aseptic technique is observed carefully. Paradoxical embolisation may occur following radiotherapy because of the well-recognised dilatation of pulmonary capillaries during radiotherapy to the lungs (Davidson, 1969).

INDICATIONS FOR LYMPHOGRAPHY

(a) **Suspected Lymph Vessel Disease.** It can be difficult to determine the cause of oedema of the extremities and demonstration of the lymph vessels and lymph nodes may help to show the presence of congenital inadequacy of lymph channels or acquired disease of the lymph nodes causing obstruction.

(b) **Diseases affecting the Lymph Nodes.** The commonest use of lymphography is to stage known malignant disease by determining the extent of lymph node involvement. Notable examples are the lymphomas and carcinomas that metastasise to the retroperitoneal nodes, e.g. cervix uteri, bladder and gonads. The presence of contrast medium in lymph nodes is sometimes helpful in checking surgical removal of glands as films can be taken in the operating theatre.

(c) **Suspected Retroperitoneal Lymph Node Disease.** Abdominal tumour of unknown aetiology is an obvious indication. An underlying occult lymphoma or occasionally carcinoma may be associated with some skin disorders, notably mycosis fungoides and persistent pruritis, exfoliative dermatitis.

(d) **Investigation of Pyrexia of Unknown Origin.** Retroperitoneal lymphoma is a well-recognised cause of this syndrome and lymphography has been a valuable method of investigation.

(e) Solution of clinical problems presented by miscellaneous conditions such as chylothorax, chyluria, lymphocoele, filariasis and the very rare lymphangiosarcomas.

Contra-Indications to Lymphography

(1) **Pulmonary disease** or impairment of lung function causing breathlessness on exertion will be exacerbated by the pulmonary reaction to oily contrast medium. In the case of lung disease it is advisable to proceed only when the investigation is essential, by cannulating first one foot and then the other after an interval of 14 days. The impairment of respiratory function can be reduced to an acceptable level in this way and the persistence of contrast in the lymph nodes enables adequate delineation to be achieved. It may be necessary even to conduct the investigation with 4 divided injections.

(2) **Breathlessness** due to cardiovascular disease is an absolute contra-indication.

(3) **Radiotherapy to the lungs** within the preceding 2 weeks, because of the consequent dilatation of pulmonary capillaries and risk of paradoxical embolus.

(4) **Proposed general anaesthesia.** The risk of general anaesthesia is increased for several days after lymphography and planned surgery should be timed carefully in relation to the lymphogram.

(5) **Known hypersensitivity** to any of the agents used in lymphography excludes its use and should lead to consideration of alternatives.

(6) **Sepsis and gross oedema** of the limb to be cannulated. Elevation and treatment of sepsis may enable a subsequent examination to be successful.

Absolute and relative contra-indications to contrast lymphography lead to an immediate consideration of alternative techniques. If the clinical need is to delineate lymph nodes, CT will be the first choice, but if a primary vessel abnormality is being investigated a radionuclide technique is more appropriate.

THE NORMAL LYMPHOGRAM

Lymphatic Vessels

These are delicate linear superficial channels, less than 1 mm in diameter, with a beaded appearance due to slight dilatation above small valves which prevent retrograde flow. They ascend the limb in relatively straight lines, without tortuosity, but with a tendency to divide and rejoin. Afferent lymphatics join their corresponding lymph node at many points on its margin (Fig. 18.03) so that they drain into its marginal sinus, which is often shown clearly around the edge of the node. As the oil passes through the node some is retained in the reticular substance whereas the remainder enters the efferent lymphatics that leave via the hilum of the node. These efferent lymphatics are larger and fewer than the afferent lymphatics and sometimes are more markedly beaded.

In the lower limb nearly all these superficial lymphatics drain along the line of the long saphenous vein receiving tributaries from adjacent regions. The exceptions are those running along the lateral side of the calf, which follow the short saphenous vein and drain into popliteal lymph nodes. Some of the efferents from the latter pathway join the deep lymphatics running along the femoral vein to the inguinal nodes. Otherwise the deep lymphatics are not demonstrated.

In the upper limb also the superficial lymphatics on the dorsal and palmar aspects follow the line of superficial veins. Those on the medial side drain into the supratrochlear glands, others accompany the basilic vein and the remainder accompany the cephalic vein.

Lymph Nodes

Typically normal lymph nodes are ovoid and measure

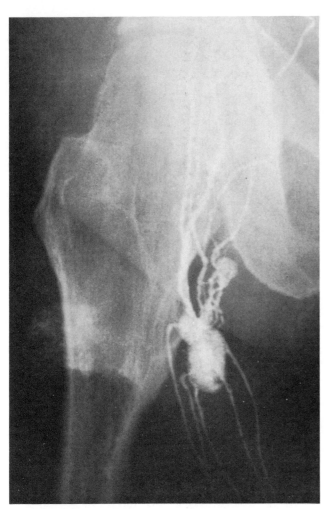

FIG. 18.03. Inguinal lymph node during filling. Afferent channels join the periphery. Efferent channels leave from the hilum.

1·5–2·0 cm. Sometimes they are spherical and may even be crescentic or irregular. Each node is outlined by its marginal sinus within which is a closely packed punctate pattern of contrast. The defects within this pattern are due to the lymphoid follicles in the node, which are sometimes large enough to give the node a reticular pattern. The hilum of the node is recognised as an identation from which the efferent channels run. Sometimes it is large because of the deposition of fibro-fatty tissue. The cardinal sign that enables it to be recognised is the demonstration of efferent lymphatics on early films in the series (Fig. 18.04 *a* & *b*).

The lymph nodes themselves are best shown at 24 hours when nearly all the contrast will have drained from the lymph vessels.

It is important to consider the *normal appearances and variations of the abdominal lymph vessels and nodes* in greater detail. In general, lymph vessels are shorter than in the limbs and range from one group to the succeeding proximal group. Thus, there is a chain from the inguinal to the external iliac nodes and another from the common iliac to the para-aortic nodes (Fig. 18.05). The internal iliac nodes and vessels drain into the common iliac but these are not shown by pedal lymphography.

From the common iliac lymph nodes a group of lymph vessels ascends on either side of the aorta overlying the vertebral bodies and transverse processes. These chains are nearly always present and in about two thirds of instances there is also a mid-line chain. These 3 chains often link with each other, the right crossing to the left more often than the converse (Fig. 18.06). They drain into the cisterna chyli, though it is surprising how infrequently the latter is shown in detail. Sometimes the chains ascend through the diaphragm to drain into the thoracic duct. Two important anomalies are worth noting. Firstly, a single large vessel to the right of the third and fourth lumbar vertebrae with no demonstration of the customary lymph node at this site. Secondly, the right lumbar chain ends abruptly at the level of L2/3 to join the middle chain. This anomaly is associated with failure to show lymph nodes to the right of L1/2. These are normal appearances that are important to note lest they should be confused with abnormal signs of lymph node obstruction or destruction (Jackson & Kinmonth, 1974).

The number, size and shape of the retroperitoneal lymph nodes is very variable. The majority are oval and lie in a vertical axis, and may be up to 3 cm long. A few small round nodes less than 0·5 cm in diameter are found. These nodes are arranged in 3 main groups, lateral groups corresponding to the lateral lymphatic chains and never extending beyond the tips of the transverse processes; and the central group that usually arises from the right iliac lymph nodes, and is projected between the aorta and vena cava. It is striking how few fibro-fatty filling defects the normal lumbar lymph nodes contain. Occasionally small filling defects up to 3 mm in diameter are found in normal nodes.

There are two notable variations in node distribution: firstly, at the level of L3/4 on the right there is a defect in the chain of nodes in about a third of instances, corresponding to the looping lymphatic already described; secondly, rather less frequently to the left of L1/2 there is a clump of smaller nodes that should not be confused with an abnormal appearance (Jackson & Kinmonth, 1974).

Filling of the left lymph node chain usually reaches a higher level (L1) than the right and middle chains (L2), possibly because of the more frequent crossover from right to left (Fig. 18.07). Failure to fill upper right lymph nodes should not be confused with neoplastic involvement. The pre-aortic nodes receive some efferents from the mesenteric lymph nodes though the greater part of lymphatic drainage from the gut is

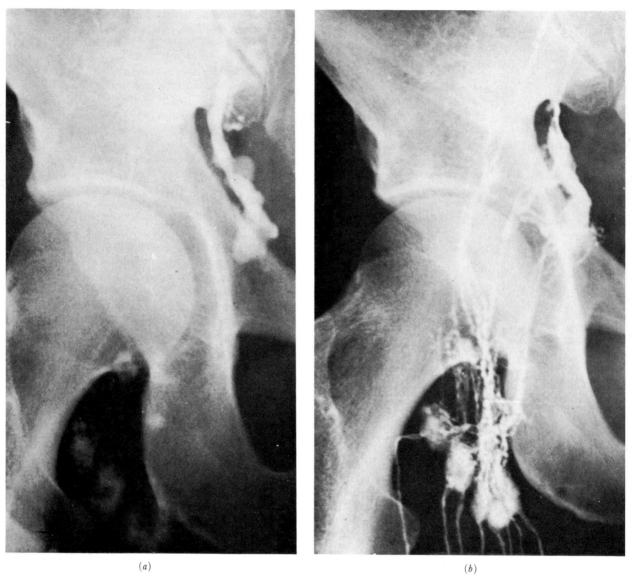

(a)   (b)

Fig. 18.04. (a) Inguinal lymph nodes containing filling defects. (b) Earlier film during filling, showing that the defects are at the hilum of each node.

directly into the cisterna chyli. Ultimately all the lymph from the abdomen and lower limbs drains into the cisterna as it lies to the right of the aorta in front of the first lumbar vertebra. It extends through the aortic opening of the diaphragm into the thorax where it becomes the thoracic duct (Fig. 18.08). Here it lies between the aorta and the azygos vein, passing to the left of the mid-line at the level of the fifth thoracic vertebra and ultimately ascending to join the junction of the left subclavian and jugular veins. The duct is beaded by its valves and its width is variable, being as much as 8 mm in some cases. Often it is slightly dilated just before its venous junction. As in the remainder of

the lymphatic system there are important variations in the radiographic appearance. The commonest variation is a division into two channels over part of its course. Occasionally the duct either fails to cross the mid-line at the level of the fifth thoracic vertebra, or divides into two terminal trunks, one draining into each brachio-cephalic system. In some normal individuals lymph nodes in the left supraclavicular fossa and in the left axilla are demonstrated by lymphography (Fig. 18.09). Less commonly para-oesophageal lymph nodes are filled and their afferent vessels return to the thoracic duct.

In children the nodes and lymphatics are, of course,

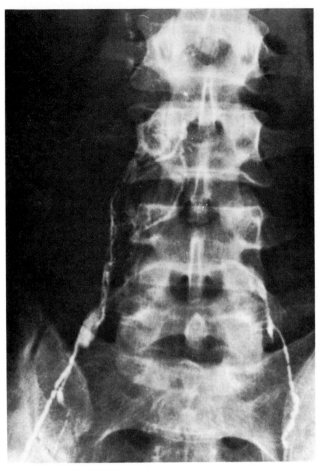

FIG. 18.05. Abdominal lymph channels during filling.

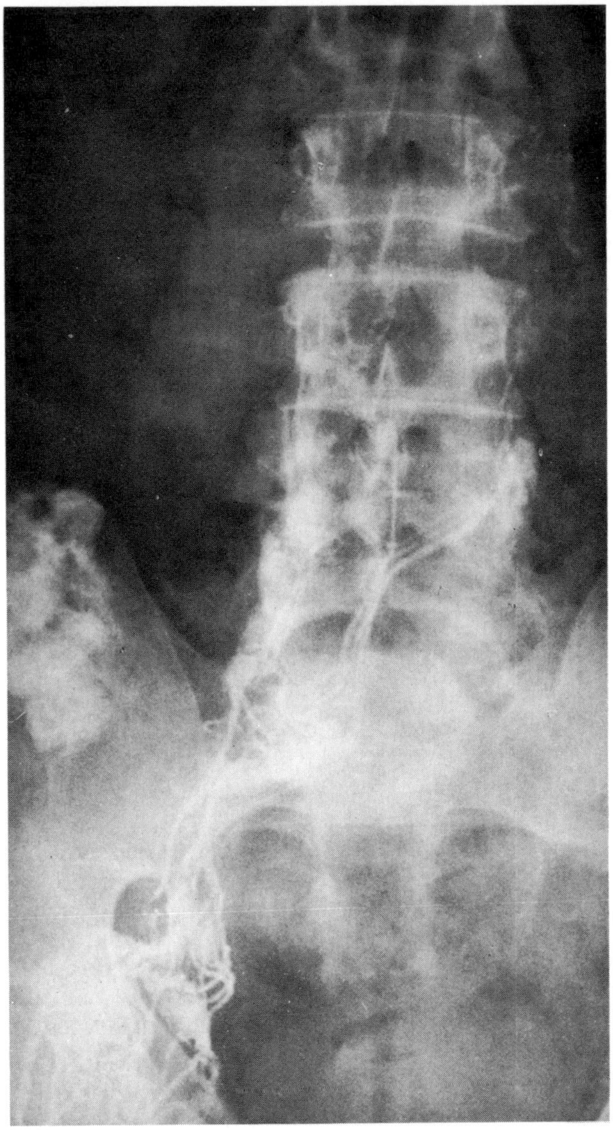

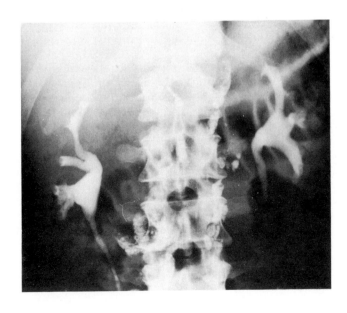

FIG. 18.06. Right to left abdominal cross-over.

FIG. 18.07. Upper abdominal lymph nodes showing better filling of
the high left para-aortic nodes than those on the right.

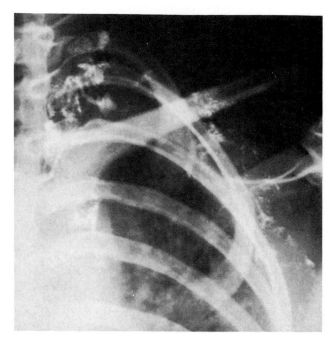

FIG. 18.09. Normal left axillary and supraclavicular nodes filled after bi-pedal lymphography.

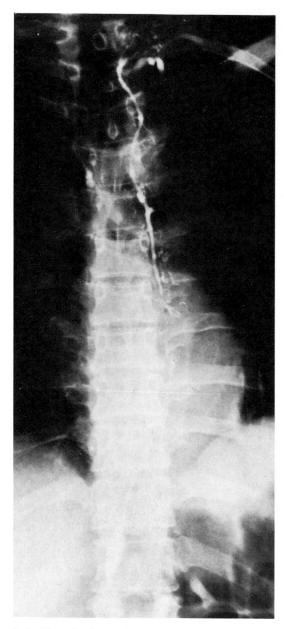

FIG. 18.08. Thoracic duct and cisterna chyli. Note that the duct crosses to the left in the lower thorax.

smaller but three other important differences merit attention: fat and fibrous tissue are usually absent from normal nodes so that normal filling defects are exceptional; the small retroperitoneal nodes can be profuse; and diffuse reactive hyperplasia is commoner than in adults so that caution is needed to avoid overdiagnosing abnormalities.

The appearances of normal lymph nodes are notably constant so that they are expected to be identified in repeated investigations. Some contrast may persist for as long as 18 months, but it is unusual to have enough residue for valid comparisons after 9 or 12 months.

COMPUTED TOMOGRAPHY

Computed Tomography (CT) is suited ideally to investigating the lymph nodes of the trunk. All these nodes can be shown by taking serial sections throughout the trunk, but it is customary to limit each investigation to those zones that are most likely to be relevant or rewarding. An understanding of the regional·lymphatic drainage of the lesion being investigated is of prime importance in determining the appropriate field of investigation.

In the lymphomas the examination should include the lower thorax and the whole abdomen as far as the iliac crests. Alternate sections of the pelvis are usually sufficient. On the other hand in pelvic and gonadal tumours serial sections from the level of the upper renal poles to the symphysis pubis are likely to be the most helpful.

Preparation

One of the major advantages of CT is its relative simplicity for the patient, but some preparation is often necessary to obtain accurate evaluation. The stomach, and more importantly the duodenum, are essential landmarks that can be outlined by giving 50 ml water-soluble contrast agent by mouth and turning the patient to the right for 5 minutes. This will outline the small bowel also and help to identify jejunal loops that resemble lymph nodes especially near the left kidney. It is not necessary to outline the urinary tract with contrast media in all cases, but it is necessary to do so when tumours of pelvic viscera are being staged, and sometimes when renal or pararenal opacities need further evaluation. 20 ml of contrast medium containing 280 mg iodine/ml is usually adequate to outline the upper urinary tract and bladder, and contrast that is too dense may obscure abnormalities in the latter. Accurate separation of the distal large bowel from pelvic masses and lymph node enlargement is helped by a small enema of dilute water-soluble contrast, but this is not required routinely. When the gut contains a lot of gas, gut movement causes artefacts that degrade the image unacceptably. It is advisable to anticipate this with a suitable paralysing agent unless there is a contraindication to its use. One of the major advantages of CT is the obligatory demonstration of all structures within the field of the sections. Thus the skeleton, liver, spleen, kidneys etc. as well as the retroperitoneal lymph nodes are viewed in serial abdominal sections and should be scrutinised carefully. Indeed it is the custom for abdominal CT to be used to stage any primary tumour that is present as well as to evaluate the extent of lymph node metastasis. Thus it is as artificial to separate CT lymphography from CT viscerography in this discussion as it would be in daily practice.

Interpretation of normal CT is centred upon the recognition of salient landmarks such as the major viscera (with or without contrast), aorta and inferior vena cava. An adequate amount of retroperitoneal fat is an advantage in distinguishinig the outline of all these structures and crucial to recognising the site of the retroperitoneal lymph chains (Fig. 18.10 a & b). The location of these is predictable from contrast lymphography except that the central chain is usually posterior to the plane of aorta and vena cava, but occasionally anterior to it. The normal lymph nodes are smooth, rounded, clearly defined, with absorption coefficient indistinguishable from that of other soft tissues. The diameter of a normal lymph node is 0·5–1·5 cm, and nodes larger than 2·0 cm are unequivocally abnormal (Ellert & Kreel, 1980). It is important to note that the following structures are not shown by contrast lymphography but can be shown quite readily by CT: internal iliac nodes, mesenteric lymph nodes, lymph nodes proximal to the origin of the cisterna chyli, (including those in the lower thorax), spleen, liver and parasplenic lymph nodes. It is not uncommon to see a small density deep to the R. crus of the diaphragm smaller than 6 mm in diameter (Fig. 18.11). It may be caused by a lymph node, or the thoracic duct, azygos vein or a small nerve. Care should be taken not to confuse the occasionally beaded smooth outline of the right crus of the diaphragm with an enlarged lymph node. The distinction is made by following the diaphragm on serial sections to its origin on the right lateral margin of the vertebrae. All para-aortic densities should be followed similarly to ensure there is not a normal structure giving rise to a

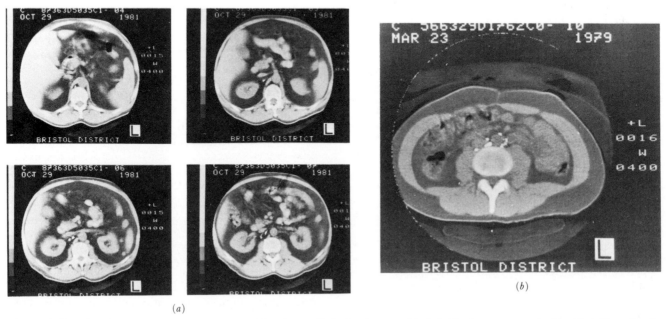

(a)

(b)

FIG. 18.10. (a) CT abdomen through the renal areas. Note how well the fat planes enable individual structures to be identified. Note also the changing profiles of the crura of the diaphragm. (b) Normal lower abdominal CT following lymphogram. Note the relationship of the lymph nodes to the aorta and vena cava.

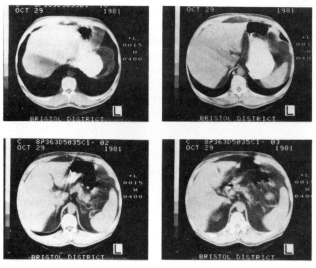

Fig. 18.11. CT upper abdomen following lymphogram. Note the normal contrast-filled lymph nodes and channels posterior to the right crus of the diaphragm.

'pseudo-tumour'. Among the important causes are: jejunum in the left para-aortic area, near the left kidney; the vena cava itself; and extrarenal pelvis. The radiologist should have a high index of suspicion, and should resolve his doubts by giving contrast medium orally or intravenously (Marincek *et al.*, 1981).

RADIONUCLIDE LYMPHOGRAPHY

Lymphatic Transport

The ideal radiopharmaceutical is a microcolloid that can be prepared consistently with suitable-sized colloid particles and can be labelled with a suitable radionuclide. $^{99}Tc^m$ *Antimony colloid* with a particle size of 4–12 μ has these characteristics (Ege, 1976, 1978) and is superior to the sulphur colloid because the particle size obtained from the commerical kit of the latter is too large for rapid absorption and lymph node retention (Dunson *et al.*, 1973).

For *abdominal lymphoscintigraphy* 40 MBq are injected in individual doses simultaneously into the medial digital webs of both feet. Walking or passive exercise promotes absorption, and serial gamma camera images of the legs are taken over the next 2 hours. Finally, scintigraphy of abdomen and pelvis are carried out at 2–3 hours (Dunson *et al.*, 1973).

The *normal appearances* are symmetrical activity in the lymph node chains. The lymph trunks are not shown and the main shortcoming of the technique is its relatively poor resolution so that individual lymph nodes are not shown reliably. Asymmetrical activity is the cardinal sign of *abnormality* (Fig. 18.12a). Usually it

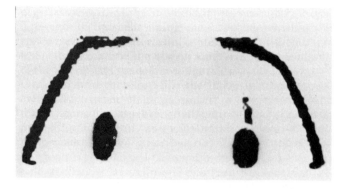
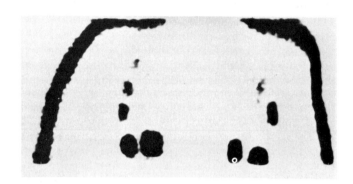
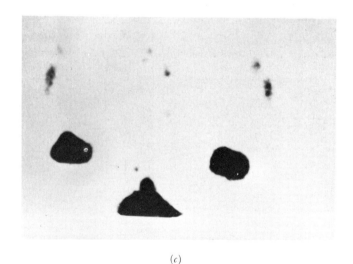

(c)

Fig. 18.12. Lymphoscintigraph. (a) Asymmetry due to unfilled right axillary nodes (the outline of the shoulders is marked). (b) Minor asymmetric filling, probably within normal limits. (c) Internal mammary scintigraph showing sites of injection and low nodal activity (*by courtesy of Dr M. V. Merrick*).

is due to absent activity in nodes destroyed by tumour but may be due to increased activity in a node distal to lymphatic obstruction. The technique offers a simple way of detecting non-specific abnormality and may help to determine the appropriate size of radiation field. In experienced hands it is reliable.

The technique of *internal mammary lymphoscintigraphy* is similar. 20 MBq are injected in two divided doses, contained in about 0·5 ml saline, subcostally just medial to the mid clavicular line. The ideal depth of injection is just superficial to the posterior rectus sheath, usually 2·0–2·5 cm below the skin (Ege, 1976). Gamma camera images are obtained at 3 hours or so. The essential features of a normal scan are bilateral parasternal chains, which come together at the levels of both the menubrium and the xiphoid. Anatomical variations in the number and symmetry of normal lymph nodes are common and increase the range of acceptable normal appearances (Fig. 18.12 *b* & *c*). A gap in filling is usually insignificant if there are normal nodes on each side of it.

Tumour Extraction

[67]*Gallium citrate* has an affinity for soft tissue neoplasms, particularly the lymphomas and has been advocated in their assessment and follow-up. 80 MBq are injected intravenously and films taken at 24 and 48

hours. Gallium citrate is excreted into the bile and also directly into the colon via the colonic mucosa. A small amount is excreted in the urinary tract and some taken up by bone marrow. Normal scan appearances reflect this distribution. Additional views or bowel clearance are needed sometimes to distinguish normal bowel activity from abnormal lymph node activity.

ULTRASOUND SCANNING

Ultrasound scanning at a frequency of 2 megahertz (2 MHz) displayed on conventional grey scale is a well established method of examining upper abdominal viscera, notably liver, pancreas, kidneys, spleen and aorta. In addition to elucidating the nature of known lesions in these viscera, the ultrasound scanning will inevitably encounter and discover retroperitoneal masses, particularly those involving lymph nodes (Fig. 18.13). Normal lymph nodes are beyond the limit of resolution of ultrasound scanning which is usually 3 cm and only exceptionally below this. Lymph nodes that are large enough to be shown are well defined and contain small echoes distributed homogeneously. The

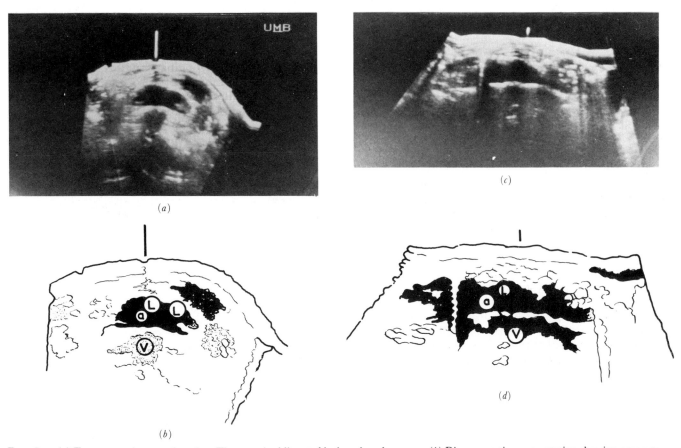

(a)

(c)

(b)

(d)

FIG. 18.13. (*a*) Transverse ultrasound section. The aorta is obliterated by lymph node masses. (*b*) Diagrammatic representation showing a = aorta, L = lymph nodes, and V = vertebra. (*c*) Longitudinal section same patient. (*d*) Diagrammatic illustration of (*c*). (*By courtesy of Dr F. G. M. Ross.*)

overall sensitivity of ultrasound in detecting retroperitoneal lymph node tumour is below 70% (Rochester, *et al.*, 1977) and this is an important restriction of its use.

ABNORMALITIES OF THE LYMPHATIC SYSTEM

The Lymph Vessels

Failure to drain interstitial fluid as fast as it is formed leads to oedema. Many causes of oedema (e.g. cardiac failure) are associated with normal lymphatic systems which are dilated but unable to cope with excessive production of interstitial fluid. The remaining causes of oedema are associated with failure of an abnormal lymphatic system to cope with normal production of interstitial fluid. This so-called lymphoedema is either primary, due to congenital lymphatic anomalies; or secondary, due to known acquired lymphatic disease (Table 18.II).

TABLE 18.II. Classification of the lymphoedemas (after Kinmonth, 1982).

(a) *Primary lymphoedema*
    Clinical classification
    (i) Congenital lymphoedema. Present at birth.   10%
    (ii) Lymphoedema praecox. Presents under 35 years.   75%
    (iii) Lymphoedema tarda. Presents over 35 years.   15%

    Radiological classification
    Aplasia 5%   Majority female
    Hypoplasia 90%   Majority female
    Hyperplasia 5%   Male and female

(b) *Secondary lymphoedema*
    (1) Trauma and wounds
    (2) Malignant disease
    (3) Filariasis
    (4) Infection and Inflammation
    (5) Radiation

Primary Lymphoedema. This form of lymphoedema is developmental. Only about 1 in 10 present at birth (congenital lymphoedema), about three quarters under the age of 35 years (lymphoedema praecox) and the remainder later in life (lymphoedema tarda) (Kinmonth *et al.*, 1957). Lymphoedema may be familial but less than 1% of cases are both congenital and familial as in the autosomal dominant condition affecting males and females and described by Milroy (1928). The typical presentation of all primary lymphoedema is with pitting oedema of the ankle or foot, initially relieved by rest and elevation, but gradually becoming more severe and progressing up the limb. Minor trauma or infection frequently precipitates deterioration in the symptoms. It is postulated that the efficiency of abnormal lymphatics deteriorates with the age of the patient because there is no reserve to allow for the effects of injuries and minor infection etc. Ultimately a critical point is reached over a range of different ages when the lymphatics are

no longer able to cope and symptoms occur (Kinmonth, 1972). In well-established cases trophic changes occur in the skin which may be hyperkeratotic. The contralateral limb is usually involved ultimately. The lower limbs are affected much oftener than the upper limbs and other sites that may be involved include the small gut leading to protein loosing enteropathy, the lung, and more rarely the head and external genitalia. Three distinct lymphographic types are recognised (Kinmonth *et al.*, 1957; Gough, 1966) and their associated features also are distinct:

i) *Aplasia.* Following injection the coloured dye permeates the subdermal layers without delineating any identifiable lymphatic trunk. It may spread to the ankle and shin, and its extent is an indication of the severity of the condition. Attempted surgical exposure is unsuccessful also. The majority are female and the condition may be a Mendelian recessive characteristic. The majority belong to the lymphoedema praecox group.

ii) *Hypoplasia.* The vast majority belong to this group. Usually these are female and have similar characteristics to the aplastic group. It may be very difficult to delineate a lymphatic with patent blue violet but in this group it is often possible with some difficulty to cannulate a fine lymphatic in the dorsum of the foot. The striking feature is the small number of lymphatics present, particularly above the knee, and their fine calibre. Usually the lymphatics are competent and there are no collateral pathways but occasionally the valves are incompetent and there is dermal backflow recognised by the appearance of a greenish blush in the skin, and a contrast filled fine network of dermal capillaries. In addition the proximal lymph nodes may be few in number, small and dense because the normal granular pattern is absent. Occasionally ectopic nodes are filled.

This group may be associated with gonadal agenesis (Turner's syndrome) and it is interesting that in these cases the oedema may resolve spontaneously.

iii) *Hyperplasia.* In this group the disease is usually congenital and affects males and females. Cutaneous angiomas may occur in the affected region. The lymphatic valves are incompetent or absent so that the lymph channels become widely dilated and tortuous, giving a characteristic appearance. The individual lymph nodes are enlarged in many instances.

A number of congenital abnormalities outside the lymphatic system are now recognised to be associated with lymphoedema. For example Down's syndrome, micrognathos, cleft palate, cardiovascular anomalies, double eyelashes, with hyperplasia of lymphatics, pes cavus. Others are the mixed vascular deformities of the limbs (Table 18.III). All these syndromes are chiefly of clinical interest, particularly as the lymphatic abnormality is often overlooked in generally well-known syndromes.

The diagnosis of lymphoedema can be made usually

TABLE 18.III. Mixed vascular deformities of the limbs (after Kinmonth, 1982)

Syndrome	Features	Lymphatics
Maffucci	Angiomas	Lymphoedema
	Dyschondroplasia	Enlarged lymph nodes
		Normal lymphatics
		Lymphoid element in angiomas
Congenital arteriovenous fistulae	Giant limbs	Hyperplastic varicose lymphatics
Klippel-Trenaunay	Hypertrophy of limb	Hypoplasia
	Naevi	
	Varices	

on clinical grounds. The indications for lymphography are:

(a) To confirm or refute the diagnosis. The management of the patient depends on a correct diagnosis.

(b) To distinguish between primary and secondary lymphoedema from an occult cause. Malignant disease within the pelvis may present with lymphoedema and lymphography and venography have been advocated in all patients over 30 with obscure lymphoedema of the lower limb (Kinmonth, 1972). CT of the pelvis is now an essential forerunner of lymphography in these circumstances.

(c) To aid the surgical management of primary lymphoedema. Several surgical techniques are available and are indicated for cosmetic, practical (wearing normal clothes) and medical (improving the state of the skin and avoiding the development of secondary angiosarcoma) reasons. The best results are obtained if the operation is done when the abnormality has ceased to progress and it is claimed that the severity of the lymphatic abnormality can aid this judgement as well as confirm the diagnosis (Kinmonth, 1972).

Lymphoscintigraphy offers a simple test of lymphatic efficiency that may help to select patients for lymphography, but reported experience is limited (Jackson & Lentle, 1977; Vieras & Body, 1977). A normal scintigram effectively excludes a lymphatic cause for oedema, whereas pedal stasis and diminished inguinal activity on the affected side are features of primary lymphoedema. On the other hand diffuse activity throughout the limb is a feature of lymphatic obstruction. The greatest potential use of this technique is in the investigation of unexplained limb oedema in childhood, because it is tolerated better than contrast lymphography, and has a lower radiation burden (Vieras & Body, 1977).

THE LYMPH NODES

Metastatic Tumours

Contrast lymphography is a well-established technique for detecting metastasis of malignant disease to regional lymph nodes. The radiographic features of a lymph node tumour depend upon its extent and rate of growth rather than its histological nature or site and are common to all tumours, where they give rise to the following signs:

Filling defects. Usually these are irregular defects at the margins of nodes (Fig. 18.14) but occasionally they are central, as in melanoma. They encroach upon the node as they grow, displacing the remaining normal node round the tumour edge, and obliterating the marginal sinus relatively early (Fig. 18.15 & 18.16). Fibro-fatty filling defects occur at the hila of inguinal nodes and are not significant. In the pelvic nodes, extra hilar defects due to inflammatory or fatty lesions may be as large as 1 cm and may give rise to falsely positive interpretation (Kolbenstvedt, 1975). Such defects are uncommon in the retroperitoneal chains, but small insignificant filling defects of 2–3 mm diameter are encountered within the substance of the nodes. Defects that are larger than this are significant.

Failed opacification. A node that is destroyed extensively by neoplasm may not be shown at all because it does not contain contrast medium. Failure to show such a node should not be confused with absence of lower

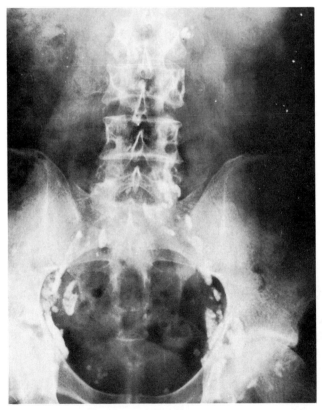

FIG. 18.14. Abdominal lymphogram. There is a large peripheral defect in a right iliac node destroying the marginal sinus.

right lumbar lymph nodes found in nearly half of normal examinations. Displacement of adjacent organs such as the kidneys and a soft tissue density are important clues to unfilled but involved nodes.

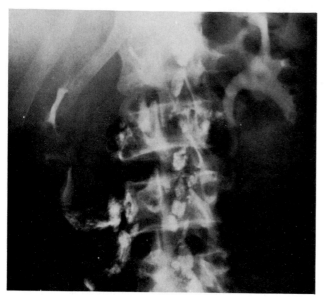

Fig. 18.15. Upper abdominal lymphogram. There is a large filling defect in a right para-renal node with poor contrast filling of its stretched margins.

Displaced nodes. Tumour in adjacent nodes may displace filled nodes from their normal position. Displacement of lumbar nodes beyond the transverse process tips is always significant whereas a lesser degree of displacement does not always indicate the presence of neoplasm.

Stasis and opacification of collateral vessels. Obstruction of lymph flow will lead to persistence of contrast in the lymph vessels beyond 24 hours and may cause the opacification of collateral lymph vessels not normally shown (Fig. 18.17 & 18.18).

Hepatic oil embolism. Rarely, hepatic oil embolus follows severe partial, or complete obstruction of the para-aortic and external iliac nodes, even if the vena cava is patent (Ngan & James, 1978). The usual primary lesion is a cervical or testicular carcinoma, and the phenomenon is rare in the lymphomas (Glazer *et al.*, 1981). The likely route is via collateral mesenteric lymphatics that anastomose with the portal circulation (Chavez *et al.*, 1965). The typical appearances are arborising densities within the liver followed by a granular pattern (Fig. 18.19). Also there is a typical CT pattern reflecting these appearances (Glazer *et al.*, 1981).

'Pseudo-lymphomatous' appearance. Occasionally nodes containing tumour are enlarged with a coarse filling pattern and preservation of marginal sinus, resembling the appearance that are found in the lymphomas. Seminoma is one of the well-recognised causes of this uncommon appearance (Wilkinson & MacDonald, 1975).

Progressive enlargement of involved nodes. In the absence of radiotherapy, metastases tend to enlarge,

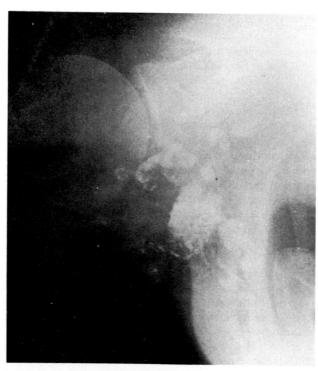

Fig. 18.16. Axial view of axillary lymph nodes showing peripheral filling defect.

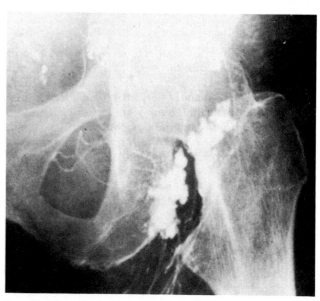

Fig. 18.17. Lymphatic obstruction. Note the collateral lymph vessels that are not normally shown.

increasing the size of the node and the size of the filling defect. The rate at which this change occurs depends on the rate of growth of the tumour and is variable. For example, in carcinoma of the cervix less than half the lesions enlarged during the period of observation (Kolbenstvedt, 1975). For this reason needle aspiration of suspected defects is now advocated, especially in pelvic tumours (Wallace *et al.*, 1977) (*vide infra*).

Follicular hyper-plasia. The response of lymph nodes to antigenic and other stimuli has been described already and its lymphographic counterpart is lymph node enlargement with a coarse pattern but without significant filling defects. There is no histological evidence of tumour and the appearances have been described in a variety of tumours including Kaposi's sarcoma (Baddeley & Bhana, 1971) and also in sarcoidosis, collagen disease and psoriasis (Viamonte *et al.*, 1963).

Differential shrinkage. Following treatment with radiotherapy, normal and abnormal lymph nodes shrink but more extensive shrinkage of abnormal nodes can be observed sometimes. This sign occasionally helps to establish the positive nature of a doubtful appearance.

In experienced hands lymphography achieves an overall accuracy approaching 90% (Koehler, 1976; Kolbenstvedt, 1975; Wallace *et al.*, 1977) in detecting retroperitoneal lymph node metastasis. The commonest source of error is inability to detect minute deposits (Castellino, 1979) and the key to identifying deposits smaller than 5 mm in diameter is to take careful and regular follow-up radiographs in order to seek evidence of enlargement.

False positive inaccuracies are usually due to inexperience in recognising the range of normal appearances. The relative infrequency of fibro-fatty filling defects in the abdominal lymph nodes is an important factor in reducing the incidence of false positive interpretations.

Marked asymmetry of a *lymphoscintigram* or decreased activity in individual nodes and delay in filling proximal nodes are signs of an abnormal lymphoscintigram. The main application of this technique is the demonstration of the internal mammary lymph node in staging breast carcinoma (Ege, 1978) (Fig. 18.12). None of the alternative techniques can offer an improved demonstration of these nodes. The relative value of the technique depends on the treatment strategy being used in individual centres and it has not gained wide acceptance yet.

The Lymphomas

In these diseases, there is a diffuse abnormality within the affected lymph nodes, causing them to enlarge and

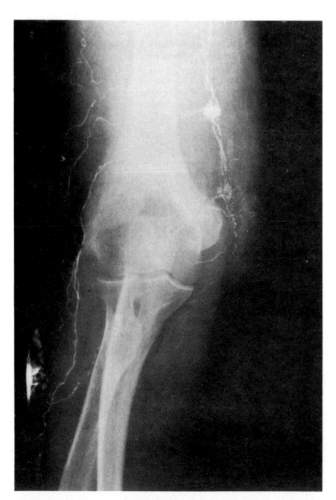

Fig. 18.18. Upper limb lymphogram. Lymphatic obstruction. Note the filling of small collateral vessels especially in the subdermal plexus.

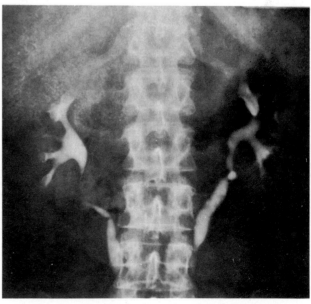

Fig. 18.19. Lymphatic obstruction. Hepatic oil emboli.

spreading the reticulum within them round the neo-plastic tissue. The following lymphographic signs are best shown at 24 hours:

Increase in size. Occasionally the increase is very dramatic, particularly in Hodgkin's disease, but adjacent nodes are often much less enlarged.

Filling defects. The striking abnormality is the presence of numerous filling defects within each node with preservation of the marginal sinus until a late stage of involvement (Fig. 18.20). This is distinct from metastasis where the tumour is usually eccentric and tends to interrupt the marginal sinus at an earlier stage. Numerous descriptive terms have been used to identify the appearances but essentially they consist of contrast-free lacunae of varying sizes pervading lymph nodes that exhibit varying degrees of enlargement. Often more nodes than usual are shown by lymphography, and nodes in unusual sites may be shown.

Delayed lymphatic transit. Overt obstruction of the vessels occurs less often than nodal abnormalities but occasionally there is striking persistence of contrast in channels adjacent to lymph nodes (Fig. 18.21). Indeed it may be the only abnormal feature and should be regarded as an important sign of disease. Globules of contrast in small veins seen during the injection of contrast are evidence of lymphovenous communication rarely shown in the lymphomas (Edwards & Kinmonth, 1969).

The possible combinations of signs in the lymphomas are numerous and do not correspond in any reliable way to the histological classifications. Thus, it is unwise to attempt to predict the histology from the radiological appearances (Gordon *et al.*, 1976).

Scrutiny of the full set of 24-hour films enables 80% or so of all lymphograms in the lymphomas to be allocated to normal or abnormal groups. The allocation of the remainder will not be clear. Usually there is uncertainty about the significance of isolated signs such as a small filling defect or filling of an unexpected lymph node. Filling defects smaller than 3 mm are not significant but larger defects may sometimes be within normal limits. Usually the difficulty can be resolved by taking follow-up films at 2, 4 and 8 week intervals. The tumour doubling time of the lymphomas is such that any genuine lesion at the time of the first films will have declared itself within 2–6 weeks. Alternatively, there is uncertainty about slight diffuse nodal enlargement with coarsening of the filling pattern. Such an appearance can be due to reactive hyperplasia, the characteristic of

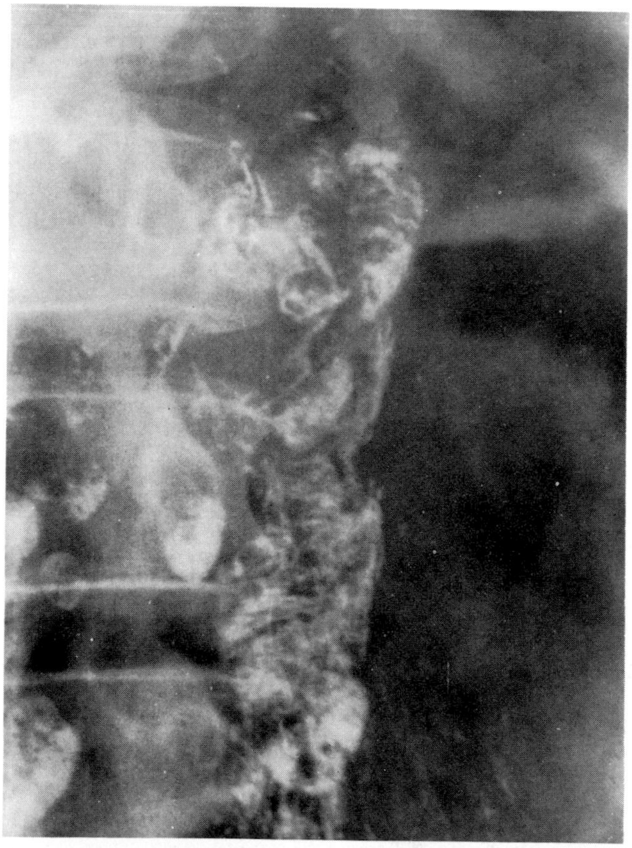

FIG. 18.20. Lymphoma. Enlarged para-aortic nodes with filling defects and late preservation of marginal outline.

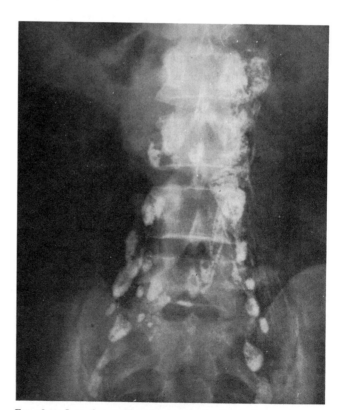

FIG. 18.21. Lymphoma. Note the lymphatic obstruction on the left, a rare occurrence in lymphoma.

which is that the abnormal signs are maximal within 1–3 days of injection and regress by the time the first interval films are taken at 2 weeks. Thus, careful assessment of the interval films enable equivocal examinations to be allocated to normal or abnormal categories and the overall accuracy of lymphography is well above 90% (Castellino *et al.*, 1974; Kadomian & Wirtconen, 1977). The errors are usually false positives due to reactive hyperplasia or fibrosis, and the specificity is high. Lymph node sampling at laparotomy is an unreliable adjunct to lymphography and the main indication for laparotomy in Hodgkin's disease is to determine if there is splenic involvement (Glees *et al.*, 1974).

Following the initial investigations further radiographs can be taken at intervals for as long as there is contrast within the lymph system, i.e. 6–18 months. The response of abnormal nodes to treatment can be recorded and recrudescence or exacerbation detected (Fig. 18.22). It is important to relate these later radiographs to radiotherapy or chemotherapy treatment which will, of course, influence the appearances. As a result of treatment abnormal lymph nodes will return towards normal, though the persistence of some abnormality is permanent. Normal nodes may become almost invisible following several courses of radiotherapy. Exceptionally, diseased nodes become smaller as the result of radiotherapy to abnormal lymph nodes in another site of the body. This abscopal regression may indicate a better prognosis in non-Hodgkin's lymphoma (Rees, 1981).

Occasionally it is necessary to repeat the lymphograph in order to restage the disease after contrast has disappeared from the nodes. The technique becomes increasingly difficult and it may not be possible to detect suitable lymphatics after 2 or 3 investigations. In any event extensive radiotherapy will lead to a rapid transit of contrast medium through the lymph nodes. It may even form globules in the thoracic duct and lead to rapid and extensive pulmonary microembolism (Kinmonth, 1972). These investigations need to be monitored very carefully.

Lymphography in paediatric oncology is taxing but rewarding with specificity and sensitivity approaching those in adults (Castellino *et al.*, 1977). Important differences from adult lymphogram appearances are: absence of fat and fibrous tissue in normal nodes; profuse small retroperitoneal nodes, and the relatively frequent occurrence of diffuse reactive hyperplasia.

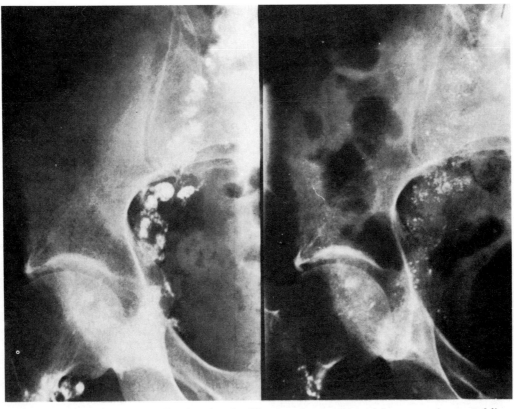

FIG. 18.22. Serial images of the right iliac lymph nodes. They have become enlarged due to recrudescence of disease.

CT Signs of Involvement

The characteristic features are similar for all tumours and at all sites, and are well illustrated in the abdomen and inguinal regions. The earliest sign of an abnormality is *enlargement of lymph nodes* (Fig. 18.23). Normal abdominal nodes may be as large as 2 cm across but any node that is larger than 1·5 cm should arouse suspicion (Blackledge *et al.*, 1980) and it is then helpful to repeat the scan in one month. The normal structures that traverse the retrocrural space are usually less than 6 mm across and opacity larger than this should be regarded as abnormal (Collen *et al.*, 1977). Enlarged retrocrural lymph nodes are nearly always associated with enlarged lymph nodes in the upper or mid abdomen. As they enlarge, lymph nodes *obliterate adjacent fat planes.* Commonly the outline of the aorta or inferior vena cava is made indistinct in this way and this may be the dominant sign of abnormality (Fig. 18.24, 18.25). Alternatively individual lymph nodes become fused, and create a *localised mass* which may enlarge very considerably. When lymph nodes adjacent to a normal organ enlarge in this way, the lesion may mimick enlargement of that organ. Thus, enlarged lymph nodes adjacent to the head of the pancreas can be indistinguishable from an intrapancreatic tumour (Fig. 18.26). Finally, the tumour may be large enough to *displace normal structures*, e.g. the kidneys, ureters and stomach.

CT provides an obligatory view of other structures in the abdomen and it is important to review these as well. In particular, lesions may be found in the vertebrae. Translucencies greater than 1·0 cm and sclerotic lesions greater than 0·5 cm are abnormal (Ellert & Kreel, 1980). Incidental hepatic deposits are difficult to detect without contrast enhancement.

The above comments apply to all malignancies and the number of additional observations should be made in the lymphomas. Firstly, enlargement of lymph nodes not shown by lymphography may occur. These include mesenteric nodes, nodes at the porta hepatis and splenic hilum. Secondly, there may be extranodal disease. Low attenuation deposits occur in the liver and spleen, but the attenuation values are unreliable indicators of involvement (Alcorn *et al.*, 1977) so that it is never

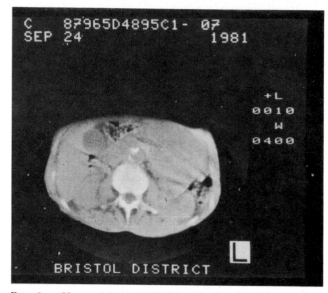

FIG. 18.24. Upper abdominal CT. There is a large left anterior mass and the outline of the retroperitoneal vessels is obliterated. Note aortic calcification.

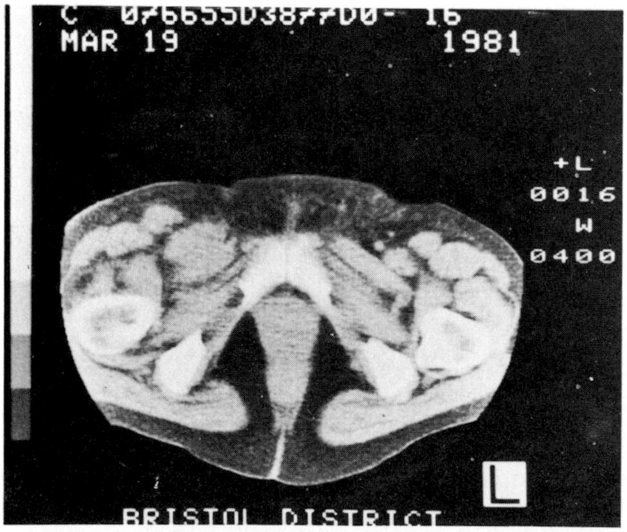

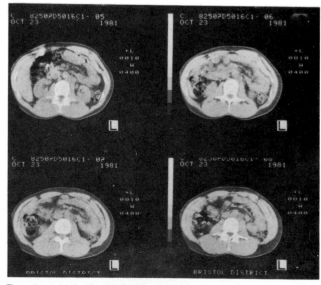

FIG. 18.25. Abdominal CT. The left posterior margin of the aorta is obliterated by a lymph node mass.

FIG. 18.23. CT inguinal nodes. The right superficial groups of nodes is markedly enlarged.

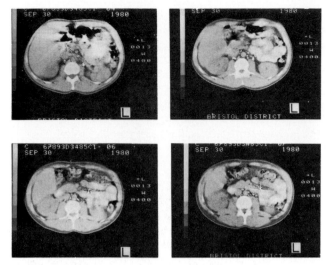

FIG. 18.26. Abdominal CT. Note contrast in the duodenum and jejunum. Enlargement of the uncinate lobe of the pancreas was found to be due to lymphoma at laparotomy.

possible to exclude involvement of these organs. Splenic and hepatic involvement usually occur in the presence of enlarged upper abdominal nodes; and hepatic involvement occurs most commonly in the presence of splenic involvement. The spleen is enlarged if it extends more than two-thirds of the distance between the posterior and anterior abdominal walls, but mere enlargement is not an indication of tumour deposit. Localised deposits in the kidneys or adrenal glands are rare. Nearly all lymphomas will have been diagnosed before abdominal CT is done, and the aim of CT is to confirm the staging of the disease (Table 18.IV). About one-third of all patients with lymphoma have unsuspected abdominal disease at the time they present. Its recognition advances the staging and this has important implications for proposed treatment.

TABLE 18.IV. Staging of the malignant lymphomas

Stage	
I	One node group, on one side of the diaphragm.
II	Two or more node groups, on same side of the diaphragm.
III	Nodes above and below diaphragm (including spleen, Waldeyer's ring and thymus).
IV	Extra-lymphatic involvement—e.g. liver, bone marrow.

Good results have been claimed with *Gallium scanning* in detecting and staging the lymphomas but there are several limiting factors: the detection rate is greater in Hodgkin's disease and the histiocytic lymphomas; superficial lesions are detected more readily than deep lesions (Johnson *et al.*, 1974), and the focal length of the collimator is critical; lesions near the liver may be difficult to separate from normal hepatic activity. Despite these limitations, ^{67}Ga citrate scanning has

many applications. In the investigation of patients with systemic symptoms before a *histological diagnosis is made*, a positive scan may indicate the optimal site for biopsy. The value of ^{67}Ga scanning in *staging lymphoma of known histology* varies with the clinical problem. For example if the probability of occult abdominal disease is low (e.g. nodular sclerosing Hodgkin's disease) a negative scan may support the decision to avoid laparotomy. On the other hand if the probability of abnormality is relatively high (e.g. mixed cellularity Hodgkin's disease) even a negative scan will not modify the clinical decision and the scan will be of little value (Turner *et al.*, 1978). If laparotomy is contraindicated or refused the combination of ^{67}Ga scan and lymphography gives valuable data. [67]Ga is also useful in evaluating known or suspected lesions of the mediastinum, which are not normally amenable to routine thoracotomy. A positive scan over a known mass makes the probability of an additional lesion well over 90%, and scanning is said to be reliable in detecting lesions too small to cause a radiographic abnormality (Levi *et al.*, 1975). Finally, in the *follow-up of treated lesions*, particularly in the mediastinum, a positive scan is a highly sensitive indicator of residual tumour. To summarise, a positive gallium scan has a sensitivity of over 90%. Unfortunately, there is significant incidence of false negative scans (Turner *et al.*, 1978). In general lymphography, CT and laparotomy will be the first line investigation. Gallium scanning is a second line investigation valuable in selected circumstances.

RELATIVE MERITS OF CONTRAST LYMPHOGRAPHY, CT, US AND RADIONUCLIDES IN ABDOMINAL EXAMINATION

Evaluation of the lymph nodes makes many important contributions to patient management (Table 18.V). The

TABLE 18.V. Contribution of lymph node evaluation to patient management

(1) Accurate staging of disease
   Showing extent of tumour
   Showing relationship to adjacent vital structures
(2) Aid to surgery
   Planning staging laparotomy and biopsies
   Selecting suitable cases for limited resection
   Confirming extent of lymph node dissection at operation
(3) Aid to radiotherapy planning
   Determining volume to be treated
   Planning therapy ports
(4) Guide to prognosis, e.g. negative lymphogram has a good prognosis in testicular tumours
(5) Follow-up
   Response to treatment
   Relapse
(6) Investigation of patients with systemic symptoms
   e.g. pyrexia of unknown origin
   CT is the investigation of choice

ultimate contribution of each technique to evaluating abdominal lymph nodes has yet to be determined, and it is likely that each will find prime place in different circumstances. In the meantime it is useful to consider their relative merits under a number of headings.

Radiation

The universal attribute of ultrasound is that it does not use ionising radiation. On the other hand, the relative hazard of the alternative technique is minimal in patients already known to have malignant disease.

Reaction to Contrast Media etc.

Lymphography and, to a lesser extent, CT carry a remote hazard of reaction to contrast agents. Genuine hypersensitivity to radiopharmaceuticals is exceptionally rare, whereas contrast agents are not used in ultrasound techniques.

Significance of Lymph Node Site

Ultrasound and CT are predominantly dependent on their ability to detect lymph node enlargement. The borderline of normality can be difficult to define, and in the iliac groups it may be necessary to rely on a discrete asymmetric mass larger than 1·5 cm if the number of false positives is to be reduced (Hodson *et al.*, 1979). The content of either normal or enlarged lymph nodes cannot be evaluated by these techniques, whereas contrast lymphography demonstrates the pattern of filling as well as the size of each node. Indeed one of its major advantages is that it can detect neoplastic filling defects in normal-sized nodes, and also show that enlarged nodes are due to reactive hyperplasia rather than tumour. Radionuclide lymphography is much less sensitive than any of the other techniques and does not reflect the size of the lymph nodes, but their failure to fill (colloid) or the avidity of tumour for gallium.

Scope of the Examination

The scope of lymphography is limited to those nodes that are filled with contrast, and is virtually constant for all investigations. The potential scope of CT includes the whole abdomen and can be varied to suit the needs of individual cases. It has the potential for detecting ascites and abnormalities of the liver as well as lymph nodes, and is more reliable than linear tomography for detecting lung metastasis (Husband *et al.*, 1979). Ultrasound has the advantage that the liver can be viewed and ascites detected, but its scope elsewhere in the abdomen is much less than that of CT.

The scope of radionuclide colloid lymphography is limited still, but gallium lymphography has the potential to demonstrate extra-lymphatic and lymphatic deposits of lymphoma.

Operator Skill

US requires skilful operation for every phase of the investigation. Lymphography requires the greatest amount of operator skill in the initial cannulation but thereafter, like CT, technical skill is required.

Influence of Other Structures

Bowel movement and bowel gas can impair CT and US images, but are much more likely to make the latter invalid.

Initial Cost and Ease of Follow-up

Contrast lymphography is probably the most expensive initial investigation but the most easy to follow up. US on the other hand is the least expensive but because of the required operator skill the most difficult in follow-up. CT and isotope lymphography occupy an intermediate position.

The sensitivity of contrast lymphography for tumour is between 80 and 90 %, and there is an important need for histological confirmation in some instances.

Aspiration Biopsy

It becomes important when there is an equivocal or unexpected filling defect on a staging lymphogram; or when an abnormality is shown during the investigation of a patient with dermatological or systemic symptoms. Successful needle aspiration has obvious advantages over surgical excision or laparotomy. A fine Chiba needle (23 gauge) is advanced under fluoroscopic control, with local anaesthetic being injected via the needle. The needle is advanced vertically over inguinal or iliac nodes and obliquely towards para-aortic nodes, as in a translumbar aortogram. Rotation of the patient in a cradle may aid accurate location of the needle, and movement of the node when the needle is moved confirms the location. The aspirate is fixed and analysed by a cytologist immediately. The results are more reliable in carcinoma than lymphoma, particularly epithelial tumours arising in pelvic viscera (Wallace *et al.*, 1975).

More recently ultrasound has been used to guide a biopsy needle. Once a mass has been displayed by means of a B-scan, a special transducer is used with a central hole through which the biopsy needle is passed along the ultrasound beam. Its precise position is best shown by an A-scan (Ross, 1981). The technique has been developed for taking biopsies of the pancreatic lesions but can be applied to other retroperitoneal lesions. It is the most elegant of the aids to biopsy and is radiation free, but lacks the precision of post-lymphogram fluoroscopy and of CT.

The precision that is lacking in ultrasound guide biopsy can be achieved more tediously with CT because of its superior resolution. A surface marker is placed at the chosen point of skin puncture, the biopsy needle is advanced perpendicularly and serial images of precisely the same section are taken to check advancement of the needle.

DIAGNOSTIC STRATEGY FOR ABDOMINAL LYMPH NODE DISEASES

Delineating the retroperitoneal lymph nodes by any technique reveals unsuspected tumour in a significant proportion of cases. The best-known examples are the lymphomas where up to 30% of all patients with extra-abdominal disease are found to have unsuspected retro-peritoneal lymph node involvement (Walker *et al.*, 1974). This advance in staging (Table 18.IV) has important implications for the management of the lymphomas. Because it delineates a wider range of lymph nodes, CT demonstrates abnormal lymph nodes in a higher proportion of subjects. However, it does not follow that the management is altered significantly in all these cases. For example, the mere presence of abdominal lymph node disease may indicate the use of systemic chemotherapy, and showing additional abdominal disease will not influence this regime of treatment. In the case of gonadal carcinomas that metastasise to the upper abdomen, the field of treatment is likely to be planned in such a way that all its common metastatic sites have been included. It is generally accepted that a negative lymphogram should not influence the treatment field of these tumours (Koehler, 1976) but demonstrating an expected distant metastasis, e.g. in carcinoma of the uterus, may lead to an enlarged field of treatment (Douglas *et al.*, 1972).

For the purpose of planning treatment it is important to consider how many investigations should be performed, and the sequence in which they should be performed. The most informative investigations are lymphography, computed tomography and excretion urography. The yield of positives from any one of these can be increased by adding any one of the remaining two. There is little, if any, further yield from doing all three. The suggested approach is that CT should be done first. If it is normal, lymphography will show the architecture of those abnormal lymph nodes that are not enlarged and therefore will increase the positive yield. If CT is abnormal it is unlikely that lymphography will yield any additional information. If CT is unavailable, lymphography will be the first line of investigation, and it does have the advantage of being more readily available if frequent follow-up is indicated (Husband *et al.*, 1979). If either is abnormal the possible contribution of urography should be considered. Usually it is not necessary. However, if there are non-specific abnormalities of the renal tract or it is necessary to locate the radiographic position of the kidneys, excretion urography is indicated. If lymphography is the first line of

investigation, urography need only be done if the position of the kidneys is not detectable by plain radiography or if it is necessary to know the influence of abnormal lymph nodes on the urinary tract. For example, the precise relationship of treatment fields to kidneys or bladder are important in planning radiation fields; and the possibility of ureteric compression or obstruction is an indication for urography, particularly in assessing tumours of pelvic origin.

Helping to stage the disease is not only the only contribution that investigating the lymphatic system makes to the management of malignant disease. The assessment of tumour volume is an important preliminary to planning treatment and determining the entry portals of radiotherapy. Once the initial programme of treatment has been planned, it is important to evaluate the response to treatment (Fig. 18.27 *a* & *b*) and to monitor and detect possible relapse of disease. In order to achieve this a comprehensive visualisation of the abdominal lymph nodes is necessary and without CT this is not possible. Therefore, even when the information is unlikely to influence the programme of treatment, there are important reasons for computed tomography of the relevant parts of the lymphatic system. With the advent of CT, cavography has been relegated from the group of radiological investigations in frequent use for assessing lymph node size.

Inflammatory Diseases

Lymphography does not play a part in the usual scheme of investigating inflammatory diseases, but many conditions may be encountered during lymphography for standard indications, and it is important to be aware of the appearances of these diseases. Lymph nodes respond in a limited number of ways, whatever the stimulus, the dominant ones being proliferation of the reticulum with enlargement, or destruction of normal architecture with enlargement. Thus, any inflammatory process will cause enlargement of relevant lymph nodes with corresponding increase in the number and size of adjacent lymph trunks. In children systemic infections may cause widespread abnormalities of this kind, which are reflected in the lymphographic appearances.

In *tuberculosis* there is often considerable lymph node enlargement, particularly in the upper abdomen, with the presence of filling defects corresponding initially to granulomata and later to regions of caseation and abscess formation. Ultimately there is non-filling of destroyed nodes with lymphatic obstruction (Beetlestone *et al.*, 1977). Thoracic *sarcoidosis* is often accompanied by abdominal lymph node enlargement with preservation of the peripheral sinus and a coarse filling pattern. These abnormalities resolve under the influence of treatment, in parallel with the thoracic abnormalities. Similar lymph node enlargement with a reticular

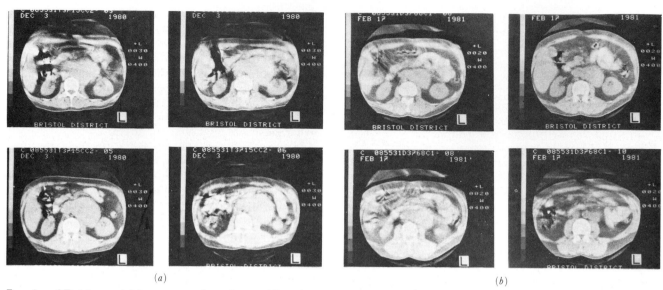

(a)   (b)

FIG. 18.27. CT abdomen. (a) Large retroperitoneal mass obliterating vascular outlines. (b) 10 weeks later the mass is much smaller and the vessels are slightly better shown.

pattern on lymphography is well recognised in *rheumatoid arthritis* (particularly in the presence of Sjorgen's syndrome).

Special consideration of *filariasis* is important, not because lymphography is the primary diagnostic test but because it is important if surgical treatment is being contemplated, and because it is important to identify the appearances in the event of investigating oedema or chyluria of uncertain origin (Middlemiss and Cockshott, 1979).

Filariasis is endemic in the tropical and subtropical regions of Africa, Asia, America and Australasia. It is caused by parasitic invasion of the lymphatics and subcutaneous tissues by the small worms W. Bancrofti and B. Malayi. Adult female filariae give birth to microfilariae that mature in an insect, usually the mosquito, and are transferred to man by an insect bite. The living worms cause inflammation of the lymphatic trunks and of the lymph nodes. Secondary infection usually supervenes and ultimately the parasite dies. Even then there is a progressing granulomatous fibrotic reaction at all the sites of infection. The site of the mosquito bite determines the maximum lymphatic involvement, which is often asymmetrical despite the systemic infection. Lymphatic drainage is seriously compromised and leads to chronic severe oedema of the legs and genitalia followed by the presence of chyluria as alternative channels for lymphatic drainage open up. The diagnosis usually is clinched by finding microfilariae in the blood at night or by complement fixation and dermal sensitivity tests.

Lymphography is often difficult in filariasis because of the severe oedema and lymphatic obstruction. In the early stages of the disease there is lymph node enlargement with punctate filling defects, which are nonspecific findings. In more advanced disease with extensive fibrosis and lymphatic obstruction the nodes are small or fail to outline. The lymph trunks are dilated, tortuous and incompetent. In the legs collateral channels open into the subdermal plexus; and in the abdomen into the renal plexuses, giving rise to chyluria (Fig. 18.28). Contrast may still be visible in the lymph trunks after some weeks. The thoracic duct can be shown by allowing contrast to drain into it, but the major abnormalities are distal to its origin. Collaterals draining into the kidney are often so fine that they are difficult to identify, but they can be shown to drain into the fornices of the minor calyces.

TUMOURS OF THE LYMPH VESSELS

Benign tumours are rare, usually congenital and slow growing. The commonest of the *lymphangiomas* is the cystic hygroma of the neck and there is no indication for lymphographic examination. Occasionally they grow in the mediastinum and in the retroperitoneum, and may cause chylothorax or chylous ascites. This is an indication for lymphography and they show as smooth rounded tumours that fill with contrast if they are in communication with the normal lymphatic drainage channels. Less common are the *lymphangiomyomas* which are also congenital, in females, giving rise to a similar clinical and lymphographic pattern to the cystic lymphangiomas.

These benign tumours may be associated with mul-

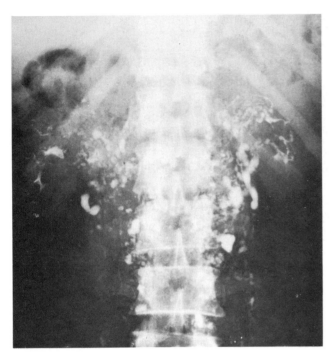

FIG. 18.28. Filariasis. Lympho-renal shunt. Note oily contrast in the right minor calyces.

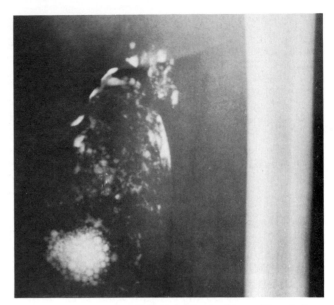

FIG. 18.29. Lymphocoele in left thigh following biopsy. Note the large oily globules.

tiple skeletal lesions giving rise to rounded translucencies, more common in the spine, pelvis and legs than in the skull, upper trunk and arms. Rarely the disease is confined to the skeleton (Castellino and Finkelstein, 1975; Gilsanz *et al.*, 1976; Beltz, 1980).

Lymphangiosarcomas occur very rarely as a complication of lymphoedema. Usually they have been described in the upper limb, secondary to radical mastectomy, the remainder being in the lower limbs, secondary to chronic oedema. Lymphography may determine the extent of the disease but the only certain evidence of malignancy is histological (Beltz, 1980).

LYMPHOCELES

An extralymphatic collection of lymph with an endothelial lining may form whenever there is an injury to a lymph vessel. The most common cause is surgical resection of regional lymph nodes, e.g. clearance of the pelvic nodes during radical hysterectomy. Usually these lymphoceles are relatively small but they may be large enough to cause symptoms due to compression of the ureters, bladder, sigmoid colon or pelvic veins. As a rule ascending pedal lymphography will enable globules of oily contrast to enter the cyst and its extent may be demonstrated fully by taking suitable radiographs in erect, supine, prone and decubitus positions.

Less commonly a lymphocele may form in a limb following lymph node biopsy (Fig. 18.29). It is uncommon for it to cause symptoms but it may be demonstrated at lymphography. Axillary lymphoceles following radical mastectomy are rare. Finally lymphoceles may follow direct trauma. The natural history of lymphoceles is to regress but very occasionally they rupture causing a fistula. Surgical treatment may be needed to relieve pressure symptoms from large intrapelvic lymphoceles.

CHYLOUS ASCITES

The commonest cause of chylous ascites is obstruction to the flow of chyle into the thoracic duct. In the neonate it is associated with atresia or hypoplasia of the lymphatic channels including the retroperitoneal nodes and cisterna, as well as lymphoedema of the lower limbs and occasionally intestinal lymphangiectasis. In a later age group the commonest cause is obstruction by enlarged lymph nodes. Less commonly obstruction may be due to tuberculous lymph node enlargement or chronic pancreatitis. Finally, penetrating injury to the mesenteric lymphatics or cisterna chyli can give rise to chylous ascites.

CHYLOTHORAX

Escape of chyle into the pleural spaces is most often due to penetrating injury of the thoracic duct. It is a rare complication of translumbar aortography. Lymphoma and other neoplasms may cause chylothorax by obstructing the flow of chyle in the thoracic duct. The remaining cases are said to be due to erosion by tuberculosis, aortic aneurysm or congenital abnormality.

The initial management of chylothorax is conservative and lymphography is indicated only when the decision has been taken to intervene surgically. The purpose of lymphography is to demonstrate the site of leakage from the thoracic duct and to show the possible cause of the abnormality by showing the retroperitoneal and sometimes intrathoracic lymph nodes (Fig. 18.30). Often it is quite difficult to demonstrate the site of leakage because it may be insidious or due to multiple small perforations. It is important to obtain a rapid filling of the thoracic duct in the erect position following completion of the lymphatic injection. This can best be achieved by moderate exercise and frequent films of the appropriate region.

CHYLOPERICARDIUM

Primary chylopericardium is rare and usually benign and asymptomatic. Sometimes it is a complication of lymphatic tumours of the mediastinum, and can give rise to cardiac tamponade. Lymphography will delineate such a tumour usually. There is a known association of this group with skeletal lymphangiomata (Gallant *et al.*, 1977).

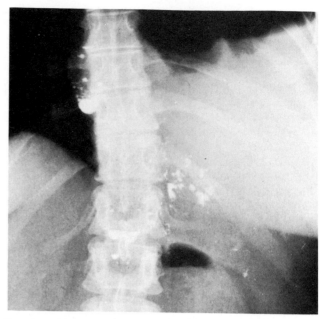

FIG. 18.30. Lymphangiogram with chylothorax. Note contrast pooling in the abnormal lymph spaces. There are some fine globules in the chylothorax.

REFERENCES

ALCORN, F. S., MATEGRAND, V. C., PETASNICK, J. P. & CLARK, J. W. (1977) Contribution of computed tomography in the staging and management of malignant lymphomas. *Radiology*, **125**, 717–723.

BADDELEY, H. & BHANA, D. (1971) Lymphography in Kaposi's sarcoma. *Clin. Radiol.*, **22**, 391–400.

BEETLESTONE, C. A., WIELAND, W., LEWIS, E. A. & ITIYOMI, S. O. (1977) The lymphogram in abdominal tuberculosis. *Clin. Radiol.*, **28**, 653–658.

BELTZ, L. (1980) In *Atlas of Lymphography*. Ed. Viamonte, M. & Ruttiman, A. New York: Thieme-Stratton, Inc. pp. 164–172.

BLACKLEDGE, A., BEST, J. J. K., CROWTHER, D., ISHERWOOD, I. (1980) Computed tomography (CT) in the staging of patients with Hodgkin's disease. *Clin. Radiol.*, **31**, 143–147.

CASTELLINO, R. A. (1979) In *CT, Ultrasound and X-Ray: an Integrated Approach*, Ed. Moss, A. A. & Goldberg, H. I. New York: Masson, pp. 106.

CASTELLINO, R. A., BILLINGHAM, M. & DORFMAN, R. F. (1974) Lymphographic accuracy in Hodgkin's disease and malignant lymphoma. *Invest. Radiol.*, **93**, 155–165.

CASTELLINO, R. A., MUSUMEA, R., MARKOVITS, P. (1977) *Lymphography in Paediatric Oncology*. St. Louis: CV Mosby.

CASTELLINO, R. A. & FINKELSTEIN, S. (1975) Lymphographic demonstration of a retroperitoneal lymphangioma. *Radiology*, **115**, 355–356.

CHAPMAN, S. & NAKIELNY, R. (1981) *A Guide to Radiological Procedures*, London: Balliere Tindall. pp. 174–182.

CHAVEZ, C. M., BERRONG, L. G. & EVERS, G. G. (1965) Hepatic oil embolism after lymphangiography. Role of the lymphaticovenous anastomosis. *Amer. J. Surg.*, **110**, 456–460.

COLLEN, P. W. KOROBLEIN, M. & ISHERWOOD, I. (1977) Computed tomographic evaluation of the retrocrural prevertebral space. *Amer. J. Roentg.*, **129**, 907–910.

DAVIDSON, J. W. (1969) Lipid embolism to the brain following lymphography *Amer. J. Roentg.*, **105**, 763–771.

DOUGLAS, B., MacDONALD, J. S. & BAKER, J. W. (1972) Lymphography in carcinoma of the uterus. *Clin. Radiol.*, **23**, 286–294.

DUNSON, G. L., THRALL, J. H., STEVENSON, J. S. & PLUSTEY, S. M. (1973) ^{99}TC^m minicolloid for radionuclide lymphography. *Radiology*, **109**, 387–392.

EDWARDS, C. L. & HAYES, R. L. (1969) Tumour scanning with ^{67}Gallium citrate. *J. Nucl. Med.*, **10**, 103–105.

EDWARDS, J. M. & KINMONTH, J. B. (1969) Lymphovenous shunts in man. *Brit. Med. J.*, **2**, 579, 581.

EGE, G. N. (1976) Internal mammary scintigraphy, the rational technique, interpretation and clinical application. *Radiology*, **118**, 101–107.

EGE, G. N. (1978) Internal mammary scintigraphy: a rational adjunct to the staging and management of breast carcinoma. *Clin. Radiol.*, **29**, 453–456.

ELLERT, J. & KREEL, L. (1980) The role of CT in the initial staging and subsequent management of the lymphomas. *J. Comput. Asstd. Tomog.*, **4**, 369–391.

GALLANT, T. E., HUNZIKER, R. S. & GIBSON, T. C. (1977) Primary Chylopericardium: The Role of Lymphography. *Amer. J. Roentg.*, **129**, 1043–1045.

GILSANZ, V., YEH, H-C. & BARON, M. G. (1976) Multiple lymphangioma of the neck, axilla, mediastinum and bones, in an adult. *Radiology*, **120**, 161–162.

GLAZER, G. M., NICOL, R. F. & MOSS, A. A. (1981) CT demonstration of hepatic oil embolism following lymphography. *J. Comput. Asstd. Tomog.*, **5**, 413–415.

GLEES, J. P., GAZET, J-C., MACDONALD, J. S. & PECKHAM, M. J. (1974) The accuracy of lymphography in Hodgkin's disease. *Clin. Radiol.*, **25**, 5–11.

GORDON, I., STOKER, D. J. & MACDONALD, J. S. (1976) The lymphographic pattern in Hodgkin's disease. A correlation with the Rye histological classification. *Clin. Radiol.*, **27**, 57–64.

GOUGH, M. H. (1966) Lymphoedema: Clinical and lymphographic studies, *Brit. J. Surg.*, **53**, 917–925.·

HODSON, N. J., HUSBAND, J. E. & MACDONALD, J. S. (1979) The role of CT in staging bladder cancer. *Clin. Radiol.*, **30**, 389–395.

HOFFER, P. B., BEKERMAN, C. & HENKIN, R. E. (1978) In *Gallium-67 Imaging*. Chichester: John Wiley and Sons.

HUSBAND, J. E., PECKHAM, M. J., MACDONALD, J. S. & HENRY, W. F. (1979) The role of CT in the management of testicular teratoma. *Clin. Radiol.*, **30**, 243–252.

JACKSON, B. T. & KINMONTH, J. B. (1974) The lumbar lymphatic crossover. *Clin. Radiol.*, **25**, 187–193.

JACKSON, B. T. & KINMONTH, J. B. (1974) The diagnosis of lumbar lymph node metastasis by lymphography. *Clin. Radiol.*, **25**, 195–201.

JACKSON, F. I. & LENTLE, B. C. (1977) The scintilymphangiographic 'Flare' sign of lymphangiotic obstructions. *Clin. Nucl. Med.*, **2**, 211–213.

JOHNSON, G., BUENA, R. S. & TEATES, C. D. (1974) [67] Gallium-citrate scanning in untreated Hodgkin's disease. *J. Nucl. Med.*, **15**, 399–403.

KADOMIAN, M. & WIRTANEN, G. (1977) Accuracy of bipedal lymphography in Hodgkin's disease. *Amer. J. Roentg.*, **129**, 1041–1042.

KINMONTH, J. B., TAYLOR, G. W. & HARPER, R. A. (1955) Lymphangiography: a technique for its use in the lower limb. *Brit. Med. J.*, **1**, 940–942.

KINMONTH, J. B., TAYLOR, G. W., TRACY, G. D. & MARSH, J. D. (1957) Primary lymphoedema. *Brit. J. Surg.*, **45**, 1–9.

KINMONTH, J. B. (1982) In *The Lymphatics: Diseases, Lymphography and Surgery*. London: Edward Arnold. pp. 114–142.

KOEHLER, P. R. (1976) Current status of lymphography in patients with cancer. *Cancer*, **37**, 503–516.

KOLBENSTVEDT, A. (1975) Lymphography in the diagnosis of metastases from carcinoma of the uterine cervix Stages I and II. *Acta Radiol.*, **16**, 81–97.

LEVI, J. A., O'CONNELL, M. J. & MURPHY, W. L. (1975) Role of

Gallium citrate scanning in the management of non-Hodgkin's lymphoma. *Cancer*, **36**, 1690–1701.

MACDONALD, J. S. (1970) Lymphography in malignant disease of the urinary tract. *Proc. Roy. Soc. Med.*, **63**, 1237–1239.

MARINCEK, B., YOUNG, D. W. & CASTELLINO, R. A. (1981) A CT scanning approach to the evaluation of left para-aortic pseudo-tumours. *J. Comput. Asstd. Tomog.*, **5**, 723–727.

MIDDLEMISS, J. H. & COCKSHOTT, P. (1979) *Clinical Radiology in the Tropics*. London: Churchill Livingstone. pp. 16–17, 210–211.

MILROY, W. F. (1928) Chronic hereditary oedema. *J. Amer. Med. Assoc.*, **91**, 1172–1175.

MORTAZAVI, S. H. & BURROWS, B. D. (1971) Allergic reaction to patent blue dye in lymphography. *Clin. Radiol.*, **22**, 389–390.

NGAN, H. & JAMES, K. W. (1978) Hepatic oil embolism following lymphography. *Brit. J. Radiol.*, **51**, 788–792.

REES, G. J. G. (1981) Abscopal regression in lymphoma. *Clinical Radiology*, **32**, 475–480.

ROCHESTER, D., BOWIE, J. D., KUZMANN, M. D. & LESTER, E. (1977) Ultrasound in the staging of lymphoma. *Radiology*, **124**, 483–487.

ROSS, F. G. M. (1981) In *Textbook of Radiology and Imaging*. Ed. Sutton, D., Edinburgh: Churchill Livingstone, p. 1369.

TURNER, D. A., FORDHAM, E., ALI, A. & SLAYTON, R. E. (1978) Gallium-67 imagining the management of Hodgkin's disease and other malignant lymphomas. *Sem. Nucl. Med.*, **8**, 205–218.

VIAMONTE, M., ALTMAN, D., PARKES, R., BLUM, E., BERILACQUA, M. & RECHLER, L. (1966) Radiographic pathologic correlation in the interpretation of lymphangioadenograms. *Radiology*, **86**, 903–916.

VIERAS, F. & BODY, C. M. (1977) Radionuclide lymphangiography in the evaluation of paediatric patients with lower extremity oedema. *J. Nucl. Med.*, **18**, 441–444.

WALKER, T. M., DAVIES, E. R. & ROYLANCE, J. (1974) The value of urography following lymphography in malignant diseases. *Brit. J. Radiol.*, **50**, 93–97.

WALLACE, S., JUNG, B. S. & ZORNOZA, J. (1977) Lymphangiography in the determination of the extent of metastatic cancer. *Cancer*, **39**, 706–718.

WALLACE, S., SCHWARTZ, P. E. & ANDERSON, J. H. (1975) A feasibility study for retroperitoneal lymph node biopsy. *Amer. J. Roentg.*, **125**, 234–239.

WHITE, R. J., WEBB, J. A. & TUCKER, A. K. (1973) Pulmonary function after lymphography. *Brit. Med. J.*, **4**, 775–777.

WILKINSON, D. J. & MACDONALD, J. S. (1975) A review of the role of lymphography in the management of testicular tumours. *Clin. Radiol.*, **26**, 89–98.

INDEX

A

Acromegaly, 173
Acute left heart failure, 59
Akinesis, 114
Alveolar flooding, 45
Amyloidosis, 173
Anaemia, 175
Aneurysm,
    aortic, 180
    arterial, 315
    dissecting, 137, 183
    left ventricle, 105
    mycotic, 181
Angiodysplasia, in aortic stenosis, 136
Angioplasty,
    of coronary arteries, 122
    of peripheral arteries, 327
Aorta,
    dilatation of, 23
    normal, 22
Aortic atresia, 228
Aortic arch,
    cervical, 258
    double, 257
    left, 255
    right, 257
Aortic incompetence. See Aortic regurgitation
Aortic interruption, 266
Aortic regurgitation,
    causes of, 136
    congenital, 232
    with VSD, 216
Aortic sclerosis, 126
Aortic stenosis,
    subvalvar, 230
    supravalvar, 266
    valvar, congenital, 229
Aortic valve, echocardiography of, 79
Aortitis, 179
    syphilitic, 137
Aortopulmonary window, 270
Arteria aberans, 265
Arteries,
    circumflex, 36
    congenital malformations of, 310
    left anterior descending, 34
    left coronary, 34
    posterior descending, 36
    pulmonary, 19, 42
    right coronary, 34
Arteriography,
    artefacts, 299
    axillary, 294

carotid, 292
    catheter, 294
    complications, 296
    direct needle, 292
    of tumours, 321
    translumbar, 293
Arteriosclerosis, 300
Asplenia syndrome, 236
Asymmetric septal hypertrophy. See
        Hypertrophic cardiomyopathy
Asynchrony, 114
Asyneresis, 114
Atheroma, 300
Atrial septal defect,
    primum, 211, 217
    secundum, 211
    sinus venosus, 211
Atrioventricular defect, 219
Atrium,
    left, enlargement of, 13
        normal, 13
    right, enlargement of, 11
        normal, 11
Austin Flint murmur, 79
Azygos vein,
    relationship to circulating blood volume,
        47
    relationship to mean right atrial pressure,
        47
    size, 47

B

Beriberi, 173
Blalock-Taussig shunt, 283
Bronchial circulation, 45
Bronchial collaterals, 243
Bronchial wall thickness, 45
Bronchovascular bundle, 43
Buerger's disease, 307, 321

C

Calcification,
    aortic valve, 127
    cardiac, 25
    coronary, 28
    in mitral annulus, 141
    in ventricular aneurysm, 107
    left atrial, 144
    metastatic vascular, 289
    pericardial, 30
    peripheral vascular, 289

Canal defect. See Atrioventricular defect
Capillary bed, 42
Carcinoid syndrome, 156, 157
Cardiac output, isotope measurement, 97
Cardiac pacemakers, 163
Cardiac volume, 4
Cardiomyopathy,
    congestive, 171
    echocardiography of, 84
    hypertrophic, 175
    post partum, 175
    restrictive, 176
Cardiothoracic ratio, 4
Carotid body tumour, 324
Cervical arch, 258
Cervical rib, 307
Chagas disease, 172
Chylopericardium, 394
Chylothorax, 393
Clubbing, with cardiac myxoma, 158
Coarctation,
    of aorta, 262
    of pulmonary arteries, 267
Collagen diseases, with cardiac involvement,
        172
Common ventricle, 250
Computed tomography,
    in arterial imaging, 290
    in lymphatic diseases, 378, 388
    of veins, 362
Contrast media, 295
    in phlebography, 331
Cor triatriatum, 278
Coronary arteries. See also Arteries
    angiography, 37, 117
    angioplasty, 122
    anomalous left, 273
    arteritis, 105
    bypass grafts, 122
    calcification, 28, 105
    ectasia, 118
    embolus, 105
    normal, 33
    spasm, 105, 121
Corrected transposition, 249
Corrigan's kink, 324
Cytotoxic heart disease, 175

D

Diastolic closure rate, of mitral valve, 76
Digital subtraction imaging, 289
Diphtheria, and heart failure, 171

Doppler echocardiography, 89
Double outlet ventricles, left and right, 252
Down's syndrome, 219
Ductus arteriosus, 268
Dyskinesis, 114

E

Ebstein's anomaly, 221
  in corrected transposition, 249
E–F slope. *See* Diastolic closure rate
Eisenmenger response, 205
Ejection fraction, 117
  isotope measurement, 98
Embolisation, 326
Embolus, peripheral arterial, 307
Embryology, cardiac, 201
Endocardial cushion defect. *See*
  Atrioventricular defect
Endocardial fibro-elastosis, 232
Endocarditis, 208
  echocardiogram in, 80, 81, 139, 153
Endothelial cell junctions, 44
Epithelial cell junctions, 44
Extravascular lung water, 57

F

Fallot's tetralogy, 239
False aneurysm, 115
Fibrinogen uptake test, 360
Fibromuscular hyperplasia, 300, 320
Filariasis, 392
Fistula,
  coronary artery, 272
  pulmonary arteriovenous, 272
  sinus of valsalva, 272
  systemic, 272
Floppy (prolapsing) mitral valve, 151
Flow inversion, 58
Fontan procedure, 283
Four chamber view, 33

G

Gallium scanning, in lymphomas, 389
Gerbode defect, 217
Glenn procedure, 287
Glycogen storage disease, 173, 232

H

Haemochromatosis, 172
Haemodynamics, 42, 43
  general principles, 204
  pathological, 204
Haemosiderosis, in mitral valve disease, 146
Heart failure, transient, of the newborn, 233
Heart size, 3, 23
  volume, 4
Howell-Jolly bodies, 236
Hurler's syndrome, 105
Hypercalcaemia, idiopathic and supra aortic
  stenosis, 266
Hypertrophic obstructive cardiomyopathy,
  175
Hypogenetic right lung syndrome, 281
Hypokinesis, 114

Hypoplastic left heart syndrome, 228

I

Idiopathic subaortic stenosis. *See*
  Hypertrophic cardiomyopathy
Ischaemic heart disease, isotope scanning, 94
Isomerism, 236

K

Klippel-Trenaunay syndrome, 347

L

Left atrial pressure assessment, 59
Left heart hypoplasia, 228
Left ventricle,
  aneurysm, 107
  angiography, 113
  echo assessment of function, 81
  false aneurysm, 115
Leriche syndrome, 306
Long axial view, 33
Lung 'erection', 62
Lutembacher's syndrome, 141
Lymphangiography,
  indications, 374
  radionuclide, 380
  technique, 371
Lymphangiomas, 392
Lymphangiomyomas, 392
Lymphangiosarcomas, 393
Lymphatic channels, 45, 57
Lymphatic system (hypertrophy), 58
Lymphocele, 393
Lymphoedema, and Down's syndrome, 382
Lymphomas, 385

M

Major aortopulmonary collateral arteries,
  243
Marfan's syndrome, 137, 183, 315
Mega-artery syndrome, 315
Mitral atresia, 228
Mitral prolapse, 151
Mitral regurgitation,
  causes of, 151
  congenital, 227
  echocardiogram of, 77
Mitral stenosis,
  acquired, 140
  congenital, 226
  echocardiogram of, 76
  parachute type, 226
  supravalvar ring, 227
Mitral valve,
  diastolic closure rate, 76
  echocardiography of, 75
  flutter, 79
  prolapse, 77
Monckeberg's sclerosis, 289
Mustard procedure, 282
Mycotic aneurysm, 181
Myocardial infarction, isotope scanning, 95
Myocarditis, viral, 171

Myxoma,
  atrial, 88
  cardiac, 158

N

Neuromuscular heart disease, 175
Noonan's syndrome, 226

O

Ochronosis, and aortic stenosis, 127
Oedema, early, 45
Ossification, pulmonary, 146

P

Paget's disease, and aortic stenosis, 126
Parachute mitral valve, 226
Parametric imaging, 101
Patent ductus arteriosus, 268
Peribronchial cuffing, 44
Pericarditis, constrictive, 196
Pericardium,
  defects of, 200
  effusion, 87, 194
  tumours of, 198
Perivascular space, 44
Phase imaging, 101
Phlebography,
  complications, 336
  intraosseous, 334
  operative, 348
  radionuclide, 358
  technique, lower limb, 331
    upper limb, 352
Physiological interpretation, 42
Pleural effusion, in mitral stenosis, 146
Pneumopericardium, 197
Polyarteritis nodosa, 320
Polysplenia syndrome, 236
Pompe's disease, 232
Post thrombotic syndrome, 343
Primitive ventricle, 250
Prolapse, of mitral valve leaflets, 151
Pseudo coarctation, 266
Pseudo shunt, 231
Pseudoachalasia, 178
Pseudoxanthoma elasticum, and coronary
  disease, 105
Pulmonary arterial hypertension, 70
Pulmonary arteries, 42
  atresia, 268
  banding of, 287
  peripheral stenosis of, 267
  stenosis in supra aortic stenosis, 266
Pulmonary artery sling, 258
Pulmonary atresia,
  Fallot type, 243
  valvar, 222
  with VSD, 243
Pulmonary blood flow, 47, 51
  distribution, 42
    effects of alveolar and interstitial
      pressure, 55, 56
    effects of gravity, 48
    effects of respiration, 48

Pulmonary blood flow—*continued*
  in mitral valve disease and left heart
    failure, 58
  mechanical factors, 48
  neurogenic factors, 48
Pulmonary blood volume, 47, 51
  effects of PEEP, 55
Pulmonary embolus, phlebography in, 335
Pulmonary haemosiderosis, 146
Pulmonary oedema, 43, 57
  distribution, 59
  effects on chronic lung disease, 59
  effects on lung volume, 58
Pulmonary ossification, in mitral valve
    disease, 146
Pulmonary regurgitation, 226
Pulmonary stenosis,
  dysplastic, 226
  valvar, 224
Pulmonary valve,
  absent, 242
  acquired diseases of, 156
Pulmonary vascular bed capacity, 49
Pulmonary vascular occlusive disease, 205
Pulmonary vascular patterns, 72
Pulmonary vascular resistance, 205
Pulmonary veins, 42
  anomalous drainage, with ASD, 211, 279
  hemianomalous, 278
  totally anomalous, 278

R

Rastelli procedure, 283
Ratio, cardiothoracic, 4
Raynaud's disease, 321
Recruitment, 49
Renal artery stenosis, 306
Replaced heart valves, 167
Resistance, pulmonary vascular, 205

S

Saddle embolus, 151
Sarcoidosis, 172, 391
Scimitar syndrome, 281
Scoliosis, 25
Screening, for LV aneurysm, 107
Seldinger technique, 294
Senning procedure, 282
Septal lines, 42
Sequestration of lung, 310

Shmoo sign, 23
Shunts,
  isotope measurement, 103
  left to right, 206
  right to left, 206
  surgical, 283
Single ventricle, 250
Situs,
  ambiguous, 236
  atrial, 235
  inversus, 236
  solitus, 236
Small vessel syndrome, 314
Sternal depression, 25
Straight back syndrome, 23
Subaortic stenosis, 230
Subclavian artery,
  aberrant left, 257
  aberrant right, 257
Subclavian steal syndrome, 303
Supra aortic stenosis, 266
Syphilis, aortic, 137
Systemic lupus erythematosus, 172
Systolic anterior motion, of anterior mitral
    leaflet, 175

T

Takayasu's disease, 180, 315
Tamponade, 88
Tetralogy of Fallot, 239
  with absent pulmonary valve, 242
Thallium-201, 92
Therapeutic angiography, 326
Thermography, in venous thrombosis, 361
Thrombosis, peripheral venous, 354
Thrombus,
  left ventricular, 111, 115
  peripheral venous, 340
Thyroid heart disease, 173
Transitional circulation, 233
Transposition,
  corrected, 249
  of the great arteries, 246
    haemodynamics, 208
  with atrioventricular discordance, 249
Trauma, arterial, 315
Tricuspid atresia, 220
Tricuspid regurgitation, congenital, 221
Tricuspid stenosis, congenital, 221
Tricuspid valve, acquired diseases of, 156
Truncus arteriosus, 270

Tuberculosis, 391
Tumour, cardiac, 157
Turner's syndrome, 183, 264

U

Uhls disease, 233
Ultrasound, of peripheral veins, 362
Univentricular heart, 250

V

Valve replacement, 167
Vascular pedicle,
  anatomy, 46
  change in width, 46
  effects of atherosclerosis, 47
  effects of projection, 46
  effects of respiration, 46
  effects of rotation, 46
  effects of supine position, 46
  width, 46
Vegetations, 139
  infective, 139, 153
Veins,
  congenital malformations, 347, 355
  pulmonary, 20, 42
  systemic, 19
  varicose, 345
Vena cava,
  inferior interrupted, 282
  superior, left, 282
Venous hypertension, 42
Ventricle,
  left, normal, 16
    enlargement of, 16
  right, normal, 11
    enlargement of, 11
Ventricular septal defect,
  complicating myocardial infarction, 111,
    115
  infundibular, 213
  muscular, 213
  perimembranous, 213
  with aortic regurgitation, 216
Viral myocarditis, 171

W

Waterston's shunt, 287